Nutritional and Metabolic Bases of Cardiovascular Disease

Companion website

This book is accompanied by a companion website:

www.wiley.com/go/mancini/cardiovascular

The website includes:

- Additional Reference lists for each chapter

Nutritional and Metabolic Bases of Cardiovascular Disease

EDITED BY

Mario Mancini MD

Emeritus Professor of Medicine
Department of Clinical and Experimental Medicine
Federico II University Medical School
Naples, Italy

José M. Ordovas PhD

Senior Scientist and Director
Nutrition and Genomics Laboratory
Jean Mayer USDA HNRCA at Tufts University
Boston, MA
USA

Gabriele Riccardi MD

Professor of Endocrine and Metabolic Disease
Department of Clinical and Experimental Medicine
Federico II University Medical School
Naples, Italy

Paolo Rubba MD

Professor of Medicine
Department of Clinical and Experimental Medicine
Federico II University Medical School
Naples, Italy

Pasquale Strazzullo MD

Professor of Medicine
Department of Clinical and Experimental Medicine
Federico II University Medical School
Naples, Italy

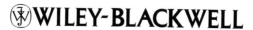

WILEY-BLACKWELL

A John Wiley & Sons, Ltd., Publication

This edition first published 2011 © 2011 by Blackwell Publishing Ltd

Blackwell Publishing was acquired by John Wiley & Sons in February 2007. Blackwell's publishing program has been merged with Wiley's global Scientific, Technical and Medical business to form Wiley-Blackwell.

Registered office: John Wiley & Sons Ltd, The Atrium, Southern Gate, Chichester, West Sussex, PO19 8SQ, UK

Editorial offices: 9600 Garsington Road, Oxford, OX4 2DQ, UK

The Atrium, Southern Gate, Chichester, West Sussex, PO19 8SQ, UK

111 River Street, Hoboken, NJ 07030-5774, USA

For details of our global editorial offices, for customer services and for information about how to apply for permission to reuse the copyright material in this book please see our website at www.wiley.com/wiley-blackwell

Library of Congress Cataloging-in-Publication Data
Nutrition, metabolism, and cardiovascular disease / edited by Mario Mancini ... [et al.].
    p. ; cm.
    Includes bibliographical references.
    ISBN 978-1-4051-8276-8
    1. Cardiovascular system–Diseases–Nutritional aspects. I. Mancini, M. (Mario)
    [DNLM: 1.   Cardiovascular Diseases–etiology. 2.   Cardiovascular Diseases–prevention & control. 3.   Metabolic Diseases–complications. 4.   Nutritional Physiological Phenomena. 5. Obesity–complications. 6.   Risk Factors. WG 120 N9765 2011]
    RC669.N88 2011
    616.1′071–dc22   2010015118

A catalogue record for this book is available from the British Library.

This book is published in the following electronic formats: ePDF 9781444318463; Wiley Online Library 9781444318456

Set in 9.5/12 pt. Minion by Aptara®, Inc., New Delhi, India
Printed and bound in Singapore by Markono Print Media Pte Ltd

1   2011

Contents

v

Section V Hemostasis and Thrombosis: From Nutritional Influences to Cardiovascular Events

Section VI Nutrition, Metabolism, and the Aging Process

Companion website

This book is accompanied by a companion website:

www.wiley.com/go/mancini/cardiovascular

The website includes:

- Additional Reference lists for each chapter

Contributor list

Chiara Viviani Anselmi, MD, MSc
Istituto Ricovero Cura Carattere Scientifico Multimedica
Milan
Italy

Lawrence J. Appel, MD
Professor, Epidemiology and International Health
Johns Hopkins Medical Institutions
Baltimore, MD
USA

Gerd Assmann, MD
President
Assmann-Stiftung für Prävention
Münster
Germany

Gianvincenzo Barba, MD
Research Associate
Institute of Food Science
National Research Council
Avellino
Italy

Pedro Bausero, MD
Professor of Physiopathology
Laboratory of Micronutrients and Cardiovascular Disease
UR4
UPMC University
Paris
France

Lydia A. Bazzano, MD, PhD
Assistant Professor of Epidemiology
Department of Epidemiology
Tulane University
School of Public Health and Tropical Medicine
New Orleans, LA
USA

Isabel Bondia Pons, PhD
Postdoctoral Research Associate
Food and Health Research Centre
Department of Clinical Nutrition
School of Public Health and Clinical Nutrition
University of Kuopio
Kuopio
Finland

George A. Bray, MD
Boyd Professor
Pennington Biomedical Research Center
Baton Rouge, LA
USA

Anne-Sophie Brazeau, PhD Candidate, MSc
Department of Nutrition
University of Montreal and
Centre de Recherche du
Centre Hospitalier de l'Université de Montréal
Quebec, QC
Canada

Ian J. Brown, PhD
Research Associate
Imperial College
London
UK

Jean-Marc Bugnicourt, MD
Department of Neurology,
Amiens University Hospital, and
Laboratory of Functional Neurosciences and Pathologies
University of Picardie Jules Verne
Amiens

Laura Calabresi, PhD
Professor of Pharmacology
Center E. Grossi Paoletti
Department of Pharmacological Sciences
University of Milan
Milan
Italy

Anna M.G. Cali, MD
Research Associate
Department of Pediatrics
Yale Clinical Center Investigation (YCCI)
Yale University School of Medicine
New Haven, CT
USA

Vito M. Campese, MD
Professor of Medicine and Chief of Nephrology
University of Southern California
Keck School of Medicine
Los Angeles, CA
USA

Brunella Capaldo, MD
Adjunct Professor of Endocrinology and Metabolism
Department of Clinical and Experimental Medicine
Federico II University
Naples
Italy

Francesco P. Cappuccio, MD, MSc,
FRCP, FFPH, FAHA
Cephalon Chair – Cardiovascular Medicine & Epidemiology
Warwick Medical School
University of Warwick
Coventry
UK

Sonia Caprio, MD
Professor of Pediatrics
Department of Pediatrics
Yale Clinical Center Investigation (YCCI)
Yale University School of Medicine
New Haven, CT
USA

Chiara Cerletti, PhD
Head of Laboratory of Cell Biology and Pharmacology of
    Thrombosis
Research Laboratories
John Paul II Center for High Technology Research and
    Education in Biomedical Sciences
Catholic University
Campobasso
Italy

Queenie Chan, MEng, MSc, MPhil
Statistician
Faculty of Medicine
Imperial College
London
UK

Jean-Marc Chillon, PharmD, PhD
Professor of Pharmacology INSERM ERI12
Faculty of Pharmacy
University of Picardie Jules Verne, and
Department of Pharmacology
Amiens University Hospital
Amiens
France

Arun Chockalingam, PhD, FACC
Professor and Director of Global Health
Faculty of Health Sciences
Simon Fraser University
Burnaby, BC
Canada

Franco Contaldo, MD
Professor of Internal Medicine
Department of Clinical and Experimental Medicine
Federico II University
Naples
Italy

Matteo Nicola Dario Di Minno, MD
Research Associate
Department of Clinical and Experimental Medicine
Federico II University
Naples
Italy

Martha L. Daviglus, MD, PhD
Professor
Preventive Medicine and Department of Medicine
Northwestern University
Chicago, IL
USA

Oreste de Divitiis, MD
Professor of Internal Medicine
Department of Clinical and Experimental Medicine
Federico II University
Naples
Italy

Elisabetta Della Valle, PhD
Associate Professor
Department of Preventive Medical Science
Unit of Occupational Medicine
Federico II University
Naples
Italy

Richard B. Devereux, MD
Professor of Medicine
Division of Cardiology
Weill Medical College of Cornell University
New York, NY
USA

Maria Benedetta Donati, MD, PhD
Scientific Coordinator of Research Laboratories
John Paul II Center for High Technology Research and
    Education in Biomedical Sciences
Catholic University
Campobasso
Italy

Alan R. Dyer, PhD
Professor, Preventive Medicine
Northwestern University
Chicago, IL
USA

Paul Elliott, PhD
Professor of Epidemiology and Public Health Medicine
Imperial College
London
UK

Stefan Engeli, MD
Senior Physician
Institute of Clinical Pharmacology
Hannover Medical School
Hannover
Germany

Eduardo Farinaro, MD
Professor of Preventive Medical Science
Head Unit of Occupational Medicine
Federico II University
Naples
Italy

Giovanni Federspil, MD
Professor of Internal Medicine
Endocrine-metabolic Unit Internal Medicine
Department of Medical and Surgical Sciences
University of Padova
Padova
Italy

L. Aldo Ferrara, MD
Professor of Internal Medicine
Department of Clinical and Experimental Medicine
Federico II University
Naples
Italy

Domnica Fotino, MD, MPH
Clinical Assistant Professor of Medicine
Department of Medicine
Tulane University
School of Medicine
New Orleans, LA
USA

Guido Franceschini, PhD
Professor of Pharmacology
Center E. Grossi Paoletti
Department of Pharmacological Sciences
University of Milano
Milan
Italy

Giovanni de Gaetano, MD, PhD
Director
Research Laboratories
John Paul II Center for High Technology Research and
    Education in Biomedical Sciences
Catholic University
Campobasso
Italy

Ferruccio Galletti, MD
Professor of Internal Medicine
Department of Clinical and Experimental Medicine
Federico II University
Naples
Italy

Claudio Galli, MD
Professor of Experimental Pharmacology
Department of Pharmacological Sciences
University of Milan
Milan
Italy

Giovanni Gallotta, MD
Research Associate
Department of Clinical and Experimental Medicine
Federico II University and ASL Napoli1
Naples
Italy

Marco Gentile, PhD
Research Associate
Department of Clinical and Experimental Medicine
Federico II University
Naples
Italy

Rosalba Giacco, MD
Research Associate
Institute of Food Science
National Research Council
Avellino
Italy

Romina di Giuseppe, PhD
Research Laboratories,
John Paul II Center for High Technology Research
and Education in Biomedical Sciences
Catholic University
Campobasso
Italy

Monica Gomaraschi, PhD
Research Fellow
Center E. Grossi Paoletti
Department of Pharmacological Sciences
University of Milano
Milan
Italy

Jørgen Gram, MD, DSc
Chief Physician
Department of Clinical Biochemistry
Faculty of Health Sciences
University of Southern Denmark
Esbjerg
Denmark

Elvira Grandone, MD
Research Associate
Unit of Thrombosis and Atherosclerosis
IRCCS "Casa Sollievo della Sofferenza"
S. Giovanni Rotondo
Foggia
Italy

Roberto Grimaldi, MD
Research Fellow
Department of Preventive Medical Science
Unit of Occupational Medicine
Federico II University
Naples
Italy

Feng J. He, PhD
Senior Research Fellow
Wolfson Institute of Preventive Medicine
Barts and The London School of Medicine & Dentistry
Queen Mary University of London
London
UK

Jiang He, MD, DrMS, PhD, MS, FAHA, FACE
Joseph S. Copes, MD Chair in Epidemiology and Professor
    of Epidemiology and Clinical Medicine
Department of Epidemiology
Tulane University
School of Public Health and Tropical Medicine and
School of Medicine
New Orleans, LA
USA

Barbara V. Howard, PhD
Senior Scientist
MedStar Research Institute
Hyattsville, MD
USA

Wm. James Howard, MD, MACP, FNLA
Director of the Lipid Clinic
Washington Hospital Center
Professor of Medicine
George Washington University
Washington, DC
USA

Licia Iacoviello, MD, PhD
Head of Laboratory of Genetic and Environmental
    Epidemiology
John Paul II Center for High Technology Research and
    Education in Biomedical Sciences
Catholic University
Campobasso
Italy

Arcangelo Iannuzzi, MD
Head of Division of Internal Medicine
A. Cardarelli Hospital
Naples
Italy

Gabriella Iannuzzo, MD, Phd
Research Associate
Department of Clinical and Experimental Medicine
Federico II University
Naples
Italy

Louis J. Ignarro, PhD
Professor of Pharmacology
Nobel Laureate for Medicine or Physiology 1998
Department of Molecular and Medical Pharmacology
David Geffen School of Medicine
University of California
Los Angeles, CA
USA

Renato Ippolito, MD
Department of Clinical and Experimental Medicine
Federico II University
Naples
Italy

W. Philip T. James, MD, DSC
Honorary Professor of Nutrition
London School of Hygiene and Tropical Medicine
International Obesity TaskForce, IASO
London
UK

Fabrizio Jossa, MD
Research Associate
Department of Clinical and Experimental Medicine
Federico II University
Naples
Italy

Mireia Junyent, MD, PhD
Nutrition and Genomics Laboratory
USDA-HNRCA
Tufts University
Boston, MA
USA

Antony Karelis, PhD
Professor of Exercise
Department of Kinanthropology
University of Quebec at Montreal
Montreal, QC
Canada

Tanika N. Kelly, PhD, MPH
Assistant Professor of Epidemiology
Department of Epidemiology
Tulane University
School of Public Health and
Tropical Medicine
New Orleans, LA
USA

Hugo Kesteloot, MD, PhD
Professor of Epidemiology
Katholieke Universiteit
Leuven
Belgium

Kay-Tee Khaw, MBBChir, FRCP, FMed Sci
Professor
School of Clinical Medicine
University of Cambridge
Cambridge
UK

Marjukka Kolehmainen, PhD, RD
Senior Scientist
Food and Health Research Centre
Department of Clinical Nutrition
School of Public Health and Clinical Nutrition
University of Kuopio
Kuopio
Finland

Elaine Ku, MD
University of Southern California
Keck School of Medicine
Los Angeles, CA
USA

Jan Kvetny, MD, DMSc
Chief Physician, Assistant Professor
Endocrinological Clinic
Department of Internal Medicine and
    Faculty of Health Sciences
University of Copenhagen
Naestved Hospital
Naestved
Denmark

Rachel Leach, MD, DSC
Policy Officer
London School of Hygiene and Tropical Medicine

International Obesity TaskForce, IASO
London
UK

Daniela Leonardis, MD
Division of Nephrology, Hypertension and Renal
    Transplantation Unit
National Research Council—IBIM Clinical Epidemiology of
    Renal Diseases and Hypertension
Reggio Calabria
Italy

Barry Lewis, MD, PhD, FRCP(London),
    FRCPath
Visiting Professor
Department of Medicine
University of Sydney
Sydney, NSW
Australia

Graham A. MacGregor, MD
Professor of Cardiovascular Medicine
Wolfson Institute of Preventive Medicine
Barts and The London School of Medicine & Dentistry
Queen Mary University of London
London
UK

Francesca Mallamaci, MD
Division of Nephrology, Hypertension and Renal
    Transplantation, and
National Research Council—IBIM Clinical Epidemiology of
    Renal Diseases and Hypertension
Reggio Calabria
Italy

Francesco P. Mancini, MD, PhD
Professor of Biochemistry
Department of Biological and Environmental Sciences
University of Sannio
Benevento
Italy

Jim Mann, CNZM, DM, PhD, FRACP, FRSNZ
Professor in Human Nutrition and Medicine
Edgar National Centre for Diabetes Research and
Department of Human Nutrition
University of Otago
Dunedin
New Zealand

Maurizio Margaglione, MD
Professor of Genetics
University of Foggia and
Unit of Thrombosis and Atherosclerosis

IRCCS "Casa Sollievo della Sofferenza"
S. Giovanni Rotondo
Foggia
Italy

Gennaro Marotta, MD
Research Associate
Department of Clinical and Experimental
    Medicine
Federico II University
Naples
Italy

Naomi M. Marrero, BSc Hons
PhD Student
Cardiac and Vascular Sciences
St. George's University of London
London
UK

Marie-Eve Mathieu, PhD
Assistant Professor
Department of Kinesiology
University of Montreal
Montreal, QC
Canada

Virginie Messier, MSc
Research Assistant
Department of Nutrition
University of Montreal
Quebec, QC
Canada

Giovanni Di Minno, MD
Professor of Internal Medicine
Department of Clinical and Experimental
    Medicine
Federico II University
Naples
Italy

Katsuyuki Miura, MD, PhD
Associate Professor
Department of Health Science
Shiga University of Medical Science
Shiga
Japan

Diana Muačević-Katanec, MD, PhD
Assistant Professor
Department of Internal Medicine
Division for Metabolic Diseases
University Hospital Center Zagreb
School of Medicine, University of Zagreb
Zagreb
Croatia

Hannu Mykkänen, PhD
Professor of Nutrition
Food and Health Research Centre
Department of Clinical Nutrition
Institute of Public Health and Clinical Nutrition
University of Kuopio
Kuopio
Finland

Claudio Napoli, MD, PhD, MBEth
Professor of Clinical Pathology
Department of General Pathology and Excellence Research
    Center on Cardiovascular Diseases
II University of Naples
Naples
Italy *and*
Adjunct Professor of Medicine
Whitaker Cardiovascular Institute
Boston University
Boston, MA
USA

Tanzina Nasreen, MD
University of Southern California
Keck School of Medicine
Los Angeles, CA
USA

Nagako Okuda, MD, PhD
Deputy Director
The First Institute for Health Promotion and Health Care
Japan Anti-Tuberculosis Association
Chiyoda-ku
Tokyo
Japan

Leiv Ose, MD PhD
Senior Consultant in Lipidology
Lipid Clinic
Department of Medicine
Oslo University Hospital
Rikshospitalet
Oslo
Norway

Claudio Pagano, MD, PhD
Assistant Professor of Internal Medicine
Endocrine-metabolic Laboratory
Internal Medicine
Department of Medical and Surgical Sciences
University of Padova
Padova
Italy

Salvatore Panico, MD
Associate Professor of Medicine
Department of Clinical and Experimental Medicine
Federico II University
Naples
Italy

Jeanie Park, MD
University of Southern California
Keck School of Medicine
Los Angeles, CA
USA

Fabrizio Pasanisi, MD, PhD
Associate Professor of Internal Medicine
Department of Clinical and Experimental Medicine
Federico II University
Naples
Italy

Roberto Paternò, MD
Research Associate
Department of Clinical and Experimental Medicine
Federico II University
Naples
Italy

Paolo Pauciullo, MD
Research Associate
Department of Clinical and Experimental Medicine
Federico II University
Naples
Italy

Thomas Perls, MD, PhD
Associate Professor
Geriatrics Section
New England Centenarian Study
Department of Medicine
Boston University Medical Center
Boston, MA
USA

Alfredo Postiglione, MD
Professor of Geriatrics
Department of Clinical and Experimental Medicine
Federico II University and
ASL Napoli I
Naples
Italy

Kaisa Poutanen, DTech
Academy Professor
Food and Health Research Centre
Department of Clinical Nutrition
School of Public Health and Clinical Nutrition
University of Eastern Finland
Kuopio
Finland

Annibale Alessandro Puca, MD
Associate Professor
IRCCS Policlinico Multimedica

Milan
Italy

Rémi Rabasa-Lhoret, MD, PhD
Assistant Professor
Department of Nutrition
University of Montreal and
Centre de Recherche du
Centre Hospitalier
de l'Université de Montréal and
Montreal Diabetes Research Center
Quebec, QC
Canada

Željko Reiner, MD, PhD, FRCP(Lond), FESC
Professor
Department of Internal Medicine
Division for Metabolic Diseases
University Hospital Center Zagreb
School of Medicine, University of Zagreb
Zagreb
Croatia

Doriane Richard, PhD
Research Associate
Laboratory of Micronutrients and Cardiovascular Disease
UR4
UPMC University
Paris
France

Angela Albarosa Rivellese, MD
Professor of Internal Medicine
Department of Clinical and Experimental Medicine
Federico II University
Naples
Italy

Albert P. Rocchini, MD
Professor of Pediatrics
Division of Pediatric Cardiology
Department of Pediatrics
University of Michigan
Ann Arbor, MI
USA

Marco Rossato, MD
Assistant Professor of Internal Medicine
Endocrine-metabolic Laboratory
Internal Medicine
Department of Medical and Surgical Sciences
University of Padova
Padova
Italy

Serenella Rotondo, PhD
Research Consultant
Laboratory of Cell Biology and Pharmacology of
    Thrombosis
John Paul II Center for High Technology Research and
    Education in Biomedical Sciences
Catholic University
Campobasso
Italy

Luca Scalfi, MD
Professor of Human Nutrition and Dietetics
Department of Food Science
Federico II University
Naples
Italy

Udo Seedorf, MD
Professor Leibniz-Institute of Arteriosclerosis Research
University of Münster
Münster
Germany

Alfonso Siani, MD
Haed Unit of Epidemiology & Population Genetics
Institute of Food Sciences
National Research Council
Avellino
Italy

Giovanni de Simone, MD, FACC, FAHA
Professor of Medicine
Department of Clinical and Experimental Medicine
Federico II University
Naples
Italy *and*
Division of Cardiology
Weill Medical College of Cornell University
New York, NY
USA

Lars Sjöström, MD, PhD
Professor of Medicine
Gothenburg University
Gothenburg
Sweden

Jeremiah Stamler, MD
Professor Emeritus
Department of Preventive Medicine
Feinberg School of Medicine
Northwestern University
Chicago, IL
USA

Saverio Stranges, MD, PhD
Associate Professor of Cardiovascular Epidemiology
Health Sciences Research Institute
University of Warwick Medical School
Coventry
UK, *and*
Executive Vice Chancellor and CEO
University of Nevada Health Sciences System
Nevada System of Higher Education
Las Vegas, NV
USA

Angelo Tremblay, PhD
Tutular Professor
Division of Kinesiology
Department of Social and Preventive Medicine
Faculty of Medicine
Laval University
Quebec, QC
Canada

Elena Tremoli, PhD
Professor of Pharmacological Sciences
Department of Pharmacological Sciences
University of Milan
Milan
Italy

Maurizio Trevisan, MD, MS
Executive Vice Chancellor and CEO
University of Nevada Health Sciences System
Nevada System of Higher Education
Las Vegas, NV
USA

Ioanna Tzoulaki, PhD
Lecturer in Epidemiology
Imperial College
London
UK

Hirotsugu Ueshima, MD, PhD
Emeritus Professor
Department of Health Science
Special Contract Professor
Lifestyle-Related Disease Prevention Center
Shiga University of Medical Science
Shiga
Japan

Olga Vaccaro, MD
Adjunct Professor of Human Nutrition
Department of Clinical and Experimental Medicine
Federico II University
Naples
Italy

Linda Van Horn, PhD, RD
Professsor of Preventive Medicine
Northwestern University
Chicago, IL
USA

Roberto Vettor, MD
President of the Italian Society of Obesity
Professor of Internal Medicine
Endocrine-metabolic Laboratory
Internal Medicine
Department of Medical and Surgical Sciences
University of Padova
Padova
Italy

Francesco Visioli, PhD
Professor of Physiopathology
Laboratory of Micronutrients and Cardiovascular Disease
UR4
UPMC University
Paris
France

Branislav Vohnout, MD, PhD
Head, Department of Physiological and Clinical Nutrition
Slovak Medical University
Bratislava
Slovakia

Liancheng Zhao, MD
Associate Professor of Cardiovascular Epidemiology and
    Nutrition
School of Public Health
Peking University
Peking
Beijing

Carmine Zoccali, MD, FASN
Director, Nephrology, Hypertension and Renal
    Transplantation Unit and
Head of Clinical Epidemiology and Pathophysiology of
    Renal Diseases and Hypertension Unit
National Research Council—IBIM Clinical Epidemiology of
    Renal Diseases and Hypertension
Ospedali Riuniti
Reggio Calabria
Italy

Foreword

Examination of trends in cardiovascular disease indicates that this is in many ways the best of times, while the worst of times may loom in the future. Fifty years after William Kannel first introduced the term "risk factor," enormous strides have been made in controlling the epidemic of cardiovascular disease in industrialized countries by preventive measures and increasingly successful treatments focused on the cardinal risk factors of dyslipidemia, hypertension and smoking and on their atherosclerotic sequelae. Age-adjusted death rates for some major cardiovascular events have been reduced by more than 50% and the relative focus of research efforts is shifting toward cancer and other conditions.

While there is cause for celebration, there is an even greater need at present to recognize the storm clouds on the horizon. The world-wide epidemics of obesity and diabetes are laying the groundwork for a new "rising tide" of cardiovascular disease stimulated by mechanistic pathways that are at present only incompletely understood, and in general poorly managed by either preventive or therapeutic strategies. To meet this challenge, there is a pressing need for those interested in cardiovascular disease to learn what is known and to identify the many gaping gaps in knowledge about the new driving forces of the future cardiovascular disease epidemic.

In this context, the present textbook entitled *Nutritional and Metabolic Bases of Cardiovascular Disease* makes a timely and extremely important contribution by bringing together in one source a comprehensive examination of the factors driving the emerging second epidemic of cardiovascular disease. The Editors, led by Professor Mario Mancini, have drawn together an international array of experts who provide up-to-date profiles of the state of the knowledge about a wide array of topics. The vast range of topics related to nutritional and metabolic aspects of cardiovascular disease are addressed with sensible grouping of chapters that consider Nutritional Habits and Obesity; the Metabolic Syndrome and Diabetes; Hypercholesterolemia and Early Atherosclerosis; Nutrition, Hypertension and Cerebrovascular Disease; Hemostasis and Thrombosis; and Nutrition, Metabolism and the Aging Process. The comprehensive nature of *Nutritional and Metabolic Bases of Cardiovascular Disease* and its thoughtful arrangement make it an outstanding source for readers who need up-to-date information on a focused topic, those who seek a multifaceted view of one or more of the above topic areas, and for others who want to be comprehensively informed about the basis of the coming wave of metabolically-driven cardiovascular disease.

Richard B. Devereux, M.D.

Preface

At the dawn of the third millennium, cardiovascular disease still represents the main cause of disability and death.

This condition is mostly mediated by atherosclerosis and the ensuing atherothrombosis that leads to ischemic heart, cerebral, and peripheral vascular disease. Our current understanding of the etiopathogenesis of atherosclerosis and the related coronary and extracoronary ischemic complications has greatly progressed, allowing us to make a strong and determined commitment to primary and secondary prevention.

Malnutrition due to excess saturated fat intake is undoubtedly the primary risk factor, as very keenly perceived and highlighted by Ancel Keys in Naples back in the 1950s. Here, he had the insight that the Mediterranean Diet played a protective role toward coronary heart disease. In fact, this was quite a rare condition in southern Italy in those days contrarily to the United States and northern European countries such as the Netherlands or Finland, where the habitual consumption of saturated fat was remarkably higher than in southern Italy. A family predisposition to cardiovascular diseases does indeed exist and is generally mediated by hyperlipidemia, high blood pressure, and thrombophilia; however, even in cases of clear family history, dietary habits contribute to improve or worsen the underlying metabolic conditions that are eventually responsible for the injury to the heart or vessels. The growing prevalence of obesity and diabetes, along with the increase in the elderly population, has further contributed to the current high trend in cardiovascular diseases worldwide.

Scientific research has made giant steps in understating the interaction between nutrition, metabolism, and molecular genetics in relation to the causes of cardiovascular diseases; we therefore felt that the most significant evidence produced in recent years deserved to be put together in a monograph. These data have been subdivided into six separate sections, spacing from nutrition to obesity (*section 1*), the metabolic syndrome to diabetes (*section 2*), hypercholesterolemia to atherogenesis (*section 3*), high blood pressure to cardio-cerebrovascular diseases (*section 4*), hemostasis to atherothrombosis (*section 5*), and diet to aging processes (*section 6*).

There is clearly a common thread in all the sections: the close relationship between type of dietary habits, metabolic processes of the nutrients, and the possibly severe pathogenic consequences on the cardiovascular system.

We are grateful to all of the authors who participated in this initiative with their scientific contributions, and to Wiley-Blackwell who welcomed our proposal to publish this book, which we dedicate to the memory of Ancel Keys, with gratitude from all his scholars.

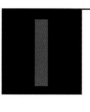

SECTION I
Nutrition and Obesity

CHAPTER 1

Basics of Energy Balance

Luca Scalfi, Fabrizio Pasanisi, & Franco Contaldo
Federico II University, Naples, Italy

Introduction

The aim of this chapter is to concisely discuss the basic concepts related to the utilization of energy in the human body. In addition, background information is provided about the practical use of these concepts. These issues are considered in more detail in chapters of books and other major publications on human nutrition to whom the reader may refer for further explanations [1–9]. Other references are indicated in the text only for more specific points. The human being needs energy to sustain life and maintain the structural and functional integrity of the body. The energy is used by cells to perform chemical work (synthesis and degradation of molecules), mechanical work (muscular contraction), and electrical work (maintenance of ionic gradients across membranes), and eventually lost in the form of heat or external work or is stored (mostly in the adipose tissue as triacylglycerols) if energy balance is positive.

The first law of thermodynamics states that energy cannot be created or destroyed, but only transformed. Human body attains energy from foods where it is stored in the chemical bonds of macronutrients (carbohydrates, fats, and proteins) and alcohol. Through biochemical transformation the energy of nutrients is made available to the body mostly as adenosine triphosphate (ATP), but this conversion into high-energy biochemical compounds is an inefficient process, with 50% of the original energy lost as heat. Furthermore, since a certain percentage of ATP is needed for the trans-port, storage, and recycling of macronutrients, actual ATP yields correspond to 90%, 75%, and 55% of those expected on the basis of pure oxidation of fats, carbohydrates, and proteins, respectively. In other words, the synthesis of one mole of ATP that can be used by the body requires about 20 kcal for fats, 24 kcal for carbohydrates, and 33 kcal for proteins.

Since all the energy used by the body is ultimately lost as heat (including that related to external work), energy is usually expressed using the calorie, which is defined as the amount of heat energy needed to raise the temperature of 1 ml of water at 15 °C by 1 °C. Actually, according to the SI system, the unit for energy is the joule (J), which measures energy in terms of the mechanical work required to accelerate a mass of 1 kg with a force of 1 newton through 1 m along the direction of the force. Because calorie and joule are small units, considering energy balance, for practical reasons, kilocalorie (kcal = 1,000 cal), kilojoule (kJ = 1,000 J), and sometimes megajoule (MJ = 1,000,000 J) are commonly used in human nutrition. The equivalence is indicated as 1 kcal = 4.184 kJ (in some texts, 4.186) with the inverse ratio of 0.239.

Food Energy

The *gross energy of food* is the energy contained in the chemical bonds of macronutrients (carbohydrates, fats, and proteins) and alcohol and can be determined using a bomb calorimeter, which is an instrument that measures heat production due to complete oxidation of organic molecules. The gross energy of food (in kcal/g: 4.10 for carbohydrates, 9.45 for fats, 5.65 for proteins, and 7.10 for

Nutritional and Metabolic Bases of Cardiovascular Disease, 1st edition.
Edited by Mario Mancini, José M. Ordovas, Gabriele Riccardi, Paolo Rubba and Pasquale Strazzullo. © 2011 Blackwell Publishing Ltd.

alcohol) is not entirely available to the body. First, some energy is lost in feces because of incomplete absorption of macronutrients from the digestive tract; the energy available after ingestion of food is termed *digestible energy*. The absorption rate of macronutrients is usually considered very high–97% for carbohydrates, 95% for fats, and 92% for proteins–but it could be much lower for high-fiber diets, especially with respect to protein digestibility. Once in the body, carbohydrates and fats are completely oxidized to water and carbon dioxide, but this is not the case for proteins. Nitrogen is not oxidized to nitrogen oxides, which are toxic, but to urea, which is much less toxic, and this molecule still contains a quarter of the chemical energy of original proteins. Small amounts of other, not completely oxidized nitrogenous molecules such as amino acids, 3-methyl-hystidine, and creatinine are also lost in the urine. The energy made available to the body after taking into account losses in feces and urine is termed *metabolizable energy*; the corresponding energy values (kcal/g) are the ones commonly used in human nutrition: 3.75 for monosaccharides, 3.94 for disaccharides, 4.13 for starch, 9.00 for fats (triglycerides composed of long-chain fatty acids), 4.00 for proteins, and 7.00 for alcohol. A figure of about 1.5 kcal/g has also been proposed for dietary fiber, as it can be metabolized (fermented) in the large bowel by bacteria to short-chain fatty acids, which can be subsequently absorbed and utilized in the body.

Components of Total Energy Expenditure

Total energy expenditure (TEE), usually expressed as 24-hour energy expenditure, comprises three main components (basal metabolic rate, thermic effect of food, and energy expenditure due to physical activity), plus a number of additional components that may be relevant in specific circumstances (Table 1.1).

Basal Metabolic Rate

Basal metabolic rate (BMR) is by far the most important component of TEE in a very large percentage (60%–75%) of individuals, and more markedly in sedentary people. BMR corresponds to the en-

Table 1.1 Components of energy expenditure.

Basal metabolic rate (BMR)
Thermic effect of food (TEF)
Energy expenditure due to physical activity (EEPA)
  Exercise activity thermogenesis (EAT)
  Nonexercise activity thermogenesis (NEAT), including fidgeting
Other thermogenic stimuli
  Psychological thermogenesis
  Cold-induced thermogenesis
  Drug-induced thermogenesis

The term *diet-Induced thermogenesis* indicates the variations in BMR and TEF due to true metabolic adaptation to chronic underfeeding or overfeeding.

ergy needed in basal conditions to sustain the metabolic activities of cells and tissues and to maintain vital functions (e.g., circulatory, respiratory, gastrointestinal and renal processes, and body temperature) when the subject is awake and alert; sleeping metabolic rate is 5%–10% lower than BMR.

BMR is determined in standard conditions avoiding any effect of food or physical activity, with the subject lying at physical and mental rest in a comfortably warm environment (thermoneutral environment) and in the post-absorptive state. In practice, according to a realistic protocol, BMR is measured in the first part of the morning after the subject has been in the supine position for 30 minutes, at least 12 hours after eating food or taking any stimulants such as coffee or smoking. Heavy physical activity should also be avoided during the day prior to the test. Resting metabolic rate (RMR) is the term used when the conditions for the measurement of BMR are substantially but not completely met (e.g., because of a shorter fasting period and heavy physical exercise the day before). RMR is, therefore, expected to be slightly higher than BMR. BMR and RMR are usually expressed in kcal/min or, if extrapolated to 24 hours to be more meaningful, in kcal/day. In the latter case, the terms basal energy expenditure (BEE) and resting energy expenditure (REE) are usually (and more appropriately) used.

A number of factors cause the BMR to vary among individuals. By far, body size (i.e., body weight) is the most important one. Heavier people have higher metabolic rates than lighter ones. As metabolic processes that require energy occur almost exclusively within the cytosol and mitochondria, BMR is strictly related to fat-free mass (i.e., body weight minus body lipids) and body cell mass. Brain, liver, kidney, and heart, which together represent 5%–6% of body weight, are the most metabolically active organs, accounting for more than 50% of BMR. For the same amount of tissue, their metabolic rate is much higher than that of skeletal muscles. Indeed, skeletal muscles contribute 20%–30% of BMR in adults because of its large mass, while adipose tissue (at least in people of average weigh) contributes to a small extent, as its metabolic rate per unit of weight is low. As far as metabolic processes are concerned, protein synthesis, Na-K ATPase pump, and gluconeogenesis account for a substantial proportion of energy utilization in basal conditions. Furthermore, BMR is subject to the control of the central nervous system and the sympathetic nervous system and is related to hormonal status (i.e., thyroid hormones and insulin).

In addition, for the same weight and height, BMR is higher in males than in females even after adjusting for body composition and, in women, is higher in the luteal compared to the follicular phase. Furthermore, BMR significantly declines with age in both genders. This trend is not entirely explained by the changes in body composition observed in older people; it may also be ascribed to a number of hormonal and metabolic changes related to senescence.

Thermic Effect of Food

The thermic effect of food (TEF) is the increase in energy expenditure occurring after the ingestion of energetic molecules (carbohydrates, fats, proteins, and alcohol) and is mostly associated with their digestion, absorption, and storage. An increase in energy expenditure can usually be observed from 4 to 6 hours after a mixed meal. Postprandial thermogenesis, specific dynamic action, thermic effect of feeding, and heat increment of feeding are other terms used to describe the same phenomenon.

TEF is influenced by the quantity and the type of macronutrients ingested. The thermogenic response is 5%–10% of ingested energy for carbohydrates, less than 5% for lipids, and 20%–30% for proteins, accounting on average for approximately 10%–15% of total energy intake (and TEE, if energy balance is neutral). The high TEF for proteins is due not only to the more complex processes of digestion and absorption but also to substantial postprandial changes in amino acid metabolism, leading to an overall increase of protein turnover.

A number of other factors have been indicated to affect TEF, for instance, overfeeding and underfeeding or physical exercise on the days prior to the test. Several studies have also shown variations due to age, genetic factors, weight changes, and physical fitness. Although these studies are relevant to metabolic and physiological knowledge, from a practical perspective, it is unlikely that in healthy individuals, and in the long term, differences in TEF may significantly influence TEE and energy balance.

Physical Activity

The third main component of TEE is the energy expenditure due to physical activity (EEPA), which is the energy expenditure for physical activities of all kinds. It is important to stress that physical activity does not always match the strict definition of muscular work, which implies external work performed on the environment. In fact, an increase in energy expenditure can also occur without any work in the case of just tensed and stretched muscles (e.g., isometric thermogenesis for standing up and dynamic thermogenesis for climbing down a ladder, respectively).

Energy expenditure due to physical activity can be further split into two components: Exercise activity thermogenesis (EAT) is the energy used during sport or fitness exercises, while non-exercise activity thermogenesis (NEAT) is due to occupational activities, leisure activities, and any other activity related to everyday life. In particular, NEAT also comprises fidgeting (spontaneous physical activity), which is a condition of restlessness, as manifested by continuous movements particularly of body segments. Finally, excess post-exercise oxygen consumption (EPOC) is an additional small increase in energy expenditure even after exercise has ceased, which is related to exercise intensity and duration.

EEPA, which widely varies among individuals as well as from day to day, depends on the type and intensity of a certain physical activity and on the combination of different physical activities over the day. It may also be influenced by the individual habits of motion, as well as the speed and dexterity with which an activity is performed. The energy cost of each physical activity is commonly expressed as a multiple of BMR, and the term correspondingly used by the World Health Organization (WHO) [1] is physical activity ratio (PAR). The term *metabolic equivalents* (METs) is often used in the same way but is somewhat different. As a matter of fact, METs are multiples of resting oxygen consumption and the latter is not measured but calculated using a fixed rate of oxygen consumption (in adults, 3.5 mL/kg of body weight per minute). This means roughly 1.0 kcal/kg of body weight per hour, or 1.2 kcal/min in a man weighing 70 kg and 1.0 kcal/min in a woman weighing 60 kg. Comprehensive tables on the energy cost of different activities are easily available [1,2]. In general, PAR (or METs) ranges from 1 to 5 (e.g., 1.4 for standing, 3.3–4.5 for walking) but can reach much higher values (>8) for jogging, running, and selected occupational activities.

The overall level of physical activity can be defined by computing the ratio of TEE to BEE, termed physical activity level (PAL), or sometimes physical activity index (PAI). PAL can be used to describe physical activity habits, or to express how sedentary is the lifestyle of individuals. The Institute of Medicine [2] identified four categories in adults: sedentary, low active, active, and very active with respective PAL ranges of 1.0–1.3, 1.3–1.6, 1.6–1.9, and >1.9. The WHO proposed alternative classification criteria [1]: sedentary or light activity lifestyle for PAL = 1.40–1.69, active or moderately active lifestyle for PAL = 1.70–1.99, and vigorous or vigorously active lifestyle for PAL >2.00. For instance, performing one hour of moderate to vigorous activity every day (brisk walking to jogging/running, aerobic dancing, cycling, etc.) is sufficient to maintain an active lifestyle. Indeed, PALs of >2.00 are uncommon in industrialized countries.

Other Components of TEE

In addition to the three components already referred to, other minor thermogenic stimuli may be mentioned: psychological thermogenesis, as anxiety and stress increase BMR; cold-induced thermogenesis, due to exposure to low temperature; and drug-induced thermogenesis, for instance, related to the consumption of caffeine, nicotine, or alcohol. The actual impact of these factors on TEE is questionable and cannot easily be evaluated in the single individual.

In terms of energy balance, additional energy needs should be considered in specific circumstances, such as growth, pregnancy, and lactation. Briefly, the energy cost of growth is very high in the first three months of life but declines rapidly to 5% of energy intake in the second year of life, and then to 1%–2% until puberty, including both the cost to synthesize new tissues and the energy deposited in those tissues. The overall energy cost of pregnancy is on average approximately 75,000 kcal, being higher in the second and third trimesters, while during the first six months postpartum, on average an additional 675 kcal/day are needed for milk production if infants are exclusively breastfed.

Variability of TEE

To a very large extent, TEE varies even in people living in developed countries, where technology, which promotes a sedentary lifestyle, is commonly and widely used. All the factors that affect BEE (e.g., body weight and composition, age, and gender) also influence TEE, whereas TEF represents a quite constant and limited component. Large differences in TEE between subjects of the same gender, age, and weight (even >2,000 kcal/day) are accounted for mostly by variance in EEPA. In particular, differences in NEAT may be of great importance since most adults are not regularly involved in sporting-like activities (EAT). The between-subject differences in NEAT may be related to environmental and biological factors affecting both occupational and leisure-time activities, with fidgeting still very difficult to assess. It should be noted that extremely high values of TEE can be observed both in individuals with high levels of physical activity and in severely obese individuals (see below).

Energy Requirements

Energy requirement is defined by the Food and Agriculture Organization of the United Nations (FAO)/WHO/United Nations University (UNU) Consultation [1] as the amount of food energy needed to balance energy expenditure in order to maintain body size, body composition, and a level of necessary and desirable physical activity consistent with long-term well-being and good health. This also includes the energy needed for growth (children and adolescents), deposition of tissues during pregnancy, and production of milk during lactation. According to this definition, energy requirement does not automatically correspond to TEE in a given individual, for instance, in underweight or obese or very sedentary people.

From a practical perspective, in order to avoid a negative outcome associated with underfeeding or overfeeding, it is crucial to assess TEE before commencing nutritional support in the single individual [9]. In this case, TEE could not correspond to energy requirement as above defined, for instance, in underweight or obese people (lower and higher than the desirable one, respectively).

Two different basic approaches may be used for the assessment of TEE [1,2,10], with an accuracy that is indeed still not completely known, especially in the single individual. In the first approach (simplified factorial method), BEE and PAL are considered [1,10]. BEE is measured by indirect calorimetry or estimated using predictive formulas including, in different combinations, easily measurable variables such as gender, age, weight, and height. As far as adult individuals are concerned, the most widely used among such formulas are still those published in 1919 by Harris and Benedict [11]. The equations proposed by Schofield et al. in 1985 [12] are frequently cited as well; they were derived for each gender and for different age ranges on the basis of a large number of data collected in several countries.

Once BEE is measured or estimated, PAL can be approximated by asking the subject to keep an activity diary or by using an appropriate questionnaire, and TEE is accordingly estimated by multiplying BEE by PAL. In the case of an activity diary, EEPA could also be calculated in absolute value (kcal/day) from recorded activities and their duration and then added to BEE.

The second approach for the assessment of TEE has been recently recommended by the Institute of Medicine as part of the Dietary Reference Intakes project [2]. In this case, BEE is neither measured nor estimated. Instead, as shown in Table 1.2, gender-specific equations for TEE are proposed, requiring four predictive variables: age, height, weight, and level of physical activity. The latter is expressed as a coefficient depending on the lifestyle category: sedentary, low active, active, and very active (see Table 1.2).

Energy Balance

The difference between the energy made available to the body (metabolizable energy) and TEE defines the energy balance. The traditional (static) energy balance equation is commonly expressed as

$$\text{Changes in energy stored in the body}$$
$$= \text{metabolizable energy intake} - \text{total}$$
$$\text{energy expenditure}$$

Neutral energy balance (or energy balance) is when the two factors are equivalent, with no changes in body energy stores. Because with common dietary habits, as observed in industrialized countries, there is little or no conversion of either proteins or carbohydrates to fatty acids, achieving neutral energy balance also means achieving neutral balance of each macronutrient.

Positive energy balance occurs when energy expenditure is low or energy intake is high, or with a combination of these two factors. The opposite is true for a negative energy balance. Short-term energy imbalance (over hours or days) is handled by the body through rapid changes in carbohydrate balance and glycogen stores, whereas over a prolonged period, there are changes in fat mass and fat-free mass. The amount of fat mass gained or lost depends on a number of factors, such as the extent of energy imbalance and the initial BMI. However, in normal conditions, fat-free mass and fat mass both increase during weight gain and decrease after weight loss.

The term adaptation describes the normal physiological responses of humans to different environmental conditions to preserve body functions and well-being as much as possible. Specifically, the maintenance of energy balance in spite of some alteration of the steady state may involve behavioral changes, variations in body composition, and true metabolic adaptation. For instance, changes of body weight per se are expected to modify different components of TEE in a direction that tends to oppose the original imbalance. Weight gain is

Table 1.2   Equations to estimate total energy expenditure (TEE) in adults as proposed by the Institute of Medicine.

TEE for normal-weight men 19 years and older

$$\text{TEE} = 662 - (9.53 \times \text{age [yr]}) + \text{PA} \times (15.91 \times \text{weight [kg]} + 539.6 \times \text{height [m]}),$$

where PA is the physical activity coefficient:
  PA = 1.00 if PAL is estimated to be ≥ 1.0 < 1.4 (sedentary)
  PA = 1.11 if PAL is estimated to be ≥ 1.4 < 1.6 (low active)
  PA = 1.25 if PAL is estimated to be ≥ 1.6 < 1.9 (active)
  PA = 1.48 if PAL is estimated to be ≥ 1.9 < 2.5 (very active)

TEE for normal-weight women aged 19 years and older

$$\text{TEE} = 354 - (6.91 \times \text{age [yr]}) + \text{PA} \times (9.36 \times \text{weight [kg]} + 726 \times \text{height [m]}),$$

where PA is the physical activity coefficient:
  PA = 1.00 if PAL is estimated to be ≥ 1.0 < 1.4 (sedentary)
  PA = 1.12 if PAL is estimated to be ≥ 1.4 < 1.6 (low active)
  PA = 1.27 if PAL is estimated to be ≥ 1.6 < 1.9 (active)
  PA = 1.45 if PAL is estimated to be ≥ 1.9 < 2.5 (very active)

Normal-weight, overweight, and obese men 19 years and older

$$\text{TEE} = 864 - (9.72 \times \text{age [yr]}) + \text{PA} \times (14.2 \times \text{weight [kg]} + 503 \times \text{height [m]}),$$

where PA is the physical activity coefficient:
  PA = 1.00 if PAL is estimated to be ≥ 1.0 < 1.4 (sedentary)
  PA = 1.12 if PAL is estimated to be ≥ 1.4 < 1.6 (low active)
  PA = 1.27 if PAL is estimated to be ≥ 1.6 < 1.9 (active)
  PA = 1.54 if PAL is estimated to be ≥ 1.9 < 2.5 (very active)

Normal-weight, overweight, and obese women 19 years and older

$$\text{TEE} = 387 - (7.31 \times \text{age [yr]}) + \text{PA} \times (10.9 \times \text{weight [kg]} + 660.7 \times \text{height [m]}),$$

where PA is the physical activity coefficient:
  PA = 1.00 if PAL is estimated to be ≥ 1.0 < 1.4 (sedentary)
  PA = 1.14 if PAL is estimated to be ≥ 1.4 < 1.6 (low active)
  PA = 1.27 if PAL is estimated to be ≥ 1.6 < 1.9 (active)
  PA = 1.45 if PAL is estimated to be ≥ 1.9 < 2.5 (very active)

TEE: estimated energy requirement (EER) in normal-weight individuals.
Adapted from Institute of Medicine [2], with permission.

associated with an increase in fat-free mass as well as metabolically active tissues, leading to an increase in both BEE and the absolute energy cost of physical activity. On the other hand, true metabolic adaptation occurs when there are biochemical changes in cellular energy metabolism that cannot be related to other factors. In this regard, the term diet-induced thermogenesis has often been used to describe possible variations in BMR and TEF that are due to true adaptation to underfeeding or overfeeding.

A convincing, consistent example regarding adaptation and energy expenditure is offered by un-derfed adult subjects. It is a universal observation [13,14] that all the components of TEE are affected by chronic energy deficiency. The decrease in TEF is due to the reduced food intake and possibly to some true metabolic adaptation. BEE and EEPA decline because of the reduction in body mass, but EEPA declines also because of possible changes in spontaneous physical activity (unconscious economy of activity). Finally, and more interestingly, there is a decrease in BEE that is greater than it would be expected from the loss of body mass and fat-free mass [13,14]. This is a major factor in the protection against further weight loss, likely to be due to both a reduction in cellular energy needs and changes in hormonal status (e.g., thyroid hormones) or in the activity of the sympathetic nervous system (leading to a true metabolic adaptation).

Much more difficult is to discuss the issue of adaptation during positive energy balance.

Since dietary energy excess may vary significantly from day to day, results obtained in experimental overfeeding studies can difficult to extrapolate to everyday life, for instance, because of peculiar characteristics of protocols such as very consistent daily energy surplus. Indeed, during short-term overfeeding, the increase in energy expenditure appears fairly small and possibly related to the type of nutrient, possibly greater for carbohydrates than fats [6].

Overall, adaptive variations in energy expenditure to contrast changes in body weight are more apparent and effective in chronic energy deficiency than chronic overfeeding, suggesting a clear priority in preventing the consequences of weight loss rather than those of excess body fat. This is in agreement with the observation that food shortages were more common than food abundance during early human evolution and more likely to be fatal in the short term.

Energy Expenditure and Obesity

Obesity is a heterogeneous disorder in which environmental, individual, and biological factors interact to influence both energy intake and energy expenditure. Long-term energy balance appears to be quite efficiently regulated in humans, with a number of sensitive mechanisms that act to oppose weight changes. In most average-weight people living in industrialized countries, body weight tends to remain quite constant despite that metabolizable energy made available to the body ranges between 600,000 and 1,000,000 kcal/yr. On the other hand, considering that even an energy surplus of only 80 kcal/day (3%–5% of total daily energy intake) is expected to cause a 4.5-kg increase in body weight over 12 months, it has been extensively discussed over the past decades whether alterations, even minor, in energy expenditure may play a role in the pathogenesis of overweight and obesity. In other words, are there abnormalities in TEE and any of its components that, at least in part, cause weight gain and lead to excess body fat?

Experimental Studies

Experimental studies in humans focus on different conditions: individuals before weight gain, already obese, or after weight loss. Few longitudinal data have indicated that low energy expenditure is a risk factor for weight gain in some groups of subjects who may be prone to obesity, such as adult Pima Indians and infants of overweight mothers, but there is no evidence of increased risk in the general population or unselected cohorts [15]. However, in pre-obese as well as post-obese subjects (i.e., subjects with a clinical predisposition to gain excess body fat), a trend toward more efficient energy storage and/or higher food intake associated with sedentarism has been suggested. In pre-obese as well as post-obese subjects, some studies have also suggested that low levels of NEAT and spontaneous physical activity represent a risk factor for weight gain, but data are still preliminary [15,16]. Taken together, these studies support a variable role of biological factors in the pathogenesis of human obesity. In fact, a positive association has been described between some genotypes and phenotypes typical of individuals predisposed to obesity. Nevertheless, nongenetic biological factors such as intrauterine factors, birth weight, and breastfeeding may facilitate the onset of obesity later in life.

Considering an achieved condition of excess body fat, it is widely accepted that BEE is increased in overweight and obese individuals. This is not surprising because not only do they have a greater fat-free mass, but in very obese people, fat mass also significantly contributes to energy expenditure, although the metabolic rate per unit of weight is low. The equations proposed by the Institute of Medicine [2] indicate an increase in BEE of 10.1 and 8.6 kcal/day for each kilogram of body weight gained in overweight/obese male and female individuals, respectively. Interestingly, after adjustment for body composition, there are no differences in BEE between overweight/obese individuals and their lean counterparts [15]. Overweight people also have a higher EEPA in absolute terms because they spend a larger amount of energy to move a greater mass, especially in weight-bearing activities. If PAL is taken into consideration, there is evidence that overweight subjects do not exhibit more sedentary lifestyles, possibly because of the low mean PAL observed in average-weight individuals living in industrialized countries [15]. On the other hand, it should be noted that excess body fat is frequently a physically incapacitating factor in morbidly obese patients, leading to a reduction in physical activity. As far as adaptive thermogenesis is concerned, while the few data available seem to suggest a similar response to short-term overfeeding in lean and overweight individuals, several studies have demonstrated that TEF is abnormal in obese individuals [15]. However, the difference, possibly due to the presence of insulin resistance, is unlikely to be due to an altered adaptive thermogenesis, is small, and is unlikely to produce significant energy imbalance. Overall, when weight stability is present, TEE is on average much higher in overweight/obese individuals than in their average-weight counterparts (energy gap) [17].

Finally, the question of whether obese individuals may have decreased energy requirements after weight loss has also been addressed. All components of TEE decline in obese individuals with weight loss, for example, due to a decrease in body mass, fat-free mass, or energy intake. On the other hand, conflicting results are available concerning the hypothesis that post-obese people have a lower BEE than would be expected on the basis of their body composition, but this difference would indeed be very small and unlikely to affect energy balance to a significant extent [15]. Indeed, it is clear that in order to maintain energy balance, post-obese people have to reduce their energy intake compared to their previous overweight condition or substantially increase EEAT.

The Epidemiological Approach

Epidemiological studies have given significant results about the role of energy expenditure in the pathogenesis of obesity, which are also somewhat in contrast with those of experimental studies [18,19]. Randomized controlled studies and cohort studies have evaluated in adults and children the relationships between weight changes and physical activity (also in combination with diet), occupational and leisure activities, and household activities. Overall, there is substantial and consistent evidence that regular and sustained physical activity may protect, at least in part, against the increase of body fat and facilitate maintenance of weight loss in the long term. Since the measurement of physical activity is complex and usually not very accurate, the actual relationship could be stronger than the observed one. It should also be mentioned that physical activity may influence energy balance in different ways, not only by increasing energy expenditure but also by affecting the regulation of food intake.

Similarly, epidemiological studies have also shown that sedentary lifestyles, which means a high level of physical inactivity, are also related to weight gain [18,19]. Several studies in children, adolescents, and young adults show a higher risk of overweight/obesity with increased television viewing (usually >3 hr/day). Indeed, television viewing is a marker of physical inactivity but may also be associated with consumption of energy-dense foods and drinks.

Main Clinical Correlates

The evaluation of energy requirements is important not only from a theoretical point of view, but also for clinical purposes. Energy requirements should be evaluated before commencing every nutritional therapy, and this is true not only for underweight and overweight patients and also for those with conditions such as metabolic syndrome, type 2 diabetes, and hyperlipidemia. Physicians should always be aware of the potential error introduced in nutritional therapy by disregarding this issue, because the diet should always be tailored to the individual's energy needs.

Standardized procedures should be used for estimating BEE and PAL with predictive equations and questionnaires. The measurement of BEE using a specific device such as the ventilated hood system should be encouraged as a standard procedure in human nutrition to improve the evaluation of energy requirements in the single individual. EEAT could be assessed with accelerometers, but the validity of this approach in the single individual is still debated.

The increase in TEE due to being overweight is not a legend, but it is real and consistent. For instance, the equations proposed by the Institute of Medicine [2] indicate that for the same age, height, and PAL, TEE is significantly affected by weight not only in average-weight but also in overweight and obese individuals. Indeed, there are overweight and obese individuals with low or very low energy requirements due to the interactions between different factors, such as age, female gender, small stature, low PAL, genetics, and weight loss. Once again, this supports the advantage of measuring energy expenditure (at least BEE) in the clinical setting.

Selected References

1. Report of a Joint FAO/WHO/UNU Expert Consultation. Human Energy Requirements. WHO technical report series UNU/WHO/FAO, Rome. 2004

2. Institute of Medicine, Food and Nutrition Board. Energy. In: Dietary Reference Intakes for Energy, Carbohydrate, Fiber, Fat, Fatty Acids, Cholesterol, Protein, and Amino Acids (Macronutrients). The National Academies Press. Washington, 2005;1:1–114.

10. Heymsfield SB, Harp JB, Rowell PN, et al. How much may I eat? Obes Rev 2006;7:361–370.

15. Prentice A. Are defects in energy expenditure involved in the causation of obesity? Obes Rev 2007;8(Suppl 1):89–91.

19. Fox KR, Hillsdon M. Physical activity and obesity. Obes Rev 2007;8(Suppl 1):115–121.

CHAPTER 2

Genotype-Phenotype Associations: Modulation by Diet and Obesity

José M. Ordovas & Mireia Junyent
Tufts University, Boston, MA, USA

Introduction

The promises of the genomic revolution have attracted a large number of scientific disciplines including nutritional sciences. The potential benefits of harnessing the power of genomics for dietary prevention of common diseases are enormous and impossible to ignore being considered as the future of nutritional research [1–5].

The major goal of nutrition research is to provide solid, science-based evidence to guide the definition of optimal dietary recommendations aimed to prevent chronic diseases and to promote health for everybody and for each stage of human life. A number of dietary guidelines have been implemented in the United States and other industrialized countries for more than 90 years to improve the health of the general population and those at high risk for specific diseases [e.g., cardiovascular disease (CVD), cancer, hypertension, and diabetes]. However, those dietary guidelines have not addressed the dramatic differences in the individual's physiological response to changes in nutrient intake. This limitation may greatly affect the efficacy of public health recommendations at the individual level.

The factors and molecular basis involved in responsiveness to diet are complex and largely unknown. A genetic component responsible for differences in dietary response was first proposed several decades ago [6], and it is clearly evident for rare inborn errors of metabolism. However, the extrapola-

tion to common phenotypes and diseases has been more challenging [5,7]. Nevertheless, the current evidence supports the notion that these diseases are triggered because of dynamic and continuous interactions between genes and environmental factors [8–10]. The concept of environment is extremely complex and broad and extends well beyond diet, tobacco smoking, drug consumption, exposures to pollutants, and educational and socioeconomic status [11]. However, among these, food intake is the environmental factor to which we are all exposed necessarily and permanently from conception to death and it has been a major driving force through species' evolution. Therefore, dietary habits may be the most important environmental factor modulating gene expression during one's lifespan but certainly is not the only one.

The concept of gene–diet interaction describes the modulation of the effect of a dietary component on a specific phenotype (e.g., plasma lipid concentrations, glycemia, or body mass index [BMI]) by a genetic variant. Importantly, this new science is changing the landscape of nutritional research [2,12,13] with the incorporation of cutting-edge technologies that have applications in the nutritional sciences [14]. In addition to genomics, techniques such as transcriptomics, proteomics, and metabolomics, coupled with bioinformatics, are already providing the tools for managing and interpreting gene–nutrient interactions at the cell, individual, and population level [1,15–17]. The development of approaches based on systems biology has transformed nutrition research from the traditional reductionism approach of studying the effect of a

Nutritional and Metabolic Bases of Cardiovascular Disease, 1st edition.
Edited by Mario Mancini, José M. Ordovas, Gabriele Riccardi,
Paolo Rubba and Pasquale Strazzullo. © 2011 Blackwell Publishing Ltd.

nutrient on a specific metabolic event into a holistic one [1,2,5,17,18], in which a significant fraction of all regulated genes and metabolites can be queried simultaneously.

Nutritional genomics has already raised high interest and expectations, and some researchers [19] have warned that genomic profiling to study the interactions between genome and environmental factors, such as diet, is not ready for prime time. It is true that the evidence supporting health outcome benefits based on such testing is still lacking, and that before this approach becomes valid and clinically useful, well-designed epidemiologic studies and clinical evaluations of recommended interventions based on genotype are required.

We describe some of the advances in nutritional genomics, with a particular emphasis on nutrigenetic approaches based on lipid levels and metabolic syndrome (MS) traits. This work is not intended by any means to be comprehensive, as several such revisions have recently been published [5,7,11,20]. Rather, the focus here will be to show a window of evidence and the challenges ahead.

Environment as a Modulator of the Effect of Genetic Variants

Dietary Intake

It is well known that nutritional environment is a powerful modulator of gene expression, as demonstrated by Jacob and Monod with the lactose repressor model in bacteria [21]. However, few examples have supported the significant effects of the nutritional environment in human evolution. One of the best known examples in human population involves the lactose gene and relates the different prevalence of lactose tolerance among worldwide populations [22], being higher in societies where dairy products are a staple in the diets of adults (e.g., Scandinavia, Switzerland) and lower in those areas in which milk is not a major nutritional resource (certain areas of Africa, Australian aboriginals). However, a more recent and exciting development came from the discovery of a positive association between copy numbers of the amylase gene with amylase activity and with the consumption of carbohydrates, regardless of ethnicity or geographical location [23]. In terms of cardiovascular diseases, the locus most consis-

tently associated with gene–diet interactions is the apolipoprotein E *(APOE)* gene. Moreover, variability at this locus has currently been implicated in the risk of other common chronic diseases such as multiple sclerosis, Alzheimer's disease, osteoporosis, and colorectal cancer [24–27].

APOE in serum is associated with chylomicrons, very-low-density lipoproteins (VLDLs), and high-density lipoproteins (HDLs), and it serves as a ligand for multiple lipoprotein receptors. The best studied genetic variation at the *APOE* locus results from three common alleles in the population, E4, E3, and E2, with frequencies in Caucasian populations of approximately 0.15, 0.77, and 0.08, respectively [28]. Population studies have shown that plasma cholesterol, LDL-cholesterol (LDL-C), and apolipoprotein B (APOB) levels are highest in subjects carrying the E4, intermediate in those with the E3, and lowest in those with the E2 allele [28]. These studies also point to the possibility that the highest LDL-C levels observed in carriers of the E4 allele were manifested primarily in the presence of an atherogenic diet, raising the notion that the response to dietary saturated fat and cholesterol may differ among individuals carrying different *APOE* alleles. Such a hypothesis has been tested numerous times under different experimental conditions and the findings have been extensively reviewed [5,11,20,29].

Furthermore, there is considerable inconsistency regarding the magnitude and significance of the reported *APOE* gene–diet associations, mainly driven by the heterogeneity of the phenotypes examined [30,31]. This heterogeneity underscores the need for more comprehensive genetic panels, combined with a better assessment of environmental factors. In general, studies differed in gender, baseline lipid levels, and dietary interventions, and all these variables are known to play an important role in the variability of dietary response [30]. In this regard, significant *APOE* gene–diet interactions have been primarily reported in men, by which male carriers of the E4 allele showed an increased response to dietary changes, suggesting a gender-specific effect. Likewise, positive studies have included subjects who were moderately hypercholesterolemic or had significant differences in baseline total cholesterol and LDL-C levels among the *APOE* genotype groups, suggesting that this gene–diet interaction is only seen in hypercholesterolemic subjects. Concerning differences in dietary interventions, significant *APOE* gene–diet interactions were more commonly observed in studies in which total dietary fat and cholesterol were modified. Importantly, some reports have also shown that cholesterol absorption is related to *APOE* genotype [32,33].

Alcohol Consumption

Similar to dietary factors implicated in gene–diet interactions affecting plasma lipid levels, the study of interactions between gene and alcohol drinking has been a topic of great interest to lipid researchers. Although the raising effect of alcohol consumption on HDL-C levels is well established, the effect on LDL-C is still unclear. It is possible that the reported variability will be due to gene–alcohol consumption interactions. Our analyses in the Framingham Study [34] showed that in male nondrinkers, LDL-C levels were not different across *APOE* groups; however, in male drinkers, there were differences in LDL-C, by which E2 subjects displayed the lowest levels. When LDL-C levels were compared among the *APOE* subgroups by drinking status, LDL-C levels in E2 male drinkers were lower than in E2 nondrinkers. Conversely, in E4 males, LDL-C was higher in drinkers than in nondrinkers. In women, the expected effect of *APOE* alleles on LDL-C levels was present in both drinkers and nondrinkers. Overall, these data suggest that in men, the variability at this locus modulates the effects of consuming alcoholic beverages on LDL-C levels.

Smoking

Smoking has also been shown to be a potentially important modulator of the effect of *APOE* on CVD risk [35,36]. In the Framingham Offspring Study [36], an *APOE*–smoking interaction was seen only in men with the overall hazard ratio (HR) for smoking of 1.95 compared to nonsmokers. Using *E3E3* as the referent group in nonsmokers, HRs for *E2* carriers (1.04) and *E4* carriers (1.04) showed no major risk increase, whereas in male smokers, these HRs were 1.96, 3.46, and 3.81 in *E3E3*, *E2*, and *E4* carriers, respectively.

Physical Activity

Physical activity is another factor that has received increased and well-deserved attention. Usually, it

is difficult to obtain reliable information about this variable in large population studies, especially when the design of the study does not include physical activity as one of the main outcomes of the study. Despite those limitations, at least two independent studies have reported a consistent interaction between *APOE* genotype and the effect of physical activity on plasma lipid concentrations. The first one, carried out in a Spanish population, reported that the direct association between HDL-C concentrations and physical activity (energy expenditure) was *APOE* dependent [37]. This interaction was confirmed and examined in more detail by Bernstein et al. [38]. As described for alcohol and smoking, these findings were also gender dependent. In this regard, male carriers of the E4 allele with increased physical activity displayed higher HDL-C and lower triglyceride levels as compared with E3 homozygotes and E2 carriers, whereas the protective effect of exercise in female carriers of the E4 allele was limited to HDL-C. Furthermore, we have to consider that the potential *APOE*–environment interactions may also differ among populations, explaining why one factor has more weight in one population and less in others. Taken together, these data highlight the complexity of these gene–environment interactions.

Obesity as a Modulating Phenotype of the Effect of the Genetic Variants

In this section, we focus on obesity, examining its effect as a modifier factor rather than a main outcome. The working hypothesis is that obesity modulates the genotype–phenotype associations for a variety of candidate genes, making necessary the stratification for this phenotype. Thus far, the best described effects are those affecting the traits of the MS. We have previously summarized more than 30 reports investigating the modulating effect of obesity on the other features of this syndrome (hypertension, dyslipidemia, and glucose intolerance) [39]. One of the main limitations of this study [39] was the lack of standardization in the definition of obesity. Most of these studies focus on BMI; however, BMI is only an incomplete surrogate marker of the body fat mass. In addition, this heterogeneity persists between the World Health Organization (WHO) and the Adult Treatment Panel III (ATP III) criteria for defining obesity. The rationale for the use of waist circumference arises from data showing that measures of BMI are relatively insensitive indicators for CVD risk as compared with measures of abdominal obesity. However, more investigation is needed, and the incorporation of novel anthropometric and biochemical measures of adipose mass and function into large epidemiological studies is clearly warranted. Another issue of discussion is the different cutoff point to define obesity depending on ethnicity. In this regard, lower cutoff points than currently recommended by the WHO (30 kg/m^2 for obesity and 25 kg/m^2 for overweight) should be recommended in some populations, especially in Asia [40]. Finally, another methodological difficulty for replication studies is the treatment of the obesity variable in the statistical analysis (i.e., continuous variable or categorical variable based on international criteria or based on the characteristics of the population). Therefore, a higher standardization for defining and analyzing obesity in the MS is needed in order to obtain valid results.

Beyond these concerns, the *APOE* locus can also be used as a model to illustrate the effect of obesity on genotype–phenotype associations. We examined the interaction between obesity and *APOE* genotype in determining fasting insulin and glucose levels in approximately 3,000 participants in the Framingham Offspring Study [41]. In this study, obese men carriers of the E4 allele displayed higher levels of insulin and glucose than other *APOE* genotype groups. These associations were not observed in non-obese men as well as in women, independently of their BMI. Therefore, although weight control is important in all people, it may be especially important in male carriers of the E4 allele in order to modify the potentially elevated fasting insulin and glucose levels.

In addition to *APOE*, genetic variants at other candidate genes have reported similar modulating effects by BMI or presence of obesity [39]. One of these genes is endothelin-1 (EDN1) Lys198Asn polymorphism and blood pressure. In this regard, several studies carried out in Caucasian and Japanese populations have shown that obesity increases the effect of the 198Asn allele on blood pressure [42,43]. Likewise, prior evidence [44,45]

supports that the effect of lipoprotein lipase (LPL) polymorphisms on plasma lipids is strongly modulated by obesity, BMI, or adiposity by which elevated adiposity or BMI is associated with a more atherogenic lipid profile. The evidence is not only relegated to *APOE, EDN1*, and *LPL* genes, showing similar interactions in several other loci such as adiponectin [46], angiotensin I–converting enzyme [47], apolipoprotein A5 [48], cholesteryl ester transfer protein [49], linkage signal on chromosome 1 [50], selectin-E [51], G-protein β_3 [52–54], interleukin-6 [55], h*epatic* lipase [56], and peroxisome-proliferator–activated receptor-γ [57] (Table 2.1). Importantly, a common basis is observed by which alleles that are deemed to be protective became deleterious in the presence of obesity.

Most of the current evidence supporting the modulating effect of diet and obesity on genotype–phenotype associations is related to cardiovascular risk factors and less information exists related to cancer risk. However, there are enough indications from the literature to support that similar interactions exist for cancer as reviewed by Gunter and Leitzmann [58]. These authors focus primarily on the association between dysregulation of energy homeostasis and colorectal carcinogenesis. It is interesting to point out how obesity-induced insulin resistance leads to elevated levels of plasma insulin, glucose, and fatty acids, which may induce a mitogenic effect on the colon cells. Inflammation is another rising CVD risk factor related to obesity that may also have an impact on colorectal carcinogenesis. Investigators are beginning to study genetic variants within these pathways in relation to colorectal cancer, but the information is still sparse.

Conclusions

Nutrition is probably the most important environmental factor that modulates the action of genes and the phenotypes being considered. This concept has been known for decades but somehow ignored. Therefore, of paramount importance is the consideration of genes in the context of nutrition as well as nutrition within the context of genes. This paradigm constitutes the basis for nutritional genomics, a fast-developing research area with tremendous potential to yield results that may

Table 2.1 Recent evidence showing the modulating effect of BMI on genotype–phenotype associations related with cardiovascular disease (CVD) risk or metabolic syndrome.

Locus/SNP	Population characteristics	Main Outcome	Reference
Adiponectin (APM1 or ADIPOQ)/(−11391G>A, −1377C>G[promoter] and +45T>G[exon2] and +276G>T[intron2])	The Prospective Second Northwick Park Heart Study (NPHS II.) European population including myocardial infarct survivors and controls	Two haplotypes GCTT/GCGG and the +276G>T SNP increased risk of T2DM in interaction with obesity	[46]
Angiotensin I-converting enzyme (ACE)/ insertion/deletion	2642 healthy middle aged Caucasian (mean age 56 years) followed for 15 years	The ACE D allele may worsen glucose metabolism which could raise the prospective T2DM risk in obese men but not in lean men.	[47]
Apolipoprotein A5 (APOA5)/(−1131T>C, −3A>G, 56C>G, IVS3+476G >A, and 1259T>C)	2,273 Framingham Offspring Study participants	The rare allele of each of the −1131T >C, −3A>G, IVS3+476G>A, and 1259T>C variants and the haplotype defined by the presence of the rare alleles in these four variants were each significantly associated with common carotid IMT only in obese participants.	[48]
Cholesteryl ester transfer protein (CETP)/TaqIB	237 hospitalized patients (185 males) with a first event of an ACS and 237 controls matched by age and sex	The protective effect of the B2B2 genotype on the likelihood of having a first event of ACS is observed only in normal-weight persons.	[49]
Chromosome 1 linkage	Subjects from the San Antonio Family Heart Study with measured Lp-PLA(2)	There is a significant genetic response to the adiposity environment in Lp-PLA(2).	[50]
E-Selectin (SELE)/Leu554Phe	478 men and 546 women were selected from the Stanislas cohort	These results suggest a BMI-specific effect of L/F554 polymorphism of the E-selectin gene on blood pressure.	[51]
G-protein beta-3 (GNB3)/(−350A>G, 657A>T, 814G>A, 825C>T and 1429C>T)	282 female Caucasian dizygotic twins aged 21–80 years	The presence of obesity reveals an association between blood pressure and the GNB3 gene in white females.	[52]
G-protein beta-3 (GNB3) 825C>T	14,716 African Americans (AAs) and whites from the Atherosclerosis Risk in Communities (ARIC) study	These findings suggest that the variation within the GNB3 gene may interact with physical activity level to influence obesity status and, together with obesity and physical activity, this SNP may influence hypertension prevalence in AAs.	[53]
G-protein beta-3 (GNB3) 825C>T	Random Brazilian population (n = 1,568)	The C825T genotype was predictive of SBP only in individuals with increased body mass index.	[54]
Interleukin-6 IL6/−174	1525 Framingham participants	Among men with the CC genotype, increased BMI was associated with higher prevalence of diabetes. The IL-6-BMI interaction was not significant in women.	[55]
Hepatic lipase (LIPC)/−514C/T	Health Professionals Follow-up Study, case control, 220 diabetes men with CHD and 641 diabetes men without CVD	These data suggest that obesity may modify the association between the LIPC C(−514)T polymorphism and CHD risk among diabetic men.	[56]
Peroxisome proliferator-activated receptor-α (PPARG)/pro12Ala	Women (Nurses' Health Study) and men (Health Professionals Follow-Up Study) in nested case control settings	This study reports a significantly increased risk associated with the A12 allele among individuals with a BMI> =25 kg/m^2, but not among those <25 kg/m^2	[57]

change the current dietary guidelines and personal recommendations in the future. The hope is that nutrigenetics will provide the basis for personalized dietary recommendations based on the individual's genetic makeup. Indeed, information provided from other environmental factors such as gender and obesity has to be considered. However, to bring all this potential to reality will probably require well-designed, adequately powered, and adequately interpreted randomized controlled studies, as well as interindividual ascertainment of all informative genetic variants or even complete sequencing of an individual's genome. Moreover, research must also investigate the molecular mechanisms involved in the gene–diet interactions reported by nutrigenetic studies. To achieve these ambitious goals, more consistent data across the different studies are needed to move toward the personalized nutrition. Importantly, the use of genetic profiling by health professionals will forecast individual genetic predisposition to multifactorial diseases as well as to predict an individual's long-term prognosis, to target preventive strategies, and to select the most efficacious treatments. Hopefully, bringing nutrigenetics to the state of becoming a practical and useful tool will take place in the near future.

In summary, nutritional genomics should be the driving force of future nutritional research, and it has the potential to change dietary disease prevention and therapy in order to have a major impact on public health. However, the complexity of the goals set for nutritional genomics is tremendous and their accomplishment will require breaking many of the molds of traditional research and seeking integration of multiple disciplines and laboratories working coordinately. Despite the difficulties described, preliminary evidence suggests that the concept will work and we will be able to harness the information contained in our genomes to achieve successful and healthy aging using behavioral changes, with nutrition being the cornerstone of this endeavor.

Acknowledgments

Supported by National Institutes of Health (NIH) grants HL54776, HL72524, and DK075030, contracts 53-K06-5–10 and 58–1950-9–001 from the U.S. Department of Agriculture Research Service.

Selected References

7. Ordovas JM, Tai ES. Why study gene-environment interactions? Curr Opin Lipidol 2008;19:158–67.

15. Gibney MJ, Walsh M, Brennan L, et al. Metabolomics in human nutrition: opportunities and challenges. Am J Clin Nutr 2005;82:497–503.

39. Corella D, Ordovas JM. The metabolic syndrome: a crossroad for genotype-phenotype associations in atherosclerosis. Curr Atheroscler Rep 2004;6:186–96.

46. Gable DR, Matin J, Whittall R, et al. Common adiponectin gene variants show different effects on risk of cardiovascular disease and type 2 diabetes in European subjects. Ann Hum Genet 2007;71:453–66.

48. Elosua R, Ordovas JM, Cupples LA, et al. Variants at the APOA5 locus, association with carotid atherosclerosis, and modification by obesity: the Framingham Study. J Lipid Res 2006;47:990–6.

CHAPTER 3

Etiopathogenesis of Obesity

Marie-Eve Mathieu[1] & Angelo Tremblay[2]

[1] University of Montreal, Montreal, QC, Canada
[2] Laval University, Quebec, QC, Canada

Introduction

Obesity is the long-term consequence of an excess energy intake over expenditure that is mostly deposited as fat in adipose tissue. Since a direct body fat measurement is generally impossible or too difficult to perform in population studies, body mass index (BMI) is used as a proxy variable to estimate variations in body fat content, be it in children or adults. As illustrated in Figure 3.1, our integration of studies documenting variation of weight status in children over time in different populations suggests that overweight prevalence has exponentially increased over the last decades. In adults, the prevalence of obesity has increased worldwide, particularly in the developing world (Asia, North Africa, and Latin America) where the increase has been 2 to 5 times faster than in the United States [1]. The increasing prevalence of obesity raises the question as to what has happened over this period to explain this obesigenic trend in most countries of the world. This chapter is aimed at providing answers to this question with particular attention on less frequently considered determinants of overweight in a context of modernity and on the potential mechanisms by which their effects might be transmitted.

Etiology of Obesity

The fact that obesity is essentially the consequence of excess energy intake over expenditure has probably led some scientists and health professionals

Nutritional and Metabolic Bases of Cardiovascular Disease, 1st edition.
Edited by Mario Mancini, José M. Ordovas, Gabriele Riccardi,
Paolo Rubba and Pasquale Strazzullo. © 2011 Blackwell Publishing Ltd.

to believe and to propose that obesity is mostly caused by gluttony and laziness. However, as discussed in this paper, our recent investigations as well as those of other scientists clearly demonstrate that factors such as suboptimal micronutrient intake, short sleep, excess knowledge-based work, and chemical pollution can also influence energy balance beyond what can be attributed to suboptimal macronutrient intake and physical inactivity.

Energy Intake

Are Variations of Energy Intake per se Predicting Overweight?

Eating a large amount of food does not necessarily lead to body fat accumulation. In fact, conquerors of the Everest who eat between 7 and 16 megajoules (MJ) daily lost between 2 and 11 kg of body weight [2] and a 3-week ski expedition through Greenland induced a loss of 8 kg of body weight in a man whose daily energy intake was 29 MJ [3]. However, in conditions where energy needs are not so pronounced, cohort studies showed that adults consuming a high total energy intake gained significantly more weight [4,5] and centimetres of waist circumference [6]. These observations are concordant with what was observed in the United States, where, in line with the documented twofold increase of obesity prevalence in the adult population between 1971 and 2000–2002, the mean energy intake increased by more than 150 kcal daily [7,8]. However, metabolizable energy intake in infants was not reported to be different between the ones who became overweight or not, by the age of one year [9]. This agrees with the absence of relation between total energy intake and weight change over a 2- to 8-year

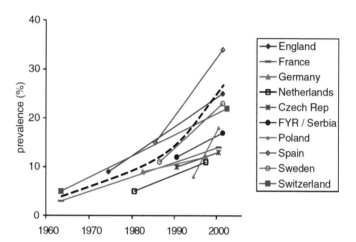

Figure 3.1 Trend in overweight prevalence in European children. (Adapted from Jackson-Leach and Lobstein [80].)

period in children [10]. Thus, it appears that variation in caloric intake per se is not systematically accompanied by concordant changes in body weight.

The Impact of Diet Composition on Energy Intake and Balance

The macronutrient composition of the diet is a factor that can exert a substantial influence on energy intake and body composition. Among 2,245 adults who were followed over a 8-year period, those who had a diet not well suited to national dietary guidelines gained significantly more weight than individuals with good quality diets, although energy intake did not appear in this case as a predictor of weight change [11]. Limited fat intake (<30% energy intake) was one of the quality markers in this study and others have reported that BMI, weight, and adiposity were greater in high- than in low-fat consumers [10,12]. The main contributor to the increase in daily energy intake was the carbohydrate intake, which increased from 42% to 49% in men and from 45% to 52% in women, corresponding to absolute changes of 62 and 68 grams in women and men, respectively. While consuming at least 50% of calories as carbohydrate was reported to help attenuate the increase in BMI in children [10], recent trends in carbohydrate consumption in the United States as well as weight gains documented after carbohydrate overconsumption [13] indicate that an increase in carbohydrate consumption over a certain level can be detrimental to adiposity status.

Among the other components of the diet that changed since the 1970s according to Na-tional Health and Nutrition Examination Survey (NHANES) studies, the significant decline from 60% to 51% in the proportion of individuals consuming a fruit the day of phone recall raises concerns regarding body weight stability [14]. Accordingly, a study conducted in our laboratory revealed that individuals who reduced their fruit consumption over a 6-year follow-up period had larger increases in body weight, adiposity, and waist circumference than subjects displaying the opposite trend. Moreover, the reduction in fruit consumption was associated with the increase in energy intake [15].

Another change in the diet that is suspected to contribute to increased adiposity is the fact that the energy density of the diet increased at the turn of the century [14] with the consequence of detrimental effects on appetite control and energy intake [16,17]. In line with those findings, the review by Rosenheck [18] showed that the frequency of meals taken in fast-food restaurants, where energy-dense foods are omnipresent, was positively associated with increases in total caloric intake and BMI in six out of seven prospective cohort studies.

Physical Properties of Diet

Apart from the diet composition, the physical properties of the diet could be a factor to consider for body weight regulation. As reviewed by Wolf et al. [19], experimental studies indicate that the consumption of liquid calories is not completely compensated by reduced caloric intake from solid food and can lead to an increase in body weight. In addition, considering that the percentage of calories from beverages almost doubled in adults between 1965 and 2002 [20] and that the amount of sweetened beverages consumed increased by 60 g/day in 10-year-old children between 1973 and 1994 [21], it is logical to expect a positive relationship between consumption of beverages and body weight or fat gains. However, most longitudinal studies failed to demonstrate such an association [21–23]. Only Dubois et al. [24] reported that a high consumption of sugar-sweetened beverages between meals more than doubled the odds for a child to become overweight. This latter finding suggests that the time of consumption might be more important than the beverage consumption in the relationship between sweetened beverages and the morphological profile of children.

Milk and the Intake of Calcium

Despite an overall increase in beverage consumption over the last decades, milk consumption now represents only half of what it was at its peak around 1945 [19]. Among the various factors that might contribute to the reduction of milk and calcium consumption, eating in fast-food restaurant was identified as a contributor [25].

Intestinal Absorption

Variations in intestinal absorption and/or fecal energy loss have been related to fluctuations in body weight and energy balance. In this regard, calcium, dairy products, and fiber intakes have been positively associated to fecal fat and energy excretion [26,27]. Accordingly, higher fiber consumption was reported to lead to lower weight gain in cohort studies [28,29]. In addition to what we eat, the gut microbial community (microbiota) could contribute to energy absorption and weight changes via their influence on factors such as the processing of dietary polysaccharides and lipoprotein lipase activity [30].

Output of Energy

Numerous studies were performed in order to determine whether variations in energy expenditure can explain a significant part of one's predisposition to gain weight. In infants and children, a low total energy expenditure (TEE) was associated with larger subsequent weight or fat gain [10,31], whereas in adults, a similar tendency was measured

for body weight [4]. As discussed in the following sections, this issue has also been frequently investigated by specifically focusing on components of daily energy expenditure.

Resting Energy Expenditure

Resting energy expenditure (REE) represents between 60% and 75% of the TEE [32] and has been reported to be positively correlated with fat-free mass and fat mass [33–34]. Thus, it is not surprising to find higher REEs in obese individuals [35], but this relationship does not indicate whether the increased REE is a cause or a consequence of fat accumulation. In opposition to studies reporting no association between REE and weight and/or body composition changes over 1- to 5-year periods, two studies have shown the possible contribution of low REE to weight and adiposity gains [34,36].

Physical Activity

Physical activity includes all body movements done for occupational work, transportation, and leisure time physical activities and represents the most variable component of energy output. These various activities have profoundly changed in the postindustrialization era in most countries of the world. If we take the example of occupational work to which a considerable amount of time is devoted, the proportion of individuals performing sedentary and low physically demanding jobs has almost doubled in the second half of the twentieth century and this occurred at the expense of physically demanding jobs [37,38]. Although this change in occupational structure might in theory explain changes in weight status, Böckerman et al. [37] estimated that it contributed to a maximum of 7% of the BMI change in males over a 30-year period. The limited influence of work is also supported by the study by Lallukka et al. [39], which showed that weight gain over 10 years was not different among the workers who had decreased, maintained, or increased their physical strain at work during that period.

The demonstration that individuals neglecting active transport were gaining more weight than the ones walking or cycling to work [40] suggests that active transportation, for example, to school or work, should be considered in body weight changes. In this regard, many investigations report that active transportation to work and to school in most cases is declining [41–43]. Consequently, it is not surprising that transportation via motorized vehicles increased by 3 times in children during the last 3 decades of the twentieth century [44] and that the proportion of workers using the automobile increased from 67% in 1960 to 88% in 2000 [38]. In China, it was even documented that acquiring a motorized vehicle was associated with a twofold increase in the odds of developing obesity in men [45].

Unlike what is documented for daily work and transportation, several studies showed that leisure-time physical activity or exercise practice was maintained or even increased recently. In Canada, the proportion of men and women considered sufficiently active during their leisure time doubled between 1980 and 2000 [45], while in the United States, recent trends showed that youth maintained their vigorous activity level and that the proportion of adults meeting the physical activity guidelines increased [38]. These recent changes could be beneficial for body weight control, as demonstrated by cohort and experimental studies showing that increases in leisure physical activity/exercise practice contribute to reduction in weight gain and body weight loss [46–49]. Increasing leisure-time physical activity would be even more important for weight management in individuals with excess weight.

Sedentary Behaviors
Despite the positive impact that leisure-time physical activity can confer to body weight regulation, it might not be sufficient to counteract the time allocated to sedentary behaviors. As recently reported, the U.S. population spends on average 15 minutes per day doing sport, exercise, and recreational activities compared to more than 150 minutes of television viewing [50]. In children younger than 10 years, most longitudinal studies have documented that television viewing was positively associated to adiposity gains, while in adolescents, about as many studies have reported a null or a positive association [51]. In adults, results are concordant with those obtained in children, with both higher baseline as well as increases in television viewing time significantly associated with subsequent weight gains [52]. Among the potential explanations of this association between television

viewing and overweight, it appears that it is not mediated by the reduction in resting or TEE, but by the increases in overall energy intake that is likely attributable to the consumption of unhealthy food and fat consumption [51,52].

Other Contributors to Increased Adiposity

Genetic Factors and Intrauterine Life
Genetics factors appear to play an important role in the adiposity status of an individual. This is true for some scarce cases of monogenic obesity such as leptin, leptin receptor, pro-opiomelanocortin, melanocortin-4 receptor, and prohormone convertase-1 gene mutations [53–56]. Moreover, genetic obesity syndromes represent another genetic cause of obesity, with high levels of adiposity characteristics of individuals having Prader-Willi, Bardet-Biedl, Alström, Borjeson-Forssman-Lehmann, or Cohen syndromes.

In addition to the genes that might explain why identical twins have a similar response when exposed to energy imbalance, the fact that they were exposed to the same milieu during intrauterine life might also play a role. In fact, a recent meta-analysis by Oken et al. [54] reported that maternal smoking during gestation increases the risk of developing overweight by 50%. Maternal diabetes, skipping breakfast, and short sleep duration are other potential prenatal programming factors of childhood overweight and obesity [55,56]. Thus, at birth, an infant already has a background that can influence subsequent adiposity gains.

Chemical Exposure
Since World War II, the important development and use of synthetic chemical products such as bisphenol A, organotins, phthalates, and organochlorines have been related to their appearance in the food chain and in the environment [57,58]. These liposoluble compounds have been identified to disturb hepatic, neurological, immune, endocrinal, and muscular functions [57,58]. Moreover, they stimulate fat accumulation by their actions on preadipocyte differentiation, stimulation of a thrifty genotype response, and reduction of resting metabolic rate and triiodothyronine plasmatic levels [57,58]. While the metabolic effects of

these compounds are not desirable, their ability to favor a storage of body fat could be seen as a way to store these liposoluble compounds and thus to reduce their presence in circulation. This hypothesis is supported by the fact that higher plasmatic levels of organochlorines are measured after weight loss [58]. Because they reduce triiodothyronine plasma levels, resting metabolic rate, and skeletal muscle oxidative capacity [58], it cannot be excluded that organochlorines might also be involved in the weight regain frequently observed after weight loss.

Moreover, some drugs such as antipsychotics, mood stabilizers, antidiabetics, and antihypertensives induce, as a side effect, a positive energy balance [59]. Thus, the growing development and use of these pharmaceutical products over the years might have contributed to increased adiposity among users.

Sleep: a Sedentary Activity that Helps Body Weight Regulation

As recently reviewed by Patel and Hu [60], most cross-sectional and all prospective cohort studies suggested that short sleep duration is associated with increased overweight/obesity risk. This emerging factor involved in body weight changes deserves a great deal of attention since the last decades corresponded to a period where sleep duration had decreased by more than 1 hour/day [61]. In children, it was reported that short sleep duration was the best predictor of overweight or obese status when compared to other factors such as parental obesity, low parental education level and family income, long hours of screen time (television, video games, and computer), and physical inactivity [62]. The main explanation pertains to increased energy intake with demonstrations that the reduction in sleep duration increases hunger, appetite, and ghrelin levels, an appetite stimulating hormone, while it decreases leptin levels, an appetite-inhibiting hormone [63]. In addition to short sleep duration, long nights of sleep in adults were shown in some cross-sectional [60] and longitudinal [64] studies to be associated to higher obesity risk and weight gains, respectively. Among potential mechanisms explaining this latter relationship, the idea that short and long sleepers can be characterized by mild hypoglycemia [65] will need to be further investigated.

This is especially relevant knowing that nocturnal hypoglycemia has been recently shown to have awakening and hyperphagic effects [66,67]. Therefore, hypoglycemia likely contributes to increases in energy intake as well as sleep disturbance that might favor extended sleep duration.

Knowledge-based Work

The growing availability of computers has been accompanied by the progressive dominance of mental work as an emerging modality of occupational work in a context of modernity. In this regard, a recent study conducted in our laboratory provides relevant observations. In comparison to a controlled situation (rest), performing knowledge-based work (reading a document and writing a summary text with a computer) induced a significantly greater spontaneous energy intake of 979 kJ while only a non-significant difference of 13 kJ was measured for energy expenditure between both tasks [68]. These authors confirmed the hyperphagic effect of mental work in another recent study that also revealed that it promotes glycemic instability [69]. In line with changes in daily labor, longer working days and increased work fatigue were documented as potential causes of weight gain [70]. This also agrees with the fact that weight gains were significantly higher for men who increased mental strain at work compared to the ones with stable or decreased mental solicitation [62,70].

Glycemic Control

According to the glucostatic theory, glycemic changes can trigger an increase in appetite [71]. Several studies indicate that glucose levels can, in addition to their acute effects on appetite, contribute to weight changes. In the Quebec Family Study, plasma glucose concentrations 2 hours after the intake of a glucose load were negatively correlated to body weight gains over a 6-year period, a finding that remained significant after correction for insulin resistance [72]. In diabetic individuals taking medication for glycemic control, the weight gains were higher for the ones having severe hypoglycemic episodes [73]. Another study showed that weight regains were more important for individuals having, after the weight loss intervention, a lower glucose area under fasting values during the oral glucose tolerance test [72]. Together, these findings support the fact that having glucose concentrations in the range of mild hypoglycemia can favor weight gain and regain.

While the importance of physical activity to favor a negative energy balance has been addressed, it appears that physical activity is more than just a calorie-burning agent. Apart from the positive impacts on metabolic heath described in Chapter 8, exercise training has been shown to reduce the hypoglycemic response to an intravenous glucose tolerance test [74]. Among the various mechanisms involved in this response, the fact that trained individuals have a higher hepatic glucose production in response to an infusion of glucagon, suggesting a better sensibility to this hyperglycemic hormone, could be one of them [75]. Using an animal model, Charbonneau et al. [76] showed that when hepatic resistance to glucagon is present, it can be considerably reduced with exercise training. In addition, exercise training contributes to increases in the muscle glycogen synthase activity and storage of glucose as muscular glycogen [14,77]. Moreover, higher insulin-stimulated glucose uptake, regulation of genetic expression, and recruitment of glucose transporter isoform-4 [77,78] can contribute to storage but also to utilization of glucose within the muscular tissues. Despite these adaptations facilitating glucose utilization and storage, muscles adapt to exercise training by increasing their utilization of lipids as an energy source and by reducing relative glucose utilization [79]. Therefore, exercise training can potentially help to prevent hypoglycemia and its deleterious effect on energy intake.

Conclusion

When identifying the causes leading to increased adiposity and weight gain, it soon became evident that it is a complex issue. While energy intake and output are the central components of energy balance, these variables are influenced by diet composition, energy absorption, genetic background, intrauterine life, sleep duration, as well as the environment and society in which an individual lives. Also, what leads to increased adiposity in one individual might greatly differ from person to person. In addition, despite that a given factor was not clearly identified as a potential cause leading to increased adiposity in a given population, it does not necessarily mean that it could not be the cause for a given individual. Thus, the individual assessment of the potential causes leading to increased weight should be encouraged when possible. Moreover, what caused weight gain in an individual might not always be an efficient target for weight loss. As a matter of fact, stopping a medication because it is inducing weight gain might not be an optimal treatment for the overall health of an individual.

Selected References

2. Reynolds RD, Lickteig JA, Howard MP, et al. Intakes of high fat and high carbohydrate foods by humans increased with exposure to increasing altitude during an expedition to Mt. Everest J Nutr 1998;128(1):50–55.

10. Skinner JD, Bounds W, Carruth BR, et al. Predictors of children's body mass index: a longitudinal study of diet and growth in children aged 2-8 y. Int J Obes Relat Metab Disord 2004;28(4):476–82.

24. Dubois L, Farmer A, Girard M, et al. Regular sugar-sweetened beverage consumption between meals increases risk of overweight among preschool-aged children. J Am Diet Assoc 2007;107(6):924–34.

39. Lallukka T, Sarlio-Lahteenkorva S, Kaila-Kangas L, et al. Working conditions and weight gain: a 28-year follow-up study of industrial employees. Eur J Epidemiol 2008; 23(4):303–10.

51. Rey-Lopez JP, Vicente-Rodriguez G, Biosca M, et al. Sedentary behaviour and obesity development in children and adolescents. Nutr Metab Cardiovasc Dis 2008;18(3):242–51.

CHAPTER 4

The Epidemiology of Obesity

W. Philip T. James & Rachel Leach

London School of Hygiene and Tropical Medicine, International Obesity TaskForce, IASO, London, UK

Introduction

Normal BMIs?

The specification of body weight in terms of the body mass index (BMI) and the range of BMIs generally classified as "normal" were set by the World Health Organization (WHO) [1]. In practice, the upper level of the "normal" range (i.e., BMI of 25.0) was set on the basis of old analyses of death rates from medical insurance data from the United States. The lower limit had to be refined because billions of people were below the original lower limit of BMI 20.0, on the basis of morbidity and mortality data and work capacity from Latin America, Africa, and Asia [2]. Thus, a BMI limit of 18.5 was accepted, below which there were physical disadvantages when working hard and BMIs < 17.0 signified increasing risks of disease and early death.

However, a BMI of 25.0 was recognized in Western adults to signify an increased prevalence of major health problems such as hypertension, glucose intolerance/diabetes, and dyslipidemia, and on the basis of medical criteria, the optimum or ideal average BMI of an adult population was set at about BMI of 21.0 [3]. Yet, Asian data already showed that the risk of diabetes, for example, occurred at much lower BMIs. Now the prevalence of diabetes in Asians has been found to be 2 to 5 times greater at each BMI level, with an absolute increase in the prevalence of diabetes even at low BMIs [4]. WHO has accepted that in practice many Asian countries will need to specify an individual BMI of 23.0 or more as disadvantageous [5]. In addition, the focus

is on the importance of the distribution of body fat with abdominal obesity, most easily measured as the waist circumference [6]. Abdominal obesity is found particularly in the developing world (now referred to as the low and middle income countries) and there is increasing evidence that this reflects a metabolic/hormonal switch that seems to involve the corticosteroid axis reprogramming in utero and perhaps the first 2 years of life. Unfortunately, there are no universally accepted criteria for waist circumference, with the original values being cited in the Scottish Intercollegiate Guidelines Network (SIGN) for obesity management [7] and then subsequently by WHO [8] for use in whites. Since then, different methodologies and criteria have been developed for different ethnic groups, so currently there is substantial confusion as to which waist circumference value to use [9]. Table 4.1 lists the current approaches to the classification of risk by the U.S. National Institutes of Health (NIH) and an Asian perspective, but when describing the epidemic, most authors follow the WHO convention of classifying according to WHO international reference points even if they also specify their own special criteria.

Children's BMIs

The original WHO reference curves available from the late 1960s for the "normal" growth of children were in practice derived from U.S. data and were used simply as a reference value for classifying low weights for age as "protein–energy malnutrition" across the world. In 1990, the WHO reference values were reassessed and were then derived from the U.S. National Center for Health Statistics

Nutritional and Metabolic Bases of Cardiovascular Disease, 1st edition.
Edited by Mario Mancini, José M. Ordovas, Gabriele Riccardi,
Paolo Rubba and Pasquale Strazzullo. © 2011 Blackwell Publishing Ltd.

Table 4.1 The implications for the risk of disease of NIH and Asian adaptations of the WHO criteria for classifying overweight and obesity.

Classification	BMI (kg/m²)	Europids Waist circumference		Asians Waist circumference	
		≤102 cm (M) ≤88 cm (W)	>102 cm (M) >88 cm(W)	<90 cm (M) <80 cm (W)	>90 cm (M) >80 cm (W)
Underweight	<18.5		—	—	
Asian normal	18.5–22.9		—	—	Increased risk
Asian overweight	23.0–24.9			Increased risk	Substantial risk
Asian obesity grade 1	25.0–29.9			Substantial risk	High risk
Europid normal	18.5–24.9		Increased risk		
Europid overweight	25–29.9	Increased risk	High risk		
Obesity	30–35	High risk	Very high risk	Very high risk	Major risk

BMI: body mass index; M: men; W: women.
Note: It is relatively unusual for appreciable increases in BMI not to be accompanied by increases in abdominal obesity identified by high waist circumferences.

(CHS) set of reference charts of 1977, which reflected the growth of predominantly bottle-fed babies. However, subsequently, the WHO established a major study involving breast-fed babies and children younger than 5 years from California, Norway, India, Oman, Ghana, and Brazil. This study showed that despite the different ethnic backgrounds, the children's growth was almost identical, different from those of bottle-fed babies and with a much smaller variability in growth across the populations. This means that if one takes the new WHO standard deviation values as the limits of normality, the estimated prevalences of underweight and overweight will now be greater, particularly in terms of overweight because in both children and adults there is an increasingly skewed distribution of weights as the average weight for age rises. Thus, overweight rates increased by one-third when the new WHO standard curves were used rather than the old NCHS data; there were also far more infants and 1 year olds classified as stunted [10].

This new set of growth curves is considered by the WHO as the ideal growth patterns for all children from any ethnic group, but in many countries, pediatricians and governments still consider that their babies grow differently for genetic or other reasons and that this particularly applies to the heights of children. The U.S. Centers for Disease Control and Prevention (CDC) also produced its own growth curves based on a selection of national studies of the growth of U.S. children. However, when these are compared with the new WHO charts of children younger than 5 years, the new CDC curves clearly relate to heavier and shorter children than the "ideal" breast-fed WHO children, particularly during the first year of life [11].

In late 2007, the WHO set out completely new estimates of the ideal growth of children from 5 to 20 years of age [12]. Remarkably, the WHO chose only U.S. data despite finding detailed growth curves from many other potentially suitable international sources. All of the world's children, if optimally fed and nurtured, should in theory now grow in line with a subset of the cohort from the U.S. children of old. However, very few countries have considered this, and the whole approach to the issue and the way these curves were developed imply that about 16% of "healthy" children (i.e., those over 1SD, equivalent in adults to a BMI of about 25.0) are at risk of disease, which is not ideal. In Asia and other parts of the world where the average adult BMI should be 21.0 at most and as few children as possible should enter adult life with a BMI > 23.0, there is medical resistance to this new approach.

When the International Obesity TaskForce (IOTF) produced its draft on obesity for the first WHO meeting on obesity in 1997, there was no robust international system for considering obesity as distinct from malnutrition in children [12]. The IOTF children's group, therefore, considered the issue in detail [13] and agreed to use BMI values for children as well as adults. Overall, the use of BMI as an indicator of adiposity appeared acceptable for children aged 6 to 7 and 17 and 18 years, but the use of the BMI value for taller children, particularly 6- to 12-year-olds, gives higher prevalence values for obesity than if the weight of the child was truly considered independent of height, which was the basis of the adult choice of BMI. Therefore, caution is needed in interpreting the long-term significance of modest increases in BMIs in tall young children.

The IOTF then developed BMI reference values [14] based on the data from nationally representative surveys of six counties: Brazil, United States, United Kingdom, The Netherlands, Singapore, and Hong Kong. These values are the mean of the percentile values at each sex and age-group, which correspond at 18 years of age to BMIs of 25.0 and 30.0. They are, therefore, based on the assumption that in general children will grow along their percentile or that the same percentile has long-term significance throughout childhood. These values are now used almost universally for quantifying the prevalence of overweight and obesity across the world [15].

The IOTF curves still need adapting for practical use in poorer countries because the reference BMIs used throughout the work are for percentiles equivalent to the adult WHO cutoff points of 25.0 and 30.0. Thus, in the low and middle income countries particularly, the overweight cutoff percentile curve values equivalent to an adult BMI of 23.0 are considered more appropriate for clinical use, with obesity percentile values equivalent to 27.5 as suggested by the Singapore WHO meeting in 2003 [5].

Prevalence of Childhood and Adult Overweight and Obesity

Table 4.2 shows the prevalence by region of childhood obesity using the standard IOTF criteria, which are the most universally used methods for

Table 4.2   The World Health Organization (WHO)–designated regions and their prevalences of excess bodyweight in school-age children in 2010 using the IOTF cutoff points for overweight and obesity. The overweight prevalences exclude both the normal and the obese categories of children's weight.

Region	Obese	Overweight
Americas	15%	31%
Middle East and North Africa	12%	30%
Europe and former USSR	10%	28%
West Pacific	7%	20%
Southeast Asia	5%	18%
Africa	>1%	>4%

Reproduced from Wang and Lobstein. Int J Pediatr Obes 2006;1:11–25, with permission.

classifying children as either overweight or obese. These regional differences highlight the fact that although the North American region (which in WHO terms includes Canada and Cuba as well as the United States), some regions such as the Middle East are not far behind. Within the regional averages are immense differences, with Russia within Europe and Mexico within Latin America having values that are close to those of the United States. Overall, however, it is clear that about half of the children in the Americas as a whole, Europe, the Middle East, and Northern Africa are in need of immediate help. In addition, the health impact of excess weight in Southeast Asia (including most of the Indian subcontinent and Indonesia) and the Western Pacific region (which includes China and Japan) is almost certainly a greater risk despite a somewhat lower prevalence of excess weight.

Figure 4.1 provides regional estimates of adult overweight and obesity where the age structures of the countries are adjusted to a WHO standard and with regional groupings according to the WHO's analyses of the global burden of disease. Note that the prevalence of overweight and obesity in the Middle East and in Latin America/Caribbean is approaching that of North America. In several Asian countries such as India, there are marked differences between the rural areas and the cities, with average BMIs in the countryside of about 18.0 but with BMIs rapidly increasing to 23.0 in average adults in many urban environments. These changes

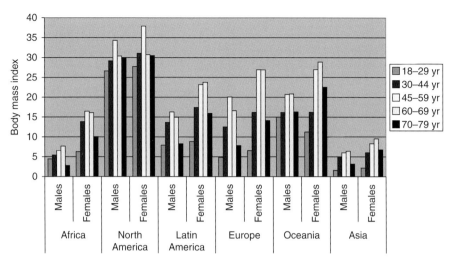

Figure 4.1 The regional prevalences are standardized by age and separated to show the age-related increases in obesity. The countries in each region comply with the World Health Organization classification.

are induced by marked reductions in physical activity and dramatic increases in fat and sugar intake. Accompanying these changes are tenfold increases in the prevalence of diabetes and hypertension. The high prevalence on excess weight in Indian cities has recently been illustrated by a five city study [16] where, using standard WHO criteria, 35% of women are overweight (BMI of 25.0–29.9) with an additional 7% obese (≥30.0)—a total of 42% of the population. However, if those BMIs that are 23.0 or higher are included, the total women's prevalence rises to 52%. In men, the comparable standard figures are 32% overweight and an extra 6% obese (i.e., a total of 38% of the population affected), but again there was an additional 14% with BMIs between 23.0 and 25.0, giving a total of 52% men at risk on a Asian basis. Even more striking is the finding that the prevalence of abdominal obesity in both women and men is higher than the rates of excess weight even when one takes the Asian criteria of BMI ≥23.0 as the value for the comparison.

Abdominal Obesity and Early Programming of Disease Sensitivity to Weight Gain

Excessive deposition of fat abdominally has been linked to early childhood stunting not only in lower income countries such as Guatemala, but also in English adults with hypertension, diabetes, and abdominal obesity in the classic analyses by Barker [17]. These characteristics of what was then called "syndrome X" and now the "metabolic syndrome" in Barker's study were linked to the subject's birth weight. This has also been shown in several countries with very different degrees of affluence, for example, from the United States [18] and Finland to poorer countries such as China and India. If the children are of low birth weight, then they are also often small and underweight in their first few years of life because few children in poor countries show accelerated growth [19]. In young Finnish adults [20], the risk of having diabetes was highest if the individual was born small but gained more weight than usual after the age of 2 years and was heavy at 12 years of age. Indian adults [21] also showed that their risk of having glucose intolerance or diabetes was highest if they were small at 2 years of age but subsequently gained excess weight so that they were heavy by the age of 12 years. The discrepancy between having a low weight and height status from birth to 2 years of age followed by faster rates of subsequent growth seems to be particularly harmful.

Micronutrient Deficiencies
More recently, Yajnik has highlighted the importance of the nutritional status of mothers during

pregnancy and has emphasized the critical role of one carbon pool metabolism. This methyl donating cycle is essential not only for synthesizing the nucleic acid, so essential for producing new cells, but the cycle also affects gene expression which therefore affects a whole range of different metabolic pathways. The one carbon pool system can only produce a plentiful supply if these methyl groups and the whole metabolic cycle of regenerating the S-adenosyl-methionine has the optimum number of enzymatic co-factors supplied by the adequate intake of folate, choline, betaine, and other methyl group donors as well as other B vitamins including riboflavin, pyridoxine, and vitamin B_{12}. These three vitamins as well as folate are in short supply because milk, meat, and eggs, as well as other rich sources of riboflavin, pyridoxine, and B_{12}, are not available to the poor, especially in Asia. Their traditional avoidance of fresh foods and reliance on vegetarian food cooked for hours in sauces also ensures that the folate as well as the pervasive contaminating bacteria are destroyed. Multiple deficiencies of these vitamins are found among the Indian rural poor and slum dwellers, but Yajnik has highlighted the problem now being amplified by the routine administration of iron and folic acid supplements to pregnant Asian women, 85% of whom are clinically anemic in pregnancy with scandalously high maternal mortality rates. Most doctors consider the use of iron and folic acid commendable, but with 75% of the Indian population B_{12} deficient as well, this use of high-dose folic acid supplements in the presence of B_{12} deficiency leads to metabolic rerouting in the one carbon pool and these women produce the smallest, fattest, and most insulin-resistant babies. Later, accelerated growth in these small babies amplifies the observed insulin resistance and higher blood pressure when assessed at 4 and 8 years of age. Thus, the propensity to diabetes and hypertension in Asia may relate to the unforeseen consequences of vegetarianism and the observed >75% prevalence of B_{12} deficiency, which is based on longstanding religious and socioeconomic reasons [22]. In India, there is also a documented link between high maternal plasma homocysteine levels and low folate, B_{12} levels, and low birth weights [23].

This issue of B_{12} and folate deficiency is not just an Asian problem but has been described in many low and middle income countries. Thus, it is not uncommon to find 50% of adults with modest folate deficiency and a quarter or more of many populations with low vitamin B_{12} levels [24].

Low Protein Intake

The association between fetal nutrition and abdominal obesity is also linked or due to low intake of appropriate protein in pregnancy. Many animal studies show that low maternal protein intake reduces the placental activity of the cortisol deactivating enzyme that normally protects the fetus from the higher normal maternal circulating concentrations of cortisol. As the fetus develops, the organization of the fetal hypothalamic/pituitary/adrenal axis is then affected because the higher maternally derived cortisol circulating in the fetus may then reset the normal sensitivity of the fetal feedback system, so the fetus is born accustomed to higher cortisol secretions. This, as in Cushing's disease, may then in part explain both increased insulin resistance and the propensity to abdominal fat deposition. If this is substantiated in humans, the low protein content of rice, the major staple for 3 billion people, when eaten without other protein sources from animal products or legumes may make these pregnant women likely to produce babies susceptible to abdominal obesity. This propensity may be amplified by the normal adaptive lower body protein turnover in response to this low protein intake, so there will be even fewer readily available amino acids and other crucial components immediately available for the fetus in the development of the essential cellular machinery needed for setting the trajectory of fetal growth, crucial cellular components, and the evolving stem cells for lean tissue growth. Indians at birth and indeed as adults have a smaller lean tissue mass for each kilogram of weight gain. Furthermore, the Chinese, Malays, and urban Thais have lean/fat ratios intermediate between the lowest ratios seen in Indians and the much higher ratios seen in British babies and adults. That this is not a racial/ethnic issue is shown by the finding that rural Thais have lean/fat ratios close to those of British individuals. Thus, the fundamental determinant of the ratio of lean and fat tissues seems in part to be set from birth and relates to the nutritional condition of the pre-pregnant woman and her nutrient intake throughout pregnancy.

Given this perspective, it may not be surprising if the majority of the world proves to have a greater propensity to both abdominal obesity and a greater sensitivity to chronic diseases than the current whites in the United States and northern Europe who have had much better diets for about two generations since the marked deprivation found throughout northern Europe in pre–World War II days. The general nutritional status of the U.S. white population has probably been better for longer.

Nutritional and Physical Activity Determinants of Weight Gain

The normal rate of excess weight gain is on average about 0.5–1.0 kg/yr in early adult life; this is equivalent to a yearly accumulation of approximately 3,500–7,000 kcal. This amounts to an average discrepancy between energy intake and energy expenditure of only 10–20 kcal/day. This is now termed the "energy" gap. The energy gap amounts to a discrepancy in energy balance of only about 0.4%–0.8% of normal food intake per day. With the major changes in activity and food habits over the last few decades, the surprising finding is how little weight gain has occurred and this in turn shows how remarkable the appetite control system is with its interplay of short, medium, and longer term regulatory mechanisms. This system is recognized to adapt as our current way of life circumvents or overwhelms these controls so that as weight gain occurs, the regulatory system adapts to the higher weights and then biologically resists the individual's attempt to return his or her weight to normal. This theory in part explains why the obesity epidemic has been maintained despite all the national efforts to slim.

Physical Inactivity and Compensatory Obesity

The substantial fall in the demand for physical exertion came with the increasing use of cars for personal transport and huge range of mechanical and electrical aids, which removed the need for physical work both at home and at work. When computers and television were introduced, it became normal for the average worker in industrialized society to earn a living without having to expend nearly as much energy as in traditional agricultural work. The number of people involved in heavy occupational physical activity has declined dramatically, with more than a 50% reduction in "heavy work" in Norwegian adults since the middle 1980s [25]. When one considers the change from mainstream agricultural work to city work as part of the so-called nutritional transition affecting most of the world, one can estimate the overall fall in energy demand for both men and women as amounting to about 300–375 kcal/day. Then if one considers the difference between commuting to work by bicycle, bus, or car, there is a further decline in energy needs with public transport by about 150 kcal and with car use by another 120 kcal. Thus, in total, the combination of substituting still moderately physically demanding work for traditional agricultural work and using cars for personal commuting totals about 500–800 kcal/day fall in the average energy needs of the population [26]. In a domestic setting, the increases in technologically sophisticated labor-saving devices, and reduced time to prepare meals and carry out household tasks have also contributed to the marked but unquantified fall in domestic energy expenditure. The overall secular reduction in food needs could be as great as a 1,000 kcal/day for many groups of adults.

This reduced demand means that we are likely to gain weight despite our appetite regulatory systems unless we eat substantially less. However, when we fail to do so, our increase in weight increases our routine energy demand to cope with the increase in metabolically active lean tissue (which inevitably accompanies the development of obesity) by about 175–250 kcal/day per 10 kg of weight gain. Thus, it then becomes evident that there may have been a decrease in total food intake, but this was not enough to compensate for the greater decrease in energy expenditure; by gaining weight, we are limiting the need to reduce intake even further. Thus, weight gain is simply an energetic mechanism that in practice balances our marked decrease in energy expenditure and slightly smaller reduction in food intake. The challenge then is how to eat appreciably fewer kilocalories, unless in some way we can once again increase our physical activity.

For some European countries, the increase in obesity was delayed by up to a decade, notably in

The Netherlands and Scandinavian countries [27] This might well relate to the high rates of active commuting, especially cycling. Nevertheless, within a country, the data are not so clear because in Finnish adults, the rates of increases in obesity were only slightly higher in the inactive adults compared with the increasing rates in the more active adults.

Dietary Change and Its Basis

Evidence for the transformation of our diets is easier to document, and it is obvious that the well-described large meals of our ancestors are no longer the norm. Over the last 30 years in relatively sophisticated European environments, the meals and portions served in restaurants have become smaller because that is what consumers seem to want. Data from national food surveys, for example, in the United Kingdom, show a progressive fall in consumption to have occurred even after allowing for the increasing use of meals outside the home. Many people now no longer have breakfast and this may also reflect the fact that we are adapting behaviorally to brain mechanisms that attempt to reduce our eating. Unfortunately, the transformation of the food chain with an increasing tendency to eat outside the home and to buy ready-to-eat meals means that populations have become far more dependent on manufactured processed foods and on decisions based on information about the nature of their food purchases.

The WHO [28] highlighted the importance of the increasing energy density of food and meals. This high density is dominated by the high fat content of the foods [29] together with additional contributions from added sugar and starch processing, which removes the water-holding property of the carbohydrates. Sugar in drinks also seems to be an energy component that tends to evade the complex regulatory systems of the brain, so sugary drinks—whether fruit juices or the heavily marketed soft drinks—are a potent contributor to the problem. In addition, food companies and supermarkets have become highly competitive and have developed with the advertising industry very pervasive and effective techniques that now use neuroimaging and tracking to both evade our normal biological restraints on eating and persuade us to buy snacks and drinks that are characterized by their obesogenic properties.

Other marketing techniques involve increasing portion size, pricing purchases to increase "value for money," and having food and drinks available everywhere. It is well recognized by business that one can alter a population's intake and thereby increase profits by three main mechanisms: adjusting the price, making the foods and drinks always available, and marketing the products intensively. In the last 10–15 years, marketing techniques have focused on vulnerable children very effectively [30], and now the priority is for Western food and commodity companies, for example, the producers of vegetable oils and sugar, to penetrate with supermarkets the developing world as part of their next phase for increasing turnover and profits. Therefore, it is no wonder that once an economy moves from one of absolute poverty, one finds both obesity rates and population blood cholesterol levels rising [31].

A Public Health Response to the Obesity Epidemic

Health Education Ineffective without Enabling, Incentivising, or Regulating Change

Financial experts are becoming increasingly concerned about the extraordinary predicted increases in the economic costs of the current obesity epidemic. They are also starting to undertake their own analyses that confirm the results of more detailed academic studies showing that health promotion through education alone is ineffective but is useful as a general background measure when one or more of three other measures are taken: a) enabling change by strategic measures that alter the way in which people gain access to food and engage in physical activity, b) providing incentives for industry to fundamentally alter their practices, and c) enforcing change by government regulation. One needs to understand, however, that the food/manufacturing industries are the largest section of the manufacturing industry in Europe and have immense power. Therefore, they routinely gain rapid access to prime ministers and presidents when they think their short-term interests are threatened.

Nevertheless, it is crucial that any action plan is not based on the idea that the professional groups such as doctors, nurses, and teachers can persuade children and adults to change their habits. There is also no point in blaming the competitive short-term media or a ministry of health, which is one of the weakest branches of government for its failure to act. Health ministries constantly use their political position to demand an ever increasing proportion of the government's budget in order to cope with the escalating costs of adult chronic diseases when these are being amplified so markedly by the overweight/obesity epidemic.

Children, the Priority?

New analyses by the U.K. government show that the politically acceptable focus on children as the key priority is misplaced if one seeks a reduction in medical costs, because these are only affected 40–50 years later if one could immediately prevent childhood obesity. The costs come in middle and old age, so older people and children are a priority for immediate action. If one can prevent or reverse the overweight/medical costs of the middle aged/older groups, then one sees much bigger cost savings much earlier.

Government-Induced Changes Affecting Spontaneous Activity

It is now clear that simply advocating more sports and leisure-time gym or other explicit exercise regimens is not the answer, as this cannot apply universally to children from the age of 2 years to the elderly in their 80s. Some aspects of modern life are inevitable, such as mechanization, transport changes, TVs, and computers, but the following general measures are increasingly seen as important in promoting physical activity:

a) Urban development policies that emphasize well-designed high-density homes and careful street planning help to promote spontaneous activity, whereas U.S.-style suburban sprawl forces people to use cars.

b) The design of roads and the layout of a community is also critical for providing ready access by pedestrian and cycle paths to important communal facilities such as shops and parks.

c) Locating offices and supermarkets in town rather than outside towns affects the quality of towns as well as whether people have to use cars for their shopping. Easy access reduces socioeconomic inequalities.

d) Road and pavement/sidewalk design is also critical. Some European countries such as the Netherlands have ample cycle paths and routinely give preference to cyclists/pedestrians rather than designing the roads to move cars as fast as possible with pedestrians excluded, as in the United Kingdom.

e) Policies on free spaces for children's play and the arrangements for lighting streets and building clean, wide sidewalks make a major difference in how parents and the elderly view the safety of their area and, therefore, the likelihood of children playing and the elderly going out at night.

f) Park, leisure, and sports facilities within school facilities made available as community centers for educational and recreational use amplify the importance of school physical activity lessons and make maximum use of publicly funded buildings, which can then also be used for adult education among other things.

These require long-term strategic changes that transport, urban planning, local government ministries need to specify in their 5- to 10-year plans, but the current problem is that doctors advising governments do not understand just how important these changes are, so the ministry of health has no backing if it proposes changes that are the responsibility of other government departments. New evidence suggests that increasing sports participation can be very useful in reducing the likelihood of diabetes but is a poor societal remedy for obesity and not easily applied to all socioeconomic groups and the full age range. Girls and women are also less amenable to competitive sports and usually enjoy other activities such as dancing. Community-wide involvement in social interactions rather than TV viewing also needs special support so that people move outside their home in the evening and do not simply retreat to their TVs for entertainment. This broader community involvement benefits childcare, reduces the isolation of people in towns and cities, and improves mental health.

Changing the Food Supply and Consumer Understanding

Many changes are needed including the following:
a) Establish catering policies including the banning of trans-fats in foods in all government-supported

organizations so that they only serve foods and meals that comply with high-quality nutritional standards and do not allow low-quality products as choices in public facilities. These include hospitals, health centers, government departments, and other publicly supported facilities such as police, military, prisons, and schools. All commercial organizations should then only gain access to these publicly supported facilities if all their products conform to the same standards. The progressive elimination of trans-fats by government specification should become the norm or they should be banned by law, as in Denmark.

b) Adopt the successful Finnish policy of requiring all catering outlets/restaurants to include vegetables, salad bar, and fruit within the cost of a main meal and not as separately priced items. This was so successful in Finland that it led to a threefold increase in the average vegetable intake of the population over a 15-year period and this was associated with a decrease in the population's average blood pressure of 10 mm Hg, which is equivalent to putting a hypotensive agent in the drinking water. Of course, the fruit and vegetable increase was not the only explanation, given the 10% decrease in the energy contribution from fat and the specific and multiple measures to reduce the population's salt intake. Nevertheless, the obesity rates in Finland slowed to a stop and the cardiovascular death rates have fallen by >80% since the early 1970s.

c) Proper food labeling is needed and the system of traffic light labeling has been shown by the U.K. government and detailed consumer surveys to be easily understood and far superior to the usual Recommended Daily Allowance labeling, which creates consumer confusion. The new scheme is valued and used sensibly by all ages and socioeconomic and education groups but of course is bitterly opposed in Europe by the food industry and many supermarkets because for the first time, consumers can understand the meaning of the food labels. Labeling requirements need to apply to all food outlets and restaurants including all the fast-food roadside outlets.

d) Limiting the density of fast-food (low-quality) outlets in towns and cities has not been considered sufficiently, particularly given the fact that the WHO Millennium analysis of the major risk factors for the world's disability and premature deaths shows that hypertension, hypercholesterolemia, and obesity induce as great a long-term disease impact as tobacco and alcohol and these medical problems are specifically promoted by the repeated frequent ingestion of fast foods currently made available everywhere despite the parallel restrictions applying to tobacco and alcohol outlets.

e) Marketing restrictions and bans on all commercial targeting of children and vulnerable adults are also essential. There is overwhelming evidence of harm from all forms of marketing to children. TV advertising as well as other new outlets (e.g., Internet, product placement, and competitions and viral marketing) are used intensely by the advertising industry and distort the understanding of both children and adults.

f) Nutritional profiling of foods is important so that all sorts of initiatives can benefit. Providing better food and handicapping the sales of energy-dense, nutrient-poor foods are essential underpinning strategies for many government policies and are being increasingly considered by many governments.

g) Adjusting the price of food is also a very effective way of changing food purchases, and the poorer the individuals, the greater the effect. Thus, governments can employ a combination of taxes and subsidies at zero cost to Treasury to progressively alter purchases, just as these measures were shown to be effective strategies when dealing with tobacco and alcohol problems. Danish Economic Institute analyses of price elasticity show that the poorer sections of the community respond extremely well to surprisingly small changes in the price of foods, so small increases in costs of sugar, fat, and salty foods with small reductions in fruit and vegetables costs should be tested.

From a medical point of view, there is of course the newly recognized need to identify glucose-intolerant adults. Many international studies now show that more than half of adults vulnerable to developing either diabetes or high blood pressure do not develop the disease for years if they adopt dietary changes and restrict fat, sugar, and salt intake, increase fruit and vegetable consumption, and become more physically active. The elderly also show even greater benefit. This then raises the possibility of developing simple medical schemes on a national basis using a set of planned interventions and simple criteria such as blood pressure screening, fasting glucose by finger-prick measures, and waist circumference. These are readily understood by the public.

National surveillance systems also need to be supported by the medical profession and again need to include simple measures such as those listed above as well as other measures to monitor the impact of the obesity epidemic and any progress in policy interventions.

These initiatives are often proposed by medical groups and academic societies as well as ministries of health, but the evidence is that one needs a national coordinating body. This should be independent and publicly transparent and involve academic/nongovernmental organizations as well as the media. Links to finance ministries are also needed if one seeks to maintain public engagement as well as supporting and exerting pressure for progressive policy development.

Selected References

3. James WPT, Jackson-Leach R, Ni Mhurchu C, et al. Overweight and obesity (high body mass index). In: Ezzati M, Lopez AD, Rodgers A, Murray CJL, editors. Comparative Quantification of Health Risks. Global and Regional Burden of Disease Attributable to Selected Major Risk Factors, Chapter 8, Volume 1. Geneva: World Health Organization; 2004.

5. WHO Expert Consultation (held in Singapore). Appropriate body-mass index for Asian populations and its implications for policy and intervention strategies. Lancet 2004;363:157–63.

6. Yusuf S, Hawken S, Ôunpuu S, et al, on behalf of the INTERHEART Study Investigators. Obesity and the risk of myocardial infarction in 27 000 participants from 52 countries: a case-control study. Lancet 2005;366: 1640–49.

7. James WPT. The fundamental drivers of the obesity epidemic. Obesity Rev 2008;9(Suppl 1):6–13.

8. Prentice AM, Jebb SA. Fast foods, energy density and obesity: a possible mechanistic link. Obesity Rev 2003;4: 187–94.

CHAPTER 5

Pre-Diabetes in Obese Adolescents: Pathophysiologic Mechanisms

Anna M.G. Cali & Sonia Caprio
Yale University School of Medicine, New Haven, CT, USA

Introduction

Obesity is one of the most serious and urgent public health problems in both developed and developing countries [1]. It has reached epidemic proportions in the United States. Among children 6 through 19 years of age in 2001 and 2002, 31.5% were at risk for overweight and 16.5% were overweight [more than 3 times the target prevalence, (5%)] [2]. Furthermore, the problem falls disproportionately on African American and Hispanic children.

Many of the metabolic and cardiovascular complications associated with obesity, namely impaired glucose tolerance (IGT), type 2 diabetes mellitus (T2DM), hypertension, dyslipidemia, and systemic "low-grade" inflammation, are already present during childhood and are closely linked to the concomitant insulin resistance/hyperinsulinemia [3] and degree of obesity [4]. Moreover, these comorbidities persist into adulthood [5,6]. Until recently, no standard definition of the metabolic syndrome (MS) for use in pediatric populations was available. Consequently, researchers have used a plethora of definitions [7]. In 2007, the International Diabetes Federation (IDF) presented a definition for use in children and adolescents, thus becoming the first major organization to do so [8]. According to the IDF definition, a child aged 10–15 years has the MS if he or she has central adiposity (≥90th waist circumference percentile or adults threshold if lower) plus two or more of the following: 1) triglycerides ≥ 150 mg/dl (1.7 mmol/l); 2) high-density lipoprotein (HDL)-cholesterol (HDL-C) < 40 mg/dl (1.03 mmol/l); 3) systolic blood pressure ≥ 130 mm Hg or diastolic blood pressure ≥ 85 mm Hg; 4) fasting plasma glucose ≥ 100 mg/dl (5.6 mmol/l), or previously diagnosed T2DM. Using data from the Third National Health and Nutrition Examination Survey (NHANES) of 1999–2004, Ford et al. [9] reported a prevalence of the MS of 4.5% among U.S. children aged 12–17 years. The prevalence increased with age, was higher among males than females, and varied by ethnicity [9]. However, among overweight children and adolescents (body mass index [BMI] >95th percentile), nearly 30% had the MS [10]. To begin to assess the impact of varying degrees of obesity on the prevalence of the MS in children and adolescents, we completed a cross-sectional analysis of our cohort of obese youth [4]. We found that the prevalence of the MS increased with severity of obesity and reached 50% in severely obese children. In particular, each half-unit increase in BMI was associated with an increase in the risk of the MS in overweight and obese children (odds ratio = 1.55) [4].

One dire prediction from the U.S. Centers for Disease Control and Prevention (CDC) estimated that if current obesity rates continue, one in three babies born in 2000 will eventually develop T2DM [11]. Several studies have reported an increasing proportion of children with apparent T2DM, especially among racial/ethnic minority populations [12,13]. T2DM is already more common than type 1 diabetes mellitus (T1DM) in Japan and Taiwan and seems to account for 7%–45% of all new diabetic patients in the United States, whereas in

Nutritional and Metabolic Bases of Cardiovascular Disease, 1st edition.
Edited by Mario Mancini, José M. Ordovas, Gabriele Riccardi,
Paolo Rubba and Pasquale Strazzullo. © 2011 Blackwell Publishing Ltd.

Europe, the reported prevalence among new diabetics is still low, on the order of 0.5%–1% [14,15].

In the present review, we describe epidemiological and pathophysiological studies of obesity and T2DM in children.

Prevalence and Natural History of IGT in Childhood Obesity

Before 1997, virtually all cases of diabetes in young individuals was thought to be autoimmune T1DM. Recently, there is a widespread recognition that T2DM can occur in childhood [16,17].

In adults, the progression from normal glucose tolerance to overt T2DM involves an intermediate stage of hyperglycemia, characterized by impaired fasting glucose (IFG) or IGT, now known as "prediabetes" [18]. Recent reports have documented a high prevalence of prediabetes among children and adolescents. Cruz et al. found that 28% of obese Hispanic children with a positive family history for T2DM had IGT but found no cases of T2DM [19]. Gruters et al. [20] reported that the prevalence of IGT was 36.3% among an obese multiethnic cohort of children and adolescents with a risk factor for T2DM. Moreover, among the children and adolescents with IGT, 86% were white and 14% were not white. High prevalence of IGT has also been reported in obese children from Thailand [21] and the Philippines [22].

Similarly, in our study of the prevalence of IGT in a multiethnic, clinic-based population of 55 obese children and 112 obese adolescents, IGT was detected in 25% of the obese children and 21% of the obese adolescents, and silent T2DM was identified in 4% of the obese adolescents, irrespective of ethnicity [23]. This was the first study to highlight the high prevalence of prediabetes in the midst of the epidemic of childhood obesity. The risk factors associated with IGT in our study were, in order of importance, a) insulin resistance (estimated by the Homeostatic Model Assessment of Insulin Resistance [HOMA-IR], b) fasting proinsulin, c) 2-hour insulin level, and d) fasting insulin. Taken together, these studies indicate that early stages of abnormal glucose metabolism may precede the full onset of clinical diabetes, as it happens in adults.

Due to the cross-sectional nature of this study, we were unable to confirm the glucose continuum in these children. Therefore, a longitudinal study was needed. We followed 117 obese children and adolescents from a pediatric weight management clinic (84 with normal glucose tolerance [NGT] and 33 with IGT) with oral glucose tolerance tests (OGTTs) repeated after 18–24 months [15]. Eight of the subjects with NGT became impaired. Eight subjects (24.2%) with IGT developed T2DM, 15 (45.5%) converted to NGT, and 10 remained impaired (30.3%). Transition from NGT to IGT and from IGT to diabetes was associated with significant increases in weight, while conversion from IGT to NGT was associated with the least amount of weight gain. The insulinogenic index, an OGTT-based estimate of insulin secretion, in subjects with IGT, specifically those who later became diabetic, was lower at baseline (2.11 [1.18–3.78]), compared to subjects with NGT (3.63 [3.12–4.26], $p = .03$). The best predictor of the change of the 2-hour glucose level was the change in insulin sensitivity.

Our data illustrate the importance of variations in weight gain on changes in glucose tolerance in childhood obesity. Most of the children grew in height and gained weight on a track consistent with their prior growth patterns, resulting in stable BMI z scores or relative adiposity. However, the children who progressed from NGT to IGT had the largest increase in body weight and an increase in relative adiposity. Even more exciting is the observation that IGT subjects who converted back to NGT had minimal increases in body weight and a reduction in BMI z score. IGT has been demonstrated to be reversible in adults who undertook significant lifestyle modifications resulting in a reduction in body weight. Our data suggest that even in the absence of frank weight loss, IGT may be reversible in obese children by lifestyle interventions that are successful in maintaining a stable body weight during a period of active growth. Nevertheless, the potential for obese children with IGT to deteriorate rapidly to T2DM makes the window of opportunity to implement such interventions very limited.

Beta-Cell Function: an Early Alteration in the Development of Type 2 Diabetes

Diabetes results from the combination of insulin resistance and impaired beta-cell function. The mechanisms whereby obesity relates to diabetes risk are not clear. Most, if not all, children and adolescents with T2DM or IGT have a significant degree of insulin resistance, which may be caused by obesity, sedentary lifestyle, ethnicity, pubertal stage of development, and family history of diabetes. Loss or reduced first-phase insulin secretion is one of the most sensitive indicators of a beta-cell dysfunction. Earlier studies from our group showed that the IGT phenotype in obese adolescents is a prediabetic state with marked peripheral insulin resistance [24] and impaired first-phase secretion [25]. More recently, we published a cross-sectional analysis of beta-cell function and tissue insulin sensitivity in a multiethnic cohort of obese adolescents with a wide range of disturbance in glucose metabolism, using state-of-art techniques. We compared the sensitivity of the beta-cell to glucose between subjects with NGT, IFG, IGT, or combined IFG/IGT [26]. Interestingly, we found that IFG, in obese adolescents, is linked primarily to alterations in glucose sensitivity of first-phase insulin secretion (Figure 5.1). The IGT group is affected by a more severe de-

gree of peripheral insulin resistance and reduction in glucose sensitivity of first-phase insulin secretion. IFG/IGT is hallmarked by a profound insulin resistance and by a new additional defect in glucose sensitivity of second-phase insulin secretion. This defect was previously described by us to be present only in childhood T2DM [25]. However, in that study, our comparator of prediabetic state was formed by children with isolated IGT, not by children with IFG/IGT. Hence, one wonders whether IFG/IGT should not be considered just as diabetes; however, the answer to this question can be found only from longitudinal studies.

Ectopic Fat Deposition and Insulin Resistance in Childhood Obesity

Controversy remains regarding the contribution of abdominal visceral and subcutaneous fat to the development of insulin resistance [27–29]. A previous study from our group showed that obese adolescents with IGT had increased visceral and

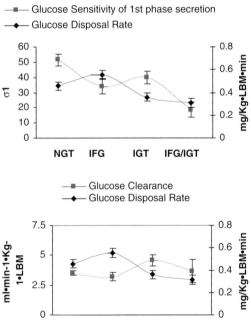

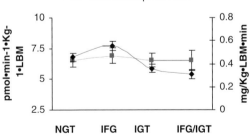

Figure 5.1 Differences in insulin secretion, insulin sensitivity, and glucose clearance among the different prediabetic phenotypes. BSR: basal secretion rate; σ^1: glucose sensitivity of first phase secretion; σ^2: glucose sensitivity of second phase secretion.

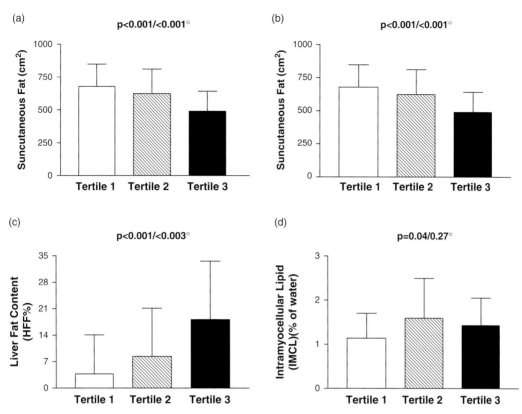

Figure 5.2 Lipid deposition: abdominal fat depots, muscle lipid, and liver fat according to visceral tertiles, adjusted for age, gender, and race/ethnicity. p values are for trend across visceral tertiles, both unadjusted and * adjusted for age, gender, and race/ethnicity.

decreased subcutaneous fat [44] (Figure 5.2). Recently, we found that a high proportion of visceral fat was associated with muscle and hepatic steatosis. Furthermore, we found that obese adolescents had high triglycerides, together with low HDL, leptin, and adiponectin levels [30]. Notably, the risk for the MS was 5 times greater in adolescents with this fat-partitioning profile. The hypothesis that inadequate subcutaneous fat results in lipid overflow into the visceral depot and nonadipose tissues, thereby modulating insulin sensitivity, was proposed by Shulman [31] and Danforth [32]. It appears that the ability of peripheral subcutaneous fat tissue to vary its storage capacity is critical for regulating insulin sensitivity and ultimately protecting against diabetes [30]. This phenotype of altered abdominal fat partitioning and its associated metabolic abnormalities have interesting parallel with partial lipodystrophy. Lipodystrophy, which is

the total or partial loss of adipose tissue mass, is often accompanied by hepatic steatosis and increased IMCL, followed by insulin resistance and T2DM [27]. Several animal models support this sequence of events. In lipoatrophic animals, transplantation of adipose tissue back into the animals reversed the phenotypes [28,29]. These studies demonstrated that inadequate adipose tissue mass leads to ectopic fat storage with its associated metabolic sequelae. Thus, in obesity, T2DM, and lipodystrophy, insulin resistance may develop because of alterations in the partitioning of fat between the adipocyte and muscle or liver [30]. Our study supports the hypothesis that the ability to retain fat in the subcutaneous depot, especially in the superficial layer, seems to be beneficial in obese adolescents since it is associated with reduced visceral and hepatic fat and, more importantly, a more favorable metabolic profile. The subcutaneous layer of adipose tissue has been proposed to act as a "sink," with the capability to accommodate excess energy in the form of triglycerides in the adipocytes and thus prevent the flow of lipid to other areas [32,33]. This hypothesis has been elegantly explored by Ravussin et al. [33]. We presented for the first time evidence that this phenotype may be present in obese adolescents. The underlying mechanism for the limited capacity in some individuals for the subcutaneous fat to expand and accommodate excess storage of fat is not clear. It may be due to an inability of the existing adipocytes to signal preadipocytes to proliferate and differentiate, instead increasing in size in response to the influx of triglycerides.

In addition to being more insulin resistant, large adipocytes have also been shown to release less adiponectin compared with small adipocytes [34]. Therefore, the lower adiponectin levels in the subjects with a high proportion of visceral fat may be due at least in part to the presence of large adipocytes in the subcutaneous fat. In addition, consistent with the reduced subcutaneous fat in these subjects, we found decreased levels of circulating leptin. Both leptin and adiponectin have antisteatosic effects [35,36]. Total adiponectin and, in particular, high-molecular-weight (HMW) adiponectin are known not only for their anti-inflammatory actions but also for activating adenosine monophosphate (AMP)–activated protein kinase (AMPK), leading to increased fat oxidation [37,38].

This pattern of abdominal fat distribution was associated with increase intramyocellular lipid (IMCL) deposition.

Lipid Droplets in the Myocyte

The lipid composition of skeletal muscle tissue, where most (70%) glucose disposal occurs, has recently attracted much attention as a major player in the development of muscle insulin resistance [39]. A strong inverse correlation between insulin resistance and IMCL has been reported in offspring of T2DM adults, suggesting that a high IMCL content might be involved in the development of insulin resistance [40,41]. Alternatively, intramuscular lipid accumulation may be caused by a reduction of fat oxidation [42], related to low aerobic capacity or reduced sympathetic tone. In particular, the tendency to accumulate lipid within muscles may be deter-

mined by the amount and functionality of mitochondria within the myocytes and by their capacity to oxidize fat.

To gain insight into the lipid composition of skeletal muscle tissue, we used ^{1}H-nuclear magnetic resonance (NMR) spectroscopy to quantify non-invasively the IMCL and extramyocellular lipid (EMCL) content of the soleus muscle [43,44] in obese children and adolescents, either with or without prediabetes. We found an excessive accumulation of IMCL content in the soleus muscle of obese adolescents with IGT compared to age- and adiposity-matched obese adolescents with NGT. Moreover, we found that whole-body insulin sensitivity, as assessed by the glucose clamp technique, varied as a function of IMCL stores (Pearson's correlation $r = -0.59$, $p < .02$) [43]. These relationships were independent of percentage of total body fat and subcutaneous abdominal fat, but not visceral fat mass. Thus, our data suggest that IMCL may play an important role in modulating insulin sensitivity, particularly in obese adolescents. The striking relationship between IMCL and insulin sensitivity in such a young population suggests that these findings are not a consequence of aging but are actually expressed early in the natural course of obesity.

Delineating mechanisms by which an increase in skeletal muscle lipid availability may confer insulin resistance in diabetes may help target specific pathways, proteins, or genes involved in insulin action. For example, excess triglyceride in insulin-resistant muscle might lead to elevated diacylglycerol (DAG) or fatty-acyl-coenzyme A (CoA) concentration, which in turn activate a serine/threonine kinase cascade involving protein kinase C, leading to phosphorylation of serine/threonine sites in insulin receptor substrate-1 (IRS-1) [45]. Serine-phosphorylated forms of these proteins fail to associate with and activate phosphoinositide 3-kinase (PI3K), resulting in decreased activation of glucose transport (mainly GLUT-4) and other downstream-associated events. If this hypothesis is correct, any perturbation that results in accumulation of intracellular fatty acyl-CoA or other fatty acid metabolites in muscle and liver, either through increased delivery or decreased metabolism, may be expected to induce insulin resistance or insulin action [45,46]. The determinants of the tendency to accumulate lipid within myocytes are strongly influenced by genetic and environmental factors.

Intrahepatic Fat Accumulation: the Hepatic Component of the Metabolic Syndrome

Concurrent with the worldwide epidemic of childhood obesity, nonalcoholic fatty liver disease (NAFLD) has become the most common cause of unexplained abnormal liver function test results in the pediatric population [47] and may encompass the entire spectrum of liver conditions, ranging from simple steatohepatitis (nonalcoholic steatohepatitis [NASH]) to advanced fibrosis and cirrhosis. It affects 2.6% of children and 22.5%–52.8% of obese children [48]. Schwimmer et al. [49] estimated that the prevalence of fatty liver is 9.6% in children 2–19 years of age in the county of San Diego, after adjusting for age, gender, race, and ethnicity. The highest rate of fatty liver was seen in obese children (38%). After controlling for the severity of obesity, Hispanic boys and girls have higher rates of fatty liver than non-Hispanic peers and they are more prone to advanced liver fibrosis. If the prevalence is similar for the entire United States, this would represent >6.5 million children and adolescents [49].

It is becoming increasingly clear that fat accumulation in the liver is not a benign condition [50]. Indeed, it is frequently associated with T2DM in both adults and children [51,52] and has been labeled as the hepatic component of the MS [50,53].

We have recently reported the metabolic consequences associated with elevations of alanine aminotransferase (ALT) and hepatic steatosis in a large multi-ethnic cohort of obese children. We showed that elevations in ALT levels, even within the normal range, were associated with deterioration in insulin sensitivity and worsening glucose tolerance assessed by OGTT [54]. Metabolic alterations were further exaggerated when ALT levels were elevated outside the normal range. Similar dose–response relationships were observed between rising ALT levels and increasing free fatty acid and triglyceride levels. These relationships persisted after controlling for age, gender, ethnicity/race, and BMI z score. In addition to demonstrating that insulin resistance is strongly and independently correlated with rising ALT levels, our study is the first

to observe that early alterations in glucose tolerance are associated with rising ALT levels in obese children. It remains unclear whether intra-hepatic fat accumulation is a consequence or cause of the observed metabolic derangements in insulin sensitivity and lipid metabolism (elevated triglycerides and free fatty acids).

The noninvasive magnetic resonance imaging (MRI) technique, fast gradient echo magnetic resonance pulse sequences (fast-MRI), used in a random subset of subjects ($n = 72$) of our cohort more firmly established the connection between fatty liver disease and altered metabolism in obese children. In our subset of obese children, steatosis was assessed as a hepatic fat fraction (HFF) >5.5% (>2.5 standard deviations [SD] above the mean for our lean controls) and was associated with subtle changes in glucose tolerance, insulin resistance, rising triglyceride levels, and the MS. In particular, 32% of our subjects had an HFF >5.5%, implying the presence of hepatic steatosis. Of note, only 48% of subjects with fatty liver had ALT levels in the abnormal range. Obese adolescents with an HFF >5.5% had a greater area under the curve (AUC) for glucose and were significantly more insulin resistant (whole-body insulin sensitivity index, WBISI), as assessed by the OGTT, compared to those with a low HFF. In addition, those with a high HFF had significantly higher triglyceride levels and significantly lower adiponectin levels.

Lipoprotein Alterations and Hepatic Steatosis

Obese children and adolescents are often diagnosed with dyslipidemia characterized by high triglycerides and low HDL-C concentrations. In addition, the presence of small dense low-density lipoprotein (LDL) particles has been shown in obese children [55,56]. Recent studies from our group reported dyslipidemia and a deterioration in glucose metabolism in obese nondiabetic adolescents with excessive intrahepatic fat accumulation. In particular, we found rising levels of triglycerides and decreasing levels of HDL-C with increasing accumulation of fat in the liver [54]. Although studies in adults have shown insulin resistance, obesity, and fatty liver playing a role in the composition of lipoproteins, there are no current studies for this comprehensive phenotype in children

[57]. NMR spectroscopy was utilized to determine lipoprotein subclass composition in fasting plasma samples, while fast-MRI was used to determine the HFF (fatty liver).

In a small group ($n = 49$) of obese adolescents with NGT, we found that the presence of hepatic steatosis was associated with a) an increase in very-low-density lipoprotein (VLDL) particle size and number, b) an increase in small dense LDL concentrations, and c) a decrease in the number of large HDL particles. These alterations were reflected by an increase in triglyceride concentrations and decreased HDL-C. It is noteworthy that, had the lipoprotein subclasses not been measured by the NMR technique, we would have missed the important finding regarding the pattern of changes in the LDL subclasses present in these children with fatty liver. Indeed, the traditional fasting lipid profile revealed normal LDL-C concentrations in both groups. In contrast, we found a significant increase in small LDL particles with increasing liver fat content. Small dense LDL is known to be proatherogenic; they are more susceptible to oxidation and may be taken up by macrophages, which eventually leads to the development of atherosclerotic plaque formation in the arterial wall. Of note, hepatic steatosis was found to predict the concentration of the large VLDL particles, independent of overall adiposity, insulin sensitivity and visceral adiposity, thereby suggesting that liver steatosis is important in the early pathogenesis of insulin resistance and T2DM in children. Hence, the atherogenic profile is fully established already at this very young age.

Childhood Obesity and Inflammation

The coexistence of obesity and a low-grade inflammatory state has been found to be present during the earliest stage of obesity and is strongly dependent on the degree of obesity [58]. One revolutionary concept is that the adipose tissue is not merely a simple reservoir of energy stored as triglycerides but also serves as an active secretory organ, releasing many peptides, complement factors, and cytokines into the circulation [59]. In the presence of obesity, the balance between these numerous molecules is altered such that enlarged adipocytes and macrophages embedded within them produce more pro-inflammatory cytokines, such as tumor necrosis factor-alpha (TNF-α) and interleukin-6 (IL-6), and fewer anti-inflammatory peptides, such as adiponectin. The dysregulated production of adipocytokines has been found to participate in the development of metabolic and vascular diseases related to obesity [60].

The role of adipocytokines in the development of altered glucose metabolism in children and adolescents is a novel and intriguing field of research. In adults, dysregulation of the expression and secretion of adiponectin may play a role in the pathogenesis of type 2 diabetes [48,61]. In fact, studies in adults have shown that hypoadiponectinemia is an independent risk factor or the progression of type 2 diabetes [49–51].

Adiponectin is the only adipocytokine that is known to be inversely related to the degree of adiposity [62]. We have recently shown that adiponectin levels differ between obese youth with NGT versus IGT, despite a similar degree of obesity [62]. In particular, we have shown that plasma adiponectin levels are positively related to whole-body insulin sensitivity, as assessed by the glucose clamp technique, whereas they are strongly inversely related to triglyceride levels, IMCL lipid content, and fasting insulin levels. These relationships are independent of total body fat percentage and central adiposity. The close association with IMCL content is consistent with the data from Yamauchi et al. [63], indicating that adiponectin acts primarily on skeletal muscle tissue to increase influx and combustion of free fatty acids, thereby reducing muscle triglyceride content in the mouse model of obesity. Thus, the modulatory effect of adiponectin on whole-body insulin sensitivity may be mediated, in part, by its effect on the IMCL lipid content.

In an attempt to understand the relationship between obesity and inflammation, we analyzed the relationship between adiponectin and C-reactive protein (CRP), the prototype inflammatory marker, in a large multiethnic cohort of obese children and adolescents. Stratifying the cohort (589 obese children and adolescents) into quartiles of serum adiponectin and adjusting for potential confounding variables, including age, gender, pubertal stage, ethnicity, BMI z score, and WBISI, we found that low adiponectin levels are associated with higher CRP levels and HDL-C. Hence, the relationship between adiponectin levels and both CRP and HDL-C appears to be independent of obesity and insulin resistance in childhood obesity and is not influenced by ethnicity (p value adjusted for ethnicity < .003). One limitation of this analysis is the fact that we measured total adiponectin levels rather than the low and high molecular forms. However, it is likely that the high molecular form is more strongly related to insulin sensitivity than is total adiponectin [64]. Whether the anti-inflammatory effects of adiponectin are also more closely related to its high molecular form remains unclear.

This study suggests that adiponectin could play a role in modulating CRP levels and thus be a potential molecular link between adiposity and inflammation. However, this link may not be entirely due to its well-known effects on insulin sensitivity. Mechanistic studies are needed to understand whether the link is indeed real and, more importantly, how these various factors interact with one another during the development of the MS and cardiovascular disease.

Conclusion

Altered glucose metabolism in obese children is an emerging phenomenon of the last two decades, strongly associated with the increase in the prevalence of childhood obesity. Childhood obesity sets the stage for multiple target organ damage and related morbidity. Prediabetes in obese children and adolescents represents a complex metabolic pheno-type, characterized by peripheral insulin resistance and altered tissue lipid partitioning. The combination of ectopic lipid deposition, an adverse lipid and adipocytokine profile, along with low-grade inflammation, may play a major role in the deterioration to overt diabetes. These events may proceed at an alarming rapid tempo and also play a role in the development of adverse cardiovascular outcomes related to the MS in these youngsters. Primary prevention of childhood obesity and tailored conservative or pharmacologic interventions for obese children with prediabetic conditions holds the promise of halting the rising prevalence of T2DM in this pediatric age-group.

Selected References

8. Zimmet P, Alberti G, Kaufman F, et al; International Diabetes Federation Task Force on Epidemiology and Prevention of Diabetes. The metabolic syndrome in children and adolescents. Lancet 2007 Jun 23; 369(9579): 2059–61.

17. Haines L, Wan KC, Lynn R, et al. Rising incidence of type 2 diabetes in children in the U.K. Diabetes Care 2007 May; 30(5):1097–101.

25. Weiss R, Caprio S, Trombetta M, et al. Beta-cell function across the spectrum of glucose tolerance in obese youth. Diabetes 2005 Jun; 54(6):1735–43.

30. Taksali SE, Caprio S, Dziura J, et al. High visceral and low abdominal subcutaneous fat stores in the obese adolescent: a determinant of an adverse metabolic phenotype. Diabetes 2008 Feb; 57(2):367–71.

44. Weiss R, Dufour S, Taksali SE, et al. Prediabetes in obese youth: a syndrome of impaired glucose tolerance, severe insulin resistance, and altered myocellular and abdominal fat partitioning. Lancet 2003 Sep 20; 362(9388): 951–7.

CHAPTER 6

Complications and Comorbidities of Obesity

Fabrizio Pasanisi, Franco Contaldo & Mario Mancini
Federico II University, Naples, Italy

Introduction

A meeting on medical complications of obesity to document the clinical relevance of excess body fat was quite innovative 30 years ago and focused mostly on metabolic complications and comorbidities of obesity [1]. The question now is what has changed the clinical relevance of obesity. Now, indeed more definite are the distinctions between overweight and obesity, the consequence of splanchnic, intraorgan, and muscle tissue fat accumulation, and the interethnic differences. New interesting aspects concerning excess body fat affecting individuals' and populations' health are the earlier onset of obesity in life, up to the present childhood obesity epidemic, and the inclusion of obesity in the metabolic syndrome (MS). It should also be mentioned that the increased prevalence, at all ages, of severe obesity, with its specific nursing and medical demands, and the definite recognition of bariatric surgery as an appropriate treatment in selected cases. Finally, it is of interest that adipose tissue has been identified not only as an energy depot but as an autocrine and endocrine organ, acting in many physiological functions, including the proinflammatory, atherogenic, and carcinogenic role. Enlarged adipose tissue also produces an increase of endoplasmic reticulum with an increased number of macrophages and other stromal cells that may contribute to the abnormal secretion of many peptides involved in several regulatory functions. Furthermore, increased secretion of free fatty acids (FFAs) from large adipocytes with abnormal peptide secretion contributes to many typical complications of obesity: type 2 diabetes, hypertension, hyperlipidemia, altered reproductive function, and some cancers. It should also be noted that increased mortality has been documented in severely obese patients and that the social health costs of obesity are now much more evident. Molecular biology, genetic, clinical, and community studies have also improved our knowledge of the etiopathogenetic determinants of excess body fat, thus giving hope for new possible pharmacological and nonpharmacological approaches to treat obesity and minimize complications and comorbidities.

Obesity is a chronic physical abnormality caused by an imbalance between energy intake and expenditure due to predisposing genetic polymorphisms and facilitating environmental factors. The excess energy is stored as triglycerides, predominantly in fat cells of adipose tissue. Triglycerides can also infiltrate hepatocytes with the consequence of fatty liver and steatohepatitis, and myocytes with insulin resistance and type 2 diabetes (see Chapter 5). The existence of obese, even severely obese, patients with no metabolic or cardiovascular complications has been described by several clinicians in populations of obese patients [2,3] and recently the topic has been rediscussed by Iacobellis and Sharma [4] (Table 6.1). The table shows summarized criteria for the definition of uncomplicated obesity. Furthermore, in the population of obese patients, the degree of excess body fat, but not fat distribution,

Nutritional and Metabolic Bases of Cardiovascular Disease, 1st edition.
Edited by Mario Mancini, José M. Ordovas, Gabriele Riccardi,
Paolo Rubba and Pasquale Strazzullo. © 2011 Blackwell Publishing Ltd.

Table 6.1 Definition of uncomplicated obesity.

- No clinically significant abnormalities on physical examination
- No lipid-lowering, hypoglycemic, or anti-hypertensive drugs
- No history of metabolic, cardiovascular, respiratory (obstructive sleep apnea), or other systemic diseases
- Normal thyroid function
- Normal resting electrocardiogram
- Normal FG (<100 mg/dL^{-1})
- Normal glucose tolerance (2-hour glucose levels <140 mg/dL^{-1} during OGTT)
- SBP <130 mm Hg and DBP < 85 mm Hg on at least three occasions
- Normal plasma lipids (TC < 200 mg/dL^{-1}, HDL > 40 mg/dL^{-1} for men and >50 mg/dL^{-1} for women, LDL <130 mg/dL^{-1}, TG < 150 mg/dL^{-1}

FG, fasting glucose; OGTT, oral glucose tolerance test; SBP and DBP, systolic and diastolic blood pressure, respectively; TC, total cholesterol; HDL, high-density lipoprotein; LDL, low-density lipoprotein; TG, triglycerides. Reproduced from Iacobellis and Sharma [4].

often is not correlated to metabolic and cardiovascular complications of obesity. Medical history, periodic clinical examination, and regular follow-up are advisable in this subgroup of obese individuals.

Autocrine and Endocrine Functions of Adipose Tissue

Adipose tissue storage and release of fatty acids, as well as the more recently studied autocrine and endocrine function [5], in fine perivascular sites [6] are related to most of the metabolic and clinical complications of obesity. In this context, excess visceral adipose tissue plays a pivotal role with an increased FFA turnover, release of glucocorticoids, beta-receptor agonist activity, increased intracellular production of cortisol from inactive cortisone, and enhanced intracellular glucocorticoid and androgen activity [7,8].

Visceral adipose tissue (VAT) is also an important source of pro-inflammatory cytokines, in particular tumor necrosis factor-alpha (TNF-α) and interleukin-6 (IL-6), and excess visceral fat induces a disequilibrium in the ratio proinflammatory/anti-inflammatory cytokines due to an overproduction of TNF-α and IL-6 with a concomitant reduced production of adiponectin [9,10].

The main relevant effects of IL-6 and TNF-α, cytokines produced either by fat cells and adipose tissue associated macrophages, is the increased liver production of acute-phase proteins such as C-reactive protein (CRP) and fibrinogen, a direct paracrine effect on fat cells [11] with effects on insulin resistance. Obesity is also frequently associated with increased production of free radicals, which may contribute to oxidative stress.

Adipokines—in particular leptin, adiponectin, and resistin—are proteins produced mainly by adipocytes.

Among the several known functions, leptin has a role in immunity, protecting T lymphocytes from apoptosis and regulating T-cell proliferation and activation; its deficiency facilitates the proinflammatory effects of specific cytokines. Adiponectin also has a protective function for the correlation with insulin sensitivity, inhibition of IL-6 production, and stimulation of anti-inflammatory cytokines as IL-10 [12].

In obesity, type 2 diabetes and other insulin-resistant states, serum adiponectin levels are low, probably also for a downregulation of its production by TNF-α. Finally, resistin, a cysteine-rich secretory protein, also produced in humans macrophages, has proinflammatory effects and has been found to be elevated in obesity.

The topic of autocrine and endocrine function of adipose tissue is discussed in Chapter 12.

Obesity and Life Expectancy

Life expectancy is reduced in obesity, and this reduction may be considered to be directly related to excess body weight [13–15].

In the United States, where obesity has surpassed smoking in 2005 as the main preventable cause of illness and premature death [16], of the 300,000 deaths due to overweight and obesity, more than 80% occur in individuals with a body mass index (BMI) > 30 kg/m^2 [17]. Prevalent splanchnic fat distribution may also affect lifespan, mostly because of the increased prevalence of metabolic, cardiovascular, and neoplastic risk factors. The present rising prevalence and severity of obesity may offset the positive influences on life expectancy, typical of developed and affluent societies, and mostly attributable to a decrease in mortality among individuals older than 50 years [18].

Negative effects of obesity on lifespan may be direct or indirect. For example, obese women with breast cancer may receive chemotherapy doses inadequate for their body weight, with reduced survival. On the other hand, obesity is associated with other negative factors such as physical inactivity and abnormal food habits directly linked to life expectancy. In conclusion, splanchnic obesity, BMI > 30 kg/m^2, and abnormal lifestyle may significantly increase mortality. Furthermore, the prevalence of sudden death, mostly due to cardiovascular events, is extremely high in severely obese patients, even at a young age.

Diabetes Mellitus and the Metabolic Syndrome

This topic will be extensively discusses in Chapter 11. Here, we summarize that the degree and duration of overweight, a more central distribution of body fat, and weight gain over the years represent well-known risk factors for type 2 diabetes, exclusively due to the excess body fat [19]. Weight gain often precedes the onset of diabetes [20], whereas weight loss, after appropriate bariatric surgery, induces a stable reversion of diabetes (see Chapter 11). The main metabolic link between excess body fat and diabetes is hyperinsulinemia with insulin resistance, a pathogenetic determinant of the MS. Hyperinsulinemia increases hepatic very-low-density lipoprotein (VLDL) synthesis and secretion, plasminogen activator inhibitor-1 (PAI-1) synthesis, sympathetic nervous system (SNS) activity, and renal sodium reabsorption, thus facilitating the onset of hypertension, hypertriglyceridemia, and fatty liver—all typical features of the MS [21].

Excess body fat simultaneously induces reduced secretion of adiponectin, while hypersecretion of TNF-α and IL-6 enhances insulin resistance. The link between adipose tissue and metabolic complications is associated with the excess visceral body fat in the MS definition [22].

Obesity and Cancer

Excess body weight is now recognized as an important risk factor in both sexes for some cancers. Two very recent papers, a report by the World Cancer Research Fund and the American Institute for Cancer Research [23], as well as a recently published meta-analysis [24], give convincing evidence that excess body fat is an important cause of most cancers. In particular, and considering only the increase of BMI due to total body fat, there is an increased risk of thyroid, renal, colon, liver, esophageal adenocarcinoma, multiple myeloma, leukemia, and non-Hodgkin's lymphoma in both sexes, with a higher prevalence of colon, liver, or rectal cancer, malignant melanoma, and prostate in men, and gallbladder, pancreas, endometrial, and postmenopausal breast cancer in women. These associations were found generally consistently across populations.

The increase in cancer risk associated with obesity, now so clearly defined, may be mediated by several factors: a) hormones such as insulin, insulin-like growth factor-1 (IGF-1), and sex steroids, which can affect the balance between cell proliferation and apoptosis; b) adipokines and increased oxidative stress, c) nonalcoholic steatohepatitis (NASH) for liver cancer, and increased gastroesophageal reflux in splanchnic obesity for esophageal adenocarcinoma, d) lipid peroxidation and hypertension for renal cancer [25].

Breast cancer risk, as far as BMI, has a J-shaped prevalence in premenopausal women, but obese women at both premenopausal and postmenopausal ages have a poorer final outcome than average-weight women. Finally, the identification of type 2 diabetes and the MS (i.e., hyperinsulinemia with insulin resistance) as risk factors for breast cancer may well be correlated to the presence of excess visceral adipose tissue [26].

Other factors facilitating breast cancer are the overstimulation of the breast epithelium by estrogens, due to an increased production from androstenedione, an altered adipokine production, that is, reduced production of protective adiponectin and increased production of leptin with a documented stimulatory effect on human breast cancer cell lines.

In conclusion, lifelong control of body weight should be part of the strategy to prevent the occurrence of some types of cancer.

Reproductive and Obstetric Complications

As the prevalence of obesity increases, the number of obese women in the reproductive age also increases. Reproductive disorders associated with obesity include fertility, a negative impact on in vitro fertilization, and increased risk of miscarriage [27].

Anovulation may be more frequent in obesity as a result of hyperandrogenism through the promotion of granulosa cell apoptosis, increased peripheral conversion of androgens to estrogen with a negative impact on gonadotrophin secretion, adverse effects of hyperandrogenism on the endometrium, and hyperleptinemia on the granulosa and theca cells [28]. Finally, polycystic ovarian syndrome (PCOS), common in obesity, is often associated with anovulatory infertility. In conclusion, obese women are at higher risk of anovulatory cycles.

It is also possible that obesity may increase the risk of miscarriage, particularly during the first trimester [29]. Obesity during pregnancy is associated with increased use of healthcare services [30] as well.

Obstetric complications of obesity have been also described. Among the most common maternal complications in obesity are hypertension, preeclampsia, venous-thromboembolism, gestational diabetes, and genital and urinary tract infections. Most frequent perinatal complications are macrosomia, intrauterine death, and some congenital anomalies [31,32].

In conclusion, regardless of the association with the PCOS, obesity may directly affect female reproductive function. Measures to reduce body weight should, therefore, be recommended before any other treatment to improve fertility in obese women.

Hypertension

Obesity is recognized as one of the most important risk factors for the development of hypertension. Blood pressure, in particular systolic, increases progressively with higher BMIs [33]. Splanchnic excess body fat, i.e., android adiposity, is much more related to high blood pressure and other components of the MS, than gynoid obesity [34]. Obesity and

hypertension contribute to the development of left ventricular hypertrophy, the onset of cardiac failure, and an increased risk of sudden death [35]. Furthermore, understanding the pathophysiology of obesity-related hypertension has useful implications for treatment. Hypertension and obesity seem to share several pathogenetic mechanisms. Starting from excess visceral adipose tissue, the renin-angiotensin system is overactivated, sympathetic nervous system activity is increased, insulin and leptin resistance are present with increased renal sodium reabsorption and extracellular volume expansion, inflammation, and endothelial dysfunction. Often the association of hypertension and obesity facilitates the onset of chronic renal failure [36]. Chronic hypercapnia, as in the obstructive sleep apnea, also facilitates the development of hypertension [37].

The frequent association of hypertension with obesity allows us in this case to also consider a direct active role of adipose tissue, in particular splanchnic adipose tissue, in the development of both hypertension and excess body fat. Studies carried out also in our department have shown that renin-angiotensin system (RAS) components are expressed by adipocytes (thus, facilitating the onset of hypertension in obesity) and that genetic variability in RAS is involved in individual susceptibility to overweight [38,39]. These pathogenetic findings might have a valuable role in the pharmacological choice of antihypertensive agents in obese individuals.

Sleep Apnea Syndrome and Pulmonary Dysfunction

Obese individuals are also more prone to respiratory problems including reduced lung volume, reduced respiratory compliance and exercise capacity, hypoxia, and hypoventilation. Obstructive sleep apnea syndrome (OSAS) is characterized by repetitive collapse of the upper airway during sleep with subsequent oxygen desaturation and sleep fragmentation [40]. Visceral obesity, with increased fat deposition in the neck and reduced diaphragm excursion, worsens OSAS risk. OSAS is associated with other comorbidities such as the MS, hypertension, transient ischemic attacks, stroke, arrhythmias, pulmonary hypertension, and sudden death [41]. Finally, hypoxia may independently stimulate the release of IL-6, with significantly higher levels in OSAS [42]. In addition to IL-6, most other studies have shown increased levels of several other inflammatory mediators in OSAS, such as CRP, leptin, TNF-α, IL-1β, reactive oxygen species (ROS) and adhesion molecules, and nuclear factor κB [41].

These findings suggest a pathogenetic link between metabolic and cardiovascular complications frequently associated with OSAS in severely obese patients or in patients with marked visceral obesity.

Nonalcoholic Fatty Liver Disease and Cholelithiasis

NAFLD describes liver abnormalities associated with obesity, in absence of other pathogenetic factors, and is represented by hepatomegaly, increased liver enzymes, steatosis, with a more complicated pattern up to steatohepatitis (i.e., NASH), fibrosis, and cirrhosis [43,44].

NAFLD is reversible after weight loss, whereas NASH has a poorer prognosis and may worsen to cirrhosis and cancer. Increased steatosis in obesity is also considered a clinical consequence of the frequent association with the MS and may reflect increased, but insufficient, VLDL production, increased FFAs associated with hyperinsulinemia, and increased secretion of proinflammatory cytokines by excess adipose tissue.

The prevalence of liver abnormalities in obesity is quite high, particularly in severely obese patients, as reported in various studies also conducted in our department [43,45].

Cholelithiasis is another frequent, often asymptomatic finding in obesity, particularly in obese premenopausal women [46]. Data from the Third National Health and Nutrition Examination Survey (NHANES III) indicate that the prevalence of cholelithiasis increases from 9.4% in the lowest quarter of BMI distribution to 23.5% in the highest quarter among women and from 4.6% to 10.6% among men [47]. Part of the explanation for the increased risk of gallstones in obesity—but also during weight loss—is the increased cholesterol turnover related to excess total body fat (or fat loss) with an increased lithogenic cholesterol flux through the biliary system, also related to large fluctuations in body weight [48].

Osteoarthritis

Epidemiological evidence suggests that obesity has a major role in the development of the osteoarthritis (OA), in particular that of the knee and hip, or the weight-bearing joints. Indeed, excess weight and the frequent varus malalignment [49] associated with obesity may well be responsible for the joint cartilage degeneration. Finally, quadriceps weakness, frequently observed in obesity, may induce a higher impact on the cartilage during gait [50,51].

Nevertheless, obesity is described also as a cofactor for the development of OA in non–weight-bearing joints such as wrists and fingers, thus suggesting the effect also of metabolic and inflammatory factors. Hyperinsulinemia may play a role, because its serum concentrations are higher in OA obese patients than in non-OA obese patients [52].

Proinflammatory cytokines may also accelerate joint cartilage degeneration [53,54]. Finally, obesity may participate in the vicious cycle predisposing to OA of diminished exercise also reported by our group in outpatients [55], decreased muscle strength, and increased joint trouble associated with the natural aging process [56].

Plantar heel pain, a symptom of enthesopathy or plantar fasciitis, is also much more frequent in obese and overweight patients than in average-weight individuals [56,57]. A possible link between excess body weight and plantar heel pain may be the impact of overweight on the subcalcaneal fat pat and on the function of the medial longitudinal arch.

Obesity may also represent a risk of wrist fracture in children [58]. The lower mineral content of obese children may reflect lifestyle factors, in particular physical inactivity, negatively affecting bone mineral density, but also general posture and muscular strength [59].

Disabilities

The prevalence of obesity and consequent disability is increasing in all developed countries. Whether being the cause or the result of disability, obesity can exacerbate the disabling condition [60]. Most common disabilities are related to the musculoskeletal system but also may regard mental health and learning capacities [61].

As already indicated in a previous paragraph of this chapter, obesity is an important modifiable risk factor for the development of OA of joint-bearing and non–joint-bearing articulations. Back pain represents one of the most prevalent disabling conditions.

Psychopathological complications of obesity seem to be elevated in clinical but not in population samples [62]. On the other hand, psychological complications of obesity, particularly in childhood, may be lower self-esteem and lower social interaction, depression, and more frequent impulse control disorders [63]. There are also some genetic syndromes such as Prader-Willi, Down's, and Bardet-Biedl where obesity is associated with severe mental disorders.

From a public health standpoint, obesity advice and health recommendations finalized to control excess body weight may be required to address the complex needs of disabled individuals.

Quality of Life in Obesity

There is a growing interest in measuring the impact of weight and weight reduction on quality of life [64]. There is also growing recognition by healthcare professionals that in some chronic illnesses, such as obesity, where it is unlikely that treatment will be frequently successful, quality of life may be an important health outcome and motivate patients for long-term treatment. In recent years, the more specific term "health-related quality of life" (HRQOL) has been used to refer to the physical, psychological, and social domains of health, seen as distinct areas that are influenced by a person's experiences, beliefs, expectations, and perceptions [65].

Obesity may have an impact on several aspects of HRQOL such as physical health, emotional well-being, and psychosocial functioning. HRQOL, in particular the one related to physical well-being, is inversely related to the degree of obesity, is more deteriorated in obese patients asking for treatment, in women than in men, and improves, in particular as far as physical health, after weight loss [66,67].

These findings have been observed with general and obesity specific HRQOL questionnaires [68].

Economic Costs of Obesity

The rapid change in food habits and the reduction in physical activity have produced a marked increase in the prevalence of diet-related chronic diseases such as obesity, hypertension, certain cancers, diabetes, stroke, and cardiovascular diseases. Nowadays, 59% of annual deaths and 46% of the global disease burden may be attributable to noncommunicable chronic diseases [69].

Direct costs of obesity are related to the costs of hospitalization, outpatients visits, and drugs prescribed. Indirect costs refer to the social costs of obesity and are calculated according to the health consequences before retirement, in relation to mortality before retirement, decreased number of years free of disability before retirement, and absenteeism [70]. Another approach to evaluating the influence of obesity on lifespan is by estimating the number of years of life lost associated with excess body fat. For example, in the Framingham Heart Study, among a group of nonsmokers 40 years of age, which included men and women with BMI > 30 kg/m^2, loss is 7.1 and 5.8 years of life, respectively [71,72].

Conclusions

Obesity is a chronic disease, currently with an epidemic uncontrolled diffusion in both developed and developing countries. It represents a major health concern whose diffusion requires, especially in childhood, proper legacy applications and national educational campaigns.

Medical complications of obesity are the consequence of long-term exposure to the excess fat, acting not only through a mass effect for the excess weight and increased FFA turnover but also through metabolic and functional derangements due to an abnormal secretion of various peptides directly secreted by enlarged adipocytes and other stromal cells of the adipose tissue.

Selected References

4. Iacobellis G, Sharma M. Obesity and the heart: redefinition of the relationship. Obesity Rev 2007;8:35–9.

10. Powell K. The two faces of fat. Nature 2007:525–7.

18. Olshansky SY, Passaro DJ, Hershow RC, et al. A potential decline in life expectancy in the United States in the 21st century. N Engl J Med 2005;352(11):1138–45.

35. Contaldo F, Pasanisi F, Finelli C, et al. Obesity, heart failure and sudden death. Nutr Metab Cardiovasc Dis 2002;12(4):190–7.

70. Popkin BM, Kim S, Rusev ER, et al. Measuring the full economic costs of diet, physical activity and obesity-related chronic diseases. Obesity Rev 2006;7:271–93.

CHAPTER 7

Cardiovascular Damage in Obesity and Metabolic Syndrome

Giovanni de Simone[1,2], *Richard B. Devereux*[2], *&*
Oreste de Divitiis[1]

[1]Federico II University, Naples, Italy
[2]Weill Medical College of Cornell University, New York, NY, USA

Introduction

The heart is substantially affected by the alteration of body composition due to disproportionate increase in fatness. Changes in central hemodynamics, alterations of neurohormonal response, and abnormalities in cytokine balance, with predominant inflammatory response, participate in the initiation and progression of cardiac modifications, ultimately precipitating heart failure, the most common end stage of obesity-associated cardiomyopathy [1–4]. In land mammals, the cardiovascular system is programmed to sustain the operational impact of skeletal dimensions, which are in turn related to muscle mass [5] needed to guarantee the two basic abilities necessary for survival: fight and escape. It is intuitive that the heart is the key organ affected by an inappropriate increase in body weight, disrupting the natural equilibrium between genetically programmed fat and nonfat tissue components of the body [5]. Changes in the arterial system related to the frequent association of obesity with other atherogenic risk factors, including hypertension, diabetes, and dyslipidemia, further alter cardiac workload and enhance structural and functional abnormalities due to obesity.

Obesity predisposes to, or is associated with, cardiovascular disease (coronary heart disease, heart failure, and sudden death) and increased all-cause

Nutritional and Metabolic Bases of Cardiovascular Disease, 1st edition.
Edited by Mario Mancini, José M. Ordovas, Gabriele Riccardi,
Paolo Rubba and Pasquale Strazzullo. © 2011 Blackwell Publishing Ltd.

mortality rate [1,6,7]. This association depends on severity of alteration of body composition. In morbid obesity, which can be identified with class III (body mass index [BMI] > 40.0 kg/m^2) obesity by National Institutes of Health (NIH) criteria [8], cardiovascular abnormalities are very evident [9].

Obesity and Systemic Hemodynamics

In obese subjects, ventricular chambers are enlarged with left ventricular (LV) and right ventricular (RV) hypertrophy [10], which may be either eccentric (with proportional increase of chamber size and wall thickness) or concentric (with disproportionate increase in ventricular wall thickness) [11]. The increased heart weight is due to the increase in all myocardial tissue components, including cardiomyocytes, fibroblasts, connective tissue, extracellular matrix, and fat cells [12]. In particular, fat accumulates at the epicardial level and infiltrates the myocardium [13].

The enlarged ventricular chambers initially maintain near-normal systolic function, with consequent enhancement of ventricular pump performance, measurable by stroke volume or stroke work [14,15]. Because heart rate is also increased due to enhanced sympathetic drive and reduced parasympathetic tone [16,17], cardiac output is almost invariably elevated [18,19], related to the increased body tissue O_2 demand, while the O_2 arteriovenous difference is within normal limits [18]. The obesity-related increase in cardiac output parallels increased blood volume and preload [18]. This enhanced LV pump performance is appropriate in relation to the increased metabolic requirements due to increased fat-free mass and visceral fat, the two components of body composition that generate the greatest metabolic demand [20–22].

Obesity-related greater blood volume is associated with reduced peripheral vascular resistance [18], but this decrease appears inadequate to maintain normal blood pressure (BP) even in subjects classifiable as normotensive. Thus, for a given cardiac output, obese individuals exhibit BP greater than that of average-weight subjects, even in the range considered average. Obese subjects are, therefore, predisposed to develop arterial hypertension, a very commonly associated cardiovascular risk factor [23–25]. The reason for the inadequate reduction of peripheral vascular resistance in the presence of the increased cardiac output is likely due to the obesity-associated endothelial dysfunction and enhanced production of vasoactive substances [26].

Signs of "preclinical cardiovascular disease," representing evidence of target organ damage in the absence of clinically overt cardiovascular disease [27], are often present at the early stages of obesity. In particular, changes of LV geometry are the hallmark of the stage of preclinical cardiovascular disease.

Several studies have provided key information on cardiac geometry and function in human obesity, using noninvasive techniques focusing on detection of preclinical cardiovascular disease and providing insights into the pathophysiology of cardiovascular changes associated with obesity.

Body Composition and LV Anatomy

Heart weight has been studied using echocardiography, focusing on LV muscle mass (which comprises roughly half of total heart weight). Echocardiographic LV mass has been found to directly correlate with BMI [28]. The accuracy of this technique has been validated in many animal and human studies [29,30], as has its reproducibility [31,32]. The technique is very reliable also when obesity is present. In the Strong Heart Study (SHS), a population-based study with nearly 80% prevalence of overweight or obesity, echocardiograms could be measured in more than 90% of population [33].

The most important body size correlate of LV mass is lean body mass [21], which can be estimated as fat-free mass by bioelectric impedance analysis, whereas adipose mass does not account significantly for interindividual variability of LV mass (Table 7.1).

In the population-based sample of the SHS, the magnitude of LV mass increases with higher fat-free mass, systolic BP, and age, with an additional contribution from diabetes [1,34] but is not influenced by adipose tissue. However, an important though little-noted effect of overweight and obesity is increased fat-free body mass, with fat-free

Table 7.1 In a multivariate analysis, LV mass is related to fat-free mass (FFM), not to adipose mass in both men and women.

Variable	Men (n = 1155)				Women (n = 1952)			
	B	SE	β	P	B	SE	β	P
FFM	1.665	0.173	0.392	<0.001	2.251	0.194	0.370	<0.001
Systolic blood pressure	0.390	0.069	0.174	<0.001	0.439	0.042	0.244	<0.001
Age	0.616	0.166	0.115	<0.001	0.412	0.112	0.088	<0.001
Diabetes	3.563	2.574	0.043	0.167	4.155	1.661	0.055	0.012
Adipose mass	0.113	0.155	0.027	0.468	0.126	0.087	0.042	0.147
Height[27]	0.005	7.310	0.001	0.987	2.085	2.505	0.021	0.405
Constant	−23.126	19.138			−52.799	12.381		

B indicates regression coefficient SE, standard error of the regression coefficient.
Reproduced from Bella et al. [21], with permission.

body mass higher by 13%, 24%, and 38% in over-weight, mildly obese, and moderately to severely obese participants, respectively, compared to those with normal BMI.

Methods of indexing LV mass for body size that take body weight into account, such as the classic indexation for body surface area (BSA), may be un-duly influenced by the increased amount of body fat in obese subjects. This is the reason for shifting from use of the traditional measure of BSA to nor-malize LV mass [35,36], in view of the increasing prevalence of overweight and obesity in virtually all populations. Normalization of LV mass for BSA underestimates the prevalence and severity of LV hypertrophy (LVH) in obese populations [11], be-cause BSA includes body weight (and in fact was not intended for obese subjects [37]). This mis-interpretation increases with increasing severity of obesity.

Use of a method of indexing LV mass that does not overadjust for effects of obesity improves the strength of LVH to predict cardiovascular events. Figure 7.1 shows that using normalization for BSA-based partition values reduces substantially the population risk attributable to LVH [38], due to the misclassification of obesity-associated LVH as nor-mal, whereas normalization of LV mass for height to the power of 2.7 or 2.13 doubles population at-tributable risk. These exponents are called allomet-ric signals and are determined in clinically-normal, normal weight reference populations to linearize the naturally curvilinear relation between a three-dimensional variable, LV mass, and a monodimen-sional measure (body height) [39,40]. Interestingly, in the SHS, partition values for clear-cut LVH ob-tained from raw values of LV mass without any normalization for body size (196.2 g) gave results very similar to those found using BSA or unadjusted heights, suggesting that normalization of LV mass for allometric measures of body size is necessary to fully estimate LVH associated cardiovascular risk.

Obesity and LVH

The exact prevalence of LVH attributable to obe-sity is difficult to determine because of the frequent coexistence of obesity with overt hypertension. As said, even in the absence of hypertension, obesity is frequently associated with nonoptimal BP val-ues, which contribute to increasing LV mass and prevalence of LVH. Using LV mass/height$^{2.7}$, the prevalence of LVH ranges between 13% in obese, normotensive individuals [11] to more than 75% in individuals with morbid obesity, in the pres-ence of hypertension [41]. In our reference pop-ulation from Italy and the United States, 12% of class I to class III, otherwise healthy, obese nor-motensive subjects exhibit LVH, a prevalence that approaches 50% when hypertension coexists, but

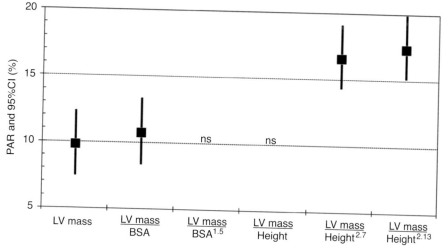

Figure 7.1 Population attributable risk (PAR) and 95% confidence interval (CI) for LVH in the Strong Heart Study hypertensive population, based on normal partition values derived from the same population. (Reproduced from de Simone et al. [38], with permission.)

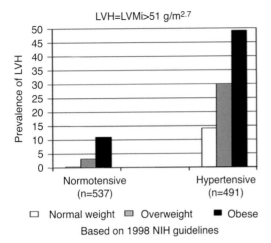

LVH=LVMi>51 g/m$^{2.7}$

☐ Normal weight   ▨ Overweight   ■ Obese

Based on 1998 NIH guidelines

Figure 7.2 Prevalence of left ventricular hypertrophy (LVH) in normotensive and hypertensive subjects, based on body size distribution.

is less than 15% among hypertensive subjects with average body weight (Figure 7.2). As suggested by these observations, obesity appears to amplify the effect of cardiovascular risk factors on systemic hemodynamics and LV mass. In the HyperGEN study, a large population of normotensive and hypertensive white and Africa American adults, the probability of LVH increased with increasing number of "metabolic" risk factors, including obesity, diabetes and dyslipemia [42] and the probability of LVH in normotensive subjects with two or more risk factors was similar to the probability of LVH in hypertensive subjects without additional risk factors [42].

In obese individuals, especially those with concomitant hypertension, LV geometry can be either eccentric or concentric. In a study of employed adults in New York [11], 18% of obese hypertensive individuals had concentric LVH, while 34% had eccentric LVH. More recently, Avelar et al. [41] reported a high prevalence of LV concentric geometry among morbidly obese subjects selected for bariatric surgery. Thus, even in the presence of severe obesity, concentric LV geometry is not rare.

There are many reasons to explain the presence of concentric LV geometry in some individuals with morbid obesity. In addition to the likely high BP load, neurohormonal activation, including sympathetic overactivity, increased expression of endothelin, reduced production of nitrous ox-

ide (made more severe because of frequent hypoxemia), and increased blood viscosity [43,44] might contribute to altered hemodynamic and local conditions, yielding concentric LV remodeling [45]. The frequent sleep apnea, increasing the BP load even during the night, also substantially contributes to produce concentric LV geometry [41,46]. Recently, the 2,058 participants in the Sleep Heart Health Study were studied to relate their sleep-disordered breathing with LV echocardiographic phenotypes, using polysomnography-derived apnea-hypopnea index and hypoxemia index [47]. LV mass index was significantly associated with both apnea-hypopnea index and hypoxemia index, independently of age, sex, ethnicity, BMI, current and prior smoking, alcohol consumption, systolic BP, antihypertensive medication use, diabetes mellitus, and prevalent myocardial infarction. A severe breathing disorder (apnea-hypopnea index ≥ 30/hr) was associated with 1.78-fold higher probability of LVH than in participants with negligible apnea-hypopnea episodes. A higher apnea-hypopnea index and higher hypoxemia index were also associated with larger LV diastolic dimension and lower LV ejection fraction, whereas LV wall thickness was significantly associated with the hypoxemia index but not with apnea-hypopnea index.

Body fat distribution might play a key role both in the prevalence of LVH and in determination of the LV geometric pattern. General adiposity, as can be assessed by BMI, is a documented predictor of LV mass [48], but central adiposity is more related to concentric LV geometry [49], even independently of effect of central BP or average 24-hour systolic BP [50].

Whereas in studies of adults, the relations between LVH and obesity can be affected by substantial confounders such as arterial hypertension and antihypertensive therapy, this limitation is less present in children and adolescents, in whom hypertension and antihypertensive therapy are much less common than among adults. The relations between obesity and LVH are confirmed also in children and adolescents [51–53]. In the Strong Heart Family Study [54], overweight adolescents exhibit high levels of LV mass that are matched with their higher hemodynamic load, but in obese adolescents the increase of LV mass exceeds this need, resulting in significant inappropriate LV mass (Table 7.2),

Table 7.2   Cardiac geometry in average weight (16.8 ± 1.3 yr), overweight (17.0 ± 1.4 yr), and obese (17.7 ± 1.4 yr) adolescents.

	Normal Weight (n = 114)	Overweight (n = 113)	Obese (n = 223)
LV diameter (cm)	5.08 ± 0.39	5.25 ± 0.37*	5.31 ± 0.44†
Aortic root (cm)	2.97 ± 0.25	3.02 ± 0.25*	3.08 ± 0.28†‡
Left atrial diameter (cm)	3.08 ± 0.32	3.34 ± 0.30	3.64 ± 0.46†‡
Relative wall thickness	0.27 ± 0.03	0.27 ± 0.03	0.28 ± 0.04†‡
LV mass (g)	131.78 ± 30.15	148.98 ± 37.40*	165.03 ± 41.07†‡
LV mass index (g/m$^{2.7}$)	30.21 ± 5.17	33.04 ± 5.57*	35.97 ± 7.60†‡
Concentric geometry (%)	0.5	1.8	4.4†‡
LV hypertrophy (%)	3.5	12.4*	33.5†‡
Inappropriate LV mass (%)	6.3	9.8	27.2†‡

Analysis of covariance with Sidak's adjustment of means of age, gender, systolic and diastolic blood pressure, heart rate, and height (as a surrogate of body growth). *P < 0.05 between normal weight and overweight; †P < 0.05 between obese and normal weight; ‡P < 0.05 between overweight and obese.
LV = left ventricular.
Reproduced from Chinali et al. [54], with permission.

associated with mild LV systolic and diastolic dysfunction.

Obesity and LV function

Whatever LV geometric remodeling occurs, either concentric or eccentric, LV chamber size is often large due to the increased preload and circulating volume, which helps maintain normal LV chamber function (i.e., ejection fraction) with usually increased LV cardiac output [14] under resting conditions. In fact, the enhanced LV performance (cardiac output and stroke volume) does not necessarily parallel increased or normal LV function (ejection fraction, midwall shortening, etc.) [55]. In normotensive obese subjects, free of cardiac or respiratory disease, the LV function curve is characterized by diminished contractile response that does not allow appropriate systolic work, despite the increased filling pressure [18,56] (Figure 7.3). The increased cardiac output in obesity is, therefore, achieved using elevated filling pressure. Similarly, the increased stroke volume, largely responsible for the increased cardiac output, is sustained by the recruitment of resting Starling forces, as evident in Figure 7.3. During stress, the utilization of the Starling forces to sustain LV performance at rest results in less ability to recruit preload reserve, leading to

impaired LV function during exercise or other stress conditions [57]. The abnormal response to exercise is also correlated with increased LV mass [58].

Similar to what is seen for LV mass, the increased LV pump performance in obesity is detectable when normalization of stroke volume or cardiac output for body size is not done using BSA, but specific allometric signals generated to linearize the relations of these hemodynamic indices with body height [15]. The increased stroke volume is due to the

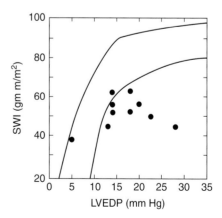

Figure 7.3 Left ventricular (LV) function (Starling) curve. The points of 8 of 10 obese subjects lie below the range of normal variability. (Reproduced from de Divitiis et al. [18], with permission.)

large LV chamber size pumping greater amount of blood with normal LV chamber function, whereas the increased cardiac output is also due to the increased heart rate, as the consequence of impaired autonomic balance in obese subjects [17].

Body fat distribution substantially influences the extent of the increase in stroke volume and cardiac output, even in the absence of obesity. In a nonobese, overweight population, central fat distribution was correlated with increased stroke volume and cardiac output, even after adjustment for fat-free mass [59]. That association was demonstrated to be due to the effect of central fat. In the SHS population, Bella et al. [60] also demonstrated that stroke volume and cardiac output are related to adipose mass as well as fat-free mass in both women and men. These results indicate that the increased LV pump performance parallels the increased metabolic requirements of central adipose tissue, consistent with the great paracrine and endocrine activity of visceral fat [61,62]. Many substances produced by visceral fat have great atherogenic potential [63], influencing arterial structure [64] and eventually LV structural response [65].

Systolic dysfunction is not easily detectable by standard indices in the obese subject [14,66], but long exposure to severe obesity can produce systolic dysfunction [67], paralleling more severe structural transformations of myocardium. In contrast, at earlier stages, obesity-associated LV geometric abnormalities are commonly accompanied by a number of abnormalities of LV filling [66,68–71], which may ultimately contribute to the development of heart failure. Most recently, an excessive increase in LV mass, especially associated with concentric LV geometry, has been demonstrated to be a strong predictor of heart failure in an elderly unselected population-based sample, independently of initial ejection fraction and incident myocardial infarction [72].

Metabolic Syndrome

Most often, obesity is not an isolated abnormality but is associated with other metabolic alterations, the most important of which is insulin resistance [73]. In many circumstances, obesity presents with the phenotype of metabolic syndrome (MetS) [74]. Although empirical, the definition of MetS

is important on both pathophysiological and epidemiological grounds [75–78]. Studies in different settings suggest that cardiovascular risk factors clustered with central obesity may amplify cardiovascular risk to an extent that cannot be predicted by consideration of single component risk factors. Of particular interest, the risk of cardiovascular events associated with the MetS remains beyond what can be predicted by individual cardiovascular risk factors, including diabetes [79].

The cardiovascular risk associated with MetS can be documented also when one of the components (arterial hypertension) is present in all individuals and initial cardiovascular risk is very high due to the concomitant presence of preclinical cardiovascular disease. In the LIFE study, in a context of very high cardiovascular risk due to electrocardiographic (ECG) evidence of LVH and hypertension in all participants, MetS was associated with twofold increased 5-year risk of cardiovascular events, an effect that was only marginally attenuated when adjusting for diabetes, obesity, low high-density lipoprotein (HDL)-cholesterol, non-HDL-cholesterol, pulse pressure and in-treatment systolic BP and heart rate [80]. These findings suggest that MetS can yield further amplification of cardiovascular risk, even in the presence of LVH.

In different contexts, when the confounding effect of arterial hypertension is minimized, MetS exhibits a strong relation with LVH. In the SHS cohort, non-hypertensive adult participants with MetS exhibited LV geometry similar to that of hypertensive participants without MetS [81]. Some of these non-hypertensive participants, however, had BP in the range defined as pre-hypertension [82] that could in part account for altered LV geometry, but the magnitude of this abnormality was comparable to that of participants with clear-cut hypertension, suggesting that abnormal LV geometry is in fact related to MetS at least in part independently of BP levels. More recently, the evidence that LV mass increases also as a consequence of non-hypertensive abnormalities gained even more evidence from the offspring of the original SHS cohort [83]. In nondiabetic adolescents (17 ± 1.5 yr) with a 25% prevalence of MetS, high prevalence of central obesity but low prevalence of hypertension (16% in the MetS group), MetS was associated with an impressive 42% prevalence of LVH, as well as with concentric LV geometry, reduced LV function, and left atrial dilatation, a worrisome cardiovascular phenotype at such a young age. In a multivariate analysis, presence of MetS was associated with 2.6-fold greater probability of LVH that was independent of the significant effects of obesity and high BP. Lipid profile and fasting glucose levels were not associated with LVH.

Whether the association of MetS with incident cardiovascular events is independent of the presence of echocardiographic LVH is an obvious question arising from these findings. A recent study in members of the SHS cohort free of prevalent cardiovascular disease [84] has shown that MetS maintained a potent predictive power also in the presence of LVH among diabetic participants, whereas in nondiabetic subjects risk related to MetS could be fully explained by prevalent LVH. In another analysis from the SHS, in adults with initial optimal BP, but high prevalence of other cardiovascular risk factors, greater LV mass was a significant risk factor for future development of arterial hypertension detected by standardized clinic BP measurements, with a 4-year incidence of hypertension >30% among individuals with LV mass in the highest decile of baseline values [85]. It is possible that obesity-associated LVH may contribute to the development of arterial hypertension in obese individuals [86,87], which may be difficult to treat when MetS coexists [88].

A bidirectional link among metabolic disorders and LVH is also observed during antihypertensive therapy. In the LIFE study, hypertensive patients with diabetes and average value of BMI of 30 kg/m^2 had less regression of ECG LVH in response to antihypertensive therapy than patients without diabetes [89]. At the same time, regression of LVH among diabetic subjects did not provide the same amount of risk reduction as in the nondiabetic participants. Also, in-treatment resolution or continued absence of ECG LVH was associated with

lower risk of incident diabetes even adjusting for confounders [90].

Many questions remain to be clarified, including hemodynamic and, perhaps even more important, non-hemodynamic mechanisms of development of LVH in the context of the complex obesity phenotypes, which would be especially important in clinical conditions in which LV mass increases beyond the values that can be explained with alteration of loading conditions. Other studies, albeit not specifically addressing this topic, have shown that myocardial structure can be profoundly altered in conditions other than arterial hypertension, and that fat infiltration can promote increase in LV mass but not necessarily in muscle mass [13]. In the Cardiovascular Health Study cohort, excessive increase in LV mass is a potent risk factor for heart failure not due to incident coronary heart disease [72]. In that study, increasing levels of excess LV mass are associated with lower BP levels, higher BMI, worse lipid profile and sharply higher C-reactive protein levels, providing other clues for future mechanistic research involving inflammatory markers [91].

Selected References

9. de Simone G. Morbid obesity and left ventricular geometry. Hypertension 2007;49:7–9.

18. de Divitiis O, Fazio S, Petitto M, et al. Obesity and cardiac function. Circulation 1981;64:477–482.

41. Avelar E, Cloward TV, Walker JM, et al. Left ventricular hypertrophy in severe obesity: interactions among blood pressure, nocturnal hypoxemia, and body mass. Hypertension 2007;49:34–39.

54. Chinali M, de Simone G, Roman MJ, et al. Impact of obesity on cardiac geometry and function in a population of adolescents: the Strong Heart Study. J Am Coll Cardiol 2006;47:2267–2273.

83. Chinali M, de Simone G, Roman MJ, et al. Cardiac markers of pre-clinical disease in adolescents with the metabolic syndrome: the strong heart study. J Am Coll Cardiol 2008;52:932–938.

CHAPTER 8

Treatment of Obesity: Beneficial Effects on Comorbidities and Lifespan

George A. Bray

Pennington Biomedical Research Center, Baton Rouge, LA, USA

Introduction

Let's begin with a brief description of the techniques that are available for the management of obesity. Obesity is the result of a long-term positive imbalance between energy intake and energy expenditure, which means that treatments can be focused on either energy intake or on energy expenditure. Figure 8.1 is an energy-balance diagram and serves as a basis for briefly reviewing therapeutic options [1].

Eating (energy intake) is a target for behavior therapy, drugs, and bariatric surgery for obesity. Physical activity and energy expenditure are targets for behavioral change and drugs, and patients who lose weight after bariatric surgery are often more physically active. When any of these therapeutic approaches is used consistently, weight loss is the expected result. In this chapter, we examine the consequences of this weight loss as they apply to the cardiovascular system. Since death from heart disease is the leading cause of death, weight loss might be expected to benefit both long-term survival and to have many intermediate effects on cardiovascular risk factors.

The metabolic syndrome (MetS) has become one way of "bundling" a group of risk factors that together point toward the risk of diabetes or cardiovascular disease (CVD) [2]. (See Chapter 11.)

Nutritional and Metabolic Bases of Cardiovascular Disease, 1st edition.
Edited by Mario Mancini, José M. Ordovas, Gabriele Riccardi,
Paolo Rubba and Pasquale Strazzullo. © 2011 Blackwell Publishing Ltd.

Weight loss is associated with significant improvement in the MetS and in the proinflammatory and pro-coagulant markers that are often present. To the extent that we are successful with weight loss, it would be the ideal approach, since it will treat many of the features of the MetS simultaneously [2].

One can view the consequences of obesity as resulting from either the mass of adipose tissue added to the body or from the metabolic consequences of enlarged fat deposits [3]. The "mass" effects of obesity depend on the specific location of the fat deposits. For the metabolic consequences, it is largely central and visceral fat that are important. Women have about 12% more body fat than men for any given body mass index (BMI) [4]. Yet women have fewer heart attacks and die, on average, at an older age than men. This implies that a significant proportion of the extra fat that women have is not "risky" fat in terms of CVD. Epidemiologic studies show that fat on the hips and lower body may, in fact, be protective in terms of mortality risks [5]. Thus, it is important to identify the "risky" fat and to not group all fat depots into a single entity.

Benefits and Potential Risks of Weight Loss

Effect on Mortality

Two groups of studies have examined weight loss and mortality. One group of observational studies suggests that weight loss is associated with

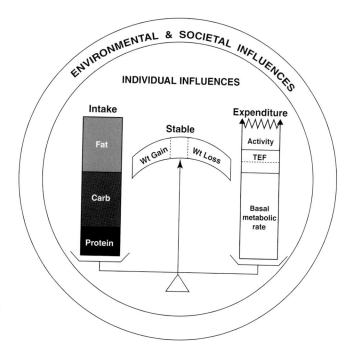

Figure 8.1 Energy balance and treatment options: influences on the development of obesity. (Copyright 1998 G.A. Bray.)

increased mortality [6]. The limitation of these studies is that, in most cases, they cannot distinguish between intentional and unintentional weight loss. We have known since the time of Hippocrates, 2,500 years ago, that unintentional weight loss is a poor prognostic sign for future health [7]. One approach to separating intentional and unintentional weight loss was taken by Allison et al. [8], who examined loss of lean body mass versus fat. When the weight loss was from lean body mass, there was an increased risk of mortality. In contrast, loss of body fat was associated with lowered risks of mortality [8].

The other approach to separating intentional and unintentional weight loss was to ask whether the weight loss was intentional. Documentation that intentional weight loss benefits mortality is scantier. In one study of intentional versus unintentional weight loss, Williamson and colleagues reported a 20% reduction in all-cause mortality among 15,069 women with health conditions who were monitored from 1959/1960 to 1972. Most of the reduction in risk was related to decrease in cancer-related deaths. Mortality related to diabetes was reduced 30%–40%. In women with no preexisting illness ($N = 28,388$), intentional weight loss

of 20 lb (9.1 kg) or more in the previous year was associated with a 25% reduction in all-cause mortality [9]. Using a different data set, Williamson et al. [10] carried out a prospective analysis of 12-year mortality among 4,970 overweight individuals with diabetes ages 40 to 64 years enrolled in the American Cancer Society Prevention Study I. Intentional weight loss was reported by 34% of the cohort and resulted in a 25% decrease in total mortality and a 28% reduction in CVD and diabetes mortality. A weight loss of 20 to 29 lb (9.1 to 13.2 kg) was associated with the largest reductions in mortality. Similar results came from a follow-up of the National Health Interview Survey that included enough subjects to link 20,439 individuals to the National Death Index. In this group with a 9-year follow-up, those reporting intentional weight loss had a 24% lower overall mortality rate when compared to individuals not trying to lose weight [11,12]. A final large study in this category was conducted in the United Kingdom by Wanamethee et al. Among individuals choosing to lose weight, the all-cause mortality was reduced 41%, but there was no association with intentional weight loss and death from cardiovascular causes [13].

Studies in the bariatric surgical literature suggest that voluntary, intentional weight loss is beneficial. In the follow-up of individuals who have had bariatric gastric-bypass surgery, Flum et al. noted a modest overall survival benefit associated with the procedure, suggesting again that "intentional" weight loss can reduce mortality [14].

Intermediate Risk Factors

A considerable body of data documents that weight loss improves a number of the intermediate risk factors that predict disease [15–24]. In a systematic review of long-term weight-loss studies and their applicability to clinical practice, Douketis et al. [17] found that dietary and lifestyle therapy provided <5 kg of weight loss after 2–4 years, and that pharmacological therapy could produce 5- to 10-kg of weight loss over 1–2 years. Weight loss of 5% or more from baseline is not consistently associated with improvements in cardiovascular risk factors, and these benefits appear primarily in the individuals with concomitant cardiovascular risk factors.

Effects on Morbidity

Hypertension and Heart Disease

One of the clearest examples of benefits from weight loss on cardiovascular risk factors comes from studies with hypertensive patients. Among these are the Trials of Hypertension Prevention (TOHP) [25,26] and the Trial of Nonpharmacologic Interventions in the Elderly (TONE) [27]. Individuals with high-normal blood pressure experienced a 21%–34% decrease in the incidence of hypertension over an interval of 1.5–4 years with a modest weight loss of only 2%–4%. Hypertensive individuals who maintained their weight loss following a weight-loss intervention were able to maintain lower blood pressure compared to the individuals who regained weight, where blood pressure returned to baseline levels [28]. Among older people, a reduction in body weight by an average of 4% produced a 30% reduction in the combined incidence of CVD and hypertension. In the Premier study, more than 800 people with borderline hypertension were enrolled into three groups: a control or advise-only group, a group who received an established behavioral intervention program, or a group who got both the behavioral intervention program along with the DASH diet [29,30]. The blood pressure was reduced by −3.7 to −4.3 mm Hg in the two intervention groups compared to the advise-only group [29]. There was also a significant reduction in the prevalence of hypertension in the two treated groups. In a follow-up study, this group has shown that over 30 months subjects can retain about 50% of an initial weight loss and still maintain the lower blood pressure [31].

Several clinical trials have shown that weight loss can improve cardiovascular risk. The Stanford Coronary Risk Intervention Project may be the most well-known of these [32]. It was a large, multicommunity project in California. Using a multifactorial program of risk reduction that involved an intensive focus on reducing saturated fat and total fat, an increase in physical activity, and a modest 4% weight loss, the investigators showed that there was an approximately 40% reduction in probability of cardiac events and a slower rate of coronary artery stenosis. A second study in this group was the Lifestyle Heart Trial, which is a landmark in the diet-heart literature, because it shows that vigorous dietary intervention can reverse the risks of CVD [33,34]. A graded reduction in cardiovascular risk was observed in still another study. A group of high-risk individuals from 50 to 75 years of age were recruited. In those who successfully lost weight over a 6-month period, the odds ratio for coronary heart disease was 0.70 over the next 3 years [35].

In addition to the data showing improvement in cardiovascular outcomes with weight loss, there is evidence that weight loss improves the function of the heart [36]. It is possible to show a reduction in blood volume with a parallel reduction in stroke volume. Cardiac output also falls, as does systemic arterial blood pressure. There is, however, little change in systemic arterial resistance after weight loss. Resting oxygen consumption declines as the size of the metabolic compartment is reduced. Possibly the most important changes are the reduction in left ventricular mass. With obesity, there is an eccentric hypertrophy of the heart, which is reduced with weight loss. There may also be a decline in heart rate, a fall in the QTc interval, and an increase in heart rate variability [36].

In addition to these positive effects, there have also been important negative effects of some weight-loss regimens on cardiac function. One of the early very-low-calorie diet formulas contained a gelatin-based protein, and a number of deaths were reported [37]. These were thought to be due to an arrhythmia called torsade de pointes, due to prolongation of the QTc interval. A second cardiac event following treatment of obesity occurred with fenfluramine and dexfenfluramine. In 1997, at the height of the use of fenfluramine/phentermine (the so-called "fen/phen craze"), Conley et al. reported 24 patients who developed aortic regurgitation while being treated with this combination [38]. The best estimates are that with treatment for longer than 6 months, the prevalence of this problem may have been 20%–30% among treated patients. In September 1997, fenfluramine and dexfenfluramine were withdrawn from the market.

Dyslipidemia

The meta-analysis by Avenell et al. [39] suggests that weight loss has significant effects on lipid profiles and blood pressure, both important predictors of future CVD. Among various types of weight-loss programs, there was a significant, but somewhat variable, effect on weight loss. In family-based intervention compared to a control group at 12 months ($N = 4$) weight loss was −2.96 kg (95% confidence interval [CI]: −5.31 to −0.60 kg). With group versus individual therapy in four studies, it was 1.59 kg (95% CI: −1.81 to 5.00 kg). When diet and behavior therapy were compared to diet alone after 12 months in four studies, weight loss was −7.67 kg (95% CI: −11.97 to −3.36 kg). Finally when diet and behavior therapy were compared against only a control group, the weight loss after 12 months was −7.21 kg (95% CI: −8.68 to −5.75 kg). With these weight losses, there was a reduction in blood pressure that averaged −4/−3 mm Hg comparing systolic and diastolic blood pressure. Cholesterol and low-density lipoprotein (LDL)-cholesterol also declined by some 5 to 8 mg/dl and triglycerides fell by 18 mg/dl. In the meta-analysis of Avenell et al. [39], the high-density lipoprotein (HDL)-cholesterol benefited at 12 months in two studies, with an increase of 0.10 nmol/L (95% CI: 0.06 to 0.14 mmol/L) and triglycerides were lowered after 12 months by −0.18 nmol/L (95% CI: −0.31 to −0.06 mmol/L). Thus, some important risk factors for CVD are improved by weight loss.

Diabetes

Diabetes is a cardiovascular risk factor; thus, reduction in the incidence of diabetes would be expected to benefit cardiovascular outcomes. The risk of diabetes is reduced by modest weight loss [40–50]. This has now been reported in several prospective trials in patients with impaired glucose tolerance. The first report was by Pan et al. from China [40]. They showed a reduction in the incidence of new cases of diabetes by 31% with diet, by 46% with exercise, and by 42% with both after 6 years of follow-up. The next was the Finnish Diabetes Study [41–43]. Incidence of diabetes was reduced by 58% over 4 years with a 5.0% weight loss and increased exercise and improved diet [41]. This was followed by the U.S. Diabetes Prevention Program (USDPP), which showed that after 2.8 years of an intensive lifestyle program and an initial weight loss of 7% of body weight, the conversion rate was reduced by 58% compared to the placebo-treated control group [44–48,51]. The Japanese Diabetes Prevention Program (JaDPP) [49] and the Indian Diabetes Prevention Program (InDPP) [50] also reported reduced rates of conversion to diabetes of 57.4% over 4 years and 28.5% over 3 years, respectively.

The USDPP participants also showed significant reductions in lipids and blood pressure in the intensive lifestyle group compared to the placebo group (Table 8.1). Similar reductions were seen in the Look AHEAD trial, which enrolled just over 5,000 individuals with established diabetes and randomized them to placebo and intensive lifestyle treatment [52]. Those in the intensive lifestyle group also showed reductions in blood pressure and lipids after the first year of treatment, when weight loss was just over 8% in the treated group.

A number of weight-loss medications also reduce the risk of developing diabetes.

Orlistat

Using data from the clinical trials of orlistat, Heymsfield et al. pooled information on 675 subjects from three of the 2-year studies described previously in which glucose tolerance tests were available [53]. During treatment, 6.6% of the patients taking orlistat converted from a normal to an impaired glucose tolerance test, compared with 10.8% in the placebo-treated group. None of the orlistat-treated patients who originally had normal glucose tolerance

Table 8.1   Changes in lipids and blood pressure with weight loss in the Diabetes Prevention Program.

Variable	Diabetes Prevention Program		Look AHEAD Trial	
	Placebo	Lifestyle	Placebo	Lifestyle
Blood pressure (SBP/DBP)	−0.90/−089	−3.4/−3.6	−2.8/−1.8	−6.8/−3.0
Cholesterol (%)	−1.2%	−2.3%	—	—
LDL-cholesterol	+1.3%	+0.7%	−4.6%	−5.0%
HDL-cholesterol (mg/dL)	−0.1%	+1.9%	+3.2%	+7.8%
Triglycerides (mg/dL)	−11.9	−25.4	−14.6	30.3
Fibrinogen (% change 1 yr)	0.6%	−2%	—	—
Tissue plasminogen activator	−5%	−20%	—	—
CRP Males	0%	−30%	—	—
Females	0%	−20%		

developed diabetes, compared with 1.2% in the placebo-treated group. Of those who initially had normal glucose tolerance, 7.6% in the placebo group and 3% in the orlistat-treated group developed diabetes. The effect of orlistat in preventing diabetes has been assessed in a 4-year study [54]. In this trial weight was reduced by 2.8 kg (95% CI: 1.1–4.5 kg) compared to placebo, and the conversion rate of diabetes was reduced from 9% to 6% for a relative risk reduction of 37% (HR = 0.63; 95% CI: 0.46–0.86) [55]. The incidence of new cases of diabetes was also reduced from 10.9% to 5.2% ($p = .041$) during a 3-year period in which overweight patients were treated with orlistat and lifestyle or lifestyle alone [56]. A meta-analysis using the pooled data shows significant overall effects after one year of treatment on lipids and blood pressure with orlistat (Table 8.2), and on lipids with sibutramine (Table 8.2).

Patients with diabetes treated with orlistat, 120 mg three times daily for 1 year, lost more weight than the placebo-treated group [57–59].

Sibutramine

A number of studies have examined the effect of sibutramine in diabetic patients.

A meta-analysis has been done of eight studies in diabetic patients receiving sibutramine [60]. In the meta-analysis, the changes in body weight, waist circumference, glucose, hemoglobin A1c, triglycerides, and HDL-cholesterol favored sibutramine. The mean weight loss was −5.53 ± 2.2 for those treated with sibutramine and −0.90 ± 0.17 for the placebo-treated patients. There was no significant change in systolic blood pressure, but diastolic blood pressure was significantly higher in the sibutramine-treated patients [60]. In the meta-analysis by Norris et al. [61], the net weight loss over 12 to 26 weeks in four trials including 391 diabetics was −4.5 kg (95% CI: −7.2 to −1.8 kg).

Table 8.2   A meta-analysis of the effects of orlistat on lipids and blood pressure.

Change in cholesterol (N = 7 studies)	−0.34 mmol/L (95% CI: −0.41 to −0.027)
Change in LDL-cholesterol (N = 7 studies)	−0.29 mmol/L (95% CI: −0.34 to −0.24)
Change in HDL-cholesterol (N = 6 studies)	−0.03 mmol/L (95% CI: −0.05 to −0.01)
Change in triglycerides (N = 6 studies)	+0.03 mmol/L (95% CI: −0.04 to 0.10)
Change in HbA1c (N = 3 studies)	−0.17% (95% CI: −0.24 to −0.10
Change in SBP (N = 7 studies)	−2.02 mm Hg (95% CI: −2.87 to −1.17)
Change in DBP (N = 7 studies)	−1.64 mm Hg (95% CI: −2.20 to −1.09)

LDL: low-density lipoprotein; HDL: high-density lipoprotein; SBP: systolic blood pressure; DBP: diastolic blood pressure; CI: confidence interval.

Table 8.3   A Meta-analysis of effects of sibutramine on lipids and blood pressure.

Change in cholesterol at 12 months ($N = 3$)	0.01 mmol/L (95% CI: −0.15 to 0.18 mmol/L)
Change in LDL cholesterol at 12 months ($N = 2$)	−0.08 mmol/L (95% CI: −0.23 to 0.07 mmol/L)
Change in HDL-cholesterol at 12 months ($N = 2$)	0.10 mmol/L (95% CI: 0.04 to 0.15 mmol/L)
Change in Triglycerides at 12 months ($N = 4$)	−0.16 mmol/L (95% CI: −0.26 to −0.05 mmol/L)
Change in SBP at 12 months ($N = 3$)	1.16 mm Hg (95% CI: −0.60 to 2.93 mm Hg)
Change in DBP at 12 months ($N = 3$)	2.04 mm Hg (95% CI: 0.89 to 3.20 mm Hg)

LDL: low-density lipoprotein; HDL: high-density lipoprotein; SBP: systolic blood pressure; DBP: diastolic blood pressure; CI: confidence interval.

Adapted from Laaksonen DE, Lindström J, Lakka TA, et al. [42], with permission.

As with other procedures for weight loss, patients treated with sibutramine experienced improvements in some lipid parameters. These are summarized in Table 8.3 from the meta-analysis of Avenell et al. [39]. There was a small but significant rise in HDL-cholesterol and a fall in triglycerides after 12 months. In contrast, cholesterol and LDL-cholesterol showed no significant responses. There was no change in systolic blood pressure, but a small rise in diastolic blood pressure at the end of one year.

Bariatric Surgery

Bariatric surgery has proven to be a very effective way to reverse the prevalence of diabetes and to reduce the incidence of new cases. Pories et al. were the first to note the marked effect on diabetes [62,63]. Although there were design issues with these retrospective studies, they showed an annual incidence of 4.5% in the control group contrasted with only 1% in the surgically operated group.

In an unblended, randomized controlled trial, Dixon et al. [64] enrolled 60 diabetic patients with a BMI between 30 and 40 kg/m^2 into either lap-band operation or a lifestyle program. At 2 years, the lap-band group had lost 20.7% of their body weight compared to 1.7% in the lifestyle group. The relative risk of remission from diabetes was 5.5 (95% CI: 2.2, 14.0) and was related to weight loss.

Metabolic Syndrome

The data for improvement in MetS come from studies with lifestyle intervention, with diet, and with medications.

Several clinical trials with weight-loss medications also show a reversal of the MetS. The MetS was present in about 50% of the subjects in several clinical trials with rimonabant. In the placebo groups after one year of treatment, the MetS was still present in 53% of the subjects in the RIO Europe study [65], 51% of those in the RIO Lipids study [66], and 38% of those in the RIO North America study [67]. Substantial decreases occurred in the rimonabant-treated groups. For the RIO-Europe and RIO Lipids groups, only 21% still had the MetS, a 60% decrease. For the RIO-North America group, it was 7.9%, a decrease of almost 60% [65–67].

Inflammatory markers

A high-sensitivity assay for circulating C-reactive protein (CRP) has brought this molecule to the forefront of markers for inflammation. There is clear evidence from the studies by Ridker et al. [68] that measurements of CRP add significantly to the prediction of whether individuals will develop CVD and do so independently of LDL-cholesterol. CRP is associated with adiposity and this does not differ significantly by age, or race. Elevated levels of CRP are associated with all the features of the MetS and it can thus serve as a measure of the response of weight loss to these inflammatory markers.

Cancer

Cancers are slow growing, and clinical trials of weight loss to affect their progression have not been performed. However, the recent evaluation of mortality in patients who underwent gastric-bypass operations for obesity has suggested that long-term weight loss can reduce the death rate from cancer. In this study, Utah residents were matched to gastric-bypass patients based on age and sex [16, 69]. Gastric bypass significantly reduced mortality rate and there was a significant 60% drop in death rate from cancer in this group compared to the controls.

Disability and Bone and Joint Diseases

Health impairments and associated healthcare costs are strongly related to degrees of excess weight, and weight loss can improve some of them. In the Health ABC study, the incidence of limitation in mobility among 70- to 79-year-olds rose as BMI rose [70]. In those with a BMI of 30.0–35.9 kg/m^2, the incidence was 18%, rising to 40% when the BMI was >35 kg/m^2. In the Nurses' Health Study, there was improved physical functioning and vitality associated with weight loss [71]. Weight loss also improves the plight of those with arthritis. In an observational study, a weight loss of 5 kg occurring over 10 years was associated with a 59% reduction in the incidence of arthritis [72]. In the Arthritis, Diet, and Activity Promotion Trial (ADAPT), 316 adults older than 60 years and a BMI >28 kg/m^2 were randomized to one of four conditions, including control, diet, exercise, or exercise plus diet. Over the next 18 months where the weight loss was 5%–6%, those in the diet and exercise group experienced the most benefit [72].

In summary, I have dealt with the approach to treating the overweight patient. Diabetes, liver disease, high blood pressure, heart disease, and some forms of cancer are among the most important complications of obesity. There are also data arguing that weight loss is beneficial.

Selected References

3. Bray GA. Medical consequences of obesity. J Clin Endocrinol Metab 2004 Jun;89(6):2583–9.

31. Svetkey LP, Stevens VJ, Brantley PJ, et al; Weight Loss Maintenance Collaborative Research Group. Comparison of strategies for sustaining weight loss: the weight loss maintenance randomized controlled trial. JAMA 2008 Mar 12;299(10):1139–48.

47. The DPP Research Group. Effect of weight loss with lifestyle intervention on risk of diabetes. Diabetes Care 2006; 29: 2102–7.

70. Lee JS, Kritchevsky SB, Tylavsky F, et al; Health ABC Study. Weight change, weight change intention, and the incidence of mobility limitation in well-functioning community-dwelling older adults. J Gerontol A Biol Sci Med Sci 2005 Aug;60(8):1007–12.

72. Felson DT, Zhang Y, Anthony JM, et al. Weight loss reduces the risk for symptomatic knee osteoarthritis in women. The Framingham Study. Ann Intern Med 1992 Apr 1;116(7):535–9.

CHAPTER 9

A Review of Results from Swedish Obese Subjects, SOS

Lars Sjöström

Gothenburg University, Gothenburg, Sweden

Introduction

The obesity prevalence has increased in all parts of the world over the last 20–30 years [1–3]. In the United States, the prevalence is now 30%. The majority of large and long-term epidemiological studies indicate that obesity is associated with increased mortality [4–10]. The life span of severely obese persons is decreased by an estimated 5–20 years [11]. Weight loss is known to be associated with improvement of intermediate risk factors for disease [12], suggesting that weight loss would also reduce mortality. However, the controlled interventional studies demonstrating that weight loss is in fact reducing mortality have been lacking. To date, most observational epidemiologic studies have indicated that overall and cardiovascular mortality are increased after weight loss [13], even in subjects who were obese at baseline [14–16]. This discrepancy concerning the effects of weight loss on risk factors as compared to mortality has been related to certain limitations inherent in observational studies, particularly the inability of such studies to distinguish intentional from unintentional weight loss. Thus, the observed weight loss might be the consequence of conditions that lead to death rather than the cause of increased mortality.

However, three observational epidemiologic reports [17–19], all based on American Cancer Society data, have suggested that intentional weight loss is in fact associated with decreased mortality,

although the information on intentionality was based on retrospective, self-reported data collected at baseline. Whether these weight losses before the baseline examination were maintained is unknown, as weight changes during the studies were not reported. Three retrospective cohort studies in obese subjects [20–22] and one in obese subjects with diabetes [23] have suggested that bariatric surgery may also result in a marked reduction in mortality.

There has been a dramatic increase in the use of bariatric surgery during the past decade. In 2003, more than 100,000 procedures were performed in the United States [24]. However, until recently, it remained unclear whether the long-term weight loss induced by bariatric surgery has favorable effects on lifespan.

In order to ascertain the effects of intentional weight loss on mortality, controlled, prospective interventional trials are needed. In the Swedish Obese Subjects (SOS) trial, we used bariatric surgery to achieve weight loss, since such surgery was and still is the only technique available with proven long-term effects on weight loss.

SOS Aims

The primary aim of SOS was to examine whether intentional weight loss induced by bariatric surgery is associated with lower mortality as compared to conventional treatment in contemporaneously matched obese controls. Several secondary aims related to the effects of bariatric surgery on diabetes and other morbidity, risk factors, health-related

Nutritional and Metabolic Bases of Cardiovascular Disease, 1st edition.
Edited by Mario Mancini, José M. Ordovas, Gabriele Riccardi,
Paolo Rubba and Pasquale Strazzullo. © 2011 Blackwell Publishing Ltd.

quality of life (HRQL), and health economics were also defined. Finally, the genetics of obesity was an additional topic for research in the SOS trial.

Study Design and Baseline Description

The ongoing SOS project consists of four substudies:

The *SOS Matching (or Registry) study* ($n = 6,905$), from which patients were recruited to the *SOS intervention study*. The intervention study consists of one surgical group ($n = 2,010$) and one obese control group ($n = 2,037$).

The *SOS reference study* ($n = 1,135$), which is a small study on randomly selected subjects from the general population examined contemporaneously with and in the same way as subjects in the reference and intervention trials.

The *SOS sibpair study* ($n = 768$) consisting of weight-discordant siblings and their biological parents [25,26]. These subjects were mainly recruited from the SOS registry and intervention studies but also from other Swedish obesity studies such as the XENDOS study. The sibpair study will be used for a genome-wide scan using expression data from adipose tissue as phenotypes, among other variables.

SOS Matching and Intervention Studies

The SOS [12,27,28] intervention trial is a prospective, matched, surgical interventional trial involving 4,047 obese subjects. Patients were recruited over 13.4 years between September 1, 1987, and January 31, 2001. The follow-up is currently (December 2009) ranging from 8 to 22 years.

As a result of recruitment campaigns, 11,453 subjects sent standardized application forms to the SOS secretariat, and 6,905 completed a matching examination (the Matching/Registry study). Among the potential subjects examined, 2,010 eligible subjects desiring surgery constituted the surgical group, and based on data from the matching examination, a contemporaneously matched control group ($n = 2,037$) was created. The matching program used 18 matching variables and the matching could not be influenced by the investigators [27].

A baseline examination for the surgical subjects and their matched controls was undertaken 4 weeks before surgery (Table 9.1).

The intervention began on the day of surgery for surgically treated subjects and their matched controls. Individual dates of all subsequent examinations and questionnaires (0.5, 1, 2, 3, 4, 6, 8, 10, 15, and 20 years) for surgically treated and control subjects were calculated based on the dates of operation. Inclusion criteria for the interventional study were age 37 to 60 years and body mass index (BMI) (weight [kg]/(height m]^2) of 34 or more for men and 38 or more for women. The BMI cutoffs corresponded to an approximate doubling in mortality rate in each gender as compared to mortality in the BMI range 20–25 kg/m^2 [29]. Exclusion criteria, described elsewhere [27], were minimal and were aimed at obtaining an operable surgical group. Identical inclusion and exclusion criteria were used for the two treatment groups.

The Matching and the Intervention studies were undertaken at 480 primary health care centers and 25 surgical departments in Sweden. At each visit, measurements of weight, height, waist circumference, other anthropometric measures (see Table 9.1), and blood pressure were obtained [27]. Biochemical variables (see Table 9.1) were measured at the matching examination, at the baseline examination (year 0 of the Intervention study), and at years 2, 10, 15, and 20 years. Blood samples were obtained in the morning after a 10- to 12-hour fast and analyzed at the Central Laboratory of Sahlgrenska University Hospital (accredited according to European Norm 45001). The baseline questionnaire included self-reported information on previous myocardial infarction (MI), stroke, and cancer, as well as questions designed to assess the likelihood of sleep apnea [30]. Psychosocial variables (Table 9.1, bottom) were also evaluated [31]. Subgroups have been examined for cardiovascular structure and function and with respect to genetic characteristics, for methodology; please see methods of the reviewed studies below.

The surgically treated subjects underwent nonadjustable or adjustable banding ($n = 376$), vertical banded gastroplasty ($n = 1,369$), or gastric bypass ($n = 265$) operations [32]. For adjustable banding, the Swedish Adjustable Gastric Band (SAGB, Obtech Medical, Stockholm) was used. The obese,

Table 9.1 Characteristics of the SOS surgery and control groups at baseline.

	Baseline examination	
Variable	Surgery N, % or mean ±SD	Controls N, % or mean ±SD
Total, n	2,010	2,037
Males, n	590	590
Females, n	1,420	1,447
Postmenopausal women, %*	37.2	41.3
Age at examination, years	47.2 ± 5.9	48.7 ± 6.3
Daily smokers, %	25.8	20.8
Diabetics, %	10.7	11.4
Sleep apnea, %	25.1	22.2
Lipid lowering mediations, %	1.8	1.6
Previous MI, n	31	29
Previous stroke, n	15	23
Previous stroke or MI, n	46	49
Previous cancer, n	24	21
Weight, kg	121.0 ± 16.6	114.7 ± 16.5
Height, m	1.69 ± 0.09	1.69 ± 0.09
BMI, kg/m^{2*}	42.4 ± 4.5	40.1 ± 4.7
Waist circumference, cm	125.8 ± 11.0	120.2 ± 11.3
Hip circumference, cm	127.1 ± 10.0	123.2 ± 10.0
Waist/hip ratio*	0.99 ± 0.08	0.98 ± 0.07
Sagittal diameter, cm	28.9 ± 3.7	27.4 ± 3.7
Neck circumference, cm	43.7 ± 4.3	42.9 ± 4.29
Upper arm circumference, cm	39.8 ± 3.8	38.7 ± 3.8
Thigh circumference, cm	75.5 ± 7.5	73.4 ± 7.5
Systolic BP, mm Hg	145.0 ± 18.8	137.9 ± 18.0
Diastolic BP, mm Hg	89.9 ± 11.1	85.2 ± 10.7
Pulse pressure, mm Hg	55.2 ± 14.5	52.8 ± 13.0
Glucose, mmol/L	5.45 ± 2.11	5.20 ± 1.92
Insulin, mU/L	21.5 ± 13.7	18.0 ± 11.4
Triglycerides, mmol/L	2.25 ± 1.54	2.02 ± 1.41
Total cholesterol, mmol/L	5.86 ± 1.12	5.61 ± 1.06
HDL cholesterol, mmol/L*	1.20 ± 0.28	1.19 ± 0.29
Uric acid, μmol/L	359.2 ± 79.8	352.3 ± 79.9
ASAT, μkat/L	0.43 ± 0.23	0.39 ± 0.21
ALAT, μkat/L	0.63 ± 0.39	0.56 ± 0.42
ALP, μkat/L	3.12 ± 0.84	3.01 ± 0.87
Bilirubin, μmol/L	9.51 ± 4.28	9.93 ± 5.27
Current health, scores	21.4 ± 6.10	22.7 ± 6.2
Monotony avoidance, scores	22.5 ± 5.1	22.6 ± 5.0
Psychasthenia, scores	23.9 ± 5.2	23.2 ± 5.3
Quantity of social support	6.02 ± 2.4	6.08 ± 2.45
Quality of social support	4.25 ± 1.32	4.28 ± 1.31
Stressful life events	2.49 ± 1.30	2.43 ± 1.28

BMI: body mass index; HDL: high-density lipoprotein; ASAT: aspartate aminotransferase; ALAT: alanine aminotransferase; ALP: alkaline phosphatase.
Adapted from Sjöström et al. [28], with permission.

contemporaneously matched controls received the customary nonsurgical obesity treatment for their given center of registration. No attempt was made to standardize the conventional treatment, which ranged from sophisticated lifestyle intervention and behavior modification to, in many practices, no treatment whatsoever.

All Social Security Numbers from the SOS database were cross-checked against the Swedish Person and Address Register (SPAR) every year on November 1. At several occasions, the SOS database has also been cross-checked against the Swedish Social Insurance System, Statistics Sweden, and the Swedish Hospital Discharge Register in order to obtain objective data on sick leave, disability pension, hospital care, and annual income for outcome and health economic studies.

SPAR provides current addresses and information on all deceased subjects. Social Security Numbers on all deceased subjects were cross-checked against the Swedish Cause of Death Register to obtain the official cause of death. In addition, all relevant case sheets and autopsy reports were adjudicated independently by two experienced clinicians blinded with respect to study arm. If the two examiners differed on a cause of death, a third, blinded physician also reviewed the case so a final decision could be made. If the study-determined cause of death did not agree with the official cause, the study-determined cause of death was used.

For statistical procedures, please see the methods sections of the reviewed publications.

The SOS Reference Study

The SOS reference study is a cross-sectional study of randomly selected individuals. The main purpose of the study was to create a reference sample to obese SOS subjects in genetic association studies and in comparative analyses of clinical conditions (see below).

Between August 1994 and December 1999, that is, during the period when the major part of patients were included in the SOS intervention study, 524 men and 611 women were included in the SOS reference study. Body composition and biochemical characteristics of the SOS reference study have been published [33–36] and are not further discussed in this review.

Follow-up Rates

In the publication on overall mortality, the vital status was known for all initial study participants except three: two who had requested to be deleted from the SOS database and one who had left the study and later obtained a secret Social Security Number. With respect to vital status on the date of analysis, the follow-up rate was 99.93%.

In the Intervention study, the participation rates of still-living subjects at the 2-, 10-, and 15-year examinations ranged between 66% and 94%. The participation rate was 100% at the baseline examination.

Baseline Characteristics in the SOS Intervention Study

The matching procedure created two largely comparable groups, although the surgically treated subjects were on average 2.3 kg heavier ($p < .001$), 1.3 years younger ($p < .001$), and smoking more frequently ($p < .001$) than the controls [28]. The higher body weight of the surgery group was associated with higher values in several anthropometric measurements and in some biochemical variables [28].

Between the matching and baseline examinations, there was an increase in weight in the surgically treated patients (1.73 kg, $p < .001$) and a decrease in weight in the control group (2.23 kg, $p < .001$). These diverging weight changes caused most variables to become significantly different between surgery and control groups at baseline (Table 9.1) [28]. However, all observed baseline differences except three (age, thigh circumference, bilirubin) constituted survival disadvantages for the surgery group in univariate analyses [28].

In an early cross-sectional analysis of 450 men and 556 women from the Matching study of SOS, it was shown that as compared to randomly selected controls, most cardiovascular risk factors were elevated in the obese [27]. The exception was total cholesterol, which was similar in obese and nonobese men and lower in obese women as compared to reference women.

Risk factors have also been analyzed in relation to baseline body composition in 1,083 men and 1,367 women from the SOS Matching study [37]. This analysis revealed one body compartment–risk

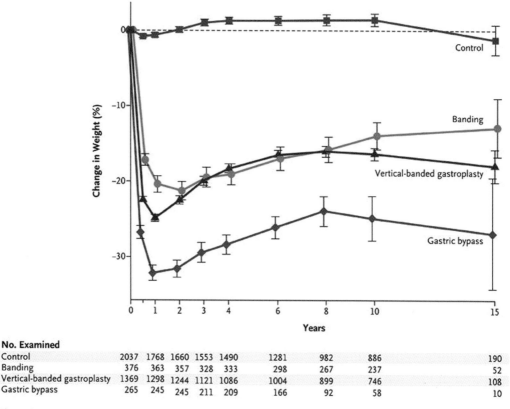

No. Examined

Control	2037	1768	1660	1553	1490	1281	982	886	190
Banding	376	363	357	328	333	298	267	237	52
Vertical-banded gastroplasty	1369	1298	1244	1121	1086	1004	899	746	108
Gastric bypass	265	245	245	211	209	166	92	58	10

Figure 9.1 Mean percentage weight change during the first 15 study years of the SOS intervention trial in the control group and the three surgical subgroups. I bars denote 95% confidence intervals. (Reproduced from Ssjöström et al. [28], with permission.)

factor pattern and one subcutaneous adipose tissue distribution–risk factor pattern. Within the first pattern, risk factors were positively and strongly related to the visceral adipose tissue mass and more weakly to the subcutaneous adipose tissue mass. Some risk factors, such as glucose and triglycerides in men and insulin in women, were negatively related to lean body mass. In addition, the subcutaneous adipose tissue distribution was related to risk factors both when and when not taking the body compartments into account statistically. A preponderance of subcutaneous adipose tissue in the upper part of the trunk, as indicated by the neck circumference, was positively related to risk factors, while the thigh circumference was negatively related to risk factors. These two risk factor patterns have also been observed longitudinally; that is, changes in risk factors and changes in body composition and adipose tissue distribution are related [38] in the same way as in the cross-sectional observations [37].

Weight Changes in SOS

Figure 9.1 shows the weight changes for up to 15 years from baseline for control and surgery subgroups [28]. The number of observations decreased over time, not only because of the 13-year-long recruitment period but also because of dropout from examinations. In the control group, average weight change remained within ±2% over the observation period. In the three surgical subgroups, weight loss was maximal after 1–2 years (gastric bypass, 32% ± 8%; vertical banded gastroplasty 25% ± 9%; and banding, 20% ± 10%, mean ± standard deviation [SD]). Weight increase was seen in all surgical subgroups in the following years, but the relapse curves leveled off after 8–10 years (Figure 9.1).

After 10 years, the weight losses were 25% ± 11% (gastric bypass), 16% ± 11% (vertical banded gastroplasty), and 14% ± 14% (banding) compared with the baseline weight. After 15 years, the corresponding weight losses were 27% ± 12%, 18% ± 11%, and 13% ± 14%, respectively.

Effects of Weight Loss on Risk Factors

The 2- and 10-year risk factor changes observed in the SOS trial were published in 2004 (Figures 9.2 and 9.3) [12]. As illustrated in Figures 9.2 and 9.3, the 2- and 10-year recovery rates from diabetes, hypertriglyceridemia, low levels of high-density lipoprotein (HDL)-cholesterol, hypertension, and hyperuricemia were more favorable in the surgery group than in the control group, whereas recovery from hypercholesterolemia did not differ between the groups. The surgery group had lower 2- and 10-year incidence rates of diabetes, hypertriglyceridemia, and hyperuricemia than the control group, whereas differences between groups in the incidence of hypercholesterolemia and hypertension were not detectable.

A number of earlier SOS reports on risk factor changes have also appeared [38–41]. In a 2-year report of 282 men and 560 women, pooled from the surgically treated group and the obese control group, risk factor changes were examined as a function of weight change [38]. A 10-kg weight loss was enough to introduce clinically significant reductions in all traditional risk factors except total cholesterol. Preliminary calculations indicate that there is a fairly linear relationship between weight loss and risk factor improvement also over 10 years, although 15 kg maintained weight loss is often required to achieve long-term risk factor improvements (Sjöström CD et al., to be published).

Effects of Weight Loss on the Cardiovascular System

In smaller subsamples of the SOS study, cardiac and vascular structure and function were examined at baseline and after 1–4 years of follow-up.

At baseline, a surgically treated group ($n = 41$) and an obese control group ($n = 31$) were com-

pared with a lean reference group ($n = 43$) [42,43]. As compared to lean subjects, the systolic and diastolic blood pressure, left ventricular mass, and relative wall thickness were increased in the obese while the systolic function (measured as left ventricular ejection fraction) and the diastolic function (estimated from the E/A ratio (i.e., the flow rate over the mitral valve early in diastole divided by the flow rate late in diastole during the atrial contraction) were impaired. After one year, all these variables had improved in the surgically treated group but not in the obese control group. When pooling the two obese groups and plotting left ventricular mass or E/A ratio as a function of quintiles of weight change, a "dose" dependency was revealed (i.e., the larger the weight reduction, the larger the reduction in left ventricular mass and the more pronounced the improvement in diastolic function). Unchanged weight was in fact associated with a measurable deterioration in diastolic function over one year.

In other small subgroups from SOS, heart rate variability from 24-hour Holter electrocardiographic (ECG) recordings and 24-hour catecholamine secretion were examined [44]. As compared to lean subjects, our examinations indicated an increased sympathetic activity and a withdrawal of vagal activity at baseline. Both these disturbances were normalized in the surgically treated group but not in the control group after one year of treatment.

The intima-media thickness of the carotid bulb was examined by means of ultrasonography at baseline and after 4 years in the SOS intervention study [45]. A randomly selected lean reference group matched for gender, age, and height was examined at baseline and after 3 years. The annual progression rate was almost 3 times higher in the obese control group as compared to lean reference subjects ($p < .05$). In the surgically treated group, the progression rate was normalized. Although results from this small study group need to be confirmed in larger trials, this study offered the first data on hard end-points after intentional weight loss.

We have also shown that the pulse pressure increases more slowly in the surgically treated group than in the obese control group after a mean follow-up of 5.5 years [46]. In individuals with gastric bypass, the pulse pressure is in fact decreasing. These observations are of interest since it has been shown that, at a given systolic blood pressure, a high pulse

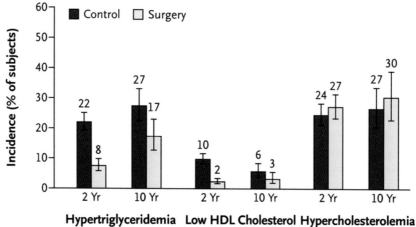

No. of subjects	801 731	281 225	1174 1293	440 431	596 504	188 135
Odds ratio	0.29	0.61	0.21	0.57	1.27	1.16
95% CI	0.21–0.41	0.39–0.95	0.14–0.32	0.29–1.15	0.95–1.69	0.69–1.95
P value	<0.001	0.03	<0.001	0.12	0.11	0.57

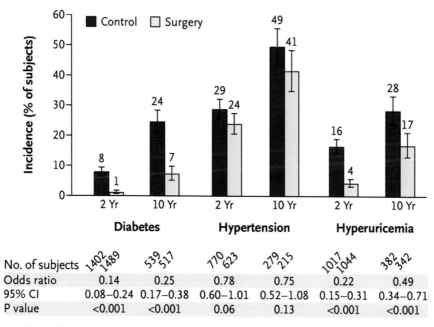

No. of subjects	1402 1489	539 517	770 623	279 215	1017 1044	382 342
Odds ratio	0.14	0.25	0.78	0.75	0.22	0.49
95% CI	0.08–0.24	0.17–0.38	0.60–1.01	0.52–1.08	0.15–0.31	0.34–0.71
P value	<0.001	<0.001	0.06	0.13	<0.001	<0.001

Figure 9.2 Incidence of diabetes, lipid disturbances, hypertension and hyperuricemia over 2- and 10-year periods among surgically treated subjects and their obese controls in the SOS intervention study. Data are for subjects who completed 2 years and 10 years of the study. The bars and the percentage values above the bars show unadjusted values for incidence. I bars represent the corresponding 95% confidence intervals. Below each panel, the odds ratios, 95% confidence interval [CI] for the odds ratios and p values have been adjusted for gender, age, and body mass index (BMI) at the time of inclusion in the intervention study. (Reproduced from Sjöström et al. [12], with permission.)

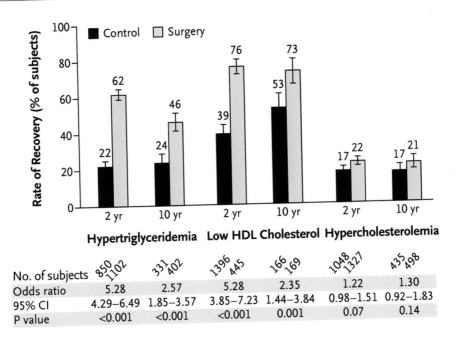

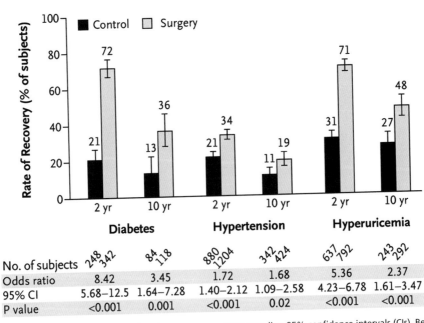

Figure 9.3 Recovery from diabetes, lipid disturbances, hypertension, and hyperuricemia over 2- and 10-year periods among surgically treated subjects and their obese controls in the SOS intervention study. Data are for subjects who completed 2 years and 10 years of the study. The bars and the percentage values above the bars show unadjusted values for incidence. I bars represent the corresponding 95% confidence intervals (CIs). Below each panel, the odds ratios, 95% CI for the odds ratios, and p values have been adjusted for gender, age, and body mass index (BMI) at the time of inclusion in the intervention study. (Reproduced from Sjöström et al. [12], with permission.)

pressure is associated with increased arterial stiffness [47], increased intima-media thickness [48], and increased cardiovascular mortality [49]. Thus, pulse pressure changes [46] as well as ultrasonographic measurements [45] indicated that bariatric surgery may slow down the accelerated atherosclerotic process in the obese.

Further support for favorable effects on the atherosclerotic process was obtained in an analysis of effort-related calf pain. This symptom was much more common in 6,328 obese subjects of the SOS Matching study than in 1,135 randomly selected subjects from the general population in the SOS reference study (men: odds ratio [OR] = 5.0; women: OR = 4.0, $p < .001$) [50]. The 6-year incidence of new cases of effort-related calf pain was lower in obese subjects undergoing bariatric surgery than in the conventionally treated control group (men: OR = .39, women: OR = .61, $p < .05$). Among subjects reporting symptoms at baseline, the 6-year recovery rate was higher in the surgical group than in the control group (men: OR = 15.3, women: OR = 5.9, $p < .001$) [50].

Questionnaire data from 1,210 surgically treated patients and 1,099 obese SOS controls examined at baseline and after 2 years were analyzed with respect to various cardiovascular symptoms [51]. At baseline, the two groups were comparable in most respects. After 2 years, dyspnea and chest discomfort were reduced in a much larger fraction of surgically treated patients as compared to controls. For instance, 87% of the surgically treated patients reported baseline dyspnea when climbing two flights of stairs while only 19% experienced such dyspnea at the 2-year follow-up. In the obese control group, the corresponding figures were 69% and 57%, respectively ($p < .001$ for difference in change between groups).

Effects of Weight Loss on Sleep Apnea

Baseline sleep apnea was examined by means of a questionnaire in 1,324 SOS men and 1,711 SOS women [30,52]. A high likelihood for sleep apnea was observed in 26% of obese men and in 9% of obese females. Sleep apnea was associated with World Health Organization (WHO) grade 4 daytime dyspnea, admission to hospital with chest

pain, MI, and elevations of blood pressure, insulin, triglycerides, and uric acid when adjusting for body fat, adipose tissue distribution, and other potential confounders [52]. In addition, sleep apnea was also associated with increased psychosocial morbidity before and after these adjustments [30].

Sleep apnea has also been investigated in the SOS intervention study [51]. A high likelihood for sleep apnea was observed in 23% of 1,210 surgically treated cases at baseline but only in 8% after 2 years postsurgery. In the control group ($n = 1,099$), the corresponding figures were 22% and 20%, respectively ($p < .001$ for difference in change between groups) [51]. In a recent follow-up, these findings were confirmed and it was also found that subjects reporting loss of obstructive sleep apnea had a lower 2-year incidence of diabetes and hypertriglyceridemia, also after adjustment for baseline central obesity and weight change over 2 years [53].

Finally, a small experimental study in obese SOS patients demonstrated an association between sleep apnea, elevated catecholamine secretion, and elevated energy expenditure, particularly during sleep [54]. Affected individuals were improved by means of nighttime treatment with continuous positive airway pressure [54].

Effects of Weight Loss on Joint Pain and Fracture Frequency

Self-reported work-restricting pain in the neck and back area and in the hip, knee, and ankle joints was more common in untreated obese men and women than in the general population, as judged from the SOS Matching and Reference studies (ORs ranging from 1.7 to 9.9, $p < .001$) [55]. Obese women treated with bariatric surgery had a lower 2- and 6-year incidence of work-restricting pain in the knee and ankle joints than conventionally treated obese women (OR: 0.51–0.71). Recovery rates from baseline symptoms in knee and ankle joints for men and in neck and back and in hip, knees, and ankle joints for women were higher after bariatric surgery than after conventional treatment (OR: 1.4–4.8) [55].

Preliminary data suggest that the fracture frequency is lower in individuals treated with bariatric surgery than in conventionally treated subjects [56].

Biliary Disease in the SOS Intervention and Reference Studies

Obese individuals had significantly higher prevalence of cholelithiasis and previous cholecystitis, cholecystectomies, and pancreatitis than randomly selected subjects from the SOS reference study [57]. BMI was related to biliary disease in both genders. Compared with conventional treatment, bariatric surgery was associated with increased incidence of biliary disease in men but not in women. Weight loss was associated with increased incidence of biliary disease in both genders [57].

Effects of Weight Loss on Lifestyle and Health Related Quality of Life

Physical inactivity was observed in 46% of the surgically treated before weight reduction but only in 17% after 2 years. Corresponding figures in the obese control group were 33% and 29%, respectively (p for difference in change $< .001$) [51]. Later, we have found increased physical activity at each observation occasion over the first 10 years of follow-up [12]. Thus, physical inactivity not only contributes to the development of obesity, but obesity favors physical inactivity. This vicious cycle is broken by surgical treatment.

At baseline, the energy intake was slightly higher in the surgery group (2,882 kcal/24 hr) than in the obese control group (2,526 kcal/24 hr), while it was significantly lower in the surgery group over the first 10 years of follow-up [12].

Cross-sectional information from 800 obese men and 943 women of the SOS Matching study demonstrated that obese patients have a much worse HRQL than age-matched reference subjects [58]. In fact, HRQL in the obese was as bad as, or even worse than, in patients with severe rheumatoid arthritis, generalized malignant melanoma, or spinal cord injuries. The measurements were performed with generic scales such as the General Health Rating Index, Hospital Anxiety and Depression Scale (HAD), Mood Adjective Checklist (MACL), and Sickness Impact Profile in original or short form [31,58] and with more obesity-specific instruments such as OP measuring obesity-related psychosocial problems [58] and Stunkard's Three-factor Eating Questionnaire (TFEQ) [59]. All scales have been validated under Swedish conditions.

Stunkard's original findings based on the TFEQ [59] (cognitive restraint, disinhibition, hunger) could not be replicated among 4,377 obese SOS patients with respect to convergent and discriminative validity of the factors. Using multitrait/multi-item analysis and factor analysis, a short revised 18-item instrument has been constructed, representing the derived factors of cognitive restrain, uncontrolled eating, and emotional eating [60].

In 2- and 4-year [61,62] reports, results from all measuring instruments improved dose dependently, that is, the larger the weight loss, the more improvement of HRQL. In subjects with weight loss $\geq 25\%$, large effects were seen for obesity-related measures reflecting eating patterns and psychosocial problems and for general health and functional health domains such as ambulation, recreation, pastimes and social interaction. Moderate effect sizes were observed for depressive symptoms (HAD-D), self-esteem and overall mood (MACL), while the effect on anxiety symptoms (HAD-A) were minor. In the obese control group, only trivial effects were seen.

Over 10 years, the HRQL was significantly more improved in the surgery group as compared to the conventionally treated obese control group in the domains current health perception, social interaction, psychosocial functioning, and depression, whereas no significant differences between groups were found for overall mood and anxiety [63]. The long-term results suggest that 10% weight loss within the surgery group is sufficient for favorable long-term effects of HRQL, a limit that is achieved by two-thirds of surgical 10-year completers [63].

In summary, HRQL is very poor in obese subjects. Large (>25%) and moderate (10%–25%) weight losses maintained over 4–10 years improve most aspects of HRQL.

Health Economic Consequences of Bariatric Surgery

In cross-sectional studies of SOS patients, it was shown that sick leave was twice as high and disability pension twice as frequent than in the general

Swedish population independent of age and gender [64]. The annual indirect costs (sick leave plus disability pension) attributable to obesity were estimated at 6 billion SEK in Sweden, or 1 million U.S. dollars per 10,000 inhabitants per year.

The number of lost days due to sick leave and disability pension the year before inclusion into the SOS intervention was almost identical in the surgically treated group and the obese control group (104 and 107 days, respectively) [65]. The year after inclusion, the number of lost days was higher in the surgically treated group but, 2–4 years after inclusion, the lost days were lower in the surgically treated group. This was particularly evident in those individuals above the median age (46.7 years) [65].

Surgical obesity treatment is associated with higher hospital costs ($10,200) than conventional treatment ($2,800) over 6 years [66]. When adjusting for the surgical intervention as such ($4,300) in the surgical group and conditions common after bariatric surgery in both groups ($2,800 in surgically treated, $400 in controls), the remaining costs were not different in the two groups. These observations from 2002 indicated that the lag time between weight loss and improvement of hard end-points requiring hospitalization was longer than 6 years. We now know that it took 13 study years until we obtained a significant effect on overall mortality (see below), but we have not yet had the possibility to examine health economic data over 10–15 years.

At baseline, the fraction of individuals on medication for various conditions was usually higher in obese subjects of the SOS Intervention study (Int) than in lean randomly selected individuals of the SOS reference (Ref) study [67]. The fraction on medication for the following conditions was significantly different between groups: diabetes (Int 6.1%, Ref 0.7%), CVD (Int 27.8%, Ref 8.2), pain (Int 10.8%, Ref 4.1%), while medication for the following conditions were not significantly different: asthma (Int 5.2%, Ref 2.3%), psychiatric disorders (Int 7.2%, Ref 4.6%) anemia (Int 1.3%, Ref 1.6%) gastrointestinal disorders(Int 4.4%, Ref 3.5%), all others (Int 20.5%, Ref 23.6%).

Among SOS intervention patients on medication at baseline, the fraction on medication dropped significantly more over 6 years in the surgically treated group than in the control group [67]. In contrast, surgery did not significantly prevent the start of medication among those who had no medication at baseline. While the average cost per individual over 6 years was lower in the surgically than the conventionally treated obese control group regarding medication for diabetes and CVD, the costs were higher for anemia and gastrointestinal disorders. The total annual cost for all medication averaged over six years was not significantly different between surgically treated individuals (1,386 Swedish crowns/yr) and obese control individuals (1,261/yr). Again it must be stressed that we do not yet have 10- to 15-year data available for costs of medication.

In a separate study on CVD and diabetes medication, we found that a weight loss $\geq$10% was necessary to reduce the costs of medication among subjects with such treatment at baseline while a $\geq$15% weight loss was required to prevent the initiation of a new treatment against the two conditions [68]. The annual average cost over six years for medication against diabetes and CVD increased by 463 SEK (96%) in subjects with weight loss <5%, and decreased by 39 SEK (8%) with weight loss $\geq$15% [68].

Modern economists are often using estimates of patients' willingness to pay for a given treatment as an expression for degree of urgency. We measured the willingness to pay for an efficient obesity treatment at baseline and found it to be twice as high as the monthly salary of the participants [69]. After inclusion, the willingness to pay for an efficient treatment increased markedly in the surgically treated group (to be published).

Taken together, the direct plus indirect costs of surgical obesity treatment seem to be only marginally higher than conventional treatment over 6 years. Taking the reduced risk factors and the improved quality of life into account, the surgical approach seemed worthwhile already as based on 6-year evaluations. As pointed out above it will now be urgent to repeat the health economic evaluations based on 10- to 15-year data in order to examine whether the reduced incidence of hard endpoints translates into reduced costs. It should be stressed that our 6-year evaluations are based on actually observed costs and are not the result of modeling from short term observations as is usually the case in health economic studies.

Genetic Findings in SOS

Segregation analysis of the SOS cohort has indicated an age-dependent major gene effect explaining up to 34% of the BMI variance [70]. This finding makes the SOS data promising for genetic association studies. So far SOS results have demonstrated that variants of the β_3-receptor [71], Prader-Willi locus [72], mitochondrial DNA D-loop polymorphism [73], MC4 receptor [25], leptin [74], and UCP1 [75]are not important in "common" obesity.

Sequencing of the ghrelin gene revealed an Arg51Gln mutation, found only in obese subjects [76]. A Leu72Met mutation tended to associate with earlier onset of weight problems in obese carriers [76]. In a larger study, the Arg51Gln was associated with lower levels of circulating ghrelin, but not with obesity [77]. Met72 carrier status was more frequent among non-obese SOS subjects while obese Met72 carriers had lower prevalence of hypertension than obese noncarriers [77].

A novel T45G polymorphism in the adiponectin gene was equally common among obese and normal weight female SOS subjects [78]. Although silent (i.e., resulting in no amino acid change), it was associated with serum cholesterol and waist circumference in the obese group, possibly due to linkage disequilibrium with a nearby functional polymorphism. An IVS2 + G62T variant was equally prevalent in obese and control subjects, but obese GG homozygotes had higher blood glucose levels, and all six diabetics in this sample were in this group. Furthermore, this polymorphism was associated with BMI, blood pressure, and sagittal diameter [78].

Spouse correlation in BMI declined over time among 8,663 spouse pairs, suggesting that spouse similarity is the result of assortative mating, rather than the sharing of a common environment [26]. The deviation from random mating occurred most frequently within the extremes of the BMI distributions of men and women. Adult offspring of obesity concordant parents had the highest BMI and an obesity prevalence being 20-fold higher than among offspring of nonobese parents. No environmental interaction could be detected in this study, which thus suggests that the globally observed increase in obesity prevalence may in part have a genetic etiology via assortative mating [26].

Surgical Complications in SOS

Of the 2,010 subjects who underwent surgery (0.25%), 5 died postoperatively (within 90 days) [28]. As reported elsewhere for 1,164 patients [32], 151 individuals (13.0%) had 193 postoperative complications (bleeding 0.5%, thrombosis and embolism 0.8%, wound complications 1.8%, deep infections 2.1%, pulmonary complications 6.1%, and other complications 4.8%). In 26 patients (2.2%), the postoperative complications were serious enough to require reoperation. The frequency of reoperations and/or conversions (excluding operations due to postoperative complications) among 1,338 subjects followed for at least 10 years in November, 2005, was 31%, 21%, and 17% for those obtaining banding, vertical banded gastroplasty, and gastric bypass, respectively [28].

Effects of Bariatric Surgery on Overall Mortality

The effect of bariatric surgery on overall mortality in SOS was recently published [28]. Figure 9.4 depicts the cumulative overall mortality up to 16 years. Surgery was associated with an unadjusted hazard ratio (HR) of 0.76 relative to conventional treatment of obese controls (95% confidence interval [CI]: 0.59–0.99, $p = .04$). Over the follow-up period, 129 subjects (6.3%) died in the control group and 101 (5.0%) in the surgery group.

The adjusted HR for treatment (surgery relative to controls) was similar when based on matching information (HR = 0.73, $p = .02$) and on baseline information (HR = 0.71, $p = .01$), although the two models did not use exactly the same variables [28]. In both models, the strongest predictors were age and smoking, while the strongest univariate predictors were plasma triglycerides and blood glucose. By using multivariate models in an iterative way, it was possible to show that it took approximately 13 study years until the favorable effect of surgery became statistically significant.

There were 53 cardiovascular deaths in the control group and 43 in the surgery group [28]. The most common cardiovascular causes of death were MI, sudden death, and cerebrovascular damage. Cancer was the most common cause of noncardiovascular death. Lack of power made it impossible

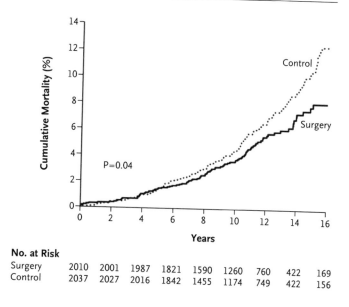

Figure 9.4 Unadjusted cumulative mortality over 16 years among surgically treated subjects and their obese controls in the SOS intervention study. The hazard ratio for subjects who underwent bariatric surgery, as compared with control subjects, was 0.76 (95% confidence interval [CI]: 0.59–0.99; $p =$ .04), with 129 deaths in the control group and 101 in the surgery group. The statistical calculations were performed on all observations, that is, up to 18 years of observation at the time of database analysis. (Reproduced from Sjöström et al. [28], with permission.)

No. at Risk									
Surgery	2010	2001	1987	1821	1590	1260	760	422	169
Control	2037	2027	2016	1842	1455	1174	749	422	156

to estimate the risk reduction for specific causes of death.

Although we have found larger improvements in risk factors, in left ventricular structure and function, and in HRQL, with increasing weight loss we failed to demonstrate an effect of weight loss on mortality. This may be related to lack of power but may also indicate that the favorable effect of bariatric surgery on mortality could be mediated by other mechanisms than weight loss. This possibility needs to be investigated.

Effects of Bariatric Surgery on the Incidence of MI, Stroke, and Cancer

Preliminary calculations indicate that the incidence rates of fatal plus nonfatal MI and cancer are more favorable in the SOS surgery group than in the obese control group obtaining nonsurgical treatment, while no significant differences between the two groups could be detected regarding incidence of stroke.

Conclusions

The prevalence of obesity is high and increasing and obesity is associated with a dramatically increased morbidity and mortality. Nonpharmacological conventional treatment at specialized

obesity units may achieve, on average, a 5% weight loss over 2–5 years of follow-up. This is not enough to keep the risk factors down long term. As illustrated by the conventionally treated obese control group of SOS, nonpharmacological obesity treatment at primary healthcare centers is not, on average, associated with any weight loss in the short or the long term. Unfortunately, most obese patients worldwide have no access to specialized obesity treatment.

Treatment with currently available anti-obesity drugs results, on average, in 7%–10% weight reduction over 2–4 years as compared to 4%–6% in the placebo groups [79–82]. This is encouraging, but more efficient drugs are clearly needed. Thus far, results of randomized drug trials with durations longer than 4 years have not been published.

Obese patients with prediabetes and type 2 diabetes deserve extra attention. It is more difficult to achieve conventional or pharmacologically induced weight loss in diabetic obese patients. Moreover, even when weight loss is achieved almost all patients relapse within a few years. Treatment with sulphonylureas or insulin causes weight increase. Thus, obesity not only causes diabetes but also is a complication of diabetes treatment. This vicious spiral must be broken.

Surgery is the only treatment of obesity resulting, on average, in more than 15% documented weight loss over 10 years. This treatment has dramatic positive effects on most but not on all cardiovascular risk factors over a 10-year period. It has excellent effects on established diabetes and prevents the development of new cases of diabetes. Large weight reductions achieved by surgery also improve left ventricular structure and function and slow down the atherosclerotic process as estimated from intima-media measurements and decreased prevalence of effort related calf pain. Quality of life is markedly improved. Finally, and most importantly, overall mortality is reduced by surgery, as recently demonstrated by the prospective controlled SOS study [28] and by four retrospective cohort studies [20–23]. Since all these positive effects are well documented, and since direct and indirect costs for bariatric surgery treatment over 6 years seem to be only moderately higher than for conventional obesity treatment, surgical treatment must become attainable for many more obese individuals.

Selected References

20. Adams TD, Gress RE, Smith SC, et al. Long-term mortality following gastric bypass surgery. New Engl J Med 2007;356.

24. Steinbrook R. Surgery for severe obesity. N Engl J Med 2004;350:1075–9.

28. Sjöström L, Narbro K, Sjöström CD, et al. Effects of bariatric surgery on mortality in Swedish Obese Subjects. New Engl J Med 2007;357:741–52.

63. Karlsson J, Taft C, Rydén A, et al. Ten year trends in health related quality of life after surgical and conventional treatment for severe obesity: the SOS intervention study. Int J Obes (Lond) 2007;31:1248–61.

68. Ågren G, Narbro K, Näslund I, et al. Long-term effects of weight loss on pharmaceutical costs in obese subjects. A report from the SOS intervention study. Int J Obes Relat Metab Disord 2002;26:184–92.

CHAPTER 10

Optimal Nutrition for Health and Longevity

Francesco P. Mancini[1] & Mario Mancini[2]
[1] University of Sannio, Benevento, Italy
[2] Federico II University, Naples, Italy

Introduction

Health and well-being associated with longevity are major goals of modern societies that reflect shared values of universal access to good healthcare and social justice. Elderly people are proportionally increasing all over the world and those aged 60 years or older are predicted to reach 1.2 billion by 2025 [1]. Interestingly, those in the oldest age-group (≥ 80 years) are experiencing the largest demographic increase. However, more than extended lifespan, it is important to increase the number of healthy life-years.

Among major factors determining such a growth of life expectancy, there are better healthcare and improved nutrition [2]. Indeed, Asian and Mediterranean diets are recognized as the best dietary styles to preserve good health and promote longevity, and the mortality for cardiovascular disease (CVD) and cancer is largely lower in the Eastern and Mediterranean regions [3,4].

Healthy Dietary Patterns

The Mediterranean Diet

Ancel Keys for the first time in 1975 [5] indicated that the eating habit of people living in southern Italy, Greece, and along the Mediterranean coasts of France and Spain is very healthy and termed it "Mediterranean Diet" (MD). MD is characterized

Nutritional and Metabolic Bases of Cardiovascular Disease, 1st edition.
Edited by Mario Mancini, José M. Ordovas, Gabriele Riccardi,
Paolo Rubba and Pasquale Strazzullo. © 2011 Blackwell Publishing Ltd.

by a high intake of vegetables and a low intake of animal food, and by olive oil as the major source of fat. Actually, this diet consists of moderate-to-high amounts of nonrefined cereal, high intake of legumes, nuts, fruits, and vegetables, a relatively high fat consumption (>30% of total energy intake, but with a minimum amount of saturated fatty acids [6%–7%] and mostly [20%] from monounsaturated fatty acids) mainly based on olive oil, a moderate-to-high fish consumption, a low intake of red meat, a small-to-moderate consumption of dairy products, and a regular, but moderate consumption of red wine, generally during meals.

After the seminal epidemiological observation of Keys et al. [6] about the beneficial effects of MD, several intervention studies have indicated that MD reduced the cardiovascular risk due to an improvement of glucose metabolism and plasma lipid profile, a reduction of blood pressure and inflammatory markers, and a better endothelial function [7,8]. Interestingly, several studies indicated that fat reduction alone is not the best choice compared to fat shift from saturated to unsaturated and particularly monounsaturated fat, in association with large amounts of fibers and micronutrients from fruit and vegetables, such as vitamins and antioxidants. A beneficial effect of the MD on the cardiovascular risk was also found in secondary prevention trials. de Lorgeril et al. observed a 70% reduction of death or recurrent coronary heart disease (CHD) in survivors of acute CHD following an MD-like regimen compared to controls after 5 years [9]. In various epidemiological studies, MD has been associated with greater longevity and better quality of life [10].

When similar recommendations were strongly implemented since the 1970s in the United States, the United Kingdom, Australia, and other countries, the intake of polysaturated and monounsaturated fat almost doubled and CHD rates declined by approximately 50% [11]. Very recently, a meta-analysis comprising more than 1.5 million subjects demonstrated the protective effect of the MD against cancer, CVD, neurological disorders, and all-cause mortality [12].

The Asian Diet

Similar to the Mediterranean countries, several Asian countries, particularly those along the Pacific Coast, have healthy dietary habits. In fact, the traditional Asian diet included mostly vegetable food and very little animal food, preferably seafood, resulting in limited fat intake (mainly unsaturated) and very little amounts of refined sugars compensated by a relatively high intake of complex carbohydrates, mainly rice and rice products (cereals and grains add up to 53% of total grams of food intake), but also legumes, potatoes, and starchy tubers. Finally, Asians drink large amounts of black or green tea. The latter contains significant amounts of epigallocathechin-3-gallate, a polyphenol with chemopreventive activity that has been shown to inhibit angiogenesis and metastasis. Therefore, the traditional Asian diet, rich in fiber, vitamins, minerals, and antioxidants and poor in fat, protects against many chronic diseases and promotes longevity.

Relationship between Specific Nutrients and Risk of CVD

CVD, comprising CHD, stroke, and peripheral vascular disease, is the leading cause of death worldwide. Understanding the causal link between diet, blood lipids, atherosclerosis, and CVD has been a major breakthrough in medicine in the last 50 years [13] and originated from the famous Seven Countries Study coordinated by Ancel Keys [7,14,15]. In this study, a striking low rate of CVD was observed in Japan and the Mediterranean region compared to northern Europe and the United States and was

associated with a lower intake of saturated fat. The amount and content of dietary fat are key determinants of serum cholesterol level given a specific genetic background, and serum cholesterol level is the most important cardiovascular risk factor explaining nearly half of the occurrence of CHD risk at population level [16].

In addition to a high saturated fat diet, high sodium intake, alcohol abuse, lack of physical exercise, and obesity are risk factors for CVD by increasing blood pressure. Hypertension, a strong risk factor not only for CHD but also for stroke, is the most important cause of excess mortality in the world [17]. Many clinical trials have demonstrated the beneficial effects on heart and blood vessels of reducing the intake of total fat, saturated fat, cholesterol, and salt [18,19]. Among others, a recent study demonstrated that the decrease in serum cholesterol levels, blood pressure, and smoking prevalence explained 53% of the CHD mortality reduction in Finland between 1982 and 1997 [16].

Fats. Fat intake must be controlled for quantity and quality, thus preferring monosaturated and polyunsaturated fats compared to saturated fats, trans-fatty acids, and cholesterol. In fact, plasma total cholesterol and low-density lipoprotein (LDL)-cholesterol decrease when the intake of saturated fatty acids was <10% of the daily kcal, and dietary cholesterol was <300 mg/day; further improvements can be obtained by reducing saturated fats to <7% of total calories and cholesterol ingestion to <200 mg/day. Thus, the diet recommended by the American Heart Association contains <7% kcal from saturated fats, <1% kcal from trans-fatty acids, ≤ 20% from monounsaturated fatty acids, and ≤10% kcal from polyunsaturated fatty acids. In order to control also plasma triglycerides, it is important to avoid an excessive carbohydrate intake; therefore, the MD is preferable than a low-fat/high-carbohydrate diet. The recommended ratio between saturated, polyunsaturated, and monounsaturated fats justifies why vegetable oils, and olive oil in particular, should be preferred to butter, other animal fats, and hardened margarine. It is also important to notice that trans-fatty acids lower high-density lipoprotein (HDL)-cholesterol, thus unfavorably changing the ratio of LDL-to-HDL cholesterol and increase plasma levels of lipoprotein(a), small dense LDL, triglyceride, and endothelial dysfunction. It is widely accepted that trans-fat is the worst type of fat.

Olive oil. It is a basic component of MD and a potential determinant of longevity [20,21]. A major component of olive oil, monounsaturated fatty acid oleic acid (18:1, ω-9), is considered the most important contributor to the heart-protecting effect of olive oil. In fact, replacing saturated fat with monounsaturated fatty acids in the diet, lowers serum cholesterol level and LDL-cholesterol in particular, without decreasing HDL-cholesterol [22]. Monounsaturated fat also stimulates insulin sensitivity and lowers blood pressure [23,24]. Endothelial activation (surface expression of leukocyte adhesion molecules and release of macrophage–colony-stimulating factor) triggered by proinflammatory stimuli is inhibited by oleic acid. Olive oil also favorably modulates platelet function, thrombogenesis, and fibrinolysis. A diet with extra-virgin olive oil reduced platelet aggregation, von Willebrand factor, thromboxane B$_2$, and factor VII plasma levels, the expression of tissue factor in mononuclear cells and finally increased fibrinolytic activity due to reduced plasma concentration of plasminogen activator inhibitor type-1 [25]. In addition to fatty acids, extra-virgin olive oil contains an array of microconstituents that are present at varying concentrations depending on the cultivar, maturation state, environmental factors, and production process. Recent studies have suggested that part of the healthy effects of extra-virgin olive oil could be attributed to these minor components, in particular to polyphenols that are especially concentrated in extra-virgin olive oil and range between 100 and 1,000 mg/kg. The most studied olive polyphenols are oleuropein and its derivative hydroxytyrosol that have shown antiatherogenic, anti-inflammatory, and antithrombotic activities.

Nuts. Nuts contain high amounts of unsaturated fats and are low in saturated fats. In particular, walnuts are rich in α-linolenic acid and are also a good source of vegetable proteins and plant sterols. This composition is likely to explain the reduced risk of CHD associated with nut consumption. In fact, consumption of 20–30 g/day of unsalted nuts, without increase of caloric intake, provides cardiovascular protection.

Soy. Soy is largely consumed in the eastern continent under different forms: soy protein, flour, and oil. Soy contains the bioactive isoflavones, genistein, and daidzein and is regarded to decrease the cardiovascular risk due to a reduction of plasma total cholesterol, LDL-cholesterol and triglycerides [26]. However, evidence is not conclusive and the LDL-cholesterol–lowering effect can be small and more pronounced in hypercholesterolemic individuals. Therefore, soy foods are considered a good source of plant protein in substitution of proteins from animal foods that are also rich in saturated fatty acids [27].

Phytosterols. Phytosterols are plant sterols that structurally resemble cholesterol, with additional methyl or ethyl groups linked to C-24 of the alkylic side chain. Phytosterols and stanols (saturated plant sterols) competitively inhibit dietary and biliary cholesterol absorption in the intestine by displacing cholesterol from micelles. β-sitosterol (and its saturated derivative sitostanol), campesterol, and stigmasterol are the most abundant phytosterols. In this way, 2–3 g/day of phytosterols can reduce total cholesterol and LDL-cholesterol plasma levels in both normocholesterolemic and hypercholesterolemic individuals by as much as 10% or more (see Chapter 29).

Fibers. Dietary fibers are a heterogeneous group of compounds, mostly carbohydrates that are indigestible by human intestinal enzymes. Dietary fiber is classified as soluble or insoluble, the former having a greater plasma LDL-cholesterol and glucose-lowering potential. An intake of >25 g/day of dietary fiber (including at least 7–13 g of soluble fiber) is associated with a reduced risk of CVD [28]. Soluble fiber (β-glucan) increases the production of bile acid, thus favoring the fecal loss of cholesterol, induces higher level of LDL receptor on cellular membranes and, consequently, decreases plasma LDL cholesterol levels. Since high intake of dietary fiber is also associated with lower body mass index, blood pressure, plasma triglyceride and glucose levels, there are various mechanisms that can reduce CVD risk following fiber ingestion.

ω-3 fatty acids. Although the protective effect of dietary ω-3 fatty acids on CVD has been appreciated since the late 1970s [29], a small number of intervention trials indicated that supplementation with very long-chain ω-3 fatty acids eicosapentaenoic acid (EPA, 20:5 ω3) and docosahexaenoic acid (DHA, 22:6 ω-3) was associated with a lower rate of mortality and sudden death. Among the proposed mechanisms there are the anti-thrombotic, anti-arrhythmic, and anti-inflammatory activities, besides a blood pressure–lowering effect, also mediated by a vasodilating activity, an endothelial function improving effect, a hypotriglyceridemic effect, and an inhibitory effect on the progression of the atherosclerotic plaque. In contrast, there is not any important effect on fasting glycemia or glycosylated hemoglobin. The primary source of EPA and DHA in the human diet is fish. Most studies, including the Seven Countries Study, have found an inverse relationship between fish consumption and risk of death from sudden and non-sudden cardiac death. Moreover, there is evidence of a protective effect of higher habitual fish and ω-3 fatty acids intake versus ischemic stroke, but not hemorrhagic stroke. Furthermore, fish consumption as low as one to three times per month may reduce the incidence of ischemic stroke, according to a meta-analysis of cohort studies [30]. In conclusion, for primary prevention, at least two or more servings/week of fish of about 150–200 g each are recommended besides the addition of ALA-rich foods like walnuts and several vegetable oils. Alternatively, dietary supplementation with 3 g/day of ω-3 fatty acids may reduce the risk of CVD (see Chapter 21 and 48).

Folate and vitamin B6. Hyperhomocysteinemia has been suggested to be an independent risk factor for CVD [31]. Although supplementation with folate or B vitamins does reduce homocysteine plasma levels, most of the available data from randomized controlled trials do not find out a relationship between such a supplementation and a reduction of the cardiovascular risk. However, a folate- and vitamin B_6-rich dietary pattern, which includes a high intake of vegetables, fruit, olive oil, mushrooms, and nuts improved homocysteine metabolism and decreased the risk of CHD [32] (see Chapter 49).

Antioxidants. Dietary antioxidants are considered a major natural aid for the prevention of most chronic degenerative diseases including CVD and premature ageing. Due also to unrestrained advertisement, this is now a common belief in the general population. Although the biological plausibility is easily demonstrated, the matter is complex. In fact, a dietary antioxidant is a food compound that neutralizes free radicals or reactive oxygen and/or nitrogen species (ROS and RNS), thus preventing the damage to biological molecules and structures. ROS and RNS can react with DNA, lipids, and proteins and, consequently, impair their function. In the cardiovascular system, besides a direct damage to heart and vessels, an excess of oxidant species (oxidative stress) can modify the LDL particle both in its lipid moiety and in its protein component, apoB. Modified, oxidized LDL then become a powerful atherogenic particle, because it is avidly taken up in the subendothelial space by scavenger receptors on the macrophage surface without any negative feedback control. Therefore, it is plausible that, if excessive oxidation is inhibited, the atherogenic process and the incidence of CVD are reduced. Although antioxidant supplementation with ascorbic acid, α-tocopherol, and β-carotene in animal models inhibits atherosclerosis progression, supplementation trials in humans provided only little, but not conclusive, evidence about the advantage on cardiovascular risk [33]. Therefore, there is no clinical evidence to support vitamin/antioxidant supplementation to prevent chronic diseases. However, people of any age are recommended to consume a diet rich in fruit and vegetable also because of their richness in antioxidants and vitamins. Food polyphenols are generating new expectation. Although heterogeneous, polyphenols have common chemical characteristics that confer the antioxidant potential such as multiple phenolic rings with several conjugated double bonds. Among polyphenols, resveratrol has focused a great deal of interest and research for its potential protective activity against CVD and cancer and also because it is present at relatively high concentration in red wine, a typical component of the MD. Resveratrol has also been indicated as the molecule responsible of the so-called "French paradox," namely the relatively low incidence of CVD despite a quite high intake of saturated fats in the French population.

Dietary electrolytes. Elevated blood pressure may be another major source of damage to heart and vessels. There is convincing evidence that an appropriate diet can reduce hypertension in men. Once again, a high intake of fruit and vegetables, combined with a low intake of saturated fat has proved to be beneficial and, in fact, reduces blood pressure. However, the reduction of sodium intake is most important to control blood pressure and its beneficial effect cumulates with that of the high-fruit, high-vegetable, low-saturated fat diet. A comprehensive overview on diet and hypertension is provided in Chapter 35.

A schematic summary of dietary recommendations to preserve cardiovascular health is provided in Table 10.1.

Nutrition and Cancer

The observation of Doll and Peto that at least 35% of all cancers could be prevented by diet dates back to almost 30 years ago [34]. On the other hand, there is a close link between total dietary fat and several cancers like colon, breast, esophageal, endometrial, and kidney cancer, thus indicating that overweight and obesity are serious cancer-prone conditions. In addition, high intakes of red meat, especially if overcooked, smoked or salted, nitrated foods, and nitrous compounds increase the odd ratios of developing cancers (particularly gastric, colon, and breast cancer).

Cancer is initiated when a multiplicity of genetic and epigenetic abnormalities accumulates in a normal cell that, consequently, acquires several new capabilities like self-sustained, unlimited growth, growth-factor independence, resistance to apoptosis, and the ability of stimulating angiogenesis and tumor invasion, and metastatization.

Solid epidemiological evidence demonstrates that people consuming large amounts of fruit, vegetable, and whole grains are at lower risk of different forms of cancer. This protection derives from the numerous bioactive compounds that are present in these foods and in 1989 the U.S. National Academy of Sciences recommended consuming daily five or more servings of vegetables and fruits in order to lower the risk of both cancer and CVD [35].

Among the wide array of bioactive compounds contained in fruit and vegetables, those that are presently regarded as the most active in the prevention of chronic degenerative diseases can be collectively grouped as antioxidants (Figure 10.1).

However, it is becoming increasingly clear that these plant antioxidants have additional remarkable properties that contribute importantly to their biological effects: they can modulate several signal transduction pathways with a resulting negative effect on inflammation, cell proliferation and survival, thus inhibiting carcinogenesis. In fact, dietary antioxidants can promote survival of differentiated cells and apoptosis of damaged, transformed cells by influencing the activities of oncogenes, tumor suppressor genes, growth factors, and hormones. In addition, anti-angiogenic and anti-inflammatory activity has also been observed in neoplastic tissues.

Finally, a recent work demonstrated life extension in cancer-prone mice fed a diet supplemented with genetically modified tomatoes expressing high levels of the antioxidant anthocyanins, thus highlighting new avenues related to the correct application of modern biotechnologies to improve food quality besides quantity [36].

It is worth recalling the cancer-protective role of some dietary hormone-like polyphenols that structurally resemble estrogens (phytoestrogens) and can therefore activate or inhibit estrogen receptors according to their potency relative to that of naturally occurring hormones. For instance, resveratrol, the antioxidant polyphenol of grapes and red wine, is classified as phytoestrogen, because it structurally resembles the synthetic estrogen diethylstilbestrol, but the most appreciated phytoestrogens derive from soybean products and therefore are most abundant in the Asian diets. Soybeans contain high amounts of glycosides of the isoflavones daidzein, genistein, and glycitein. A protective role of phytoestrogens has been postulated in the prevention of several types of cancer, especially breast, prostate, and colorectal cancer. Indeed Asians have a lower incidence of prostate and breast cancer (25- and 10-fold lower, respectively) than western people, but this advantage dramatically decreases when Asians move to the western countries [37]. However, besides soybeans, dietary chemoprevention

Table 10.1 Dietary advises for the prevention of cardiovascular disease.[1]

To be preferred		
Food type (frequency or other notes)	Nutrient	Advantages
Whole grains (daily)	Complex, unrefined carbohydrates, B vitamins, fibers	Lower glycemic index, better intestinal function
Legumes	Protein, vitamins, minerals, fibers	Low-fat protein source, stimulate intestinal function
Soy	Protein, phytosterols	Low-fat protein source, lowers LDL-cholesterol and triglycerides[2]
Fruit and vegetables (5 times/day)	Vitamins, minerals, fibers, phytosterols, antioxidants	Low caloric density, low fat, lower LDL oxidation, better intestinal function
Fish (150–200 g, 2 times/wk)	Protein, ω-3 fatty acids (EPA, DHA)	Low-saturated fat protein source, lowers triglycerides, antithrombotic, anti-inflammatory
White meat (chicken, turkey, etc., 150 g, 2 times/wk)	Protein, low-fat	Low-fat protein source
Nuts[3] (unsalted)	ω-3 fatty acid (ALA)	Anti-thrombotic, anti-inflammatory
Extra-virgin olive oil[3] (daily for cooking and dressing)	Monounsaturated fatty acids; antioxidant polyphenols	Increases HDL/LDL cholesterol ratio, insulin sensitivity, plaque stability; decreases blood pressure, endothelial activation, platelet aggregation, LDL oxidation
Other vegetable oils[3]	Polyunsaturated fatty acids	Lower LDL-cholesterol
Skim/low-fat milk, yogurt and other low fat dairy products	Calcium and vitamins (especially vitamin D and vitamin A)	Increase bone mass, relatively low-fat protein source
To be limited		
Food type (frequency or other notes)	Nutrient	Disadvantages
Red meat (150 g, once a week)	Saturated fatty acids	Increases LDL-cholesterol
Butter and other high fat dairy product	Saturated fatty acids	Increase LDL-cholesterol, high energy density
Hard margarine	Trans fatty acids	Increases LDL-cholesterol, high energy density
Processed meat (e.g., salami, sausages; consume sparingly)	Saturated fatty acids, high-sodium content	Increases LDL-cholesterol, high-fat protein source, raise blood pressure
Sweets and candies (consume sparingly)	Simple sugars	High energy density, increase adiposity and plasma triglycerides
Salty foods	NaCl	Increase blood pressure

[1] Eating well with an optimal diet must be paralleled by regular, moderate physical exercise at any age.
[2] Evidence not conclusive, LDL-C lowering more pronounced in hypercholesterolemic individuals.
[3] Consume frequently, but in controlled amounts, because of high-energy density.
LDL: low-density lipoprotein; HDL: high-density lipoprotein; EPA: eicosapentaenoic acid; DHA: docosahexanoic acid; ALA: α-linolenic acid.

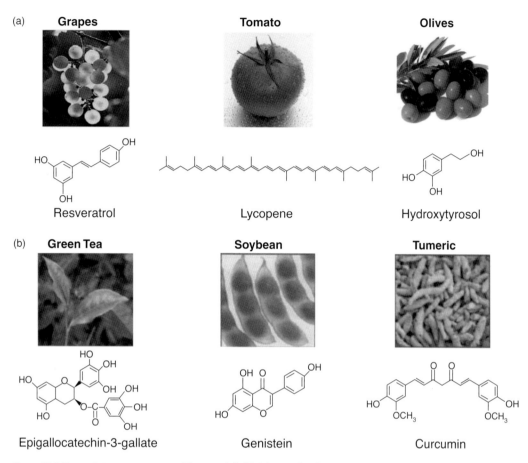

Figure 10.1 Some dietary components with potentially high impact for disease prevention and their major bioactive chemical compounds. (a) Food items mostly common in the MD. (b) Food items mostly common in the Asian diet.

has been associated with elevated intake of food of plant origin: vegetables, fruit, legumes, whole grains, nuts, seeds, and tea [38]. Apart from tea, these food items are hallmarks of the MD, together with an elevated intake of monounsaturated fat from olive oil, moderate consumption of fish, dairy products, and red wine and a low intake of red meat. In comparison with a western-type diet, rich in saturated fat, MD provides a remarkable protection from various cancers including colorectal (−25% incidence), breast (−15% incidence), prostate, pancreas, and endometrial cancer (−10% incidence) [39]. Also pharynx, esophagus, and larynx are less prone to develop cancer in people adopting the MD [40]. Among the chemical components that are present in a plant food-rich diet, and besides the already mentioned polyphenolic

antioxidants, β-carotene, vitamin C, D, and E, calcium, and riboflavin are indicated as the most active compounds in the prevention of cancer, especially of the digestive tract. Also a diminished folate status has been associated with an increased risk of colorectal cancer. Dietary fiber, including the indigestible carbohydrates from fruit, vegetables, and whole grains, has also a remarkable anticancer potential. A high intake of fiber has been shown to protect from colorectal cancer, but not all data are consistent [40]. Among proposed mechanisms to explain this effect, there are the reduced transit time of feces, which lowers the contact time between carcinogens and the colon epithelium, and the production of the short-chain fatty acid, butyric acid, which has been shown to inhibit mitosis and promote apoptosis of enterocytes [41].

Table 10.2   Association of particular food components, dietary styles or nutritional statuses and increased or decreased risk of several types of cancer.

Food compound, dietary style, or nutritional status	Increased cancer risk	Decreased cancer risk
Overweight or obesity	Esophagus, stomach, colon, rectum, liver, kidney, thyroid, myeloma, leukemia, non-Hodgkin's lymphoma in both sexes; pancreas, breast (postmenopausal), endometrium, gallbladder in women; prostate, melanoma in men	
High intake of total dietary fat	Esophagus, colon, breast, prostate, endometrium, kidney	
High intake of red meat (especially if overcooked, smoked, or salted)	Stomach, colon, breast	
High intake of nitrite/nitrate containing foods	Esophagus, stomach, colon, nasal cavity, brain, leukemia	
Alcohol	Liver, breast	
β-carotene, vitamin A, C, E, calcium, riboflavin (i.e., fruit and vegetables)		Esophagus, stomach, colon, rectum, larynx, and lung
High folate status		Colon, rectum
High intake of dietary fiber		Colon, rectum
High intake of phytoestrogen		Breast*, prostate*, ovary*, endometrium*
Fish		Breast*, prostate*, ovary*, endometrium*
Mediterranean Diet		Pharynx, esophagus, stomach colon, rectum, pancreas, larynx, breast, prostate, endometrium, kidney
Asian Diet		Breast, prostate, ovary, endometrium

*Weak association or controversial issue.

Several studies suggest that the interaction between diet and genomic background play a central role in controlling health. For example, only those with a less active variant of the peroxisome proliferator-activated receptor-γ (PPARγ) develop colorectal cancer with lower frequency when ingesting high amounts of lutein, low amounts of refined grain or when assigned a high prudent score diet [42].

A synthetic view of all the associations reported in this chapter is reported in Table 10.2.

Although in this chapter the importance of the quality of the diet in CVD and cancer prevention has been highlighted, it is necessary to remark that also the quantity of the diet affects the odds of developing cancer: eating more than needed causes overweight and obesity, which are reaching epidemic proportion in the developed countries and increase the risk of cancer (Table 10.2). Obesity and overweight is a complex matter affecting about two-thirds of the population in the United States and Europe. The understanding of the neurohormonal control of food intake is becoming better elucidated, and it is appreciated that high-calorie, low-nutrient, processed food is much easier to consume than healthier alternatives. However, fighting the obesity epidemic requires advances in research coupled with public education programs, but, more importantly, the action of policymakers to make possible for a larger proportion of the population to eat healthy food and to practice physical activity.

Calorie Restriction and Longevity

Longevity is the capacity of live long, beyond the average life expectancy and close to the maximum lifespan. Life expectancy is the age reached by 50% of the population and has increased dramatically in the last 100 years, rising from about 45 years at the beginning of the twentieth century to about 80 years for women and 75 years for men at the beginning of the twenty-first century [43]. Japan has the longest life expectancy in the world: 85.6 yrs for women and 78.6 for men in 2004. Currently, about 600 million persons around the world are 60 years or older, and it has been estimated that this number will double in the next 2 decades [1]. Maximum lifespan is the average lifespan of the longest-lived decile of a population sample. What is the optimal nutrition to extend lifespan? Of course, optimal nutrition is also a quantitative besides a qualitative concept. To keep a lean body, nutrition should not provide more calories than what is consumed, thus leading to an energy balance equal to zero. Therefore, if physical activity is to be kept to the optimal minimum necessary level, then also calorie intake should be restricted to favor longevity. This is the basis of the striking observation that calorie restriction (CR) without malnutrition prolongs lifespan in many species from yeasts to flies, worms, fish, and rodents [44]. Indeed, since the first evidence provided many decades ago [45], several studies have demonstrated that life-long reduction of energy intake prolongs the life of laboratory rats by about 25% [46]. Moreover, accumulating data show the brain as the common ground to sense CR and promote longevity in metazoans [47]. The remarkable effect of CR on lifespan extension in mammals is supported by several findings, both in rodents and in nonhuman primates that have been subjected to limited food supply: lower body and fat mass, lower body temperature and basal metabolic rate, and amelioration of the cardiovascular risk profile. The latter refers to better indices of lipid and glucose metabolism, including a reduced insulin resistance and plasma concentration. Furthermore, CR decreases inflammatory response,

glycation of proteins, oxidative stress, and preserves the immune function. Even more strikingly, it has been observed in animal models that CR prevents or retards the progression and onset of several chronic, age-related diseases, including CVD, a number of different cancers, neurodegenerative disorders and diabetes. On these premises, it should not be at surprise that short-term CR protects from coronary disease and stroke also in humans and that there is some epidemiological data showing association between decreased calorie intake from one side and lower incidence of CVD, cancer, and prolonged survival from the other side [46]. Indeed, data from intentional or accidental intervention human studies on calorie restriction are available [46], and perhaps the first one was reported by Keys et al., back in 1950 [48]. However, these are not lifelong studies, but short-term trials lasting from a few months to a few years. In contrast, a natural trial is provided by the people from the Japanese island of Okinawa that have been subjected to calorie restriction and exhibit long and healthy lives with low death rates from heart disease, cerebrovascular disease and cancer [49]. With aging DNA damage and mutations accumulate and damaged DNA favors the onset and progression of chronic degenerative diseases, particularly cancer. Interestingly, CR increases genomic stability, particularly by enhancing repair of oxidatively damaged DNA, and this may protect against chronic diseases and favor longevity [50]. As far as neurodegeneration and neuronal loss, it has been proposed that CR, alone or in association with physical exercise, can preserve brain function by enhancing adult neurogenesis [51]. Interestingly, CR and intermittent fasting can prolong the health-span of the nervous system by impinging upon fundamental metabolic and cellular signaling pathways that regulate lifespan [52].

Is CR expected to be always beneficial in humans? When CR is severe in non-obese individuals and is associated with physical inactivity, decreased muscle mass and work capacity, associated with weakness and reduced bone mineral density, were observed. It is not known whether CR extends maximum lifespan in lean humans and excessive CR causes malnutrition and has adverse clinical effects in persons with minimal body fat [46].

Can we predict how longer human beings can live if they undergo a 20% CR since the childhood?

It has been estimated that, based on the reduction of the risk factors for CVD, type 2 diabetes, and cancer, an extra 3–13 years of life could be gained, which is still highly desirable but is significantly less than could have been predicted from the experimental results obtained in rodents, and certainly smaller than achieved by medical and public health interventions which have extended life by about 30 years in developed countries in the twentieth century by reducing deaths from infections, accidents and CVD [53].

Because maintaining long-term CR is difficult in modern society, there is a strong interest in the search and development of chemical compounds that could mimic the beneficial physiological, metabolic, and hormonal effects of calorie restriction without having to reduce food intake. These chemicals are called CR mimetics, and resveratrol might be one of these because it directly stimulates the sirtuin/Sir2 family of NAD(+)-dependent deacetylases known to mediate the effects of CR (see Chapter 51).

Therefore, eating less and eating well increase the odds of live longer and healtier.

Conclusions

The goal of improving health and longevity, particularly through adoption of optimal nutrition, requires a concerted action by many different sectors of the society. Agricultural and food public policies, regulating manufacturing, marketing, and trading of foods, profoundly influence the diet of a population. To promote health and longevity people must reduce the intake of high-fat meat and dairy products, while preferring vegetable oils, vegetables, fruit, and fiber-rich cereals in combination with regular physical exercise. This requires public education campaigns and industrial policies to make healthy food easily available, adequately marketed and labeled, and reasonably priced. However, we should recall that individuals are not identical due to genomic variations. Although only a small dec-

imal fraction of the human genome differs among individuals, that minimal variation is sufficient to confer difference not only in the susceptibility to almost every disease, but also in any complex trait, from body height or weight to lifespan. Differences of genetic background interact in a combinatorial fashion with differences of the environmental factors, thus originating the full expression of the complexity of life. In fact, genetic heritage influences the way each individual responds to environmental stimuli, including food. In the near future it will be possible to pinpoint single individuals or subgroups of population that would fit a particular variant of a dietary pattern or that would perfectly tolerate saturated fat or energy dense foods. Although this will be a tremendous advantage at the individual level, it is likely that, at the population level, it will still be correct to recommend a dietary style that has already emerged as optimal for health and longevity and that reflects the evolutionary modification of human genome in response to the environmental conditioning through millions of years. Aging is an unavoidable consequence of life, but healthy aging is a major possible target for biomedical research and healthcare systems.

Selected References

5. Keys A, Keys M. How to eat well and stay well, the Mediterranean way. Garden City: Doubleday; 1975.

12. Sofi F, Cesari F, Abbate R, et al. Adherence to Mediterranean diet and health status: meta-analysis. BMJ 2008 Sep 11; 337:a1344.

15. Mancini M, Stamler J. Diet for preventing cardiovascular diseases: light from Ancel Keys, Distinguished Centenarian Scientist. Nutr Metab Cardiovasc Dis 2004;14: 52–57.

40. Rubba P, Mancini FP, Gentile M, et al. The Mediterranean diet in Italy: an update. World Rev Nutr Diet 2007;85–113.

52. Martin B, Mattson MP, Maudsley S. Caloric restriction and intermittent fasting: two potential diets for successful brain aging. Ageing Res Rev 2006;5:332–353.

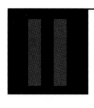

SECTION II
Metabolic Syndrome and Diabetes

CHAPTER 11

Definition and Diagnostic Criteria for Metabolic Syndrome

Wm. James Howard[1,2], Giovanni de Simone[3,4], & Barbara V. Howard[5,6]

[1]Washington Hospital Center, Washington, DC, USA
[2]George Washington University, Washington, DC, USA
[3]Federico II University, Naples, Italy
[4]Weill Medical College of Cornell University, New York, NY, USA
[5]MedStar Health Research Institute, Hyattsville, MD, USA
[6]Professor of Medicine, Georgetown University, Washington, DC, USA

Introduction

A syndrome that is characterized by a cluster of risk factors for coronary heart disease (CHD) has been recognized for almost 90 years. In 1923, Kylin described a group of patients with hypertension, hyperglycemia, and gout [1]. In 1947, Vague suggested upper body obesity as a risk factor for CHD [2], and in 1955, Adelsberg described five cases of patients with mild diabetes, hyperlipidemia, and severe vascular damage [3]. Additional description of this syndrome was provided by Avogaro et al., in 1967, in a publication outlining six cases of patients with maturity onset diabetes, hyperlipidemia, and obesity [4]. In 1988, Reaven recognized insulin resistance (IR) as an additional component of these concordant risk factors and labeled the cluster of factors (dyslipidemia, hypertension, and hyperglycemia) that is frequently observed in individuals who develop diabetes and cardiovascular disease (CVD) *Syndrome X* [5]. Since that time, the concept of a constellation of cardiometabolic risk factors has received much attention [6]. Over time, these factors have been further studied and refined and are now often referred to as IR syndrome or metabolic syndrome (MetS)

[7]. Although the underlying cause of MetS is unclear, it is thought to result from obesity and IR, which often are the result of an unhealthy lifestyle [6].

IR is characterized by a diminished response to the biological effect of insulin and is associated with obesity with a predominantly abdominal fat distribution, elevated blood pressure and triglyceride levels, low high-density lipoprotein–cholesterol (HDL-C), an increased number of small low-density lipoprotein–cholesterol (LDL-C) particles, and elevations in inflammatory cytokines [8]. IR is a known predictor of type 2 diabetes in many populations [9]. The prevalence of MetS is increasing worldwide, and MetS is a strong predictor of diabetes [10–12]. Hyperglycemia, diabetes, and other aspects of MetS, such as abdominal obesity, increased concentrations of plasma insulin, and atherogenic dyslipidemia (consisting of low concentrations of HDL-C, increased triglycerides, and an increased number of small LDL-C particles), have all been significantly and independently related to increased risk of CVD [13]. CVD is the major cause of death in all developed and in many emerging countries. Thus, in an effort to prevent diabetes and CHD, it is important to identify MetS and treat the individual risk factors for this syndrome.

Nutritional and Metabolic Bases of Cardiovascular Disease, 1st edition.
Edited by Mario Mancini, José M. Ordovas, Gabriele Riccardi,
Paolo Rubba and Pasquale Strazzullo. © 2011 Blackwell Publishing Ltd.

Table 11.1 Definitions of MetS

Factor	WHO (main criterion plus two factors)	ATP III (any combination of three factors)	IDF (main criterion + 2 factors)
Body mass index	>30 kg/m^2 or waist/	—	———
Abdominal obesity	hip > 0.9/0.85 (M/W)	> 102/88 cm waist (M/W)	> 94/80 cm (M/W)†
Triglycerides	≥ 150 mg/L	≥150 mg/dl	≥ 150 mg/dL
HDL-cholesterol	< 35/39 mg/L (M/W)	<40/50 mg/dl (M/W)	< 40/50 mg/dL (M/W)
Blood pressure	Hypertension	≥130/≥ 85 mm Hg	Hypertension or > 130/85 mmHg
HOMA	> 4.3 or	—	—
Type 2 diabetes	present or	—	present or
Fasting glucose	≥110 mg/dl	≥110 mg/dl	> 100 mg/dl
Fasting insulin	—	—	—
Urinary albumin excretion	≥ 20 μg/min or ≥30 mg/g creatinine	—	—

WHO: World Health Organization; ATP III: Adult Treatment Panel III; IDF: International Diabetes Federation.
Reproduced from de Simone G et al. Diabetes Care 2007;7:1851–6, with permission.

Definition of MetS

Since the syndrome was first postulated, different names have been proposed, and multiple definitions have been promoted by various medical organizations. All of these definitions share a number of common factors, including the presence of hypertension, atherogenic dyslipidemia, and obesity, but each differs slightly. The World Health Organization (WHO) [14] and the European Group for the Study of Insulin Resistance (EGIR) [15] definitions both emphasize the requirement for IR. The International Diabetes Federation (IDF) definition [16,17] requires the presence of central obesity as measured by an increased waist circumference, and the ATP III definition [18] is based on the presence of at least three of the risk factors outlined above [11,19]. The ATP III attempted to make the MetS definition more clinically useful by choosing diagnostic criteria of proven cardiac risk factors that can be determined during a routine office examination (Table 11.1) [19]. The criteria for waist circumference in both the IDF and the most recent update of the ATP III criteria by the American Heart Association and the National Heart, Lung, and Blood Institute of the U.S. National Institutes of Health [20] recognize ethnic differences, with the threshold for an increased waist circumference being lower for certain Asian and other ethnic populations. The IDF [16] and ATP III [20] definitions are now virtually identical and represent the most widely used criteria for defining MetS (Table 11.1) [21].

Metabolic Syndrome Components

Obesity

With the exception of individuals from southeast Asia, the majority of individuals with MetS are overweight or obese. It has been recognized that there is a significant correlation between abdominal obesity and MetS components [21]. For this reason, anthropometric measurements that emphasize this type of fat distribution, such as waist circumference, are more predictive of diabetes and CHD than nonspecific measures of obesity, such as body mass index (BMI) [22].

Atherogenic dyslipidemia

A typical pattern of atherogenic lipid disturbance is seen in patients with MetS and diabetes, namely elevated triglycerides, decreased HDL-C, and an increased number of small, dense LDL-C particles [18,20]. One of the earliest of these lipid abnormalities is the increase in triglycerides. Borderline triglyceride elevations (150–199 mg/dl) are primarily markers for other components of MetS: small LDL-C particles, low HDL-C, central obesity, and hyperglycemia. High triglycerides (200–499 mg/dl) are predictive of the presence of atherogenic remnant lipoproteins. Very high triglycerides (>500) may represent the presence of atherogenic remnants as well as other atherogenic and nonatherogenic lipoprotein abnormalities [20,21]. Individuals with very high triglycerides are at risk for pancreatitis, particularly when the triglyceride level exceeds 1,000 mg/dl [18]. An additional atherogenic lipid abnormality results from the reduction in HDL-C as triglycerides increase.

HDL-C has long been recognized as an "anti-atherosclerotic" lipoprotein. Framingham and other epidemiologic studies have demonstrated an increased risk for CHD as HDL-C decreases [18]. The ATP III [18] designated an HDL-C below 40 mg/dl as a risk factor for CHD in both sexes and defined an HDL-C below 50 mg/dl in women and below 40 mg/dl in men as a component of atherogenic dyslipidemia, one of the diagnostic criteria for MetS. Although part of the decreased HDL-C observed in individuals with MetS is secondary to the increase in triglycerides, HDL-C often remains low even after triglycerides are reduced [21].

LDL-C has been demonstrated in observational and interventional trials to be the primary contributor to the formation of atherosclerotic plaque [18]. Although the LDL-C concentration in MetS is often not significantly increased, the presence of an increased number of small, dense LDL-C particles as indicated by an increase in the Apo B100 concentration and/or increased LDL-C particle number as measured by nuclear magnetic resonance (NMR) lipid analysis represents a significant component of the atherogenic dyslipidemia of MetS. The primary goal of therapy in MetS is reduction of the LDL-C concentration [20].

Non-HDL-C (total cholesterol minus HDL-C) is the secondary goal of therapy for patients with MetS and type 2 diabetes [18]. Non-HDL-C represents the sum of all the Apo B containing atherogenic lipoproteins (LDL-C + IDL-C, + VLDL-C + Lp[a]). A continued elevation in non-HDL-C after LDL-C has been reduced to target has been demonstrated in interventional trials [18] to represent the continued presence of atherogenic triglyceride-rich lipoproteins.

Hypertension

Hypertension has long been recognized as a reversible risk factor for CHD as well as other forms of CVD. The ATP III has recognized the most recent report of the Joint National Council on the Detection and Treatment of Hypertension (JNC 7) as the definitive set of recommendations on the topic of hypertension.

Elevated Fasting Insulin

MetS has generally been assumed to be a reflection of IR, because many of the components of MetS—dyslipidemia, abdominal obesity, and impaired fasting glucose (IFG)—are observed in individuals with IR. This assumption has been reinforced by factor analyses using several datasets [23]. A single underlying factor that can be generalized across sex and ethnicity was found using National Health and Nutrition Examination Survey (NHANES) data [23]. However, full concordance was not found; for example, elevated blood pressure is not always associated with IR and has multiple other etiologies. Similarly, elevated triglycerides or low HDL-C may be due to genetic dyslipidemias. Analyses show that many patients with IR do not have MetS [24]. Because of the close association, some of the criteria for MetS include measures of fasting insulin. Measurement of insulin can be problematic, however, because these measures are expensive in the clinical setting and are not rigorously standardized. There are no universally accepted criteria for elevated insulin levels.

Elevated Glucose

Glucose concentration is included in all major definitions of MetS. Criteria are based on the definition of IFG, originally 110 mg/dl (6.1 mmol/L) but more recently 100 mg/dl (5.6 mmol/L) [20]. A progressive increase in glycemia accompanies increasing IR. IFG is an established predictor of diabetes, and a number of analyses have shown that individuals with IFG begin to show increased risk for CVD. The lowering of the threshold for IFG has resulted in increasing numbers of persons being diagnosed with IFG and MetS; presumably this will result in earlier recognition and preventive strategies in individuals at risk for diabetes and CVD. Some debate has centered on whether MetS should be assessed in individuals with diabetes. The WHO criteria specify that diabetes can be a criterion. In the ATP III definition, on the other hand, individuals with diabetes are already classified as having a CVD risk equivalent for the purposes of determining therapeutic strategies. Therefore, screening for MetS has been proposed as a tool for identifying individuals who do not yet have diabetes but are at elevated risk for diabetes.

Prothrombotic State

One of the unique features of the ATP III definition of MetS is the inclusion of a hypercoagulable state, characterized by increases in certain procoagulant factors which contribute to the risk of CHD and CVD. According to the ATP III definition, fibrinogen, factor VII, and plasminogen activator inhibitor 1 are increased in MetS and are accompanied by increased platelet aggregation and endothelial dysfunction, all of which promote thrombosis [18].

Proinflammatory State

With the onset of MetS, components of the adipose tissue secrete circulating cytokines and acute phase reactants, such as interleukin-6 (IL-6) and C-reactive protein. Some speculate that these inflammatory markers play a role in the progression of MetS to type 2 diabetes. One additional consequence of these circulating inflammatory markers is that their presence in individuals with abdominal obesity is not indicative of a more malignant form of CHD, as is the case in lean individuals without diabetes.

Diagnosis of MetS and its Implications

The Strong Heart Study: A Population with High Prevalences of IR and Diabetes

IR and diabetes are highly prevalent in American Indians, and heart disease has increased rapidly in recent decades to become the leading cause of death in most American Indian populations [29]. The Strong Heart Study (SHS) [25], a longitudinal study of CVD in American Indians, has collected data on CHD, diabetes, and potential risk factors since 1989 [25–27]. The cohort consists of a population-based sample of 4,549 men and women 45–74 years of age at baseline from 13 communities in Arizona, southwestern Oklahoma, and South and North Dakota. SHS methods have been described previously [25–28]. Because this population shows the same trends of increasing prevalence of obesity and diabetes observed worldwide, the SHS data provide an excellent opportunity to examine risk factors for diabetes and CVD. Data on MetS and its relation to diabetes and CVD in this population may, thus, provide insight into the utility of MetS diagnosis in disease prevention.

Although MetS prevalence differs according to the definition of MetS used (Table 11.2), MetS in American Indians [16] is high by any criteria, ranging from 44% to 59% (men) and 53% to 73% (women) in those ages 45–74 years [29]. The WHO definition yields similar prevalence rates among American Indian men and women, because it is not

Table 11.2   Prevalence of MetS in AI, per WHO, ATP III, and IDF definitions of MetS: blood pressure and urinary albumin/creatinine ratio.

Prevalence of metabolic syndrome			Systolic blood pressure (mm Hg)		Diastolic blood pressure (mm Hg)		Log$_{10}$ of urinary albumin/creatinine ratio	
	Men (%)	Women (%)	No MetS	MetS	No MetS	MetS	No MetS	MetS
WHO	48	53	122 ± 16	133 ± 20	75 ± 9	79 ± 10	0.80 ± 0.59	1.57 ± 0.98
ATPIII	44	63	121 ± 17	132 ± 20	75 ± 9	78 ± 10	0.91 ± 0.73	1.42 ± 0.96
IDF	59	73	120 ± 16	131 ± 19	74 ± 9	78 ± 10	0.92 ± 0.75	1.33 ± 0.93

AI: American Indian; WHO: World Health Organization; ATP III: Adult Treatment Panel III; IDF: International Diabetes Federation; MetS: metabolic syndrome.
Reproduced from de Simone G et al. Diabetes Care 2007;7:1851–6, with permission.

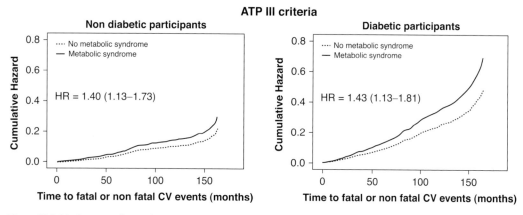

Figure 11.1 MetS as a predictor of CVD, per ATP criteria (Strong Heart Study population). (Reproduced from Russell M, de Simone G, Resnick HE, Howard BV. J CardioMetabolic Syndrome 2007;4:283–7, with permission.)

based on sex-specific values for the main criterion, whereas the ATP III and IDF definitions yield higher prevalence rates in women, because a frequently occurring component (and the main criterion in the IDF definition) is sex specific, with substantially lower cutoff points for women (Table 11.2).

The prevalence rates for the components of MetS, such as hypertension and albuminuria, also vary by the definition of MetS used. MetS prevalence among American Indians is much higher than among the general U.S. population as sampled in the NHANES [30,31]. In the third NHANES cohort (8,608 participants older than 20 years), the age-adjusted MetS prevalence rate was 23.9% per the ATP III definition and 25.1% per the WHO definition [29].

MetS as a Predictor of Diabetes

Diabetes is a major public health concern among American Indians. Fifteen percent of American Indians have diabetes, compared with 8.1% of U.S. non-Hispanic whites [14]. MetS is a strong predictor of type 2 diabetes in American Indians. In the SHS [8], 35% of the nondiabetic participants had MetS at baseline [29]. After nearly 8 years, 25% of those with MetS at baseline had developed type 2 diabetes with a relative risk (RR) for CVD of about 2. The RR associated with MetS in this population, however, is lower than that seen in the San Antonio Heart Study (RR = 6) [32] and in the fourth Framingham cohort (RR = 7) [11]. Additionally, in American Indians, there is a clear link between incident arterial hypertension and development of

diabetes, as well as prevalence and worsening of central fat distribution, which suggests that early interventions to reduce metabolic risk factors may help prevent both hypertension and diabetes [19].

MetS as a predictor of CVD

In an early analysis of the SHS cohort, at 4.2 years of follow-up, no significant association was found between MetS and incidence of CHD [8]. After more than 8 years of follow-up, significantly increased risk for fatal and nonfatal cardiovascular events (e.g., CHD, stroke, and congestive heart failure) and cardiovascular mortality were observed in nondiabetic and diabetic participants with MetS [31]. In the later analysis, participants without diabetes but with MetS per ATP III criteria had a 40% increased cardiovascular risk (Figure 11.1), similar to participants with diabetes and MetS. Using WHO criteria for MetS slightly reduced the hazard ratio (HR) observed in nondiabetic participants but amplified the HR of participants with both diabetes and MetS. IDF criteria yielded lower HRs, which were not statistically significant in nondiabetic participants [29].

Conclusion

The definition of MetS has progressed from early descriptions of an association of obesity, diabetes, and hyperlipidemia to a meaningful medical syndrome recognizing the clustering of concordant metabolic risk factors for diabetes and CHD. Since

Reaven [5] first recognized IR to be an essential component of this syndrome, which he called Syndrome X, MetS has been described by various names, including the deadly quartet and IR syndrome, and has been defined by various criteria. The ATP III attempted to make the diagnosis of MetS an office procedure by using diagnostic criteria easily obtained in a health care provider's office. The ATP III also focused on the role of lifestyle in the development of MetS and recommended that therapeutic life change be the initial approach to therapy. Some medical experts have questioned the utility of this diagnosis [33]. Others have compared the various definitions for the MetS, examining the frequency with which each definition identifies MetS in various populations. A significant amount of study has been directed at determining the value of MetS in predicting the development of type 2 diabetes and/or CHD. Questions have been raised as to whether the diagnosis of MetS offers an advantage in predicting the development of CHD over an evaluation of the individual risk factors comprising this syndrome. With the reconciliation of the definitions of MetS by the ATP III and IDF, the diagnosis of MetS has become truly useful. It is well recognized that MetS predicts type 2 diabetes and precedes the development of this form of diabetes in > 85% of individuals. A number of studies have demonstrated that MetS is a reliable predictor of CHD, and as a syndrome exceeds the predictive value of its individual risk factors. However, one of the most useful contributions offered to the clinician by the diagnosis of MetS is the ability to immediately recognize an individual who is at risk for developing type 2 diabetes and CHD by simply observing that the individual has central obesity. Although the presence of central obesity is no longer an absolute requirement for MetS and may not be present in certain ethnic groups, the increased frequency of this form of adiposity in most populations with MetS allows the clinician to immediately recognize a patient who needs further evaluation. As some have observed, if the "patient's belly enters the examining room before the patient," the clinician should screen for the risk factors comprising MetS and for signs of atherosclerotic CVD. Therapeutic life changes should be immediately instituted and pharmacologic management of critical

risk factors should be considered. With the significant increase in the prevalence of MetS in Western populations, its recognition as a predictor of diabetes and CHD has made MetS a public health issue and increased resources have been directed toward its prevention. In addition, new pharmacologic agents are being developed to treat MetS in its entirety and to prevent the obesity which comprises the initial phase of MetS. It is our hope that the information in this chapter and subsequent chapters of this book will be of benefit to clinicians in helping patients deal with this important medical problem.

Acknowledgments

Gratitude is expressed to the tribal leadership and members, without whose support this study would not have been possible. We thank the Indian Health Service hospitals and clinics at each center, the directors, and their staffs. We gratefully acknowledge Rachel Schaperow, MedStar Health Research Institute, Hyattsville, MD, for editing the manuscript. The opinions expressed in this paper are those of the authors and do not necessarily reflect the views of the Indian Health Service. The Strong Heart Study was supported by cooperative agreement grants (Nos. U01HL-41642, U01HL-41652, and U01HL-41654) from the National Heart, Lung and Blood Institute.

Selected References

18. Expert Panel on Detection, Evaluation, and Treatment of High Blood Cholesterol in Adults: Executive summary of the Third Report of the National Cholesterol Education Program [NCEP] Expert Panel on Detection, Evaluation, and treatment of high blood cholesterol in Adults [Adult Treatment Panel II]. JAMA 2001;285:2486–97)

20. Grundy SM, Cleeman JI, Daniels SR, et al. Diagnosis and management of the metabolic syndrome: an American Heart Association/National Heart, Lung, and Blood Institute Scientific Statement. Circulation 2005;112:2735–52.

22. Yusuf S, Hawken S, Ounpuu S, et al., and the INTERHEART Study Investigators. Effect of potentially modifiable risk factors associated with myocardial infarction in 52 countries (the INTERHEART study):

case-control study. Lancet 2004 Sep 11–17;364(9438): 937–52.

27. Howard BV, Lee ET, Cowan LD, et al. Rising tide of cardiovascular disease in American Indians. The Strong Heart Study. Circulation 1999 May 11;99(18):2389–95.

33. Kahn R, Buse J, Ferrannini E, et al., and the American Diabetes Association; European Association for the Study of Diabetes. The metabolic syndrome: time for a critical appraisal: joint statement from the American Diabetes Association and the European Association for the Study of Diabetes. Diabetes Care 2005 Sep;28(9):2289–304.

CHAPTER 12

Cardiac and Vascular Effects of Adipocytokines in Normal and Obese Individuals: The Concept of Cardiometabolic Risk

Roberto Vettor, Claudio Pagano, Marco Rossato, & Giovanni Federspil
University of Padova, Padova, Italy

Adipose Tissue and "Cardiometabolic Risk"

Among the causes of the metabolic syndrome and its susceptibility to be linked with the development of a number of cardiovascular complications, visceral obesity and a dysfunctional adipose tissue almost certainly represent the key factors leading to endothelial dysfunction, promoting oxidative stress, and inducing a low-grade chronic inflammation, which represent the pathophysiological basis for progression of atherosclerotic lesions and the increase in the rate of cardiovascular events. Adipose tissue is now considered an active endocrine and paracrine organ, secreting a number of mediators, known as adipokines, which are implicated in different metabolic processes that may have an impact on the cardiovascular system [1]. There is evidence to suggest that current risk-assessment algorithms may not accurately estimate the global risk of cardiovascular disease (CVD) in patients with visceral obesity and with a dysfunctional adipose organ. In light of this, better methods are needed to assess the global risk of CVD and type 2 diabetes in the presence of traditional risk factors and emerging markers found in individuals with excess

Nutritional and Metabolic Bases of Cardiovascular Disease, 1st edition.
Edited by Mario Mancini, José M. Ordovas, Gabriele Riccardi, Paolo Rubba and Pasquale Strazzullo. © 2011 Blackwell Publishing Ltd.

intra-abdominal adiposity and a dysfunctional adipose tissue phenotype. This global risk including the classic and these emerging risk factors is defined as cardiometabolic risk.

The Concept of Dysfunctional Adipose Tissue: "Adiposopathy"

Since the role of the adipose organ is primarily devoted to the storage of lipids as fuel to be utilized by the working muscles, in conditions characterized by food excess and energy overflow, the simple presence of excess adipose tissue per se is unlikely to be responsible for peripheral insulin resistance. In fact, the lack of adipose tissue worsens insulin resistance because of the limitation in triglyceride storage capacity and the consequent leakage of lipids and their accumulation in the peripheral organs (lipotoxicity). This limitation in adipose tissue expansion could be due to its failure to develop new adipocytes with their differentiation and growth into mature adipocytes or to the appearance of fat cell insulin resistance. The maintenance of adequate insulin sensitivity and the capacity to increase its glucose uptake is a fundamental prerequisite for fat cell growth and for the maintenance of peripheral insulin sensitivity and glucose tolerance [2]. Thus, the disruption of insulin-stimulated glucose uptake

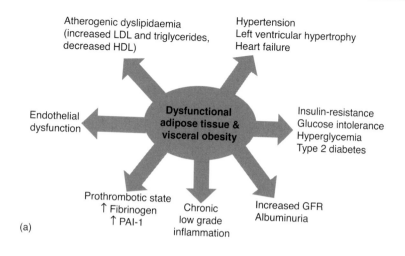

(a)

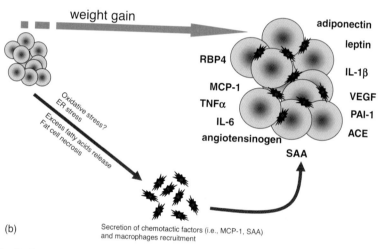

(b)

Figure 12.1 (a) Qualitative alterations of adipose tissue (adiposopathy) and their pathophysiological consequences. (b) The increase in adipose tissue mass and fat cell size leads to fat cell insulin resistance, excess fatty acid release, oxidative stress and fat cell necrosis. All these events are accompanied by macrophage infiltration of adipose tissue and changes in the pattern of adipocytokines synthesis and release.

specifically in adipocytes is able to induce type 2 diabetes even if adipose tissue mass remains constant [3]. These observations put forward the concept of adiposopathy, which denotes the functional failure of the adipose organ and the mechanism linking obesity to insulin resistance [4] (Figure 12.1a). Moreover, the energy fuel overload on the adipose tissue triggers qualitative and quantitative changes in adipokine production, which are able to affect both local and systemic insulin sensitivity, thus regulating whole-body glucose homeostasis. They also act locally affecting adipose tissue functions and

growth. In obesity, the inappropriate but chronic increase in proinflammatory cytokine production in adipose tissue can have a profound impact on whole-body energy balance [5,6]. On the contrary, the actions of the insulin-sensitizing adipokines, such as adiponectin and leptin, are also relevant to impairing adipose tissue function and plasticity (Figure 12.1b). However, in obese insulin-resistant states, the activities of adiponectin and leptin are reduced substantially, through either decreased levels or decreased activity, respectively. Finally, a in recent research work, the systemic lipid profiling also

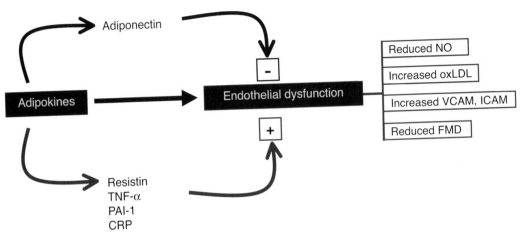

Figure 12.2 Role of adipocytokines in promoting the atherogenic process.

led to the identification of C16:1n7-palmitoleate as an adipose tissue-derived lipid hormone that significantly stimulates muscle insulin action and suppresses hepatosteatosis. These data extend the concept of the existence of lipid mediators (prostaglandins, endocannabinoids, etc.), which could act as true hormones at not only the paracrine and autocrine levels but also at the endocrine level. These data also reveal the existence of a lipid-mediated endocrine network and demonstrate that adipose tissue uses lipokines such as C16:1n7-palmitoleate to communicate with distant organs and regulate systemic metabolic homeostasis [7].

Leptin

Leptin is a 16-kD peptide hormone coded by the ob gene and specifically produced and released by adipocytes. Leptin acts as a satiety signal, acting on the hypothalamus to suppress food intake and stimulate energy expenditure; thus, leptin plays an important role in controlling body fat stores [8]. Leptin exerts its effects by binding to specific receptors that belong to the class I cytokine receptor superfamily and whose signal transduction involves JAK/STAT pathways and adenosine monophosphate (AMP)–activated protein kinase (AMPK) [9]. Different isoforms of the leptin receptors were cloned, but the most important is Ob-Rb, which is abundantly expressed in hypothalamic nuclei involved in the regulation of food intake and energy balance. Apart from adipose tissue, several

studies have reported that leptin may be produced also by other tissues, namely muscle, blood vessels, and cardiomyocytes, in which the leptin receptors have also been identified [10,11], thus, suggesting a paracrine role of leptin in modulating local homeostasis. Leptin secretion is regulated by and controls food intake, energy status, and several hormones. However, leptin deficiency is not the cause of common human obesity, since leptin circulating levels increase in obesity and directly correlate with adipose tissue mass [12]. However, rare families with a deficient leptin production due to mutations of leptin gene or a deficient leptin action due to mutation of leptin receptor show severe obesity and diabetes [13,14]. It was suggested that hyperleptinemia induces leptin resistance via an increase in the levels of suppressor of cytokine signaling. However, the mechanisms inducing leptin resistance are far from being fully elucidated. Circulating leptin levels are elevated both in obese individuals and in patients with type 2 diabetes and are associated with increased coronary artery calcification, a measure of coronary atherosclerosis [15]. Furthermore, leptin appears to promote a proinflammatory milieu, by increasing the secretion of tumor necrosis factor (TNF), interleukin-6 (IL-6), and activating neutrophils, and increasing the generation of reactive oxygen species (ROS), all of which promote endothelial dysfunction and vascular inflammation, prerequisites for atherogenesis [16] (Figure 12.2). Clinically, in patients with angiographically confirmed coronary atherosclerosis, plasma leptin

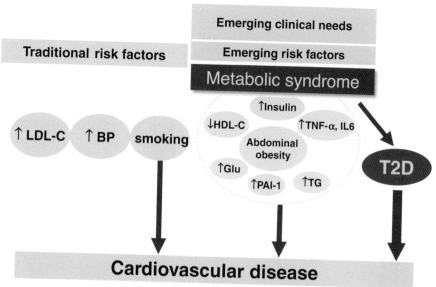

Figure 12.3 Classical and emerging risk factors in the progression from obesity to type 2 diabetes and cardiovascular disease.

serves as a predictor of future cardiovascular events independent of other risk factors such as lipid or C-reactive protein (CRP) levels [17].

Increased leptin is associated with myocardial infarction and stroke independently of other cardiovascular risk factors and obesity [18]. Moreover, increased leptin is also associated with insulin resistance, inflammation, disturbances in hemostasis, and hypertension, as well as with coronary artery calcification in women [19–22]. Leptin induces vasodilation in humans with coronary artery disease and increases nitric oxide release [23,24]. In fact, in leptin-deficient (ob/ob) mice, endothelial function is impaired [10]. In addition to its role in atherosclerosis, leptin induces cardiomyocytes hypertrophy [19] and affects heart cell metabolism and function [25,26].

It has been proposed that leptin could play a role in the pathogenesis of atherosclerosis in combination with other inflammatory cytokines [27]. This hypothesis is supported by several observations *in vitro*. Leptin stimulates the proliferation of vascular smooth muscle cells and activates the production of matrix metalloproteinase-2, promotes vascular production of inflammatory cytokines, enhances platelet aggregation, and induces CRP in human endothelial cells [10,28]. Leptin stimulates monocyte chemotactic protein-1

(MCP-1) expression in aortic endothelial cells, suggesting a role in monocyte/macrophage recruitment to the vessel wall in early atherosclerosis. Leptin-deficient ob/ob mice and leptin-resistant db/db mice are resistant to atherosclerosis [10].

Resistin

Resistin, also known as "found in inflammatory zone-3" (FIZZ3), was first identified as a fat cell–secreted protein by Steppan et al. in 2001 [29]. It is a 108 amino acid protein expressed in white adipose tissue and immune cells. It is a member of the resistin-like molecules family that can be secreted in two different multimeric forms, whose primary sources differ between rodents (adipocytes) and humans (stromal vascular cells in adipose tissue) and whose receptors have not yet been identified. In rodents, its main action is to impair insulin signaling and insulin sensitivity [30]. Resistin has relevant effects on hepatic glucose and lipid metabolism and seems to be a major determinant of hepatic insulin resistance induced by high fat feeding [31].

Although the role of resistin in insulin resistance has been well established in rodents, its role in humans is still under debate. Conflicting results on resistin in human obesity, insulin resistance, and diabetes have been reported [9,32–34].

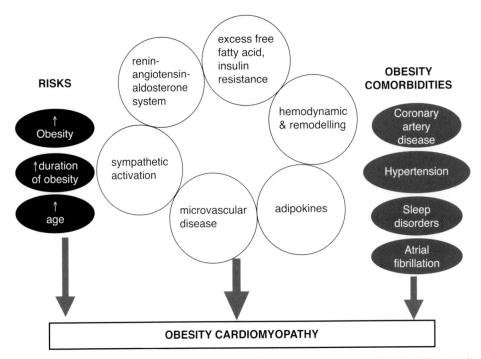

Figure 12.4 The contribution of pathophysiologic mechanisms, risk factors, and obesity comorbidities in the genesis of obesity cardiomyopathy

Increased resistin is related to proatherogenic inflammatory markers, metabolic syndrome, nonalcoholic fatty liver disease, increased cardiovascular risk, unstable angina, and poor prognosis in coronary artery disease [35–37]. In human vascular endothelial cells, resistin increases the production of proinflammatory markers and induces the release of endothelin-1, vascular cell adhesion molecule-1, and MCP-1. Resistin protein is present in atheromas of animal models of atherosclerosis and its levels are related to the severity of the lesion [38]. Moreover, resistin induces endothelial dysfunction in isolated coronary artery rings [39]. In mouse cardiomyocytes, resistin impairs glucose metabolism [40] and worsens cardiac ischemia-reperfusion injury in isolated perfused rat hearts [41].

Several pieces of evidence indicate that resistin interacts with other adipokines in inflammation and metabolic regulation. Opposite effects of resistin and adiponectin on the inflammatory status of endothelial cells were found. Resistin induces the expression of adhesion molecules vascular cell adhesion molecule-1 (VCAM-1) and intercellular

adhesion molecule-1 (ICAM-1), and pentraxin-3, a marker of inflammation. The induction of VCAM-1 and ICAM-1 by resistin was inhibited by adiponectin [42]. A link between leptin and resistin was also suggested, since resistin messenger RNA (mRNA) expression and protein levels in ob/ob mice are regulated by leptin [43].

Apelin

Apelin is a secreted protein produced by adipocytes, stroma-vascular cells and heart muscle. Its circulating levels are elevated in obesity [44]. It is produced as a 77 amino acid prepropeptide that can be cleaved into fragments that activate APJ receptors (i.e., apelin receptors) [45,46]. Apelin has been shown to increase cardiac contractility, while exogenous apelin administration induces nitric oxide release by endothelial cells, produces vasodilation, and lowers blood pressure in mice and rats [44,47,48]. The cardiac apelin system is down-regulated by angiotensin II in heart failure, and it is restored by treatment with angiotensin type 1 receptor blocker [49]. Hypoxia and ischemic heart disease up-regulate apelin expression in cardiovascular tissues [50,51]. Adipocytes synthesize and release apelin [52], and its production is higher in adipocytes from obese insulin-resistant mice and humans [52,53]. A positive correlation between adipocyte apelin mRNA and plasma insulin was also reported, thus supporting a link between production of apelin by fat cells and insulin resistance. Adipocyte apelin expression is stimulated by insulin and TNF-α [52,54]. The aorta of db/db mice expresses less apelin and apelin receptor APJ, and apelin improved the impaired endothelium-dependent relaxation in db/db mouse aortic rings. However, despite some evidence linking obesity to increased apelin production by adipose tissue and cardiovascular dysfunction [53], the exact mechanism of this relationship still needs to be clarified.

Tumor Necrosis Factor-α and Interleukin-6

It is well known that obesity is characterized by elevated levels of TNF-α and IL-6, two well-known proinflammatory cytokines. Elevated levels of these proteins were also associated with cardiometabolic risk factors, as well as obesity, diabetes mellitus, and angina pectoris [55]. Elevated levels of these inflammatory proteins are also associated with cardiovascular risk, but this increase in the systemic inflammation was generally thought to be the result of multiple local atheromatous inflammations. Nowadays, it has been demonstrated that the main origin of the systemic inflammatory response is located within the adipose tissue and that the systemic inflammation plays a primary role in the pathogenesis of CVDs, and it is not only a mere epiphenomenon [55].

Since 1993, it has been demonstrated that TNF-α is overexpressed in the adipose tissue of obese mice, providing the first association between obesity, insulin resistance, and inflammation [56]. It has been shown that in obese mouse models lacking TNF-α function, there was an improvement in insulin sensitivity and glucose homeostasis, confirming that the inflammatory response has a critical role in the regulation of insulin action in obesity [57]. Furthermore, therapy of inflammatory diseases such as rheumatoid arthritis with monoclonal antibody anti-TNF-α treatments has indirectly confirmed these observations [58].

As for TNF-α, obesity is associated with elevated IL-6 concentrations and it has been shown that adipocytes contribute, together with other inflammatory cells resident within the adipose tissue, to the production of this cytokine, with adipose tissue contributing up to 30% of circulating IL-6 and with visceral producing higher levels of IL-6 than subcutaneous adipose tissue [59]. IL-6 plasma levels correlate with body mass and with the degree of insulin resistance [60]. IL-6 directly affect insulin signaling by the induction of suppressor of cytokine signaling-3 (SOCS-3), which inhibits insulin-dependent insulin receptor autophosphorylation [61]. IL-6 might also act centrally, influencing body weight and insulin sensitivity [62]. Furthermore, IL-6 increases lipolysis and decreases lipoprotein lipase activity [63], resulting in increased macrophage uptake of lipids and transformation in foam cells at the early stages of atheromatous plaque formation, confirming an important role for this cytokine in atherosclerosis development (Figure 12.3).

Adiponectin

Despite the fact that most adipokines seem to be linked with the development of the metabolic and cardiovascular complication of obesity, adiponectin possesses a favorable effect because of its insulin-sensitizing, anti-inflammatory, and antiatherogenic properties. Adiponectin is the most abundant known secreted protein produced by adipocytes and, in human subjects, accounts for 0.01% of total plasma protein [64–67] and is only slightly synthesized and secreted by human cardiomyocytes [68]. Of note are the structural characteristics with similarities to the complement 1q family and a collagen-like fibrous domain at the NH_2-terminus and a COOH-terminal globular region. Once in the blood circulation, adiponectin forms low-molecular-weight trimers, middle-molecular-weight hexamers, and high-molecular-weight multimers [69]. At present, there are no conclusive statements about the physiopathological meaning and the clinical relevance of the different molecular complexes [70]. The adiponectin receptor system seems to be tissue specific, with AdipoR1 mostly present in skeletal muscle and AdipoR2 mostly expressed in the liver [71]. The post-receptor signaling pathway involves the activation of the AMPK, the peroxisome proliferator–activated receptor-α (PPAR-α), and the p38 mitogen-activated protein kinase (MAPK)-signaling pathways [72]. The adiponectin signaling pathway, however, can stimulate mitochondrial biogenesis by activating the peroxisome proliferator–activated receptor coactivator 1A (PGC1A), which regulates mitochondrial biogenesis and function.

In rodents, the obese phenotype is characterized by lower adipose tissue adioponectin mRNA levels and plasma concentrations of adiponectin negatively correlate to body mass index (BMI) [73]. The plasma adiponectin level is paradoxically reduced in obese individuals also, with plasma adiponectin concentrations being correlated more negatively with visceral fat than BMI [74–76]. This phenomenon is at present far to be clarified, but the increase in proinflammatory adipokines, fat cell size, and insulin sensitivity [77] could account for the decrease in adiponectin expression and secretion. It is possible to speculate that some of the metabolic benefits induced by caloric restriction may result from improved secretion of adiponectin. Among these beneficial effects, caloric restriction improves mitochondrial biogenesis [78] and oxidative phosphorylation [79], with an induction in human skeletal muscle of PGC1A mRNA and mitochondrial biogenesis of "efficient" mitochondria as an adaptive mechanism, which in turn lowers oxidative stress. Increased signaling through an adiponectin-AMPK interaction stimulates PGC1A protein expression and mitochondrial biogenesis and lowers ROS production in human skeletal muscle [80]. It has been clearly shown that mitochondrial function is linked to adiponectin synthesis in adipocytes, and mitochondrial dysfunction in adipose tissue may explain decreased plasma adiponectin levels in obesity. Impaired mitochondrial function activates a series of mechanisms involving endoplasmic reticulum (ER) stress, c-Jun NH$_2$-terminal kinase (JNK), and activating transcription factor 3 (ATF3) to decrease adiponectin synthesis. Adiponectin expression and mitochondrial content in adipose tissue were reduced in

obese db/db mice, and these changes were reversed by the administration of rosiglitazone. In cultured adipocytes, induction of increased mitochondrial biogenesis (via adenoviral overexpression of nuclear respiratory factor-1) increased adiponectin synthesis, whereas impairment in mitochondrial function decreased it. Impaired mitochondrial function increased ER stress, and agents causing mitochondrial or ER stress reduced adiponectin transcription via activation of JNK and consequent induction of ATF3. Increased mitochondrial biogenesis reversed all of these changes [81].

Type 2 diabetes is a condition characterized by a reduction of adiponectin concentrations independently from age and the degree of adiposity [82] and strongly related to the presence of macrovascular disease [82]. Since it has been reported that subjects carrying variants of the adiponectin gene are particularly prone to present with hypertriglyceridemia, low high-density lipoprotein (HDL)-cholesterol levels, insulin resistance, type 2 diabetes and hypertension, and a faster progression toward coronary artery disease [83–85], it is possible to conclude that adiponectin could be directly involved in the progression from obesity to type 2 diabetes, playing also a fundamental pathogenic role in their cardiovascular complications.

Adipocytes secrete several biologically active substances that are presumed to be involved in obesity-related hypertension. A significant negative correlation was found between plasma adiponectin concentration and mean, systolic, and diastolic blood pressure (BP), suggesting that adiponectin contributes to the clinical course of essential hypertension [86,87]. We studied the relationship between adiponectin levels and insulin sensitivity in newly diagnosed never-treated patients with essential hypertension. In the absence of major cardiovascular risk factors, essential hypertensive patients with a normal nighttime pressure decrease (i.e., dippers) show more prominent insulin resistance and lower adiponectin levels compared to patients with BP persistently elevated throughout the 24-hour period (i.e., nondippers) [88]. In mice, it has been shown that adiponectin could influence the development of hypertensive cardiomyopathy since in adiponectin-knockout mice, pressure overload led to a concentric cardiac hypertrophy [89], which can be reverted with the addition of adiponectin.

In addition, in mice, adiponectin was also shown to protect against overload-induced and adrenergically induced cardiac myocyte hypertrophy, specifically by inhibiting hypertrophic signals via AMPK [90]. However, in humans, the available evidence suggests that the impact of adiponectin on the development of hypertensive cardiomyopathy is quite negligible [88].

Adiponectin as a Protective Factor against Atherosclerosis and the Cardiometabolic Risk

Adipose tissue secretes metabolic hormones, enzymes, anti-fibrinolytic proteins, and inflammatory cytokines [91,92]. These secretory proteins, which have been collectively named adipokines [91], include leptin, TNF-α, plasminogen activator inhibitor type-1 (PAI-1), adipsin, resistin, and adiponectin [73]. There is a substantial body of evidence that focuses on the role of adiponectin in the atherosclerotic process and related disorders [93]. All the conditions in which adiponectin concentrations in the blood are decreased also exhibit an atherogenic profile with smaller and more dense low-density lipoprotein (LDL) particles, lower HDL-cholesterol levels, and higher triglyceride levels [72]. This fact explains why patients with low levels of adiponectin had a significant increase in peripheral and coronary artery disease [94], along with a significantly increased risk of myocardial infarction [95] or stroke [96], independent of other cardiac risk factors.

A state of low-grade chronic inflammation is an important co-determinant for atherosclerotic CVD [97]. A number of studies have shown direct effects of adiponectin on endothelial and vascular smooth muscle cells [98]. It has also been hypothesized that adiponectin has inflammatory-modulating activities, and clinical studies have demonstrated inverse associations between adiponectin levels and markers of inflammation [99]. The anti-inflammatory effects of adiponectin are mostly directed to endothelium and macrophages [100]. Thus, there is evidence that some of the proven antiatheromatous effects of adiponectin may be mediated by anti-inflammatory activities acting directly on the vasculature. It is important to emphasize the influence of systemic inflammation on adiponectin production by adipocytes. In fact, it has been shown that it is inhibited by inflammatory cytokines such as TNF-α [101] via activation of nuclear factor (NF)-κ B signaling [55]. Moreover, reduction or complete exclusion of adiponectin binding and actions, through the disruption of both AdipoR1 and AdipR2 in mice, leads to clear manifestations of an increased inflammation in addition to the appearance of metabolic alterations [102], suggesting a role of both receptors in also mediating the anti-inflammatory effects of adiponectin.

The importance of adiponectin on cardiovascular function starts from the presence of the two receptors in endothelial cells [103] and the AdipoR1 in cardiomyocytes [68]. Hypoadiponectinemia appears to be associated with early biomarkers for vascular disease as the impaired endothelium-dependent vasorelaxation [93,104] and the intima-media thickness. This assumption has been further supported by a series of other important findings. However, it has recently been reported that in high-risk patients with coronary artery disease, plasma adiponectin levels above the median (6.38 µg/ml) imply a paradoxical higher risk of cardiovascular death [105].

Adiponectin opposes endothelial dysfunction and inflammatory activation by promoting NO generation. *In vitro* studies reported that adiponectin enhances endothelial NO synthase (eNOS) mRNA, protein expression, and NO production by endothelial cells [106]. Adiponectin attenuates the progression from endothelial dysfunction to atherosclerosis by reducing the expression of ICAM-1, VCAM-1, and E-selectin provoked by locally secreted cytokines. All the effects on the very early stages of the atherogenetic process result in a clear reduction of the adhesion and migration of the monocytes throughout the intima endothelial cells, the expression of macrophage scavenger receptors-A, and their conversion into foam cells [99]. It is important to note that after adiponectin-expressing adenovirus infection, the adipokine co-localizes with foam cells in the fatty streak lesions [107]. Adiponectin is also able to inhibit the synthesis and release of proinflammatory cytokines from foam cells, while the release of the anti-inflammatory cytokine IL-10 from macrophages leads to an increased synthesis and release of proinflammatory cytokines from foam cells [100]. Adiponectin controls the proliferation of smooth muscle cells within the intima, therefore influencing the plaque stabilization and its propensity to rupture [108]. Adiponectin could be considered a potential endogenous antithrombotic factor, as suggested by the results obtained in knockout mice showing a particular susceptibility to thrombus formation after vascular injury [109].

Adiponectin as a Preferential Target to Treat Cardiometabolic Disease

Weight reduction, an increase in physical activity, and a hypocaloric diet are commonly followed by a significant beneficial increase in plasma adiponectin levels [110,111], which is tightly related to the subsequent metabolic and cardiovascular improvements. At present, we are far from a therapeutic use of recombinant adiponectin, but drug manufacturers are working intensively on drugs acting on adiponectin receptors. However, thiazolidinediones (TZDs) increase the expression of AdipoR1 and AdipoR2 in skeletal muscle and adipose tissue, thereby enhancing adiponectin action [112], and moreover, increase adiponectin mRNA expression and secretion in adipose tissue [102,113]. Recently, endocannabinoid blockade with rimonabant resulted in a significant increase in plasma adiponectin [114].

Conclusions

Obesity often co-presents with other cardiometabolic risk factors such as hypertriglyceridemia, low HDL-cholesterol, insulin resistance, type 2 diabetes, and hypertension. It is becoming clearer that an altered pattern of adipokine production by a dysregulated adipose tissue promotes a state of low-grade systemic chronic inflammation and a prothrombotic state that is involved in the development of both atherosclerosis and subsequently cardiovascular events (Figure 12.4). Adiponectin has appeared as an anti-inflammatory, antiatherogenic, insulin-sensitizing adipokine that appears to protect against obesity-related metabolic diseases and CVDs. A series of experimental and clinical studies have highlighted the biological roles of adipose organ products and their circulating levels. To shut down the hypersecretion and to antagonize the molecular signaling of the proinflammatory adipokines and enhance adiponectin secretion and action represent the pathophysiological rationale for future treatment of obesity and the related metabolic diseases and CVDs.

Selected References

5. Hotamisligil GS. Inflammation and metabolic disorders. Nature 2006;444:860–7.
22. Wannamethee SG, Tchernova J, Whincup P, et al. Plasma leptin: associations with metabolic, inflammatory and haemostatic risk factors for cardiovascular disease. Atherosclerosis 2007;191(2):418–26.
30. Trujillo ME, Scherer PE Adipose tissue-derived factors: impact on health and disease. Endocr Rev 2006;27:762–78.
37. Pagano C, Soardo G, Pilon C, et al. Increased serum resistin in nonalcoholic fatty liver disease is related to liver disease severity and not to insulin resistance. J Clin Endocrinol Metab 2006;91:1081–6.
55. Berg AH, Scherer PE. Adipose tissue, inflammation, and cardiovascular disease. Circ Res 2005;96:939–49.

CHAPTER 13

Dietary Carbohydrates, Overweight and Metabolic Syndrome: The Role of Glycemic Index in a Healthy Diet

Angela Albarosa Rivellese[1] *& Rosalba Giacco*[2]

[1] Federico II University, Naples, Italy
[2] Institute of Food Science, National Research Council, Avellino, Italy

Dietary Carbohydrates: Quantity/Quality

Dietary carbohydrates are a heterogeneous family of nutrients with different metabolic effects depending not only on their amount but also particularly on their quality. In the last decades in the attempt to take into account the quality of carbohydrates and their nutritional and metabolic effects, different classifications have been formulated, and furthermore, new concepts, such as glycemic index (GI) of foods and glycemic load (GL) have been introduced.

Dietary Carbohydrate Classification

Chemical classification divides carbohydrates in three main groups: 1) sugar (mono-disaccharides and polyol), 2) oligosaccharides (malto-oligosaccharides occurring from the hydrolysis of starch, raffinose and stachyose) and 3) polysaccharides [1]. Polysaccharides may be divided into starch (α-1:4 and 1:6 glucans) and non-starch polysaccharides (NSPs), of which the major components are the polysaccharides of the plant cell wall such as cellulose, hemicellulose, and pectine, and also plant gums, mucillages, and hydro-colloids; these NSPs are known as "fiber." Some carbohydrates, such as inulin, do not fit in this classification because they exist in nature in multiple molecular forms. However, a classification based purely on their chemistry is essential for estimation of carbohydrate intake but does not allow a simple translation into nutritional benefits since each of major chemical class of carbohydrates has a variety of overlapping physiological effects. This has led to the use of a number of terms to describe carbohydrates in foods, for example, prebiotic, resistant starch, dietary fiber, available and unavailable carbohydrates, complex carbohydrates, glycemic carbohydrates, and whole grain. With regard to human nutrition, it is more important to classify carbohydrates on their ability to be digested and absorbed in the small intestine, thereby contributing directly or indirectly to the body carbohydrate pool (glycemic carbohydrates) [1]. In this classification, carbohydrates that are not digested and absorbed in the small intestine, namely dietary fiber, are kept separate from glycemic carbohydrates. In turn, on the basis of the velocity of their digestion, glycemic carbohydrates (monosaccharides and disaccharides, some oligosaccharides, and starches) may be classified based on the speed at which they are digested (i.e., slowly or fast). However, most unprocessed carbohydrate-rich foods contain both glycemic and nonglycemic carbohydrates. The extent to which

Nutritional and Metabolic Bases of Cardiovascular Disease, 1st edition.
Edited by Mario Mancini, José M. Ordovas, Gabriele Riccardi,
Paolo Rubba and Pasquale Strazzullo. © 2011 Blackwell Publishing Ltd.

Table 13.1 Glycemic index (GI) of carbohydrate-rich foods widely consumed in the human diet.

	GI (glucose = 100)		GI (glucose = 100)
Sugars		**Potatoes**	
Glucose	100	New potato (boiled)	78
Sucrose	68	French fries	75
Pure honey	58	Baked potatoes	60
Fructose	20	**Legumes**	
Cereals		Beans dried boiled	29
White wheat bread (baguette)	95	Chickpeas dried boiled	28
Special K (Kellogg's)	84	Lentils red, dried, boiled	26
Pizza	80	**Fruit**	
Crackers	70	Pineapple	59
Sourdough bread	66	Banana	52
Rusk	64	Oranges	42
Polished rice	64	Apple juice	40
Parboiled rice	56	Apple	38
Sweet corn	53	Pears	38
Potato-dumplings	52	**Beverages**	
Spaghetti	44	Orange soft drink	68
Barley	25	Coca-cola soft drink	58

carbohydrates in foods raises blood glucose levels compared with an equivalent amount of reference carbohydrates permits us to classify carbohydrate-rich foods on the basis of glycemic response, indicated as GI.

Glycemic Index

GI is a measure of the blood glucose–raising ability of the available carbohydrate in foods. This is calculated by dividing the incremental areas under the curve (AUCs) of blood glucose concentrations measured after the ingestion of a portion of a test food containing 50 g of available carbohydrates by the incremental blood glucose area achieved with a portion of a reference food (glucose or white bread) containing the same amount (50 g) of carbohydrates in the same subject and expressed as a percentage. This index was proposed for the first time in 1981 by Jenkins as an alternative system for classifying carbohydrate-containing foods.

Since several factors can influence the accuracy and precision of food GI, its evaluation requires standardized methodology. Factors affecting the accuracy of GI essentially are errors in the calculation of AUC, outliers more than 2 standard deviations from the mean and within individual variability of AUC of more than 30%. Since the precision of

GI depends also on analytic methods and subject preparation, glucose analysis should be performed in duplicate and, the evening before the test, the patient should consume a normal meal and avoid unusual physical activity [2]. Among carbohydrate-rich foods, those rich in soluble fiber generally have a low GI, in general less than 50% compared with starch-rich foods (Table 13.1). Legumes (beans, chickpeas, lentils, green peas), some kinds of fruits (apples, oranges, pears, plums), several vegetables (artichokes, carrots, etc.), and some cereals (barley, oat etc.) belong to this class of fiber-rich foods [3]. Their low glycemic potential is due to several mechanisms that are able to prolong nutrient digestion and absorption in the small intestine: viscosity, delayed gastric emptying, increased colonic fermentation, and limited access of starch to digestive enzymes owing to the physical structure of the food. However, not all foods with a low GI necessarily have a high fiber content. In fact, spaghetti, potato dumplings, corn, and high-amylose rice are starch-rich foods with a low fiber content and a lower GI compared to bread, pizza, and other cereals (Table 13.1). Low GI of these products is consistent with a reduction of the rate of starch accessibility owing either to physical structure or to high amylose content, a kind of starch less rapidly digested than amylopectin [4]. However, the clinical relevance of GI also remains the subject of a debate centered on two points. First, how does glycemic response change when several foods are eaten in combination? Some studies report that the GI of individual food eaten alone does not predict blood glucose response after these are eaten as part of mixed meal, whereas others argue that GI predicts glycemic response with excellent accuracy when appropriate methodology is used. In fact, when white bread was replaced by an equivalent portion of spaghetti (in terms of carbohydrates) within a mixed meal in type 2 diabetic patients, postprandial plasma glucose response after 5 hours decreased by 40% [5]. The second question is whether a low-GI diet is able to improve health in the long term. This point is addressed later in this chapter.

Glycemic Load

Postprandial blood glucose response is influenced not only by the GI of the food, but also by the amount of ingested carbohydrates. For this reason, in 1997 the concept of "glycemic load" (GL) was introduced to quantify the overall glycemic effect of a portion of food. GL is calculated indirectly as the product of the GI of a specific food and the amount of available carbohydrates contained in an average portion of the food consumed, divided by 100. Each unit of dietary GL represents the equivalent glycemic effect of 1 g of carbohydrates from white bread, which is used as a reference food. This index can be used only when foods have been already selected on the basis of their GI and carbohydrate content. At present, international tables are available that report both the GI and the GL of several foods [6].

Dietary Carbohydrates and Overweight

Overweight and obesity are increasing all over the world. Therefore, sound strategies to reduce this epidemic are needed. Although it is well known that excess calorie intake is the primary dietary cause, the composition of the diet is of relevance. Within this context, attention has been paid to fat and carbohydrates with alternate luck among scientists and in particular among the public going

from one extreme (very low fat, high-carbohydrate diets are the best one for controlling body weight) to the other (only very low carbohydrate, high-fat diets are able to induce hunger-free weight loss). Reasons for the different opinions are many, and in relation to carbohydrates, one of the most important relies on the fact that carbohydrates are a heterogeneous category whose differences are not always properly taken into consideration. In fact, the relationship between carbohydrate intake and body weight should be considered taking into account the proportion of total carbohydrates, the amount of free sugars, and sugar–sweetened beverages, the GI, the amount of dietary fiber, and finally, the GL of the diet, which attempts to consider both the amount and the quality of carbohydrates [7–8]. Moreover, even if data based on epidemiological evidence are of paramount importance, it is also important to understand that they have to be reinforced and proven by results from well-conducted, controlled intervention trials.

Epidemiologic Evidence

Most epidemiologic studies show an inverse association between carbohydrate consumption and body mass index (BMI). In particular, in women cohorts, a BMI of 0.5–3.0 units lower is reported for the group with the highest carbohydrate intake in comparison to that with the lowest carbohydrate intake [7–11]. For men, this difference is less evident, being of 0.6–1.3 BMI units. The results of the few prospective studies are much more inconsistent. Of course, from these epidemiologic data, a casual relationship may not be established, and moreover, some bias and methodological considerations should be emphasized, such as under-reporting of food intake—particularly evident in overweight people—higher reported physical activity in high- carbohydrate/energy consumers, and higher intake of dietary fiber, generally associated with high carbohydrate consumption.

In relation to body weight gain, particular attention has been paid in the last decades to the amount of free sugars, defined as any added sugar plus concentrated sugars in honey, syrups, and fruit juices. In fact, foods high in free sugars may contribute to weight gain in different ways:
1) For their very high energy density;
2) For the lack of dietary fiber;

3) For their higher palatability;

4) For possible unique effects of fructose on satiety;

5) Because they are often consumed in the form of high-calorie liquids instead of solid foods with very low satiating effects.

Most of the prospective studies looking at the relationship between sugar-sweetened beverages and weight gain have supported the possible negative influence of these dietary components showing that increases in the consumption of these beverages was associated with a significant increase in body weight [12]. The relationship between the GI of foods and body weight is very controversial, since some studies show a direct association while others show none [7,8,13,14]. The same is true for the relationship with GL. Many factors may explain this extreme variability, and one of the most important may be the lack of uniformity in determining the GI of foods and, therefore, the GL of the diet. Moreover, it is important to emphasize that the association found in some studies between the GI and body weight (the lower the GI, the lower the body weight) should, at least in part, be explained by the higher intake of dietary fiber, generally associated with a low-GI diet. In fact, the inverse association between higher intake of dietary fiber, in particular cereal fiber, as well as of whole grain, and body weight is quite consistent in all the epidemiologic studies.

Intervention Studies

The role of carbohydrates on weight loss and weight maintenance has been extensively studied by means of intervention studies, and several systematic reviews and meta-analyses have been published about this topic. Nonetheless, the amount of studies, definitive and firm conclusions are difficult to draw since the data are very contrasting. The reasons for that are many, and among them, two of the most important are 1) very few studies are really of long-term duration and we know how difficult it is not only to lose weight, but also to maintain the weight lost in the long run; 2) in many of the intervention trials performed, the differences between different types of carbohydrates have not been taken in consideration.

Trying to summarize the main points, it is important to emphasize that in trials with strictly controlled energy intakes, where participants are instructed to restrict total energy intake first, the macronutrient composition of the diet does not seem to greatly influence body weight loss [7,8,15]. More important seems to be the composition of the diet in trials where energy restriction is not the first end-point. Regarding strategies to lose weight, the very low carbohydrate/very high fat approach (Atkins-type diet) became very popular in the last decade because some intervention trials showed a significantly larger weight reduction in obese people with this kind of diet in comparison to the low-fat/high-carbohydrate diet. A recent meta-analysis of all of these studies reported a pooled 3.3-kg greater weight loss with the high-fat diet vs. the high-carbohydrate diet [16]. However, from the same meta-analysis, it was clear that there was a substantial weight regain with the high-fat diet after the first 6 months, leading to a lack of differences in weight between the two approaches after 12 months. Therefore, while very low carbohydrate/high-fat diets could be considered more effective in the short term, their effectiveness decreases in the long term and the body weight reduction after only one year is equal in the two approaches. The ketogenic effect of the very low carbohydrate diet, leading to a more satiating effect, the simplicity of the diet, and the restriction of food choices have been considered possible explanations for the greater weight loss achieved with this diet in the short term. However, the simplicity of the diet becomes one of the reasons for the decreased effect of this diet in the long term due to a reduction in compliance. Two other considerations should be done for this kind of diet: 1) a very low carbohydrate diet is difficult to be accepted, even only for a short period, in countries where there is a large consumption of carbohydrates, and in fact, intervention trials with this diet have been performed, mainly in the United States and New Zealand; 2) advice to consume foods rich in fat may lead to a higher intake of saturated fat with adverse effects on low-density lipoprotein (LDL)-cholesterol and other cardiovascular risk factors. This may surely be detrimental, especially if this behavior is maintained in the long run.

In addition to a high-fat diet, a high-protein diet has been utilized in the treatment of obesity and compared to a high-carbohydrate diet. The data from intervention trials suggest that the high-protein diet, probably because of a higher satiating effect, induces greater weight loss in the short term (6 months) with a less pronounced weight regain in the subsequent 6 months, even if the difference in the weight between the two diets after one year is not always statistically significant [17]. In any case, the possible more positive effect of high-protein diets on body weight reduction should be confirmed by other log-term trials.

Until now, only amount of carbohydrates have been considered but no attention has been given to the influence of quality of carbohydrates on body weight. What about the effects on body weight of sugar-sweetened beverages in intervention studies, and what about the effect of GI, GL, and dietary fiber?

For what concerns sugar-sweetened beverages, short- and mid-term controlled studies suggest that reduction of their consumption may have beneficial effects on weight management [18]. More complex and contrasting are the data regarding GI and GL. Very recently, a meta-analysis and a systematic review have been published on the topic. In the first, 6 randomized controlled trials (202 participants), lasting from 5 weeks to 6 months and comparing a low GI or GL diet with a higher GI or GL diet in obese or overweight people, were considered [19]. The decrease in BMI was significantly greater (-1.3 units, $p < .05$) with the first approach compared to the other, and the same happened for total fat mass. On the basis of these results, it is possible to say that the reduction of the GI and GL of the diet seems to promote a greater weight loss, at least in the midterm (6 months). Of course, longer term studies are needed to verify whether this effect is maintained in the long run. More recently, a systematic review has been published, in which the authors have tried to evaluate the independent role on body weight reduction and other metabolic parameters of GI, GL, and available and unavailable carbohydrates [20]. In this case, 23 studies performed in different populations—healthy subjects, glucose intolerant subjects, type 1 and type 2 diabetic patients, subjects at higher cardiovascular risk—have been identified. Body weight reduction was significantly associated with the GI of the diet and still more with its GL. In particular, reduction in body weight occurs when GL is reduced by at least 17 g glucose equivalent/day and this reduction is mostly consistent when the

reduction of GL is more marked (>42 g glucose equivalent/day). Dietary fiber is certainly one of the main factors influencing the GI and GL of the foods. In fact, foods rich in fiber are also the foods with the lower GI. Therefore, some of the effects of low GI/GL diets may also be due to independent effects of fiber. While the association between high dietary fiber intake, in particular cereal fiber, and lower body weight is quite consistent on the basis of the epidemiologic evidence, the results of the few intervention studies are less convincing [21,22].

Dietary Carbohydrates and Metabolic Syndrome

Data on the possible influence of quantity and/or quality of dietary carbohydrates on the metabolic syndrome as a whole are lacking, while more information is available on their influence on some of the individual components of the metabolic syndrome, in particular type 2 diabetes and its risk and dyslipidemia.

Epidemiologic Evidence

Among the different types of carbohydrates, the positive association between consumption of sweetened beverages and incidence of metabolic syndrome seems to be the most consistent at the population level. In fact, studies in different age-groups—children, adolescents, and middle-aged people—have shown that increased intake of soft drinks is associated with an increased risk of the incidence of metabolic syndrome and its individual components [23].

Regarding the prevention of type 2 diabetes, epidemiologic evidence suggests that a diet with a low GI and rich in fiber contributes to diabetes prevention. In fact, two large prospective studies (the Nurses Health Study and the Health Professional Follow-up Study) have reported an increased incidence of diabetes in those consuming a diet with a higher GL, especially if consumed with a low intake of cereal fiber [24,25]. In another large prospective study, the Iowa Women's Health Study, no association was found between GL and the risk of diabetes, while an inverse association was found between fiber intake and incidence of diabetes, reinforcing the protective role of high-fiber intake [26].

Also in relation of other cardiovascular risk factors, such as hypertriglyceridemia and low high-density lipoprotein (HDL)-cholesterol levels, observational studies show that triglyceride concentrations tend to rise and HDL-cholesterol concentrations decline when the GI or the GL of the diet increase [27]. In line with these studies on cardiovascular risk factors, some, but not all, epidemiological studies show an inverse relationship between the GI or GL of the habitual diet and the incidence of cardiovascular events [28]. More consistent is the epidemiologic evidence regarding the inverse association between fiber intake, both soluble and insoluble, and the incidence of cardiovascular events.

The association between low GI or GL and a reduced risk of type 2 diabetes as well as of cardiovascular events might be mediated by an improvement in insulin resistance, the main pathogenetic mechanism of this form of diabetes and cardiovascular diseases. However, in relation to this variable, again the data are not so convincing, since in two studies no relation between either GI or GL and insulin-resistance was observed, whereas in another one a direct association was found.

Intervention Studies

The beneficial effects of low GI foods on blood glucose control and other metabolic parameters are particularly evident in intervention studies performed in diabetic patients and in other high-risk individuals compared to healthy subjects [29]. Particularly in relation to blood glucose control, the data show clearly that low GI/high-fiber diets improve, both in type 1 and type 2 diabetes, blood glucose concentrations, especially in the postprandial state, and reduce the number of hypoglycemic events and glycosylated proteins by 2% [30,31]. Moreover, this kind of diet also reduces LDL-cholesterol levels [32].

In these intervention studies, the low GI diet was also rich in fiber. Therefore, the beneficial effects on blood glucose control and other cardiovascular risk factors may be due, in large part, to these dietary components. Less information is available on the effects of a low GI diet independent of fiber content, because few starchy foods with low GI and low fiber content are available. To this regard, only one study has been performed in type 2 diabetic patients with the aim to evaluate two diets differing only in GI but with the same content of dietary fiber and other nutrients. The diet with low GI foods, obtained with appropriate food technologies, improved not only blood glucose control but also insulin sensitivity, LDL-cholesterol, and plasminogen activation ihinibitor-1 activity, suggesting a possible role of low GI foods, independent of fiber content, in the treatment of diabetic patients [33]. The independent role of dietary fiber and low GI foods on blood glucose control and insulin sensitivity seems to be reinforced also by a recent meta-analysis, in which authors have tried to evaluate the independent role of GI and unavailable carbohydrates [20]. In fact, from this meta-analysis, it is quite clear that both blood glucose control and insulin sensitivity are significantly improved either by reducing the GI of the diet or by increasing the consumption of unavailable carbohydrates.

Conclusions

Both epidemiologic and intervention studies, though not conclusive, suggest that low GI diets may be useful in weight regulation, are useful for blood glucose control and improvement in coronary heart disease risk factor profiles in diabetic patients, and even to a lesser extent, also in high-risk subjects, such as those with insulin resistance/metabolic syndrome (Table 13.2). It is important to emphasize that a major contributor to a low GI diet is given by foods rich also in dietary fiber, whose independent effects on body weight regulation, blood glucose control, and other metabolic parameters is much more established (Table 13.2). Low GI foods not rich in fiber are not abundant; therefore, in order to increase the real impact of these foods on health status, it is important to try to find appropriate technologies able to reduce the GI of some starchy foods, in particular those more largely used at the population level, such as bread, rice, and potatoes. Other points to emphasize in regard to the GI of foods and their possible health effects is that the GI should not be considered alone but in relation to the other properties of foods, that it should be used to classify carbohydrate-rich foods, and is only meaningful when comparing foods within a comparable food group, that is, breads, fruit, and different types of cereal foods.

Table 13.2 Impact of specific feature of carbohydrate-rich foods on body weight regulation, metabolic and cardiovascular risk.

	Low GI	Soluble fiber	Insoluble fiber
Epidemiologic observations			
Body weight loss	+/−	+/−	+
Reduced risk of diabetes	+/−	+	+
Reduced risk of CHD	+/−	+	+
Controlled clinical trials			
Body weight loss	−	−	−
Reduced risk of diabetes	−	+/−	+/−
Reduced risk of CHD	−	+/−	+/−
Plausible mechanisms			
Satiating effect	+/−	+/−	+/−
Blood glucose regulation	+	+	+/−
CHD risk factor profile	+/−	+	+/−

GI: glycemic index; CHD: coronary heart disease.

Taking all these aspects into consideration, the adoption of a low GI, low GL, high-fiber diet could be relevant at the population level in order to reduce the risk of diabetes, other metabolic diseases, and cardiovascular events and to help in the reduction and maintenance of body weight.

Selected References

2. Wolever TM, Brand-Miller JC, Abernethy J, et al. Measuring the glycemic index of foods: interlaboratory study. Am J Clin Nutr 2008;87(Suppl 1):247–57.

5. Riccardi G, Clemente G, Giacco R. Glycemic index of local foods and diets: the Mediterranean experience. Nutr Rev 2003;61:S56–60.

19. Thomas DE, Elliott EJ, Baur L. Low glycaemic index or low glycaemic load diets for overweight and obesity. Cochrane Database Syst Rev 2007;18; (3): CD005105.

20. Livesey G, Taylor R, Hulshof T, et al. Glycemic response and health–a systematic review and meta-analysis: relations between dietary glycemic properties and health outcomes. Am J Clin Nutr 2008;87(Suppl 1):258–68.

29. Riccardi G, Rivellese AA, Giacco R. Role of glycemic index and glycemic load in the healthy state, in prediabetes, and in diabetes. Am J Clin Nutr 2008;87(Suppl 1):269–74.

CHAPTER 14

Metabolic Effects of Wholegrain Foods in Relation to Composition, Structure and Type of Food

Hannu Mykkänen, Marjukka Kolehmainen, Isabel Bondia Pons, & Kaisa Poutanen

Food and Health Research Centre, Department of Clinical Nutrition, School of Public Health and Clinical Nutrition, University of Kuopio, Kuopio, Finland

Introduction

Cereals constitute a major part of the daily diet in many countries and provide almost half of the total intake of carbohydrates and more than one-fourth of the total intake of energy for many world populations (FAO Statistical Yearbook 2005–2006). In the less developed areas of Asia and Africa, cereals can provide more than 70% of energy intake and are also a major source of protein, B vitamins, and minerals. The most consumed grains worldwide are wheat and rice, which together provide more than half of the total cereal food intake. Barley, oats, and rye are minority crops, accounting less than 2% of world grain production, and are consumed mainly in northern and eastern Europe and Canada.

Cereals are consumed as refined-grain products, in which the outer layers of the grain (bran and germ) are removed during milling. This will significantly influence the nutritional content of the final product. Whole-grain products containing intact, flaked, or broken kernels or flour ground from whole grains are a good source of dietary fiber, minerals, vitamins, lignans, and other phytochemicals. Epidemiological and cohort studies show that intake of whole-grain cereal foods reduces the risk of type 2 diabetes [1] and cardiovascular disease [2,3]. The bran component seems to play an important role in this association [2,4], and it has been suggested that grains should be consumed in a minimally refined form to achieve the benefit [5,6]. The metabolic link between the consumption of cereal foods and diseases risk is not clear, and there is a lack of controlled intervention trials demonstrating the mechanisms by which whole-grain cereals might produce these effects.

This chapter reviews the metabolic effects of whole-grain cereal foods with respect of their potential in reducing the risk of type 2 diabetes. The role of factors related to food structure and composition, especially fiber, in controlling carbohydrate digestibility and absorption, is discussed, and evidence based on intervention studies with whole-grain cereals will be presented.

Postprandial Glucose and Insulin Responses in Relation to Structure and Type of Cereal Foods

Dietary fiber and food structure are well-established factors affecting starch digestion and consequently the postprandial glucose and insulin responses, but rye bread, rich in fiber, appears to display a pattern of glycemic response different from other cereal foods.

Nutritional and Metabolic Bases of Cardiovascular Disease, 1st edition. Edited by Mario Mancini, José M. Ordovas, Gabriele Riccardi, Paolo Rubba and Pasquale Strazzullo. © 2011 Blackwell Publishing Ltd.

Dietary Fiber

Native wheat, rye, and oat grains contain about 15 % dietary fiber, which in addition to large intestine–mediated physiological signals may also have an important effect on food structure and postprandial absorption. The major fiber components in cereals are the nonstarch polysaccharides (NSPs), cellulose, β-glucans, and arabinoxylans, as well as some oligosaccharides. Water-extractable NSPs such as β-glucan may increase viscosity in the intestine, slowing intestinal transit, delaying gastric emptying, and slowing glucose and sterol absorption in the intestine [7]. Oat β-glucan [8] and barley β-glucan [9] are known to reduce postprandial glucose and insulin responses after an oral load. This functionality depends on their ability to increase viscosity, as reviewed recently by Wood [10].

Another major component of dietary fiber in cereal grains, arabinoxylan (AX), consists of a chain of β-1,4-linked D-xylopyranosyl units to which O-2 and/or O-3-L-arabinofuranosyl units are linked. AX behaves physiologically like a soluble, viscous fiber [11]. AX-rich fiber from wheat has been shown to improve glycemic control in patients with type 2 diabetes [12], and AX concentrates decrease postprandial serum glucose, serum insulin, and plasma total ghrelin response in subjects with impaired glucose tolerance [13]. The effect of soluble fiber is, however, dependent on viscosity and may be lost if viscosity is reduced during processing. The amounts of soluble fiber needed to achieve the beneficial effects on glycemic response are 4–14 g/meal [14,15]. Such amounts are seldom received in conventional meals.

Insoluble cereal fiber contains lignin, a lipophilic, phenolic polymer, as well as NSPs. Insoluble dietary fiber usually has high water-holding capacity, which contributes to increased fecal bulk [16].

Role of Food Structure

Food structure influences starch digestion and therefore the postprandial glucose and insulin responses. Digestion of cereal foods starts in the mouth by chewing and salivary excretion and continues in the stomach, where pieces of food are subjected to pepsin, acid conditions, and vigorous grinding by gastric motility. The partly digested foods are passed from the stomach to the small intestine via the pylorus, which acts as a sieve for the food particles allowing through pieces smaller than 2-mm diameter [17]. The rate of gastric emptying regulates the carbohydrate digestion and absorption, and subsequent blood glucose rise and insulin release. The rate of gastric emptying varies between foods depending on the particle size; the half-time is longer (75 minutes) for spaghetti forming larger coherent particles than for mashed potato (35 minutes) [18]. Food structure can affect both the accessibility of digestive enzymes and the gastric emptying of the partly digested foods [17,18], and preserving the structure of foods is an important determinant of the glycemic response [19]. However, a recent study showed that gastric emptying, measured indirectly with paracetamol baked into breads, was not affected after meals composed of whole-kernel rye bread or whole-meal rye bread compared to white wheat bread [20]. There were no significant differences in the glucose responses between these products, although insulin response to rye bread was lower.

The rate of starch hydrolysis in the upper intestinal tract is dependent on the maintenance of the tissue structures in cereal grains during processing. Milling of the barley kernels to flour increases the glycemic response of barley bread to the level observed after white wheat bread [21]. Similar results have also been shown with wheat, rye, and oats. The intact botanical grain structure protects the encapsulated starch of the kernel against the hydrolysis by gastrointestinal amylolytic enzymes [22].

In addition, the physical state of starch itself is an important determinant of the glycemic response of starch-containing foods. Native starch granules are digested slowly by α-amylase, and during gelatinization the *in vitro* rate of amylolysis increases remarkably [23,24]. Bread baked from a high-amylose barley genotype by using long-time/low-temperature baking conditions produces a lower glycemic response and contains more resistant starch [25]. Retrograded amylose, one form of resistant starch, is formed in heat processing due to recrystallized amylose. Resistant starch content can be increased by prolonging the wet stage after cooking and heating or freezing the cooked food.

It has been suggested that presence of lactic acid during thermal processing promotes interactions between starch and gluten, hence reducing starch bioavailability. Addition of acid in baking of barley bread has reduced the rate of gastric emptying and starch digestion in comparison to white wheat breads [26]. Acid will also make the bread structure very firm and less porous, which retards digestion [27]. The structure of breads is generally porous, while that of pasta and other low glycemic products such as potato dumpling is dense and firm [28,29]. Consequently, the glycemic responses to breads are variable depending on the structural characteristics, with many breads having, however, high GI values in comparison to unprocessed grains and pasta, which have low values [30].

The "Rye Factor"

It has been repeatedly shown that rye breads produce lower responses of insulin and the incretin hormones, but not of glucose both in healthy humans [20,31,32] and in subjects of the metabolic syndrome [33]. The results suggest that with rye breads, less insulin is needed to regulate the level of blood sugar after the same amount of starch than in white wheat bread. Interestingly, foods such as high-amylose rice [34] and barley-pasta containing β-glucan [35] have also been shown to decrease insulin responses of healthy subjects while having small or no effect on glucose responses.

The low insulin response after rye bread appears to be associated with an interesting pattern in the glucose curve; 3 hours after the wheat bread meal the plasma glucose level declines below the fasting level, whereas glucose level is maintained above the fasting level after the rye bread meal [20]. This difference in late postprandial glycemic response may produce other metabolic consequences; rapid decrease of blood glucose may increase the feeling of hunger and may cause more frequent snacking, which may be of relevance to weight gain. A decrease in blood glucose at later postprandial phase may stimulate the release of counter-regulatory stress hormones such as cortisol and catecholamines, which restore glucose levels and increase nonesterified fatty acid concentrations [36]. The latter suggestion is supported by the results of the postprandial challenge, comparing the responses of insulin, glucose, catecholamines, and nonesterified fatty acids to rye bread versus oat and wheat bread meals in subjects with the metabolic syndrome [33]. The insulin response to the rye bread meal was lower than that to the oat and wheat bread meal and

there were no differences in the early postprandial glucose response, but plasma glucose concentrations decreased more below fasting concentrations 2.5–3.0 hours after the oat and wheat bread meal than after the rye bread meal, and a late postprandial rebound of free fatty acids was detected after the oat and wheat bread meal [33].

The difference in the postprandial insulin response after rye products as compared to other cereals cannot be explained solely by the amount of fiber, since no difference was observed in postprandial insulin and C-peptide responses between different types of rye breads ranging in fiber content from 6.1 to 29 g per portion [32]. The lower C-peptide response after ingestion of rye breads, as compared to wheat bread, indicates that diminished pancreatic secretion of insulin rather than enhanced liver extraction explains the lower postprandial insulin response after rye bread. Structural differences in breads may explain this phenomenon, since rye breads have a less porous and mechanically firmer structure than wheat bread [27], and the gelatinized starch in wheat is more available to hydrolytic enzymes than the starch granules from rye [32].

Metabolic Effects Associated with Fermentation of the Cereal Fiber Complex

Whole-grain foods are rich in dietary fiber, which by definition is an important substrate for the conversions in the large intestine. The rate of fermentation of different fiber forms by the gut microbiota is physiologically important. The fermentability of fiber is influenced by several factors, such as the chemical composition, solubility, physical form and the presence of lignin and other compounds [37]. Extractable dietary fiber, resistant starch (RS). and oligosaccharides are more readily fermented than insoluble cell wall structures and non-extractable polysaccharides such as cellulose and certain forms of arabinoxylan.

Fermentation Products of Cereal Fiber and Their Metabolic Effects

Undigested carbohydrates that reach the colon are anaerobically fermented by intestinal microflora to short-chain fatty acids (SCFAs) and gases. The rate and amount of SCFA production depends on the species and amounts of microflora present in the colon, the substrate source and gut transit time [38,39]. A study carried out in pigs fed diets with a similar dietary fiber content but with different proportions of the main dietary fiber compounds (cellulose added in refined wheat bread versus natural AX in rye bread), resulted in moister feces and significantly enhanced gut production and plasma concentrations of butyrate when pigs consumed the rye diet compared with the wheat diet. The quantitative degradation of fiber in the large intestine was more than twice as high in the rye diet [40]. However, a previous study in humans did not show any difference in absolute or relative levels of butyrate in the peripheral blood of human subjects after a high-fiber rye bread based diet compared with a low-fiber wheat bread based diet [41].

SCFAs, which include acetate, butyrate, and propionate, have shown a variety of biological effects [42]. SCFAs are readily absorbed and account for <10% of daily energy. Butyrate is mainly metabolized by the colonic epithelium, propionate by the liver, and acetate partly by the liver and partly by the muscle and other peripheral tissues [43]. SCFAs lower the pH of digesta contents, leading to the ionization of potentially cytotoxic compounds such as biogenic amines and ammonia [44]. The reduction of the luminal pH inhibits the conversion of primary bile acids to secondary bile acids and makes the free bile acids less available, thereby reducing carcinogenic activity [45]. Fermentation of soluble dietary fiber may also produce potential anti-inflammatory effects via butyrate [16]. The reported reductions in inflammatory markers due to soluble fiber are comparable with both insoluble dietary fiber and more readily fermentable soluble dietary fiber [46].

Recent studies have also pointed out the role of the fermentable dietary fiber in the management of appetite and food intake control in humans as a potential tool to help control obesity and other related metabolic diseases [47,48]. Fiber fermentation might promote L-cell differentiation in the proximal colon, contributing to a higher endogenous GLP-1 production and suggesting a new mechanism by which dietary fiber may lower food intake and fat mass development [49]. Prebiotic fructo-oligosaccharides have been shown to improve glu-

cose tolerance, insulin secretion and lower food intake in both animals and humans [39,49]. The manipulation of the microbiotic environment could therefore open a new area in nutrition to treat or prevent diseases such as type 2 diabetes.

Arabinoxylo-oligosaccharides (AXOSs), which are fragments products of AX [50] may also have an interest as prebiotic compounds. Unlike AX, which is poorly fermented in the colon, AXOSs have been shown to be selectively fermented by bifidobacteria in *in vitro* studies [51]. The physiological effects of AXOS preparations in humans are currently under research. In their recent review on metabolic effects of fiber consumption and its relation to diabetes, Weickert and Pfeiffer [52] proposed, based on animal data, that the shift in gut microbiotic communities is a potential mechanism linking dietary fiber with reduced diabetes risk.

Phenolic Compounds, Their Conversions, and Absorption

The presence of unique phytochemicals, not present in fruits and vegetables in such quantities, may also contribute to the observed health benefits of whole-grain cereals in epidemiologic studies. These phytochemicals include phenolic acids, lignans and alkylresorcinols. The potential health benefits of phenolic acids have been related mostly to their effective antioxidant activity while lignans are thought protect against hormonally mediated diseases [53,54].

Most phenolic compounds in cereals are present in bound form and are typically components of complex structures. Ferulic acid is the most abundant phenolic acid in cereal grains, and is found mainly in the *trans* form, which is esterified to AX and hemicelluloses in the aleurone and pericarp of the grain [55]. Several dimers of ferulic acid are also found in cereals and form bridge structures between chains of hemicellulose. A crossover study in healthy subjects given whole-grain wheat or wheat bran revealed that whole-grain wheat can exert a pronounced prebiotic effect on gut microbiota composition and increases the ferulic acid concentration in fasting plasma, suggesting that the whole-grain intake can produce a continuous release of antioxidant into the bloodstream [56].

Lignans are metabolized to enterodiol and enterolactone by the intestinal microflora and, as recently reviewed by Adlercreutz [57], may exert many biological activities. In healthy humans, the intake of whole-grain rye bread clearly increased plasma and urinary enterolactone levels as compared to white wheat bread [58]. Cereal grains also contain lignans, which may appear in circulation in their original form, such as syringaresinol and hydroxyl-mataresinol, which are not converted to enterolactone *in vitro* [59].

Alkylresorcinols are phenolic lipids unique to the outer layers of wheat and rye grains. The specific homologue profile for both cereals makes alkylresorcinols to be considered as potential biomarkers of the intake of rye and wheat. Their presence in intact form in human plasma has been confirmed in different crossover studies, indicating that they are absorbed in humans [60,61]. Alkylresorcinols have been also found to be incorporated into human erythrocyte membranes [62], and they have recently been shown to be almost exclusively transported in lipoproteins in plasma, with very low-density lipoprotein and HDL being the main carriers [63].

To fully understand the implications of dietary phenolic compounds in human health, it is essential to determine their bioavailability to tissues and *in vivo* effects. The metabolites formed in the colon circulate in plasma and are excreted via urine. The enterohepatic circulation plays an important role as it ensures that the residence time of the phytochemical metabolites in plasma is extended compared to that of their parent compounds [64]. The microbial metabolites of phenolic compounds are thought to exert systemic effects, but more research is needed to elucidate and evaluate their health implications.

Evidence Based on Intervention Studies

Even though the findings from epidemiologic studies show convincingly that the intake of whole grain is inversely associated with reduced risk of type 2 diabetes, there are only a few controlled interventions carried out to elucidate possible mechanisms and to demonstrate the effects of whole-grain foods on biomarkers related to improved insulin economy.

Leinonen et al. [65] studied the effects of rye bread containing diet on glucose metabolism in 40 healthy nondiabetic subjects using a 2- × 4-week crossover design (using white wheat bread as control) and found no difference in fasting glucose and insulin levels. Similarly, controlled trials on feeding wheat bran, oats and barley breads resulted in no improvement in insulin sensitivity [28,66,67]. All these studies used fasting glucose and insulin measurements which are perhaps not sensitive indicators of the changes in glucose and insulin metabolism. However, Pereira et al. [68], using the euglycemic hyperinsulinemic clamp test and measurements of fasting glucose and insulin and postprandial response to a mixed meal, were able to demonstrate the beneficial effects of whole grains on insulin sensitivity in hyperinsulinemic overweight adults consuming diets containing 6–10 servings/day of either whole-grain or refined grains cereals. Approximately 80% of the whole-grain products were wheat, the rest were oats, rice, corn, barley, and rye.

Using a randomized crossover study design, Andersson et al. [69] evaluated the effects of a diet rich in whole grains compared with a diet containing the same amount of refined grains on insulin sensitivity and markers of lipid peroxidation and inflammation in 30 moderately overweight subjects. The subjects substituted whole-grain products (mainly milled wheat) for refined-grain products for two 6-week periods. Peripheral insulin sensitivity was determined by the euglycemic hyperinsulinemic clamp test, and markers of lipid peroxidation and inflammation were measured. They found no effects by whole whole grains on insulin sensitivity or markers of lipid peroxidation and inflammation.

Juntunen et al. [70] studied the effect of high-fiber rye bread on glucose and insulin metabolism in 20 hypercholesterolemic, moderately overweight postmenopausal women using a randomized crossover trial (2 × 8 weeks, white wheat bread as a control). The test breads, high-fiber rye bread and white wheat bread, provided 23%–27% of the daily energy intake. Although this modification of the carbohydrate intake did not significantly affect the insulin sensitivity measured by the intravenous glucose-tolerance test, acute insulin secretion was significantly enhanced, indicating an improvement of the β-cell function.

Laaksonen et al. [71] assessed the effect of carbohydrate modification on insulin and glucose metabolism in 72 overweight or obese men and women with the metabolic syndrome, as determined according to the National Cholesterol Education Program criteria. The subjects were randomly assigned to 12-week diets in which either rye bread and pasta or oat and wheat bread and potato were the main carbohydrate sources (34% and 37% of energy intake, respectively). No significant difference was observed in the changes in fasting glucose and insulin concentrations or in glucose and insulin AUCs between the groups during a 2-hour oral glucose-tolerance test. However, the insulinogenic index (an index of early insulin secretion) increased more in the rye bread and pasta group than in the oat and wheat bread and potato group. These effects are not explained by the higher fiber content of the rye diet, since the control diet included the same amount of fiber-rich bread, but as whole wheat and oat breads. The reduced first-phase insulin response is often a prerequisite for the development of impaired glucose tolerance and type 2 diabetes and seems to be a primary determinant of those persons with insulin resistance who will eventually develop impaired glucose tolerance or diabetes [72].

To investigate in more detail the mechanism behind this effect, the gene expression in adipose tissue was examined using genomewide transcriptomic analyses [73]. It appeared that in the adipose tissue of those subjects whose glucose metabolism was improved, the genes related to insulin signaling were down-regulated [73]. This was speculated to be caused by the improved peripheral insulin sensitivity. However, the control diet caused the increase in expression of genes related to inflammation and metabolic stress [33]. This evidence indicates that there are potentially beneficial health effects when consuming rye products in prevention of insulin resistance and type 2 diabetes, which are complications most often caused by the obesity.

More well-controlled intervention studies are needed on effects of defined cereal diets on metabolic changes at different levels of physiology. Differences in cereal foods should be studied in terms of their influence on serum metabolomic and proteomic profiles in order to detect the small changes leading to differences in clinical end-points during long exposure. New analytical technologies combined with bioinformatics will reveal new biomarkers and may thereby assist in identifying protective food factors and mechanisms of wholegrain foods.

Future Outlook

It is obvious that the quality of diet is a key lifestyle factor in the battle against development of metabolic syndrome–related chronic diseases. Cereal foods are a major energy source, and recent evidence clearly shows that we should pay more attention to the composition and digestibility of cereal foods. The sound epidemiologic evidence already gives a basis to nutrition recommendations to increase the consumption of whole-grain foods and foods rich in outer grain layers. Grains are gradually recognized as one of the important plant foods providing protective food factors. In addition, cereal foods provide energy in the form of carbohydrates and protein. Food structure has especially been shown to play an important role in the digestibility and bioavailability of glucose and also of phytochemicals present in cereal foods. Food structure also influences digestibility and fermentability of the dietary fiber complex in the large intestine.

There is a large gap between recommended and actual consumption of whole-grain foods and dietary fiber. To overcome this, improved consumer education and communication, as well as availability and accessibility of cereal foods rich in whole-grain ingredients, should be achieved. Development of consumer-appealing food concepts with good sensory perception and high in whole grain and bran is an important challenge of food technologists and the cereal industry. At the same time, more research is needed in elucidating the factors relevant for delivery of cereal macronutrients and micronutrients and non-nutrients into the circulation, and to show the relationship between cereal food-induced physiological changes and biomarkers of early pathogenesis of insulin resistance and other metabolic disorders.

Selected References

1. de Munter JSL, Hu FB, Spiegelman D, et al. Whole grain, bran, and germ intake and risk of type 2 diabetes: a prospective cohort study and systematic review. PLOS Medicine 2007;4:1385–1395.

2. Jensen MK, Koh-Banerjee P, Hu FB, et al. Intakes of whole grains, bran, and germ and the risk of coronary heart disease in men. Am J Clin Nutr 2004;80:1492–1499.

6. Venn BJ, Mann JI. Cereal grains, legumes and diabetes. Eur J Clin Nutr 2004;58:1443–61.

32. Juntunen KS, Laaksonen DE, Autio K, et al. Structural differences between rye and wheat breads but not total fiber content may explain the lower postprandial insulin response to rye bread. Am J Clin Nutr 2003;78:957–964.

33. Kallio P, Kolehmainen M, Laaksonen DE, et al. Inflammation markers are modulated by responses to diets differing in postprandial insulin responses in individuals with the metabolic syndrome. Am J Clin Nutr 2008;87:1497–1503.

CHAPTER 15

Complex Dietary Patterns (Mediterranean Diet, Vegetarian/ Vegan Dietary Models): Impact on Carbohydrate and Lipid Metabolism

Jim Mann

Edgar National Centre for Diabetes Research and University of Otago, Dunedin, New Zealand

Introduction

Nutrition recommendations have traditionally focused on ensuring adequacy of human diets, hence, the emphasis on total energy and intake of vitamins and minerals. More recently, since the realization that nutritional factors are important in the etiology of chronic diseases, recommendations have also included advice on macronutrient distribution [1]. Obesity, cardiovascular disease, diabetes, and cancer have now reached epidemic proportions in many, if not most, developing countries as well as affluent societies [2]. This has led to particular emphasis on the importance of reducing the intake of energy-dense foods and saturated fatty acids and increasing vegetables, fruit, and whole-grain cereals, generally rich sources of dietary fiber as well as micronutrients [2,3]. A substantial number of intervention studies have suggested that supplementation with several micronutrients may not confer the benefit suggested in observational studies where the nutrients were derived principally from food rather than supplements [4]. As a result, it is generally accepted that advice regarding optimum nutrition should be offered in terms of food in addition to recommendations concerning nutrient intake. The concept that dietary patterns may be even more relevant than individual foods in determining human health is not particularly new but has aroused increasing interest [5]. Much attention has centered around the Mediterranean and vegetarian (or vegan) dietary patterns.

Mediterranean Diet

Epidemiologic Aspects

Some 50 years ago, Ancel Keys initiated the Seven Country Study, which confirmed earlier clinical observations that rates of coronary heart disease (CHD) were exceptionally low in the Mediterranean region, compared with countries in northern Europe and North America [6]. There is considerable variation in the dietary patterns across the Mediterranean region, especially with regard to total fat consumption, which may range from fairly low (approximately 30% total energy) to fairly high (approximately 40% total energy). However, Mediterranean-type diets do have a number of features in common: a high consumption of foods of vegetable origin, including fruits, vegetables, legumes, nuts, and cereals, and a relatively low consumption of meat and animal products.

Nutritional and Metabolic Bases of Cardiovascular Disease, 1st edition. Edited by Mario Mancini, José M. Ordovas, Gabriele Riccardi, Paolo Rubba and Pasquale Strazzullo. © 2011 Blackwell Publishing Ltd.

Fat is derived much more from olive oil than animal sources, leading to a relatively high ratio of monounsaturated to saturated fatty acids. In some Mediterranean communities, fish forms an important component of diet. Keys considered that variation in intake of saturated fatty acids explained much but not all of the variation in CHD rates.

More recently, the association between attributes of the Mediterranean diet and CHD and diabetes has been examined in longitudinal studies within Mediterranean countries using a diet score created by Trichopoulou et al. [7]. The whole index includes nine attributes of the Mediterranean diet: high ratio of monounsaturated:saturated fatty acids, moderate intakes of alcohol, high intake of legumes, high intake of grains, high intake of fruits and nuts, high intake of vegetables, high intake of fish, low intake of meat and meat products, and moderate intake of milk and dairy products. Using a very simple scoring system, increasing adherence to these dietary attributes has been associated with progressive reduction in risk of both CHD and diabetes [8]. For example, in the SUN project carried out in Spain, those with a low score (zero to two of the nine attributes) had an incidence rate ratio of 1 compared with 0.41 for those with a moderate score (three to six of the attributes) and 0.17 for those with a high score (seven to nine of the attributes) [9].

Similar studies have been undertaken by the Harvard group in the United States. Low-risk groups, defined according to similar dietary attributes, plus other healthy lifestyle–related behaviors (not smoking, regular physical activity, not overweight), were at dramatically reduced risk of both CHD and diabetes [10,11]. Recently, the Mediterranean diet has also been characterized by low intakes of transfatty acids [12]. However, epidemiologic data, even when derived from larger prospective studies, do not enable the reliable determination of the extent to which benefit might be attributed to the complex dietary pattern per se, rather than one or more of its component attributes that could be constituted in an alternative dietary pattern.

Intervention Studies

Relatively few intervention studies have examined the potential of the Mediterranean diet to reduce the risk of developing clinical cardiovascular disease or diabetes, although several studies have examined the effects of diets with many similar nutritional attributes. There are also studies in which the effects of the Mediterranean diet have been considered in relation to risk indicators. The Lyon Diet Heart Study reported a dramatic 70% reduction in the risk of death or recurrent cardiovascular disease in individuals with established CHD randomized to receive "Mediterranean dietary advice" compared with a control group [13]. The experimental diet was high in α-linolenic acid (primarily from rapeseed oil) and olive oil; the amounts of red meat and diary products were low. The control diet was based on the low-fat diet recommended by the American Heart Association. Interestingly, the difference between the groups started to emerge within just months after randomization, suggesting that benefit was primarily due to the antithrombotic and antidysrhythmic effects of the diet. The Finnish Diabetes Prevention Study involved randomization of people with impaired glucose tolerance (IGT) to intervention and control groups. The former received intensive advice regarding reduction of energy intakes and increase in physical activity as well as specific dietary messages compatible with attributes of the Mediterranean diet: reduction of saturated fat, increase in fruit and vegetables, and increase in whole-grain cereals. Individuals in the control group were referred back to their general practitioners. Rate of progression from IGT to diabetes was some 60% lower among those in the intervention group compared with those in the control group, and among those who complied with all five intervention recommendations, very few progressed to diabetes during the follow-up period [14]. The findings depend, to a considerable extent, upon the comparison diet.

Innumerable studies have examined the effects of a Mediterranean diet on indicators of lipid and carbohydrate metabolism and other cardiovascular risk factors in healthy individuals as well as those with diabetes and prediabetic states, including the metabolic syndrome. However, a Mediterranean type of diet has been shown to be associated with weight loss [15], improvement in insulin sensitivity [16], reduction in blood glucose levels [15,17], and improved lipid profile (reduced low-density lipoprotein [LDL]-cholesterol and triglyceride, increased high-density lipoprotein (HDL)-cholesterol) [17,18]. The changes appear more marked in those with diabetes than in healthy individuals [15]. The Mediterranean diet also has the potential to improve endothelial dysfunction and reduce levels of a range of inflammatory markers [19]. These observations provide ample explanation for the observed reduction in cardiovascular and diabetes risk conferred by the Mediterranean diet.

Interpretation

The observations described above provide clear evidence for the suitability of the Mediterranean dietary pattern in the management of cardiovascular risk and the prevention and treatment of diabetes. What is less clear is whether there are unique attributes of the Mediterranean diet that confer the benefits or whether similar benefits are likely to occur from food choices that result in comparable intakes of macronutrients and micronutrients. Furthermore, it has not been established whether the Mediterranean diet or a comparable dietary pattern has advantages beyond those of an appropriate low-fat, high-carbohydrate diet.

Evidence-based European recommendations for the prevention and treatment of diabetes include reduced intakes of saturated fat and sugars, a range of acceptable intakes of mono and cis-polyunsaturated fats and carbohydrates, provided the latter are derived from intact fruits and vegetables and whole-grain cereals rich in dietary fiber [20]. Diets fulfilling these attributes have been shown to be associated with many, if not all, of the benefits attributed to the Mediterranean diet, even when the foods have been consumed in the context of other dietary patterns. Furthermore, diets much higher in carbohydrate and lower in fat, but still within the recommended ranges, have also been associated with beneficial effects on measures of lipid and carbohydrate metabolism and other measures of cardiovascular risk.

When optimal benefits have been attributed to the Mediterranean diet beyond those observed on comparison diets, most frequently a low-fat, high-carbohydrate diet, the comparison diet has often not complied with the criteria specified in the recommendations. In particular, the carbohydrate consumed at the expense of fat may not have been high in dietary fiber and characterized by a low glycemic index. Thus, while it is conceivable that a particular aspect of the Mediterranean dietary pattern (e.g., the nature of the dietary fat or the blend of Mediterranean fruits and vegetables) explains unique benefit, it seems more likely that the Mediterranean diet affords a means of achieving nutrient and food goals. Only a direct comparison of dietary patterns with identical nutrient compositions could answer this question with any certainty. The question about whether a Mediterranean or comparable dietary pattern confers benefit over and above an appropriate low-fat, high-carbohydrate diet requires comparison with a diet where most of the dietary carbohydrate is derived from intact fruit and vegetables and whole-grain cereals rich in dietary fiber and with a low glycemic index.

Vegetarian and Vegan Diets

Epidemiological Aspects

In the United States, the first Adventist Health Study was established in the late 1950s. Early reports suggested that Adventists, who were vegetarian, had much lower rates of mortality due to CHD than those who were meat eaters [21]. The second cohort of Adventists was assembled about 15 years later and examined fatal and nonfatal events [22]. This confirmed lower rates of CHD and diabetes among vegetarians compared with nonvegetarian Adventists [23,24]. Subsequent cohort studies have attempted to compare mortality and health outcomes of vegetarians who were not necessarily members of a single religious denomination with comparable healthy cohorts who were meat eaters. For example, the Oxford Vegetarian Study compared volunteers, most of whom were members of the British Vegetarian Study with a cohort made up of their friends, family members, and colleagues who were meat eaters [25]. This approach did indeed generate cohorts that were well matched in terms of socioeconomic status, smoking habits, and other lifestyle practices, but not surprisingly, the healthy lifestyles of both cohorts resulted in remarkably low standardized mortality rates (SMRs) in respect to both total and most cause-specific mortality. The small number of deaths and associated relatively wide confidence intervals made comparisons between the cohorts difficult; however, several studies and a meta-analysis did suggest reduced rates of ischemic heart disease among vegetarians compared with healthy controls [26].

There is a considerable body of data, based on cross-sectional comparisons between vegetarians and meat eaters, relating to risk factors for cardiovascular disease and diabetes. Much attention has centered around lipid levels with significantly lower levels of total and LDL-cholesterol reported among vegetarians [27]. In addition, vegetarians tend to be less overweight [28], have lower levels of blood pressure [29] and blood glucose (even among nondiabetics) [30], and are more insulin sensitive compared with comparable groups of meat eaters [31]. Given that these are important risk factors for cardiovascular disease and diabetes, it might be expected that disease rates would be low among vegetarians. Where data for vegans (those who refrain from eating eggs and dairy products, in addition to avoidance of meat, meat products and fish) have been considered separately from vegetarians, differences between vegans and meat eaters with regard to all of these risk factors is more striking [27]. Epidemiologic approaches have also been used in attempts to disentangle the extent to which avoidance of meat rather than other aspects of the vegetarian or vegan diets explain the improved risk factor status and probable reduced risk of cardiovascular disease and diabetes. In addition to the total avoidance of meat, fish, and products derived from them, the vegetarian diet is generally characterized by high intakes of grain, vegetables, fruits, and nuts. Thus, it tends to be very low in saturated fat, though not necessarily total fat since vegetable oils are not necessarily restricted. Consumption of eggs, milk, and dairy products tends to be variable with some vegetarians eating substantial quantities, whereas "strict" vegetarians and vegans eat, respectively, little or none of these foods. (Note that many of these attributes are shared with the Mediterranean dietary pattern.) Several of these attributes, notably high consumption of whole-grain cereals [31] and nuts [32] have been shown in cohort studies, including both vegetarians and nonvegetarians, to be protective against ischemic heart disease and diabetes. A high ratio of dietary unsaturated to saturated fatty acids (a consistent feature of vegetarian diets) is also associated with a reduced risk of CHD [33].

Thus far, none of the epidemiologic studies has provided convincing evidence that avoidance of meat and meat products are associated with advantages to human health beyond those conferred by the other attributes of the vegetarian and vegan dietary patterns. The data certainly do not exclude a small protective effect and it is quite conceivable that the risk reduction conferred on both vegetarian and healthy control groups by the aggregated effect of protective dietary and other lifestyle-related factors overwhelm any specific advantageous effect of vegetarianism per se. Our own, admittedly limited, data suggest that the most striking difference between vegetarians and health conscious meat eating controls is the appreciably lower intake of saturated fat and consequently increased ratio of unsaturated to saturated fatty acids and that this, rather than meat avoidance is likely to explain the benefit in terms of lipid profile and reduced risk of cardiovascular disease [33,34].

Intervention Studies

There have been no randomized controlled trials that have examined the effects of vegetarianism or veganism on risk of developing coronary heart disease or diabetes but a series of carefully conducted randomized studies in western Australia confirmed the potential of a vegetarian diet to reduce blood pressure. Of particular relevance was the fact that none of the readily identifiable individual elements, including meat avoidance, generated blood pressure lowering; levels were reduced only with implementation of the whole dietary package [35].

Barnard et al. compared the effects of a very low fat vegan diet and a standard American Diabetes Association diet in individuals with type 2 diabetes [36]. There appeared to be a greater improvement in glycemic control as well as LDL-cholesterol in those randomized to the vegan diet, compared with those advised to follow the American Diabetes Association diet, especially among those whose hypoglycemic and lipid-lowering medications were not altered. Weight loss was appreciably greater on the vegan diet and this appeared to explain the differences in both glycemic control and lipid levels. While this study confirms the suitability of a vegan dietary pattern in the management of type 2 diabetes, it does not demonstrate benefit in terms of meat avoidance since many of the other attributes of vegetarianism and veganism have been shown to improve measures of carbohydrate and lipid metabolism and other indicators of cardiovascular and diabetes risk in healthy individuals and those with diabetes.

Interpretation

Epidemiologic and intervention studies confirm the potential of vegetarian and vegan diets to reduce the risk of diabetes and cardiovascular disease and the suitability of these dietary patterns in the treatment of diabetes. However, as is the case with the Mediterranean dietary pattern, it is not possible to say what, if any, benefit accrues from avoidance of meat and animal products as distinct from the many other cardioprotective attributes of vegetarian and vegan diets, which have also been clearly demonstrated to reduce the risk of diabetes and improve glycemia and cardiovascular risk factors in those with the condition. However, it is important to note, given that many vegetarians have high carbohydrate intakes, that high fiber, low glycemic index carbohydrates derived from intact fruit and vegetables and whole-grain cereals should form the bulk of total dietary carbohydrate. If diets are high in sugars and rapidly digested starches, similar benefits will probably not occur. Indeed, it is likely that triglycerides will rise and HDL levels fall.

Conclusion

Mediterranean and vegetarian (including vegan) dietary patterns are suitable for reducing the risk of cardiovascular disease and diabetes, as well as in the treatment of diabetes. The improvement in cardiovascular risk factors and diabetes risk and the reduction in glycemia is undoubtedly considerably due to the fact that both dietary patterns are conducive to weight loss in the overweight and obese and to the maintenance of weight loss. It is clearly established that many of the attributes of these dietary patterns (low ratio of saturated to cis-unsaturated fatty acids, high intake of fiber-rich vegetables, fruit and whole-grain cereals) have the potential to further reduce risk and improve measures of lipid and carbohydrate metabolism independently of any effect on body weight. Whether avoidance of meat, fish, and products derived from them or the unique blend of foods involved in the Mediterranean or vegetarian dietary pattern provides specific benefit independently of the other attributes remains unanswered and likely to remain so for the foreseeable future. In order to achieve the maximum benefit from these dietary patterns, it is important that carbohydrate should be derived principally from vegetables, fruit, and whole-grain cereals. Carbohydrate-containing foods should be high in dietary fiber and have a low glycemic index. Sugars and rapidly digested starches confer little benefit other than as energy sources. Vegetarian and vegan diets, previously considered by some to be nutritionally inadequate, have the potential to provide adequate intake of energy, micronutrients, and essential macronutrients. However, those following a vegan or very strict vegetarian diet may require specialist advice.

Selected References

2. World Health Organization. Diet, nutrition and the prevention of chronic diseases. Report of a Joint WHO/FAO Expert Consultation. WHO Technical Report Series 916, Geneva: WHO; 2003.

3. Nutrition and your health. Dietary Guidelines for American Home and Garden Bulletin No.228. Washington: US Department of Agriculture and Department of Health and Human Services; 2005.

12. Willett WC. The Mediterranean diet: science and practice. Public Health Nutr 2006;9(1A):105–110.

20. Mann JI, De Leeuw I, Hermansen K, et al. Evidence-based nutritional approaches to the treatment and prevention of diabetes mellitus. Nutr Metab Cardiovasc 2004;14:373–94.

34. Mann JI, Appleby PN, Key TJ, et al. Dietary determinants of ischaemic heart disease in health conscious individuals. Heart 1997;78s:450–5.

CHAPTER 16

Physical Activity and Risk of Cardiovascular Diseases

Eduardo Farinaro, Elisabetta Della Valle, & Roberto Grimaldi
Federico II University, Naples, Italy

Introduction

For more than 2 million years, humans have evolved throughout hundreds of thousands of generations and their genes have changed very little over time. Originally, genes were designed for men and women to live in caves, to eat plants they gathered and animals they killed, and moreover, to run around naked. During ancient times, it could have been an advantage to have a thrifty gene pattern that allowed them to store glucose and lipids. The saved energy could have been used in case of lack of food consumption [1–2].

Nowadays, lifestyle has changed dramatically; civilization and education have helped people become flexible and adapt to different foods and biological mechanisms that allow a balance between caloric intake and energy expenditure (EE). Only in the past few decades, human genes have needed to figure out how to metabolize a very rich diet high in calories, in lipids, particularly saturated fats, in salt, and in refined sugars. On the other hand, a lack of exercise within the frame of a sedentary lifestyle elicits an abnormal phenotype expression. New technologies and the automation of many daily activities in modern societies have greatly contributed to reduced physical activity (PA) at work and home; therefore, reduced EE together with a greater availability of food has led to a positive energy balance and a consequent increase in body weight.

As a result of a greater body weight, mean plasma lipids, blood pressure, and heart rate values can increase and have a substantial impact on carbohydrate absorption and insulin metabolism [3–8]. The modern genome has evolved within a frame of a physically active lifestyle and is programmed to settle in the body with an adequate amount of PA. Contrary to ancient occupations, jobs in industrialized societies demand less physical energy. In other words, our genes expect the body to be in a physically active state to function normally, and consequently chronic inactivity is abnormal from a physiological point of view. Practically, ancient human genes have collided with a modern affluent environment, causing the human phenotype to change.

Many epidemiological observations support the thesis that chronic degenerative diseases, particularly cardiovascular diseases (CVDs), are not prevalent in societies where PA is largely represented in daily life [9–11].

Along with the amount and quality of caloric intake, reduced PA can be considered one of the factors that determine CVD. Its role is extremely important for energy balance in humans.

In the fourth century B.C., the importance of food and exercise to achieve positive health was first documented by Hippocrates. In one of his writings titled, "About Regimen" [12], he states that it was essential to understand one's own primary constitution and the influence of different foods. He believed that food consumption was not enough to accomplish a long-term healthy life. He considered exercise to be crucial, and that one should be aware of the effects; nevertheless, he wrote that if the body

Nutritional and Metabolic Bases of Cardiovascular Disease, 1st edition.
Edited by Mario Mancini, José M. Ordovas, Gabriele Riccardi,
Paolo Rubba and Pasquale Strazzullo. © 2011 Blackwell Publishing Ltd.

lacked in either food or exercise, it would become ill. Finally, he strongly suggested that although a good diet was key for humans, physical exercise was even more vital to thwart off excessive nutrition and achieve a healthy long-term life expectancy.

In the last century, and in a more scientific fashion, some comprehensive reviews of the relationship between PA and all-cause mortality support the suggestion of an inverse linear relationship with level of activity. Moderate levels of regular PA are associated with lower mortality rates: EE of about 1,000 calories/wk is associated with a 30% reduction of all-cause mortality [13–19].

The very close association of hypertension, hyperlipidemia, overweight, diabetes, and coronary heart diseases (CHDs) with lack of physical exercise at work and during leisure time has made the sedentary lifestyle a significant risk factor for CVDs [20–23].

Currently, intense PA during occupations throughout industrialized societies has almost vanished; therefore, leisure-time PA is now an important factor in the prevention of CVDs. A relationship between physical inactivity and coronary artery disease has been clearly demonstrated. The lack of regular exercise is a factor contributing to the process of heart disease in a cause–effect manner; a sedentary person is almost twice as likely to develop heart disease compared to a very active individual. A number of studies have demonstrated that holding all the risk factors constant, there is a lower mortality rate among persons engaging regularly in PA than those with a sedentary lifestyle [24–26].

Definitions

Physical activity is usually defined as the movement of the body produced by skeletal muscles that results in EE.

Physical exercise is a structured, programmed, and repetitive movement and is finalized to maintain or improve physical fitness.

Physical fitness is the ability to perform physical activities that require aerobic fitness, endurance, strength, or flexibility without undue fatigue and is determined by a combination of regular activity and genetically inherited ability.

Health is physical, mental, and social well-being, not simply absence of disease.

A sedentary lifestyle is defined as engaging in no leisure-time PA in 2-week period.

Physical inactivity is a level of activity not sufficient to maintain good health.

Measures

PA shares many aspects with diet, and the methods required to assess regular PA encounter the same difficulties.

The intensity of PA indicates the level of physical exertion while executing the activity. Absolute intensity represents the overall rate of EE performing the PA. Metabolic equivalents (METs) are units used to express EE. One MET is the rate at which a person burns kilocalories at rest: This is approximately 1 kcal/kg of body weight/hr (expressed as 1 kcal/kg/hr). A MET also is defined as oxygen uptake in ml/kg/min and one MET is 3.5 ml/kg/min.

Any activity that burns less than 3 METs is considered light PA (walking or housekeeping).

Any activity that burns 3–6 METs is considered moderate-intensity PA; these levels are equal to the effort for an individual while walking briskly, dancing, swimming, or bicycling.

Any activity that burns 6–9 METs is considered vigorous-intensity PA; these levels are equal to the effort for an individual while participating in high-impact aerobic dancing, jogging, or uphill bicycling.

A second way of monitoring PA intensity is to determine whether a person's heart rate is within the target zone during PA. The maximum heart rate is based on the person's age; an estimate of maximum age-related heart rate can be obtained by subtracting the person's age from 220. For example, for a 35-year-old person, the estimated maximum age-related heart rate would be calculated as $220 - 35$ years $= 185$ beats per minute (bpm). For moderate-intensity PA, a person's target heart rate should be 65%–74% of his or her maximum heart rate. The 65% and 74% levels would be for a 35-year-old person:

65% level: $185 \times 0.65 = 120.25$

74% level: $185 \times 0.74 = 136.9$

For vigorous-intensity PA, a person's target heart rate should be more than 75% of his or her maximum heart rate.

Another method to asses PA intensity is oxygen requirement in ml/kg/min (%VO_2 max). VO_2 max is the maximum amount of oxygen in milliliters that one can use in one minute per kilogram of body weight during intense, whole-body exercise. Since oxygen consumption is linearly related to EE, when we measure oxygen consumption, we are indirectly measuring an individual's maximal capacity to do aerobic work.

Those who are fit have higher VO_2 max values and can exercise more intensely than those who are not as well conditioned. For light PA, a person's target VO_2 should be 20% to 39% of his or her VO_2 reserve % (VO_2 reserve $= VO_2$ max $- VO_2$ at rest); for moderate-intensity PA, VO_2 should be 40%–59% of VO_2 reserve %; for vigorous-intensity PA, VO_2 should be more than 60% of VO_2 reserve %.

Epidemiologic Evidence

The epidemiology of CHD during the mid-1900s did not take account of hearty PA as a means of prevention. In 1953, Morris et al. carried out a study on bus drivers and conductors, postal clerks, and postmen in London. They discovered that the postmen and conductors, who led a more active daily lifestyle, had 73% the rate of recurrence of CHD that was observed in the other two less active occupations [27,28]. Although these early findings could have been influenced by various factors and that the study approach was obviously not the same as today, the positive results deriving from PA since then have gained important recognition.

In 1960, Paffenbarger began investigating the exercise habits of more than 50,000 University of Pennsylvania and Harvard University alumni. In his report, on a subsample of 17,000 male alumni who entered college between 1916 and 1950, he found that moderate aerobic exercise, equivalent to about a 5-km jog per day, promotes good health and may increase life expectancy. In 1986 he showed that people who exercised more had an improved health profile; for example, the mortality rates were 21% lower for men who walked 9 km or more per week than for men who walked 5 km or less. Furthermore, lifespan was increased in men practicing a light sport activity compared to their sedentary counterparts.

The extent of decreased risk of CHD attributable to regular PA is similar to that of other lifestyle factors, such as abstaining from cigarette smoking [29]. Regular PA prevents or delays the development of high blood pressure [30], and exercise reduces blood pressure in people with hypertension; it can also lower blood cholesterol with the possibility of decreasing the risk of developing CVD [31]. The following mechanisms are considered to be important in understanding why PA positively affects cardiovascular risk: First, PA increases myocardial oxygen supply, improves myocardial contraction, and improves myocardial electrical stability. Second, PA increases HDL levels, decreases LDL and very-LDL levels, and blood coagulability, lowers blood pressure, increases insulin sensitivity, ameliorates endothelial function, and lowers heart rate [30–34].

Regular PA, fitness, and exercise are critically important for the health and well being of people of all ages. Research has demonstrated that virtually all individuals can benefit from regular PA, whether they participate in vigorous exercise or some type of moderate health-enhancing PA. Even among very old adults, mobility can be improved through PA. Recent studies have demonstrated that a moderate or high level of PA is also associated with a reduced risk of total and cardiovascular mortality among patients with type 2 diabetes [35]. The power of PA to predict CHD or all-cause mortality was investigated in the Seven Countries Study in 1980 by Keys in a cohort of men 40–59 years of age at study baseline between 1958 and 1964. In this report [36], PA of participants was basically at work with almost no significant activity during leisure time. The findings indicated that in Italian rural cohorts, in railroad workers from Rome and in a Greek sample, higher mortality was related to a higher prevalence of sedentary lifestyle. However, the report failed to demonstrate that levels of PA have a great magnitude on the wide range in population rate of mortality or morbidity for CHD.

The Women's Health Study [37] presents a comprehensive assessment of established risk factors and inflammatory/hemostatic biomarkers to lower cardiovascular risk at different degrees of PA in more than 27,000 women. Although the details of the process are still unknown, investigators have discovered that elevated levels of PA are linked to fewer CVD accidents.

Subsequently, in a recent report, light activities (<3 METs) were not associated with reduced mortality rates, moderate activities (3–6 METs) appeared somewhat beneficial, and vigorous activities (≥6 METs) clearly predicted lower mortality rates. These data fairly support current recommendations that emphasize moderate intensity activity; they also clearly indicate a benefit from vigorous activity [38].

It is possible to evaluate the effect of leisure-time PA in a number of anthropometric, metabolic and cardiovascular variables known to be involved in the etiology of CHD.

A dose–response correlation between CHD risk factors and physical exercise at vigorous intensity was assessed in 8,283 male runners in the National Runners' Health Study [39]. Long-distance runners (≥80 km/wk) revealed a 2.5-fold augmented prevalence of clinically established excessive levels of HDL-cholesterol, compared to their counterparts who ran less than 16 km/wk. To disrupt the development of coronary artery disease, researchers have discovered that it is important to consume about 1,600 kcal/wk. Moreover, patients with heart disease who burned 2,200 kcal/wk were found to have reduced plaque [33,40].

In the Duncan study [41], results have supported findings that have already been reported: Considerable improvements in cardiorespiratory fitness were obtained in a group that performed approximately 60–90 min/wk of brisk walking or 90 min/wk of leisurely paced walking; significant improvements in fitness and lipoprotein outcomes at 6 months were achieved only by the group practicing the higher intensity and frequency volume of exercise. In this study, the high-intensity, high-frequency prescription was the only intervention that produced a significant effect on HDL-C level compared with the level of PA of the other group. These findings are similar to those of Kraus et al. [42] who observed significant increases in HDL-C level over 8 months for high-intensity, high-volume exercise, but not for high-intensity, low-volume or for low-intensity, low-volume exercise. Another interesting study on 73,743 postmenopausal women enrolled in the Women's Health Initiative Observational Study demonstrated a relation between hours spent sitting and the risk of cardiovascular events [43], and both walking and

hardy exercise were key elements in reducing CVDs.

Recent studies have demonstrated that regular PA may have beneficial effects on a number of metabolic parameters clustered in the insulin resistance syndrome; any intervention aimed at increasing PA could help reduce cardiovascular risk and play a role in decreasing the specific cause of mortality.

In the 22-year follow-up of the Olivetti Heart Study, participants were divided into two subgroups: Group 1 consisted of 588 men who did not practice any sport or spend less than 1 hr/wk of PA during their leisure time; group 2 consisted of 146 men who spent 1–4 hr/wk on sporting activities (an average of 2.5 hr/wk, the most frequent activities being soccer, tennis, cycling, and jogging). The sedentary group had frequently higher mean values for all of the anthropometric and metabolic variables: namely umbilicus circumference, subscapular and triceps skinfold, heart rate, blood pressure, serum cholesterol, serum triglyceride, serum glucose, serum insulin, and homeostasis model assessment (HOMA). Even in overweight and obese men, physical exercise seemed to have a favorable influence on the risk factor levels [44,45].

Recommendation

In industrialized countries, almost half of the population does not participate in leisure-time activities and, as a possible consequence, has a lower life expectancy and an increased risk of premature death from heart disease and other chronic conditions. It is obvious that healthcare costs for prevention, diagnosis, and treatment of related diseases have an important impact on the economy of a country. In addition, the expenses associated with lack of working days for illness and disability should also be considered, as well as the value of premature deaths [46]. Together with diet modification, no single intervention has greater promise than physical exercise for reducing the risk of all chronic diseases, CVDs included.

The American College of Sport Medicine (ACSM) was an early leader in providing specific exercise recommendations, especially on the development of frequency, intensity, time and type of exercise. Before 1995, PA guidelines had stated a frequency of 3 days a week at vigorous intensity to improve body composition and physical fitness.

The Centers for Disease Control and Prevention (CDC) and the ACSM report published in 1995 has been the next major development in public health recommendations for PA: It was established that the frequency should be at least 5 days/wk of moderate-intensity PA for 30 minutes, even if performed more than once (at least 10 minutes); moreover, it was reported that engaging in extra physical activities would provide additional health benefits. Although the optimal intensity of activity remains unclear, there is evidence that the intensity of PA is inversely and linearly associated with mortality [47].

The question is how much PA is important to have a positive effect on CVD. What intensity, and at what frequency?

Frequency expresses how many days per week PA should be done; duration is the time spent working out; intensity is the effort required for a specific activity.

The product of intensity, duration, and frequency gives the amount the activity; the measure of this amount is the total EE expressed in calories per week.

Recently, many reviews have emphasized that, in evaluating the effects on the health, total amount of PA is more important rather than intensity, frequency, and duration.

The findings of the Harvard Alumni Study [19,38] could be a fundamental milestone to give a reasonable answer to many of these questions. This study shows that the death rate drops when walking 1 mi/day and continues to go down after a distance of 2 or 3 mi/day. After 3 mi, the death rate reaches a plateau.

One mile per day or any other aerobic activity with almost 700 calories cumulatively spent per week is proven to be beneficial to the health, two miles (1,400 calories) is better still, and three (2,100 calories) is better yet.

In conclusion, positive health benefits are achieved when moderate levels of PA are performed on a regular basis. There are also many advantages for people who have always led a sedentary lifestyle and decide to change; however, many people find it difficult to include PA in their daily lives.

A possible successful approach should involve mass information and education strategies; in schools, worksites, and community centers, adoption and maintenance of healthy lifestyle behaviors should be emphasized in order to help anyone understand the importance of and implement recommendations on physical exercise for better health.

Selected References

13. Thompson PD. Exercise and physical activity in the prevention and treatment of atherosclerotic cardiovascular disease. Arterioscler Thromb Vasc Biol 2003;23: 1319–21.

25. Fletcher GF, Balady G, Blair SN, et al. Statement on exercise. Benefits and recommendations for physical activity programs for all Americans. A statement for health professionals by the Committee on Exercise and Cardiac Rehabilitation of the Council on Clinical Cardiology, American Heart association. Circulation 1996;94:857–62.

33. Warburton DE, Nicol CW, Bredin SS. Health benefits of physical activity: the evidence. CMAJ 2006;174:801–9.

37. Mora S, Cook N, Buring JE, et al. Physical activity and reduced risk of cardiovascular events: potential mediating mechanisms. Circulation 2007;116:2110–8.

44. Della Valle E, Stranges S, Trevisan M, et al. Self-rated measures of physical activity and cardiovascular risk in a sample of Southern Italian male workers: the Olivetti heart study. Nutr Metab Cardiovasc Dis 2004;14: 143–9.

CHAPTER 17

Physical Exercise in the Prevention and Treatment of Obesity, Diabetes, and Metabolic Syndrome

Virginie Messier[1], *Anne-Sophie Brazeau*[1,2],
Rémi Rabasa-Lhoret[1,2,3], *& Antony Karelis*[4]

[1]University of Montreal, Montreal, QC, Canada
[2]Centre de Recherche du Centre Hospitalier de l'Université de Montréal, Montreal, QC, Canada
[3]Montreal Diabetes Research Center, Montreal, QC, Canada
[4]University of Quebec at Montreal, Montreal, QC, Canada

Introduction

During the past half century, there has been a dramatic increase in the incidence of obesity [1], the metabolic syndrome [2], and type 2 diabetes [3]. There is no doubt that physical inactivity is directly linked to this rising incidence of obesity [4], the metabolic syndrome [5], and type 2 diabetes [6]. Accordingly, it has been shown that higher levels of physical activity decreases the risk of developing obesity [7], the metabolic syndrome, and type 2 diabetes [8]. Moreover, aerobic exercise (walking, jogging, or cycling) produces beneficial effects on glycemic control, insulin sensitivity, lipid abnormalities, hypertension [9], and cardiorespiratory fitness [4,10]. Furthermore, resistance training has been shown to increase muscle mass and muscle strength (up to 60%), which may induce beneficial changes in insulin sensitivity [11–14], resting metabolic rate [14], and total energy expenditure [15]. Collectively, exercise, whether aerobic, and resistance training could be used as a non harmacological therapeutic approach for the prevention and treatment of obesity, the metabolic syndrome, and type 2

diabetes. Therefore, in this chapter, we review the effects of aerobic and/or resistance training on the prevention and treatment of obesity, the metabolic syndrome, and type 2 diabetes (Table 17.1).

Obesity

Over the past 20 years, the prevalence of obesity has increased significantly in North America and Europe, a trend that now appears to be increasing at an alarming rate across most age groups [16]. Moreover, obesity is associated with increased risk of developing dyslipidemia, hypertension, joint disorders, digestive disease, diabetes, and cardiovascular disease. Finally, obesity has now been recognized as a serious public health problem. Thus, strategies for the prevention and treatment of obesity such as exercise training must be a high public health priority.

Role of Physical Activity in the Prevention of Obesity

Using data from the Coronary Artery Risk Development in Young Adults (CARDIA) and the National Health and Nutrition Examination Surveys, it was reported that in average Americans gained 0.45–0.90 kg/yr [1]. Results of epidemiologic studies are consistent in that those who are physically active are less likely to gain weight over

Nutritional and Metabolic Bases of Cardiovascular Disease, 1st edition.
Edited by Mario Mancini, José M. Ordovas, Gabriele Riccardi,
Paolo Rubba and Pasquale Strazzullo. © 2011 Blackwell Publishing Ltd.

Table 17.1 Comparison of the effects of aerobic and resistance training on obesity, metabolic syndrome and type 2 diabetes.

Variables	Obesity		Metabolic syndrome		Type 2 diabetes	
	Aerobic training	Resistance training	Aerobic training	Resistance training	Aerobic training	Resistance training
Body composition						
Body weight	↓	↓	↓↔	↔	↓↔	↔
Muscle mass	↑↔	↑	↔	↔	↔	↑
Fat mass	↓	↓	↓↔	↔	↓	↓↔
Abdominal obesity	↓	↓↔	↓	↔	↓	↓
Serum lipids						
High-density lipoprotein	↑↔	↔	↔	↔	↑↔	↔
Low-density lipoprotein	↔	↔	↔	↔	↔	↔
Blood pressure						
Diastolic blood pressure	↓	↓	↓↔	↔	↓↔	↓↔
Systolic blood pressure	↓	↓	↓↔	↔	↓↔	↓↔
Glucose metabolism						
Fasting glucose	↔	↔	↓↔	↔	↓	↓
Fasting insulin	↔	↔	↓↔	↓↔	↓	↔
Insulin sensitivity	↑	↔	↔	↔	↑	↑
HbA$_{1c}$	N/A	N/A	N/A	N/A	↓	↓
Cardiorespiratory fitness	↑	↔	↑	↔	↑	↔
Muscle strength	↑	↑	↔	↑	↑	↑

↑ indicates increased; ↓, decreased; and ↔, negligible effect.

time than those who are not [7]. Accordingly, it was previously shown that individuals who were either inactive [17], reduced their physical activity [17], or presented lower levels of cardiorespiratory fitness [18], an objective measure of recent physical activity patterns, gained weight over time, whereas those who were physically active maintained or lost weight.

However, there is a lack of studies that address the question of how much, what type, what intensity and what frequency of physical activity are required to prevent weight gain. It was proposed that increasing physical activity by 100 kcal/day could prevent weight gain in most of the population [1]. This is comparable to 1.0–1.5 mi of walking (15–20 minutes) or an additional 2,000 steps/day [1].

Role of Aerobic Exercise in the Treatment of Obesity

Weight loss can be achieved by reducing energy intake, increasing energy expenditure by practicing physical activity, or both. In the past decade, intensive research was undertaken to determine if exercise without caloric restriction could induce weight loss and decrease the metabolic risks associated with obesity [10,19,20]. For example, a 14-week randomized, controlled trial was conducted to determine the independent effect of diet or exercise weight loss on obesity and insulin resistance in moderately obese women [20]. Participants were randomized to one of the following groups: control, diet weight loss, exercise weight loss, and exercise without weight loss. Weight loss occurred only in the diet-induced weight loss and exercise-induced weight loss groups and represented approximately 6.5% of initial body weight. The reduction in total fat and the increase in skeletal muscle mass were greater in the exercise-induced weight-loss group. Moreover, the reduction in total abdominal fat and abdominal subcutaneous fat within the exercise-induced weight loss was more important than within all other groups. Visceral fat was also decreased in the three interventions groups, but there was no difference between the groups. Interestingly, glucose disposal improved only within the exercise-induced weight-loss group. The results of this study demonstrate that 1) in comparison with a diet-induced weight loss, equivalent exercise-induced weight loss is associated with greater reduction in total fat and abdominal fat; 2) exercise without weight loss was associated with significant reductions in total, abdominal, and visceral fat. Furthermore, it was reported that 12 months of moderate-intensity aerobic exercise reduced body weight (-1.3 kg), body fat (-1.4 kg), and increased cardiorespiratory fitness by 11.7% (19). In addition, this study showed that individuals who were highly active (>195 min/wk) lost 4.2% of total body fat compared to 0.6% in low-active individuals ($\leq$135 min/wk). A similar trend of total body fat loss with increasing cardiorespiratory levels was observed.

Furthermore, the separate and combined effects of the amount of exercise and exercise intensity on weight loss in overweight and mildly obese men and women were investigated in the Studies of Targeted Risk Reduction Interventions through Defined Exercise (STTRIDE) [21]. In this 8-month aerobic exercise program, subjects were randomized to one of three exercise training groups: high amount/vigorous intensity, low amount/vigorous intensity, and low amount/moderate intensity. The results of this study showed that the high-amount/vigorous-intensity group had better changes in weight, fat mass, skinfolds (abdominal, suprailiac, and thigh), and waist circumference. These results suggest that exercise amount and intensity could determine total body weight change and fat mass loss in obese individuals.

Even though studies show no weight loss after aerobic training, there is an improvement in fat mass loss [4,22]. For example, it was reported that 13 weeks of aerobic exercise was not associated with a change in body weight in middle-age men [4]. However, there was a decrease in waist circumference, total fat mass, and visceral fat content. Moreover, in the same study, an increase in cardiorespiratory fitness and muscle mass as well as a decrease in muscle lipid infiltration was observed. These results suggest that, despite the absence of weight loss, a moderate-intensity aerobic program decreases the

metabolic risk associated with obesity. Finally, aerobic training is associated with improvement in high-density lipoprotein (HDL)-cholesterol [22], blood pressure [22], and cardiorespiratory fitness [10] in obese individuals. Thus, these observations provide strong support for the recommendation of aerobic exercise with or without weight loss as an effective strategy for the treatment of obesity.

While examining the role of exercise in the treatment of obesity, it is also important to consider at the effects of different exercise intensity. The fuel used as a source of energy during exercise depends on the exercise intensity [23]. It has been reported that plasma free fatty acids are the primary fuel source when exercise is perform at low intensity (25%–40% of $VO_{2\,peak}$). Moderate-intensity exercise ($\sim$65% of $VO_{2\,peak}$) uses plasma free fatty acids in addition to glycogen and possibly intramuscular fat. At high-intensity, exercise relies more on glycogen stores than on fat. Thus, it would be reasonable to suggest that exercise intensity may influence weight loss by altering which substrates provide the predominant fuel [23]. Moreover, exercise intensity could also affect the total energy expended in physical activity, with higher-intensity exercise expending more energy. Given that total energy expended is positively associated with weight loss, high-intensity exercise should have a larger impact on the composition of weight loss [23]. Furthermore, higher amounts of exercise training and intensity may have a positive impact on resting metabolism. That is, energy expenditure after exercise will last longer than the physical activity itself.

As described earlier, aerobic exercise is associated with improvements in cardiorespiratory fitness ($\sim$20%) [4,10]. Adequate levels of cardiorespiratory fitness in overweight and obese individuals are associated with lower risk of morbidity and mortality [24]. Moreover, studies have shown that higher levels of cardiorespiratory fitness are associated with lower insulin resistance in adults [25]. Accordingly, Gerson and Braun [25] observed that insulin resistance was 50% higher in obese women than in obese fit women. Furthermore, there was no difference in insulin resistance between lean fit and obese fit women suggesting that the deleterious consequences of high body fatness could be counteracted by high levels of cardiorespiratory fitness.

Role of Resistance Training in the Treatment of Obesity

Resistance training, which involves the voluntary activation of specific skeletal muscles against some form of external resistance, is an effective mode of exercise to increase muscle mass and strength. However, few studies have examined the role of resistance training without caloric restriction in the treatment of obesity [10,22]. For example, it was reported that 10 weeks of resistance training decreased the waist-to-hip ratio and percentage of body fat without any change in body weight in obese men [22]. Furthermore, resistance training was associated with an increase in fat-free mass. This increase in fat-free mass may increase resting metabolic rate and thus total energy expenditure.

However, if the goal is to produce weight loss, weight-lifting programs without caloric restriction are maybe not an effective strategy due to the increase in muscle mass associated with resistance training. Accordingly, it has been previously reported that individuals using resistance training programs as a weight-loss intervention actually gained weight [26].

Aerobic Versus Resistance Training in the Treatment of Obesity

In the previous paragraphs, we described the role of aerobic and resistance training in the treatment of obesity. However, is there a difference in the benefits of aerobic versus resistance training in the treatment of obesity? Banz et al. [22] observed that both resistance and aerobic training induced a decrease in waist-to-hip ratio after 10 weeks of training in obese men. However, in this study, only resistance training was associated with a decrease in percentage of body fat and an increase in fat-free mass. A second study showed that neither aerobic or resistance training alone reduced body weight, abdominal obesity, and blood pressure in obese women [10]. However, both aerobic and resistance training without caloric restriction resulted in improved performance and exercise capacity. While resistance training is more effective in improving muscle strength, aerobic training is effective in improving cardiorespiratory fitness. These results suggest that an optimal training program for the treatment of obesity may require both resistance and aerobic components [22].

Metabolic Syndrome

The metabolic syndrome is a cluster of metabolic risk factors that comprises hyperglycemia, dyslipidemia, abdominal obesity, and hypertension. Interestingly, a recent study reported that approximately 35% of U.S. adults have the metabolic syndrome according to the National Cholesterol Education Program and approximately 40% according to the International Diabetes Federation [27]. Furthermore, the metabolic syndrome increases the risk of type 2 diabetes, coronary artery disease, and premature mortality.

Association of Physical Components with the Metabolic Syndrome

It was previously shown that cardiorespiratory fitness was inversely associated with the prevalence of the metabolic syndrome after adjustment for potential confounding variables such as macronutrient intake [28]. Moreover, Lakka et al. [5] investigated the association of leisure-time physical activity and cardiorespiratory fitness with the metabolic syndrome in a sample of healthy middle-age men. The results of this study showed that a sedentary lifestyle and poor cardiorespiratory fitness were associated with the metabolic syndrome. Furthermore, it was reported that men in the lowest fitness category had a 6.4-fold increased risk for having the metabolic syndrome compared to men in the highest fitness category [5]. In addition, Jurca et al. [29] showed that muscular strength and cardiorespiratory fitness were inversely associated with the prevalence of the metabolic syndrome. Finally, results from the ATTICA study [30] showed that light-to-moderate leisure time physical activity was associated with a considerable decrease in the prevalence of the metabolic syndrome in men and women.

Role of Aerobic and Resistance Training in the Treatment of the Metabolic Syndrome

Currently, there is a lack of studies investigating specifically the role of exercise training in the treatment of the metabolic syndrome. To our knowledge, the effect of aerobic or resistance training on the metabolic syndrome characteristics was evaluated in three studies [31–33]. For example, the efficacy of aerobic training in treating the metabolic syndrome (based on the NCEP ATP III guidelines) in men and women was investigated in the HERITAGE Family Study [31]. The results of this study showed that 20 weeks of aerobic training decreased the percentage of participants with high triglycerides, high blood pressure, high glucose and high waist circumference. In addition, of the 105 participants with the metabolic syndrome before the intervention, 32 participants (30.5%) were no longer classified has having the metabolic syndrome after the aerobic training. Furthermore, of the participants who were no longer classified has having the metabolic syndrome, 43% reduced their triglycerides, 16% increased their HDL-C, 38% reduced their blood pressure, 9% reduced their blood glucose, and 28% reduced their waist circumference below the threshold values used to diagnose the metabolic syndrome.

Moreover, a study reported that 20 weeks of resistance or aerobic training improved glucose tolerance and reduced insulin responses to an oral glucose tolerance test in overweight sedentary men at high risk for coronary heart disease [32]. However, neither resistance nor aerobic training had an effect on lipoprotein lipids and blood pressure. Similarly, Watkins et al. [33] observed that hyperinsulinemic responses to an oral glucose tolerance test were improved following a 6-month aerobic training intervention in adults with the metabolic syndrome. In contrast, there was no change in blood pressure and lipoprotein-lipid responses. Taken together, these results suggest that exercise training is an effective strategy to treat the metabolic syndrome, which could decrease the risk of cardiovascular disease and type 2 diabetes.

It should be noted that there is no consensus on the amount of exercise and exercise intensity required to improve the characteristics of the metabolic syndrome. However, it has been previously reported that metabolic benefits are observed when regular exercise is performed frequently (3–5 times/wk), for a duration up to 60 minutes and at a low intensity (40%–60% of cardiorespiratory fitness) [2].

Diabetes

Even though exercise plays a major role in the treatment of type 1 diabetes, this section focuses on the effects of exercise training in the prevention and treatment of type 2 diabetes. Type 2 diabetes is a complex metabolic disorder characterized by fasting hyperglycemia and by elevated, normal, or low levels of insulin [6]. These metabolic abnormalities are caused mainly by defects at 3 major sites: altered insulin secretion from the β-cell, elevated hepatic glucose production, due to hepatic insulin resistance, and decreased peripheral glucose utilization due to skeletal muscle insulin resistance [6]. Moreover, type 2 diabetes can lead to various complications such as nephropathy, retinopathy, cerebrovascular and cardiovascular diseases.

Role of Physical Activity in the Prevention of Type 2 Diabetes

It is well established that physical inactivity is directly linked to the rising incidence of type 2 diabetes. Accordingly, it was demonstrated that every 2-hour/day increment in television watching was associated with a 14% increased risk of developing type 2 diabetes [34]. Conversely, each 1-hour/day spent doing brisk walking was associated with a 34% decreased risk of developing type 2 diabetes [34]. Moreover, it was previously reported that each 500 kcal/wk of self-reported leisure-time physical activity decreased the risk of diabetes by 6% [35]. Similarly, Manson et al. [8] showed that women who reported vigorous exercise at least once per week had a 33% lower risk of developing diabetes compared to women reporting no exercise. Finally, additional prospective observational studies have indicated a graded inverse association between levels of self-reported physical activity and the prevalence of type 2 diabetes [3]. However, cardiorespiratory fitness is stronger than self-reported physical activity as a predictor of several health outcomes. Accordingly, it is now well known that higher levels of fitness protect against the development of type 2 diabetes in men and women [36]. Although observational studies suggest that higher levels of physical activity or fitness are associated with reduced risk of developing diabetes, experimental studies are required to determine if higher levels of physical activity delay the progression of type 2 diabetes. Pan et al. [37] conducted a randomized trial in a group of Chinese individuals with impaired glucose tolerance to study the progression of type 2 diabetes over a 6-year period. Participants were randomized to one of these four intervention groups: control, diet, exercise, or diet plus exercise. The results of this study showed that participants in the exercise group were 46% less likely to develop diabetes than those in the control group and this was better than the risk reduction observed in the diet group (31%). Taken together, these results suggest that regular physical activity and higher levels of fitness may be a potential tool to prevent the development and delay the apparition of type 2 diabetes.

Role of Aerobic Exercise in the Treatment of Type 2 Diabetes

It has been previously shown that cardiorespiratory fitness is positively associated with insulin-stimulated glucose uptake in type 2 diabetic individuals. Therefore, aerobic exercise, by increasing cardiorespiratory fitness, could be a non pharmacological treatment for type 2 diabetes that may improve insulin sensitivity and glucose tolerance. Accordingly, Winnick et al. [38] studied the effects of short-term aerobic exercise on insulin sensitivity in obese individuals with type 2 diabetes. This study showed that while seven days of aerobic exercise did not affect endogenous glucose production and hepatic insulin sensitivity, it did increase whole-body insulin sensitivity. Moreover, it was reported that six months of supervised aerobic exercise decreased body mass index, body weight, total body fat and trunk fat in obese type 2 diabetic individuals [39]. Furthermore, a decrease in percent glycosylated hemoglobin (HbA$_{1c}$), fasting insulin, fasting glucose, insulin resistance, and plasma triglycerides and an increase in HDL-C were observed after the intervention. Similarly, 8 weeks of aerobic exercise was associated with a decreased HbA$_{1c}$ from 8.5% to 6.2% and a 46% increase in insulin sensitivity [40]. The acute effect of aerobic exercise on insulin sensitivity lasts 24–72 hours depending on the intensity and duration of exercise [3]. Therefore, physical activity should be performed on a daily basis.

Role of Resistance Training in the Treatment of Type 2 Diabetes

Traditionally, aerobic training has been recommended as the most suitable mode of exercise in the treatment of type 2 diabetes due to its effect on weight loss, improved glucose tolerance, and cardiorespiratory fitness. However, the American College of Sports Medicine [41] has recently recommended the use of progressive resistance training as part of an exercise program for individuals with type 2 diabetes. Therefore, several studies investigated the effect of resistance training on the metabolic profile, insulin sensitivity and glycemic control of patients with type 2 diabetes [12,13,26, 42,43]. Accordingly, it was reported that 16 weeks of prolonged resistance training at intensities of 50%–80% of 1-RM (one-repetition maximum) improved insulin sensitivity by 46.3% and decreased fasting blood glucose by 7.1% in older men with type 2 diabetes [13]. Moreover, increases in muscle strength and decreases in abdominal fat were observed after 16 weeks of prolonged resistance training. Furthermore, one study showed that a 3-month individualized progressive resistance training program improved HbA$_{1c}$ (8.8% to 8.2%) and increased muscle strength in patients with type 2 diabetes [43]. Noteworthy, reductions in HbA$_{1c}$ were strongly associated with muscle size suggesting that increases in muscle mass improve glycemic control. In addition, it was shown that 10 weeks of moderate-intensity resistance training improved glycemic control, decreased fasting insulin, and increased lean body mass in obese type 2 diabetic men [42]. However, 2-hour glucose, 2-hour insulin, and insulin sensitivity were not changed following the intervention. The authors explained the absence of change in insulin sensitivity by the fact that fasting and 2-hour samples were used to assess insulin sensitivity. In contrast, Honkola et al. [12] reported improvements in total cholesterol (−12%), LDL-cholesterol (−14%), and triglycerides (−20%) following 5 months of progressive resistance training in type 2 diabetic individuals.

Moreover, a randomized controlled trial was undertaken to determine the efficacy of high-intensity progressive resistance training on glycemic control in older adults with type 2 diabetes [26]. Sixty-two men and women with type 2 diabetes were randomized to 16 weeks of standard care (control group) or standard care plus resistance training. The results of this study showed that subjects in the resistance training group improved their plasma glycosylated hemoglobin levels by 12.6%. Furthermore, diabetic medication regimens were reduced in 22 of 31 (72%) subjects in the resistance training group. However, fasting plasma glucose, total cholesterol,

HDL-C, LDL-C, and triglycerides did not change following the intervention. Interestingly, this study also reported that the change in HbA_{1c} was associated with the change in lean tissue mass, trunk fat, and muscle strength, suggesting that resistance training reduces hyperglycemia by eliciting glucose uptake at the cellular level in skeletal muscle, where the largest proportion of glucose uptake takes place.

Collectively, these results suggest that resistance training could be a potential adjunct therapy in the management of type 2 diabetes. However, further studies are needed to determine the optimal volume and intensity of training required to induce changes in the metabolic profile of individuals with type 2 diabetes.

Role of Aerobic Training Versus Resistance Training in the Treatment of Type 2 Diabetes

Aerobic exercise has been advocated as the most suitable form of exercise for the treatment of type 2 diabetes, with many positive effects on glycemic control, insulin sensitivity, and lipid abnormalities [38–40]. However, recent evidence suggests that resistance training could also be a potential therapy for the management of type 2 diabetes [12,13,26, 43]. Cauza et al. [11] investigated the potential beneficial effects of strength training versus endurance training on insulin resistance, muscular mass and cardiorespiratory fitness in type 2 diabetic. This study showed that 4 months of strength training improved fasting blood glucose, HbA_{1c}, and insulin sensitivity, whereas 4 months of endurance training had no effects on these variables. Moreover, only strength training was associated with decreases in cholesterol, LDL-C, and triglycerides and increases in HDL-C. In addition, a reduction in systolic and diastolic blood pressure was observed in both groups. Furthermore, it was previously reported that 5 months of strength training improved glucose tolerance by 12% and insulin action by 22%, while 5 months of aerobic exercise increased glucose tolerance by 16% and insulin action by 16% [44]. Collectively, these results suggest that resistance or aerobic training are effective in the management of type 2 diabetes; however, resistance training alone appears to be a better therapeutic approach than aerobic training for the treatment of type 2 diabetes.

Combined Aerobic and Resistance Training in the Treatment of Type 2 Diabetes

The American Diabetes Association [3] and the American College of Sports Medicine [41] have recently recommended that a complete rehabilitation program for patients with diabetes should include both aerobic and resistance training. Therefore, studies were undertaken to determine the effects of a combined strength and aerobic exercise program on glycemic control and insulin sensitivity in type 2 diabetes. Accordingly, Tokmakidis et al. [45] reported that 4 months of strength and aerobic exercise improved glucose tolerance by 12.5% and insulin sensitivity by 38% in sedentary women with type 2 diabetes. Moreover, HbA_{1c} was reduced by 10.4% after 4 months of training. Improvements in upper-body strength (31.4%), lower-body strength (39.7%), and exercise tolerance (10.9%) were also observed after 4 months of training. Furthermore, it has been shown that 1 year of aerobic and resistance training was associated with decreased fasting blood glucose, total cholesterol, LDL-C, triglycerides, systolic blood pressure, and diastolic blood pressure and increased HDL-C [9]. Finally, the effects of aerobic and resistance training alone versus a sedentary control group, and the incremental effects of practicing both types of exercise versus aerobic or resistance training alone on glycemic control were assessed in the DARE study [46]. The primary findings of this study were that aerobic training and resistance training alone both improved glycemic control, and that the combination of these two forms of exercise further improved glycemic control. Thus, these results suggest that a proper exercise program for individuals with type 2 diabetes should combine aerobic and resistance training.

Proposed Physiological Mechanisms

Proposed physiological mechanisms by which aerobic and resistance training improve the metabolic profile and reduce the risk of obesity, the metabolic syndrome, and type 2 diabetes are summarized in Figure 17.1.

Aerobic training is a strong stimulus for mitochondrial biogenesis. Moreover, aerobic training

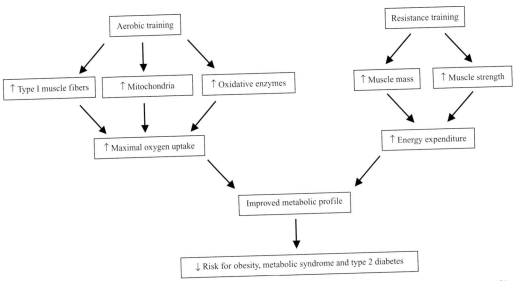

Figure 17.1 Proposed physiological mechanisms by which aerobic and resistance training improves the metabolic profile.

could increase oxidative enzymes and type I muscle fibers. The increase in mitochondria, oxidative enzymes along with increases in type I fibers are a potential mechanism by which aerobic training improves maximal oxygen uptake ($VO_{2\,max}$). Resistance training increases muscle mass and muscle strength, which could result in increased energy expenditure. Furthermore, increases in $VO_{2\,max}$ and energy expenditure could improve the metabolic profile of individuals, which could lead to a reduce risk for obesity, the metabolic syndrome and type 2 diabetes.

Conclusion

Evidence suggests that aerobic and resistance training are effective in the prevention and treatment of obesity, the metabolic syndrome, and type 2 diabetes. It should be noted that most of the studies described in this chapter were performed in a laboratory-based setting. It would be interesting to investigate whether physical activity practiced at home or in community facilities is also associated with metabolic improvements. In support of this hypothesis, it has been previously reported that center-based training was effective for maintaining improved glycemic control. In contrast, home-based training was not effective for maintaining improved glycemic control [47]. Furthermore, ad-

ditional work may be required to determine the appropriateness of physical activity for patients with type 2 diabetes patients who have ischemic heart disease or advanced diabetes complications such as neuropathy and retinopathy.

Finally, obesity, which has been linked to various chronic diseases, results in 300,000 deaths each year and causes $117 billion dollars worth of direct and indirect annual costs in the United States [10]. In addition, nearly 1 million deaths were attributed to type 2 diabetes worldwide in 2002 [48]. The American Diabetes Association estimates that the direct medical costs associated to diabetes were $92 billion and the indirect costs (disability, work loss, premature mortality) were $40 billion [48]. Thus, effective strategy such as exercise training for preventing and treating obesity and type 2 diabetes could provide important economic benefits for the healthcare system in addition to improving quality of life.

Selected References

16. World Health Organization: Obesity. Preventing and managing the global epidemic. Geneva: WHO; 1998.
19. Irwin ML, Yasui Y, Ulrich CM, et al. Effect of exercise on total and intra-abdominal body fat in postmenopausal women: a randomized controlled trial. JAMA 2003 Jan 15;289(3):323–30.

23. Votruba SB, Horvitz MA, Schoeller DA. The role of exercise in the treatment of obesity. Nutrition 2000 Mar;16(3):179–88.

34. Hu FB, Li TY, Colditz GA, Willett WC, Manson JE. Television watching and other sedentary behaviors in relation to risk of obesity and type 2 diabetes mellitus in women. JAMA 2003 Apr 9;289(14):1785–91.

48. LaMonte MJ, Blair SN, Church TS. Physical activity and diabetes prevention. J Applied Physiol 2005;99(3):1205–13.

CHAPTER 18

Functional Foods for Diabetes and Obesity

Gabriele Riccardi, Brunella Capaldo, & Olga Vaccaro

Federico II University, Naples, Italy

Introduction

Overweight and low physical activity are thought to be important risk factors for type 2 diabetes, cardiovascular diseases, and many other diseases highly prevalent in affluent societies; therefore, any strategy to prevent or treat these conditions should consider lifestyle modifications, including not only weight reduction and regular physical exercise but also changes in the nutrient composition of the diet [1]. However, sustained behavioral changes are difficult to achieve; as a matter of fact, the general trend in the last decades has been toward an increased prevalence of overweight and obesity in many populations, especially among children and adolescents, followed by a dramatic rise in the incidence of type 2 diabetes and other cardiovascular risk factors clustering in individuals with impaired insulin sensitivity. This represents the most plausible pathophysiological link between overweight (particularly with an abdominal localization of adiposity) on the one hand and type 2 diabetes or cardiovascular diseases on the other hand. The identification of food properties able to influence specific physiological functions relevant for fat accumulation, insulin sensitivity, and glucose control may be helpful in achieving long-term lifestyle changes aimed at the prevention or the management of overweight and type 2 diabetes. Once the health effects of foods have been identified, they should be communicated to the general public,

to help consumers benefit from this important information [2].

In affluent societies, nutrition science is at a new frontier since it is progressing from the concept of "adequate nutrition" (for survival) to that of "optimal nutrition" (for improving health). Plausible reasons are as follows:

- The increasing cost of healthcare
- The continuing increase in life expectancy
- The increase in the number of elderly people
- The pursuit of improved quality of life

In this respect functional foods able to influence body fat accumulation, insulin sensitivity, or blood glucose control may be helpful for the prevention and management of overweight and type 2 diabetes.

Foods can be regarded as functional if proven to affect beneficially one or more target functions in the body, beyond adequate nutritional effects, in a way relevant to improved state of health and well-being, reduction of risk of diseases, or both. The development of functional foods should be based on a sound scientific knowledge of the target function in the body and the demonstration of effects relevant to improved health or reduction of disease risk Table 18.1). The substantiation of health claims should be based primarily on human intervention data that show demonstrable effects consistent with the claim. They should have a scientifically valid design compatible with the purpose of the study [3].

In the field of weight regulation, the criteria for a valid design of an intervention trial aiming to evaluate the health impact of a food are largely the same as for testing a drug. In most cases (whenever

Nutritional and Metabolic Bases of Cardiovascular Disease, 1st edition. Edited by Mario Mancini, José M. Ordovas, Gabriele Riccardi, Paolo Rubba and Pasquale Strazzullo. © 2011 Blackwell Publishing Ltd.

Table 18.1 Categories of evidence that may be used in the substantiation process (PASSCLAIM Consensus).

Intervention
  Randomized controlled trials
  Clinical trials
  Physiological and psychological trials
Observational
  Prospective (cohort)
  Cross-sectional (analytical)
  Case-control
Supporting
  Animal
  In vitro cell and molecular
  Studies of genotype
  Modeling (of mechanism)

possible), the study has to be controlled (with a control group not exposed to the test food, with similar characteristics of the study participants) and randomized (the assignment to the test or to the control group are casual) (Table 18.2) [3–5].

Obviously, a food is much more complex than a drug, since it has more than one active ingredient and, moreover, carries a significant amount of energy; therefore, dietary studies often require that in order to compensate for the extra calories of the test food, other dietary components need to be reduced. In addition, it is very seldom possible to adopt a "double-blind" type of intervention, since both the patient and the investigator can identify who is in the experimental or in the control arm of the study. This makes the interpretation of the study results not as straightforward as for placebo-controlled pharmacological studies; however, these difficulties do not preclude the possibility of performing dietary intervention studies, with a valid design, able to support health claims at the highest level of scientific evidence [6,7].

A crucial aspect of human intervention studies is the number of participants. It should be high enough to allow the detection of a difference in the end-point, between the test and the control group that is statistically significant. Moreover, the difference in the end-point also has to be biologically meaningful. In other words, the magnitude of a difference in the end-point considered biologically meaningful has to be decided a priori; then, the sample size of the study group is calculated on the basis of the variability of the end-point within the population (which is known from previous studies). Obviously, the smaller the difference considered as biologically meaningful, the larger the

Table 18.2 Criteria for the scientific substantiation of claims (PASSCLAIM Consensus).

1 The food component to which the claimed effect is attributed should be characterized.
2 Substantiation of a claim should be based on human data, primarily from intervention studies the design of which should include the following considerations:
  (a) Study groups that are representative of the target group.
  (b) Appropriate controls.
  (c) An adequate duration of exposure and follow up to demonstrate the intended effect.
  (d) Characterization of the study groups' background diet and other relevant aspects of lifestyle.
  (e) An amount of the food or food component consistent with its intended pattern of consumption.
  (f) The influence of the food matrix and dietary context on the functional effect of the component.
  (g) Monitoring of subjects' compliance concerning intake of food or food component under test.
  (h) The statistical power to test the hypothesis.
3 When the true endpoint of a claimed benefit cannot be measured directly, studies should use markers.
4 Markers should be:
  — biologically valid in that they have a known relationship to the final outcome and their variability within the target population is known;
  — methodologically valid with respect to their analytical characteristics.
5 Within a study the target variable should change in a statistically significant way and the change should be biologically meaningful for the target group consistent with the claim to be supported.
6 A claim should be scientifically substantiated by taking into account the totality of the available data and by weighing the evidence.

sample size should be. Often, this is on the order of a magnitude of several hundreds. Also, the length of the trial represents a crucial aspect of a valid design, since the impact of nutrition on health is a long-term phenomenon [3].

According to the current definition for functional foods, different types of foods could be included in this category: 1) unmodified whole foods like fruit, vegetables, and whole-grain products rich in physiologically active components like fiber, β-carotene, and lycopene; 2) modified foods such as low-fat dairy products or "light foods" in which sugars have been replaced by sugar alcohols; 3) fortified foods such as those that have been enriched with nutrients or enhanced with phytochemicals or botanicals such as folate-enriched cereals or margarines additioned with plant sterols. However, by the appropriate use of food technology, more and more new functional foods will be developed and made available to consumers [8].

Functional Foods for Obesity

Obesity is now recognized as a chronic disease with a significant impact on quality and duration of people's life, globally producing major public health problems and thereby contributing significantly to health care costs. It represents the most important risk factor for type 2 diabetes; moreover, it impairs relevant body functions that eventually lead to dysfunctions involving the cardiovascular system, bones and joints, the reproductive system, and the gastrointestinal tract. However, there is strong evidence that weight loss in overweight and obese individuals reduces the risk for diseases and improves life expectancy at all ages [9–11].

In most European countries, the prevalence of obesity has increased by up to 40% in the past 10 years and is currently in the range of 10%–20% in men and 10%–25% in women. Any strategy to prevent or treat this disease should consider lifestyle modifications based on diet and regular physical exercise [9].

Functional foods might have a particularly high impact for prevention and/or treatment of overweight and obesity where, more than in many other fields, the link between nutrition, biological responses, and diseases is clearly established. Functional foods for obesity should be able to influence

the energy balance equation regulated by the control of energy intake and/or of energy dissipated as heat (thermogenesis). Overall, the available evidence on functional foods so far identified in this field is incomplete. The major gap is the lack of diet-based intervention trials of sufficient duration to be relevant for the natural history of overweight and obesity [12].

On this aspect, through an iterative process of discussion among expert groups and workshops supported by the Fifth European Community Framework Program for Research and Technological Development and coordinated by ILSI Europe, scientists and representatives of regulatory bodies or food industries, have outlined the critical steps in the Process for the Assessment of Scientific Support for Claims on Foods (PASSCLAIM), finally reaching a consensus on the criteria for the scientific substantiation of claims (Table 18.1) [3].

In this context, the area covering body weight regulation, insulin sensitivity, and diabetes was identified as one in which health claims are likely to be made; therefore, an Individual Theme Group was established to specifically elaborate on the links between diet and health in this field. The group reviewed the scientific basis for existing and potential health claims based not only on modifications of target body functions (for obesity: body fat deposition), but also of other relevant associated functions (for obesity: energy intake, energy expenditure and fat storage) and evaluated methodologies and markers that can be used to substantiate claims [2].

Functions Associated with Body Fat Deposition

Excess body fat deposition is a consequence of an energy imbalance between calorie intake and energy expenditure; the energy that the body derives from foods is required to match that expended not only by physical activity, but also by all body functions essential for growth, survival, and reproduction. When energy intake exceeds expenditure, energy is stored in the form of adipose tissue to be utilized in conditions of food scarcity or increased energy demand; key elements in this system are a) the control of energy intake, regulated, at the simplest level, by sensations of hunger and satiety; and b) the control of energy efficiency that influences the amount of

Table 18.3 Examples of foods or food ingredients that may potentially be considered as "functional" in the field of body weight regulation.

Food/ingredient	Target functions	Measurements
Fiber-rich foods	Energy intake	a) Satiety, hunger (visual analogue scale)
Low-glycemic-index starchy foods		b) Dietary records, nutrient intake
Fat replacers/trappers		
Noncaloric sweeteners		
Caffeine, capsaicin, green tea	Energy expenditure	Indirect calorimetry
Medium-chain triglycerides		
Conjugated linoleic acid		
N-3 polyunsaturated fat		
Calcium		
Chromium		

Modified from Riccardi et al. [12], with permission.

energy dissipated as heat (thermogenesis) instead of being stored as fat (adipogenesis) [2].

Energy Intake

Among the strategies that could be used to influence energy intake, some could be implemented at meal time, for example, decreasing the energy density of foods by adding water or "fiber," others after the meal has been terminated, such as during the satiety period. The "satiety cascade" proposed by Blundell suggests many possible approaches; for example, evidence suggests that nutrient metabolism is directly or indirectly related to postingestive satiety: protein, carbohydrate, and fat exert hierarchical effects on satiety in the order protein > carbohydrate > fat [12].

However, to lower energy intake, it seems more promising to substitute high-energy with low-energy food components; fat replacement, for instance, could be achieved by several polysaccharides, such as inulin, modified starches, or sucrose polyesters, which act to partly or totally mimic fat in food without the negative aspects of the high caloric value of fat. The position of the American Dietetic Association is that the majority of fat replacers, when used in moderation by adults, can be safe and useful adjuncts for lowering the fat content of foods and may play a role in decreasing total dietary energy and fat intake. Replacement of carbohydrates, for example, sucrose or glucose, in foods can be achieved using a carbohydrate of similar sweetness and taste but with different phys-

iological and energy properties like polyols (sugar alcohols) or using non nutritive sweeteners (Table 18.3) [13].

To substantiate claims made on reduction of energy intake, there is need for markers able to record the energy intake and its reduction. There are accurate tables for converting food eaten into energy consumed that might be helpful to determine energy intake under conditions of a controlled diet. However, under free-living conditions, the measurement of energy intake seems more difficult, particularly in relation to an accurate evaluation of the amount of a food consumed by an individual. There are several methods that are usually applied to estimate energy intake in individuals, they are based on either a retrospective or a prospective evaluation or a combination of the two [2].

Claims that a given food increases satiety should be supported by demonstrating that post-meal events are indeed modified in a significant way following intake of that specific food product. Many indices have been proposed to assess satiety effects. A tool frequently used for assessing the intensity and duration of satiety is the visual analogue scale (VAS). Commonly, the effect of food or dietary treatment on satiety is determined in preload studies. In these studies a fixed amount of a test food (a preload) is consumed and after an interval of time, the effect of the preload on subsequent food intake (e.g., subsequent meal or the remainder of the day) is measured [2].

However, the amount of food eaten is not always a good marker of energy intake since foods differ for their energy density; therefore, diet composition may have a stronger influence on body weight than the amount of foods eaten. In addition, the composition of the diet may influence satiety, thus regulating food intake, and energy expenditure; both represent important mechanisms of long-term weight changes. There is no clear evidence that altering the proportion of fat and total carbohydrate in the diet has any major effect in modifying body weight; conversely, there is clear evidence that carbohydrate rich foods are a heterogeneous group in relation to their impact on body weight. In particular, an increased consumption of sugar-sweetened soft drinks is associated with weight gain, particularly in children, since beverages induce less satiety than solid forms of carbohydrate. On the other hand, the intake of fiber-rich foods such as whole-grain cereals, vegetables, legumes, and fruits is associated with a lower risk of weight gain in observational studies (Table 18.3). A moderately elevated protein intake, in association with controlled energy intake, may represent an effective and practical weight-loss strategy since it induces 1) increased satiety, 2) increased thermogenesis, and 3) the stimulation of lean muscle mass, which in turn is able to stimulate energy expenditure in the long term [12].

Energy Expenditure

The role of energy expenditure in energy regulation remains controversial. Low energy expenditure seems to cause obesity, although direct evidence of this hypothesis has been difficult to obtain in humans. Energy expenditure includes several components: resting metabolic rate (RMR), the thermogenic effect of exercise, the thermogenic effect of food, and facultative thermogenesis. RMR is usually the greatest contribution (60%–75%) to total daily energy expenditure and is due to energy expenditure for maintaining normal body functions and homeostasis, plus a component due to activation of the sympathetic nervous system. The energy expended by an individual, especially under resting conditions, can be assessed by indirect calorimetry, a technique based on the measurement of oxygen consumption and carbon dioxide production. In addition, the most commonly used method to assess total energy expenditure in humans in natural living conditions is the doubly labeled water measurement [2].

Several foods or food components are supposed to influence energy expenditure, e.g. caffeine, capsaicin, gingerols, and shogaols (the pungent principle of ginger and spices) or green tea extract. Therefore, in theory, including such ingredients could be a viable approach to stimulate energy expenditure and reduce body weight. Also, medium-chain triacylglycerols (MCTs), diacylglycerols, low-fat dairy products, and nuts have been associated with increased thermogenesis and reduced body weight. In addition, they may also have a role in cardiovascular disease prevention (Table 18.3) [12]. However, claims on increasing energy expenditure need to be supported by measurements in humans, using reliable methods and appropriate study designs and, therefore, by much more research work.

Lifestyle is a Risk Factor for Type 2 for Diabetes

Diabetes mellitus is a metabolic disorder of multiple etiologies characterized by chronic hyperglycemia associated with impaired carbohydrate, fat, and protein metabolism. These abnormalities are the consequences of either inadequate insulin secretion or impaired insulin action, or both. Type 2 diabetes mellitus accounts for almost 85%–95% of all disease cases. In western countries, the estimated prevalence in the population is 4%–6%. Half of these are diagnosed, while a similar number remains unrecognized. The disease is observed much more frequently in older people and in some ethnic communities (up to 40% of Pima Indians). The importance of lifestyle modifications for the prevention of type 2 diabetes has long been recognized. Several observational studies suggest that diabetes is primarily a life-style disorder. As a matter of fact, the highest prevalence rates occur in developing countries and in populations undergoing "westernization" or modernization. Under such circumstances, genetic susceptibility seems to interact with environmental changes, such as sedentary life and overnutrition, leading to type 2 diabetes. In the last decade, nutritional research on diabetes has improved dramatically in terms of both number of studies produced and quality of methodologies employed. Therefore, it is now possible to attempt to provide the evidence on which nutritional recommendations for the prevention of type 2 diabetes could be based [1].

Lifestyle factors that have, so far, been consistently associated with increased risk of type 2 diabetes are overweight and physical inactivity. However, recent evidence from epidemiologic studies has shown that the risk of type 2 diabetes is also associated with diet composition, particularly with 1) low fiber intake, 2) a high trans-fatty acid intake, and a low ratio of unsaturated-to-saturated fat intake, and 3) absence of or excess alcohol consumption. All these factors are extremely common in western populations, so the potential impact of any intervention on them is large. Indeed, more than 90% of the general population has one or more of these risk factors. The ability to correct these unhealthy behaviors in the population is estimated to reduce the incidence of diabetes by as much as 87% [1].

Recent intervention studies have shown that type 2 diabetes can be prevented by lifestyle changes aimed at body weight reduction, increased physical activity, and multiple changes in the composition of the diet (in particular, reduction in total and saturated fat intake and increase in the consumption of foods rich in fiber and with a low glycemic index [GI]) [14,15]. Within this context, the average amount of weight loss needed is not large, about 5% of initial weight, which is much less than the weight loss traditionally considered to be clinically significant for prevention of type 2 diabetes [10,11]. New emphasis on prevention by multiple lifestyle modifications, including moderate changes in the composition of the habitual diet, might hopefully limit the dramatic increase in incidence of type 2 diabetes envisaged worldwide for the coming decades.

Functions Associated with Insulin Sensitivity and Blood Glucose Control

Blood glucose levels are very stringently regulated to provide a steady fuel supply to the brain, which relies almost exclusively on glucose for its energy needs. In the brain, like in all non–insulin-dependent tissues, glucose uptake is regulated by glucose concentrations in arterial blood and, since the ability of neural cells to store glucose is minimal, optimal brain function depends on stable glucose levels, with a very narrow range of fluctuations in the postprandial period as well as in the fasting state. A complex hormonal system, which involves insulin and other hormones with anti-insulin actions, is able to regulate glucose production and disposal keeping blood glucose concentrations between 4 and 8 mmol/L almost all day long, irrespectively of the size and composition of the meals or the duration of the fasting period [2].

In the presence of insulin resistance, peripheral glucose utilization is impaired, which leads to a slight increase in plasma glucose levels. This occurs in all individuals—with or without diabetes—with insulin resistance, who represent as much as one-quarter of the general population; however, when impaired insulin secretion is also present stable hyperglycemia develops.

Since insulin resistance is selective, in the presence of this condition high plasma insulin levels are associated with subnormal metabolic effects (leading to hyperglycemia, hypertriglyceridemia, low high-density lipoprotein, high blood pressure, impaired fibrinolysis, and all other conditions clustering in the metabolic syndrome) but also with an excessive stimulation of cell growth, which may facilitate the occurrence of arteriosclerosis and cancer. In addition, hyperinsulinemia facilitates the occurrence of overweight and may aggravate insulin resistance as a consequence of a down regulation of the transduction system of the insulin receptor signal. Therefore, high plasma insulin levels might be not only a marker of a metabolic derangement but they may also contribute directly to the development of diseases with a widespread diffusion, such as type 2 diabetes, the metabolic syndrome, ischemic vascular disease, and cancer [15].

Hyperglycemia is not only the cause of most symptoms affecting the quality of life of diabetic patients but represents also the cause of the long-term specific complications of diabetes (retinopathy, nephropathy, neuropathy); in addition, high plasma glucose levels contribute to the excess risk of cardiovascular disease associated with this disease. High plasma glucose concentrations below the diagnostic cutoff level for diabetes may also predispose to ischemic cardiovascular disease in the nondiabetic population, but since this condition is often asymptomatic, it may go unrecognized and untreated for years while its ill effects on the arteries persist [16]. Various mechanisms have been proposed to link high plasma glucose concentrations, but below the diagnostic threshold for diabetes, with the occurrence of angiopathy at the level of small or large arteries. Glycosylation of proteins in the arterial wall is most probably one of the key mechanism, since this process is able to modify many of the physicochemical properties of these molecules, thus facilitating the occurrence of ischemic processes. The arteries progressively lose their elasticity and increase the thickness of their wall, which eventually leads to significant reduction of blood flow. Other mechanisms involve accelerated arterial cell proliferation, alterations of lipid metabolism and hemostasis, endothelial dysfunction, and many other abnormalities triggered by hyperglycemia [17].

Chronically elevated plasma glucose levels impair both glucose utilization and insulin secretion and, therefore, may contribute to self-perpetuation or, even, worsening of the metabolic abnormalities responsible for the impaired glucose homeostasis.

In the presence of insulin resistance and/or impaired glucose regulation, both the amount of carbohydrate in the meal and the rate of digestion of carbohydrate foods play a relevant role in the regulation of the postprandial blood glucose rise (Figure 18.1) [18].

Functional Foods for Diabetes

Carbohydrates are traditionally classified on the basis of their chemical structure; however, in order to provide a true guide to their importance for health a classification based on their ability to influence postprandial glycemia (GI) seems more relevant. This is calculated dividing the incremental area under the curve of blood glucose concentrations measured after the ingestion of a portion of a test food containing 50 g of carbohydrate by the incremental blood glucose area achieved with a portion of reference food (glucose or white bread) containing the same amount (50 g) of carbohydrate and expressed as a percentage. Fiber-rich foods generally have a low GI, although not all foods with a low GI necessarily have a high fiber content. Since postprandial blood glucose response is influenced not only by the GI of the food, but also by the amount of ingested carbohydrate, in epidemiologic studies, the concept of glycemic load (GL) (the GI of a specific food multiplied by the amount of carbohydrate contained in an average portion of the food consumed) has been developed to better represent both quantity and quality of the carbohydrate consumed. Each unit of dietary GL represents the equivalent glycemic effect of 1 g of carbohydrate from white bread, which is used as the reference food [18].

Several beneficial effects of low GI/high-fiber (LGI/HF) diets have been shown including lower postprandial glucose and insulin responses,

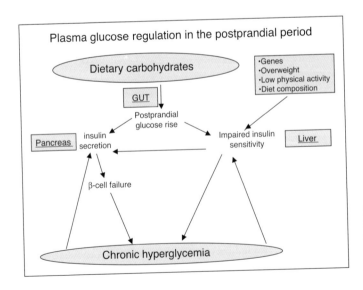

Figure 18.1 Impact of glycemic carbohydrates on metabolic derangements leading to impaired insulin sensitivity and type 2 diabetes.

Table 18.4 Evidence-based evaluation of the impact of specific features of carbohydrate-rich foods on the risk of type 2 diabetes.

Diabetes risk	Low GI	Soluble fiber	Insoluble fiber
Epidemiological observations	+−	+	+
Controlled clinical trials	−	+−	+−
Plausible mechanisms	+	+	+−

+, strong evidence; +−, weak evidence; −, no evidence (not tested).

improved lipid profile, and possibly, reduced insulin resistance. Epidemiologic studies have provided very suggestive evidence that a diet in which carbohydrate-rich foods with high fiber and low GI are predominant may contribute to diabetes prevention (Table 18.4).

The association between low GI/GL and reduced risk of type 2 diabetes might be mediated by an improvement of insulin resistance, since this condition is recognized as a metabolic derangement predisposing to diabetes in the large majority of individuals at risk. However, in relation to this parameter the available evidence on GI/GL fails to be convincing. No intervention studies have so far evaluated the effect of fiber and/or GI on prevention of diabetes, although the most important intervention studies aiming at lifestyle modifications also included an increase in fiber consumption (most probably associated with a lower GI) in the intervention group (Table 18.4).

The best evidence of the clinical usefulness of GI is available in diabetic patients in whom low GI foods have consistently shown beneficial effects on blood glucose control in both the short and the long term. In these patients, low GI foods are suitable as carbohydrate-rich choices, provided other attributes of the foods are appropriate [18].

The available evidence on functional foods for the prevention of diabetes supports the use of whole grain foods, vegetables, fruit, low GI starchy products, low saturated fat foods as natural, unmodified products (Table 18.5) [12,14,19].

Among other foods with possibly inherent functional properties linked with the prevention of type 2 diabetes, are dairy products, particularly the ones with a low fat content, which have been recently reported to be strong predictors of reduced diabetes risk in men, independently of any effect on body weight and other known risk factors. Previous studies have suggested that dairy products might have favorable effects not only on excess body weight but also on other features of the metabolic syndrome. The mechanisms have not yet been elucidated, but electrolytes in dairy products, such as calcium and magnesium, may play a role [12,20,22].

The diet for the management of type 2 diabetes does not significantly differ from that recommended for diabetes prevention. However, also in people with diabetes, compliance to dietary recommendations is poor even in countries where the background diet of the population is not particularly unhealthy and therefore the goals of dietary recommendations are, in theory, more easily achievable. Therefore, the potential benefits of functional foods may well extend from prevention to treatment. However, although there are many products with potentially relevant functional effects, the European Guidelines highlight the need for longer term evaluation in formal clinical trials

Table 18.5 Examples of foods or food ingredients that may potentially be considered as "functional" in the field of blood glucose control.

Food/ingredient	Target functions	Measurements
Low glycemic index starchy foods Low-saturated fat foods Whole grains Low-fat dairy products	Insulin sensitivity	Plasma insulin, HOMA index, glucose clamp
Low-glycemic-index starchy foods Fruit and vegetables	Glucose metabolism	Postprandial plasma glucose

Modified from Riccardi et al. [12], with permission.

before offering firm recommendations on their use. Obviously, this caveat does not apply to natural unmodified foods with functional properties for which the available evidence is sufficient to make recommendations [14].

Conclusions

It is now generally accepted that a food can have health-promoting properties that go beyond its traditional nutritional value; this is particularly true in the field of overweight and diabetes, where, more than in many other fields, the link between nutrition, biological responses, and diseases is clearly established, and therefore, there is a strong potential to set up a functional food science. However, despite these great promises, the evidence supporting the functionality of foods for prevention of overweight and diabetes is, so far, weak. The major gap is the lack of diet-based intervention trials of sufficient duration to be relevant for the natural history of diseases.

For most claims related to overweight and energy balance, the available markers of relevant biological functions seem to be sufficiently reliable and valid [4].

Moreover, the link between the markers of energy intake and expenditure and the end-point (change in body fat) seems well established. Nevertheless, properly controlled intervention studies in humans are needed to evaluate the long-term effects of foods, food ingredients, and diets on markers of the target functions and, particularly, body weight.

As for type 2 diabetes, on the basis of the available evidence, it seems reasonable to attempt a multifactorial rather than a monofactorial intervention because it allows more flexibility and thus accounts for the individual's capacity to act on and modify one or more lifestyle behaviors at risk. Moreover, since lifestyle modifications have an additive effect on diabetes prevention, a multifactorial approach might also amplify the efficacy of the intervention [19]. The lifestyle factors that have been consistently associated with increased risk of type 2 diabetes are overweight and physical inactivity. However the recent evidence from epidemiological studies has shown that the risk of type 2 diabetes is also associated with 1) low fiber intake, 2) a high trans-fatty acid intake and a low ratio of unsaturated-to-saturated fat intake, and 3) absence of or excess alcohol consumption [2]. All these factors are extremely common in western populations and therefore the potential impact of any intervention on them is large; indeed, taking into account these risk factors for type 2 diabetes, only 9.5% of women recruited in an observational study in the United States were in the low-risk category. The ability to correct these unhealthy behaviors in the rest of the population was estimated to reduce the incidence of diabetes by as much as 87% [23]. However, incontrovertible evidence that each of these lifestyle modifications can reduce the risk of diabetes is not available since for these measures controlled intervention studies with a monofactorial design have not been produced.

Acknowledgments

PASSCLAIM is a European Commission Concerted Action Programme supported by the European Commission and coordinated by the European branch of the International Life Sciences Institute –ILSI Europe. The expert linguistic revision by Rosanna Scala is gratefully acknowledged.

Selected References

3. PASSCLAIM Consensus on Criteria. A European Commission Concerted Action Project. Eur J Nutr 2005;44(Suppl 1):5–30.

8. Saris WH, Asp NG, Bjorck I, et al. Functional food science and substrate metabolism. Br J Nutr 1998; (80 Suppl 1): S47–S75.

12. Riccardi G, Capaldo B, Vaccaro O. Functional foods in the management of obesity and type 2 diabetes. Curr Opin Clin Nutr Metab Care 2005 Nov;8(6): 630–5.

20. St-Onge MP. Dietary fats, teas, dairy, and nuts: potential functional foods for weight control? Am J Clin Nutr 2005;81(1):7–15.

22. Mann J, Cummings JH, Englyst HN, et al. FAO/WHO scientific update on carbohydrates in human nutrition: conclusions. Eur J Clin Nutr 2007;Dec;61(Suppl 1):S132–7.

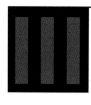

SECTION III

Hypercholesterolemia and Early Atherosclerosis

CHAPTER 19

Familial Dyslipidemias: From Genetics to Clinical Picture

Paolo Rubba, Marco Gentile, Salvatore Panico, &
Paolo Pauciullo
Federico II University, Naples, Italy

Familial Hypercholesterolemia

Definition

Familial hypercholesterolemia (FH) is a clinical definition for a pronounced increase of cholesterol serum concentration, presence of xanthomas, and an autosomal dominant trait of increased serum cholesterol and premature coronary artery disease (CAD). The identification of the low-density lipoprotein (LDL)-receptor (LDLR) mutations as the underlying cause and their genetic characterization in FH patients revealed more insights in the trafficking of LDL, which primarily transports cholesterol to hepatic and peripheral cells. Mutations within LDLR result in hypercholesterolemia and, subsequently, cholesterol deposition in humans to a variable degree. This confirms the pathogenetic role of LDLR and highlights the existence of additional factors in determining the phenotype [1–3].

Autosomal dominant FH is caused by LDLR deficiency and defective apolipoprotein B-100 (ApoB), respectively [1,3]. Heterozygosity of the LDLR is relatively common (1:500). Clinical diagnosis is highly important and genetic diagnosis may be helpful, since treatment is usually effective for this otherwise fatal disease. Recently, mutations in PCSK9 have been also shown to cause autosomal dominant hypercholesterolemia [4,5]. For autosomal recessive hypercholesterolemia (ARH), mutations within the

so-called ARH gene [6,7] encoding a cellular adaptor protein required for LDL transport have been identified. These insights emphasize the crucial importance of LDL metabolism intracellulary and extracellularly in determining LDL-cholesterol (LDL-C) serum concentration .

Although the cause of FH is monogenic, there is wide variation in the onset and severity of atherosclerotic disease in these patients. Additional atherogenic risk factors of environmental, metabolic, and genetic origin are presumed to influence the clinical phenotype in FH [1,3]. Criteria used to identify individuals with FH include a combination of clinical characteristics, personal and family history of early CAD, and biochemical parameters. Since the introduction in 1989 of statins, which have been shown to be effective and to delay or prevent the onset of cardiovascular disease (CVD), drug treatment of FH has greatly improved [3].

New lipid-lowering agents are presently being developed for clinical use. People with FH have dramatically high levels of LDL-C, which can lead to accelerated atherosclerosis and, if untreated, early cardiovascular death. Although the heterozygous form of FH is often unrecognized, detecting it early can enable risk reduction before premature coronary heart disease (CHD) occurs.

Pathophysiology

Uptake of cholesterol, mediated by LDLR [8], plays a crucial role in lipoprotein metabolism. The LDLR is responsible for the binding and subsequent

Nutritional and Metabolic Bases of Cardiovascular Disease, 1st edition.
Edited by Mario Mancini, José M. Ordovas, Gabriele Riccardi,
Paolo Rubba and Pasquale Strazzullo. © 2011 Blackwell Publishing Ltd.

cellular uptake of ApoB- and ApoE-containing lipoproteins. To accomplish this, the receptor is transported from the site of synthesis, the membranes of the rough endoplasmic reticulum, through the Golgi apparatus, to its position on the surface of the cellular membrane. The translation of LDLR messenger RNA into the polypeptide chain for the receptor protein takes place on the surface-bound ribosomes of the rough endoplasmic reticulum. Immature O-linked carbohydrate chains are attached to this integral precursor membrane protein. The molecular weight of the receptor at this stage is 120,000 d. The precursor-protein is transported from the rough endoplasmic reticulum to the Golgi apparatus, where the O-linked sugar chains are elongated until their final size is reached. The molecular weight has then increased to 160,000 d. The mature LDLR is subsequently guided to the "coated pits" on the cell surface. These specialized areas of the cell membrane are rich in clathrin and interact with the LDLR protein. Only here, the LDLR binds LDL particles. Within 3–5 minutes from its formation, the LDL-particle-receptor complex is internalized through endocytosis and is further metabolized through the receptor-mediated endocytosis pathway.

Mutations in the gene coding for the LDLR can interfere to a varying extent with all the different stages of the posttranslational processing, binding, uptake, and subsequent dissociation of the LDL-particle-LDLR complex, but invariably the mutations lead to FH. Thus, mutations in the LDLR [2] gene give rise to a substantially varying clinical expression of FH.

The characterization of a rare genetic defect causing ARH has provided new insights into the underlying mechanism of clathrin-mediated internalization of the LDLR [6,7]. Mutations in ARH on chromosome 1p35-36.1 prevent normal internalization of the LDLR by cultured lymphocytes and monocyte-derived macrophages but not by skin fibroblasts. In affected cells, LDLR protein accumulates at the cell surface; this also occurs in the livers of recombinant mice lacking ARH gene, thereby providing an explanation for the failure of clearance of LDL from the plasma in subjects lacking a functional ARH gene. The approximately 50 known affected individuals are mostly of Sardinian or Middle Eastern origin. The clinical phenotype of ARH

is similar to that of classic homozygous FH caused by defects in the LDLR gene, but it is more variable, generally less severe, and more responsive to lipid-lowering therapy [6,7].

Genetics

FH results from defects in the hepatic uptake and degradation of LDL via the LDLR pathway, commonly caused by a loss-of-function mutation in the LDLR gene or by a mutation in the gene encoding ApoB. FH is primarily an autosomal dominant disorder with a gene-dosage effect. FH can result from mutations in the LDLR gene, the ApoB-100 gene, and the recently identified proprotein convertasi subtilisin/kexin type 9 gene (PCSK9). To date, more than 800 variants have been identified in the LDLR gene. With the exception of a small number of founder populations where one or two mutations predominate, most geography-based surveys of FH subjects show a large number of mutations segregating in a given population [2,4,5].

An autosomal recessive form of FH caused by loss-of-function mutations in LDLRAP1, which encodes a protein required for clathrin-mediated internalization of the LDLR by liver cells, has also been documented [6,7]. The most recent addition to the database of genes in which defects cause FH is one encoding a member of the proprotein convertase family, PCSK9 [2,5]. Rare dominant gain-of-function mutations in PCSK9 cosegregate with hypercholesterolemia, and one mutation is associated with a particularly severe FH phenotype. Expression of PCSK9 normally down-regulates the LDLR pathway by indirectly causing degradation of LDLR protein, and loss-of-function mutations in PCSK9 result in low plasma LDL levels.

The wide variety of mutations and phenotypic variability have made it difficult to establish definite diagnostic criteria, but three sets of clinical criteria commonly used are the Simon Broome criteria, the Dutch Lipid Clinic criteria, and the American criteria. Screening could be carried out on a population basis, in a clinical setting or by application to relatives of probands. This latter approach, termed *cascade testing*, is generally preferred [1].

Clinical Picture

Heterozygous FH [1,3,9,10] is among the most common inherited dominant disorders and is characterized by severely elevated LDL-C levels and premature CVD. Although the cause of FH is monogenic, there is a substantial variation in the onset and severity of atherosclerotic disease symptoms. Additional atherogenic risk factors of environmental, metabolic, and genetic origin, in conjunction with the LDLR defect, are presumed to influence the clinical phenotype in familial hypercholesterolemia.

In homozygous FH [11], both genes for the LDLR are mutated and LDL levels are markedly elevated. High-density lipoprotein-cholesterol (HDL-C) concentration is often reduced and lipoprotein(a) levels are high when corrected for apolipoprotein(a) isoforms. Cutaneous and tendinous xanthomas develop in childhood and are the most common reason for initial presentation. The diagnosis can be confirmed by analysis of LDLR genes or studies of LDLR function in cultured cells. Severe aortic and coronary atherosclerosis usually occurs within the first or second decades of life. Left ventricular outflow tract obstruction may be at the level of the aortic valve or the supravalvar aorta.

A clinical diagnosis of FH is widely used, but a definitive diagnosis can be made by genetic screening, although mutations are currently only detected in 30%–50% of patients with a clinical diagnosis. Underdiagnosis of FH has been reported worldwide ranging from less than 1% to 44% [10].

Mutations in the LDLR gene can result in the FH phenotype, and there is evidence that receptor-negative mutations result in a more severe phenotype than do receptor-defective mutations. Mutations in the ApoB-100 gene can result in a phenotype that is clinically indistinguishable from FH, and mutations in this gene have also been shown to be associated with CHD.

Early identification of persons with FH and their relatives, and the early start of treatment are essential issues in the prevention of premature CVD and death in this population. The FH clinical phenotype has been shown to be associated with increased CHD [12] and premature death. FH is a public health problem throughout the world. FH affects approximately 1 in 500 people (10 million worldwide) and the elevated serum cholesterol concentrations lead to a more than 50% risk of fatal or nonfatal CHD by age 50 years in men and at least 30% in women aged 60 years.

Since increased cholesterol levels lead to atherosclerosis, FH has also been proposed as a risk factor for peripheral vascular and ischemic cerebrovascular disease [13]. Currently, the association between clinical FH and risk of stroke is unclear. Two studies conducted in the 1980s indicated an increased risk of stroke in FH subjects. However, two others found no higher risk, and all had methodological limitations. A prospective study of FH by the United Kingdom–based Simon Broome Register Group did not find an excess risk of stroke mortality for subjects with clinical FH. By contrast, the prevalence of peripheral arterial disease is increased from five- to 10-fold in FH subjects compared with non-FH controls. In addition, the intima-media thickness (IMT) of the carotid and/or femoral artery is increased in FH subjects. Better understanding of the association between FH and the incidence of ischemic stroke events could have a public health impact by improving the diagnosis, prognosis, and treatment of individuals with FH and their relatives and by elucidating the relation between cholesterol levels and ischemic cerebrovascular disease.

A study assessed the role of a new LDLR mutation [14] for the development of early atherosclerotic lesions, independently of plasma cholesterol levels and other risk factors. LDLR gene was sequenced in 102 patients with clinical features of heterozygous FH. Sixteen different mutations (five never described) were found in 82 patients (49 families, mean age 39 years, 53% women). One of the newly described mutations, the 2312-3 C>A, was found in 24 patients (13 families). Carotid artery IMT was measured by B-mode ultrasound. The mean of maximum thicknesses was significantly higher in the 2312-3 C>A group than in patients with other LDLR mutations ($p = .004$ after adjustment for major cardiovascular risk factors). Similar results were obtained in the 6- to 55-year age-group, and in the comparisons of probands. This study supports the role of the LDLR mutation 2312-3 C>A as a predictor of cardiovascular damage, independently of, and in addition to, serum cholesterol and other traditional risk factors [15].

Tendon xanthomatosis [16] often accompanies FH, but it can also occur in other pathologic states. Achilles tendons are the most common sites of tendon xanthomas. LDL derived from the circulation accumulates into tendons. The next steps leading to the formation of Achilles tendon xanthomas (ATXs) are the transformation of LDL into oxidized LDL (oxLDL) and the active uptake of oxLDL by macrophages within the tendons. Although physical examination may reveal ATXs, there are several imaging methods for their detection. It is worth mentioning that ultrasonography is the method of choice in everyday clinical practice. Although several treatments for ATXs have been proposed (LDL apheresis, statins, etc.), they target mostly in the treatment of the basic metabolic disorder of lipid metabolism, which is the main cause of these lesions.

Management

The relative risk of death of FH patients not treated with statins is between threefold and fourfold, but treatment is effective and delays or prevents the onset of CHD. Early detection and treatment are important [9,10].

In the presence of FH, dietary and lifestyle advice should be offered and supported. According to current guidelines on cardiovascular disease prevention [17], patients with FH should be aggressively treated with statins, up to a daily dosage of 80 mg of atorvastatin and rosuvastatin [18]. Aggressive statin therapy is more effective in preventing vascular damage than conventional LDL therapy.

In FH patients, combined therapy of statin with either ezetimibe or torcetrapib did not result in a significant difference in changes in IMT, as compared with statin alone, despite additional decreases in levels of LDL-C or increase in HDL-C [19,20].

In homozygous FH, a high dosage of atorvastatin and rosuvastatin has been prescribed. Mean LDL reductions from baseline after crossover treatment with rosuvastatin 80 mg and atorvastatin 80 mg were 19% and 18%, respectively. All treatments were well tolerated [21].

The type of mutation in the LDLR gene has been associated with different phenotype expression and response to statins [22]. Several studies have been undertaken to assess the efficacy of statins and evaluate the influence of mutations on the response to treatment with statins. Not all patients respond in the same way to statin therapy.

Other Interventions

Premature CHD can result from high LDL-C levels even in the absence of any other risk factors.

A striking example is found in children who have the homozygous form of FH with extremely high levels of LDL-C, and severe atherosclerosis and CHD often develop during the first decades of life. LDL apheresis [23,24] was developed for the treatment of severe type of FH patients who are resistant to lipid-lowering drug therapy. Clinical efficacy and safety of the therapeutic tool that directly removes LDL from circulation have already been established in the treatment for refractory hypercholesterolemia in FH patients. The most recently developed method enables lipoproteins to be adsorbed directly from whole blood, using polyacrylate column. A systematic review [23] concluded that LDL apheresis reduces cardiovascular events in hypercholesterolemic patients and may be a useful treatment for other vascular diseases.

Liver transplantation [25] in homozygous FH provides the missing functional LDLRs and thus partially restores LDLR activity to more than 50% of normal. Combined heart and liver transplantation was successfully performed in a homozygous FH patient with end-stage heart failure. Liver transplantation reverses the metabolic defect but requires chronic immunosupression, and rejection may still occur. Liver transplantation is indicated if cardiac transplantation becomes necessary. Portocaval shunt may still play a role in patients with CAD who do not have access to plasmaphoresis.

Somatic gene therapy [26] is considered to be a potential approach to the therapy of several of these lipid disorders. In many cases preclinical proof-of-principle studies have already been performed, and in one (homozygous FH) a clinical trial has been conducted. Other clinical gene therapy trials for dyslipidemia are likely to be initiated within the next several years.

A review focused [27] on advances in the management of patients with homozygous FH, autosomal recessive hypercholesterolemia, and familial defective ApoB. Apheresis is still the treatment of choice in homozygous FH and in autosomal recessive hypercholesterolemia patients in whom maximal drug therapy does not achieve adequate control. In addition to the profound cholesterol-lowering effects of apheresis, other potentially beneficial phenomena have been documented: improved vascular endothelial function and hemorheology, reduction in lipoprotein(a) and procoagulatory status, and a decrease in adhesion molecules and C-reactive protein (CRP). Patients with severe homozygous hypercholesterolemia illustrate the natural history of atherosclerosis within a condensed timeframe. Effective cholesterol-lowering treatment started in early childhood is essential to prevent onset of life-threatening atherosclerotic involvement of the aortic root and valve, and the coronary arteries. Noninvasive methods for regular monitoring of the major sites involved in the atherosclerotic process are necessary in patients with no symptoms or signs of ischemia. Management of patients with severe homozygous hypercholesterolemia continues to be a major challenge.

Familial Combined Hyperlipidemia

Definition

Familial combined hyperlipidemia (FCHL) is a common inherited hyperlipidemia, with a prevalence of 1–2% in the Western World [28]. FCHL is a metabolically and genetically heterogeneous disorder [29,30]. Affected individuals have elevated cholesterol or triglyceride concentrations or both. Such a lipid profile is frequently associated with an unfavourable decrease in HDL concentration, an elevated apolipoprotein (apo) B and an increased prevalence of atherogenic, sd-LDL subfractions. Although several metabolic abnormalities have been suggested to be relevant to the FCHL phenotype, such as an overproduction of very LDL (VLDL) apo B, reduced insulin sensitivity, altered metabolism of fatty acids in adipose tissue, impaired hydrolytic activity of lipoprotein lipase (LPL), the exact cause of this metabolic disorder is presently unknown [28,31].

Furthermore, no model proposed so far is able to fully explain the genetic bases of FCHL. Due to the absence of a specific genetic or metabolic marker for the disorder and to the characteristic variability in the presenting lipid phenotype, family studies are necessary to establish the diagnosis of FCHL in each patient. Recently, diagnostic criteria with a high degree of sensitivity and specificity to discriminate affected/non-affected subjects in the individual families, have been proposed [32,33].

Pathophysiology

The most founded pathogenetic hypothesis of FCHL [29] suggests an hepatic hyperproduction of ApoB and VLDL, associated or not to reduced clearance of triglyceride-rich lipoproteins (TGRLs). *In vivo* and *in vitro* studies demonstrated that in FCHL patients, in the postprandial phase, the capacity of adipocytes to incorporate and esterify free fatty acids (FFAs) is impaired, due to a reduced activity of acylation-stimulating protein (ASP). This may be responsible for the enhanced flux of FFA to the liver and a consequent increased production of ApoB and VLDL [34].

TGRLs derive from the absorption of dietary lipids, from the consequent assembly of chilomycrons, and from hepatic synthesis of VLDL. TGRL can be atherogenic via several mechanisms. It has been shown that lipoprotein remnants accumulate into the arterial wall, suggesting a role for an excess of these particles, as in the postprandial state, for the development of atherosclerosis. At variance of native chilomycrons, remnant lipoproteins have a plasma half-life of several hours, similar to that of VLDL. Their residence time is, therefore, sufficient for atherogenic interactions with endothelial and circulating cells. TGRLs of intestinal origin contain ApoB-48, an apoprotein that results from the ApoB synthesis in the enterocytes, while VLDLs of hepatic origin contain ApoB-100. The determination of the presence of the two forms of the ApoB is taken as an estimate of the relative contributions of the intestinal and liver source to the hyperlipidemia of the postprandial phase.

Genetics

Several candidate genes, such as those coding for ApoB, the LPL, the hepatic lipase (HL), and the ApoAI/CIII/AIV gene cluster, and more recently, the tumor necrosis factor receptor (TNFR) gene have been studied [28,35,36], but the results have been mostly inconclusive. Linkage of FCHL to upstream stimulatory factor-1 remains controversial [31].

The complexity of inheritance of FCHL suggests that alternative strategies need to be used to identify the susceptibility loci for this highly atherogenic lipid disorder and requires a genome-wide search. The characterization of microsatellite markers loci by polymerase chain reaction (PCR) and the application of fluorescent-based, automated fragment-sizing technology have been proved to be a successful approach in identifying susceptibility loci for common human polygenic disorders. Another promising tool to tackle the molecular problems of FCHL is now the DNA microarrays technique, one of the most powerful approaches of the post-genomic era. Finally, an accurate analysis of the expression profiles may help to define in a more accurate and comprehensive way the whole of the regulatory interconnections among the different genes involved (regulomics), providing us with useful hints to understand the multigenic basis of FCHL.

Clinical Picture

FCHL diagnostic [30] criteria include evaluation of phenotype variability:
• Intrafamilial phenotype variability at a certain time, that is, different phenotypes within the same family and/or phenotype of mixed hyperlipidemia (hypercholesterolemia + hypertriglyceridemia) in more than one subject in the same family,
• exclusion of families with hypercholesterolemia or hypertriglyceridemia alone in all dyslipidemic members,

together with exclusion of secondary dyslipidemias, of iatrogenic interference, of major dietary changes, but not of fairly compensated diabetes (HbA1 less than 7%), since FCHL is often complicated by this disease. In all cases described in the previous point, and particularly in patients with mixed hyperlipidemia phenotype but no available family data, the presence of one of the following conditions will constitute a reinforcing or additional diagnostic criterion:
• Former aortocoronary, aortoiliac, aortorenal bypass, endarterectomy, or other surgical revascularization procedure (in the proband);
• Former major cerebrovascular accident (reversible ischemic neurological disorders, thromboembolic stroke) and/or obliterating vasculopathy of the lower limbs (in the proband);
• Previous episode of ischemic heart disease (410-414 code of ICD) in the proband;
• Premature atherosclerotic CVD (men younger than 60 years, women younger than 65 years) in a first-degree relative.

• Instrumental evidence (ultrasound, angiography) of severe atheromasia of any vascular district (e.g., carotid artery IMT > 2 mm, and/or ankle/arm ratio of systolic blood pressure less than 0.90).

Laboratory analyses in FCHL are performed after withdrawing all lipid-lowering therapy for at least 4–6 weeks. Blood glucose values are often borderline in this disease and HDL-C concentration is reduced (<40 mg/dl in women, less than 35 mg/dl in men). The following lipid cutoff points are used for FCHL diagnosis: LDL-C > 160 mg/dl and/or triglyceride > 200 mg/dl. In addition, a level of plasma ApoB > 120 mg/dl has been suggested [32] as a third biochemical criterion. The presence of an increased ApoB/non-HDL-C ratio, particularly in patients with prevalent hypertriglyceridemia or when a "normal" lipid phenotype is present, could constitute an additional diagnostic criterion.

The sd-LDL particles have been considered a risk marker in FCHL [37–40]. Compared with a prevalence of 5% for a high score of the sd-LDL particles in the general population, the score is high in approximately 80% of patients with FCHL [41].

Obesity and overweight, which are key features of the so-called metabolic syndrome (MetS), are highly prevalent in FCHL [42]. Abdominal obesity enhances the expression of FCHL [43]. FCHL and MetS share several metabolic abnormalities, including central obesity, hypertension, insulin resistance, and hypertriglyceridemic dyslipidemia. FCHL and MetS are complex metabolic disorders that are associated with increased CVD risk [37,42]. The sd-LDL particles have been considered a risk marker in FCHL and MetS [37,38].

A general pattern of activated blood coagulation and endothelial activation has been demonstrated in patients with FCHL. In the case of FCHL patients with hypertriglyceridemia and other components of the MetS, impaired fibrinolysis might contribute to additional thrombotic risk [44].

Nonalcoholic fatty liver, as evaluated by ultrasonography, was found in approximately in three-fourths of cases of FCHL as compared to 10% in comparable clinically healthy controls [45]. It is suggested that hepatic steatosis is part of the clinical picture of FCHL, especially in the presence of a hypertriglyceridemic phenotype.

The main clinical feature of FCHL is the development of premature atherosclerotic lesions, with a very high cardiovascular mortality. Cohort studies involving survivors of premature myocardial infarction (MI) have indicated that FCHL carries at least a 10-fold increased risk of such events [46].

High resolution B-mode ultrasound is a relatively inexpensive, safe, and validated technique that can be used to assess the presence of initial structural atherosclerotic changes of the arterial wall in superficial arteries, such as carotid, femoral, and aorta, which are favored sites for the development of atherosclerosis. An increase in carotid IMT has been found in subjects with FCHL [47].

The B-mode ultrasound technique can be used to study endothelial dysfunction (ED) (loss of endothelium-dependent vasodilation). This dysfunction occurs early in vascular disease and may be caused by a decreased production, an increased degradation or a less sensitivity to nitric oxide (NO). Major risk factors for atherosclerotic vascular disease (e.g., hypertension, smoking, diabetes, obesity, and hypercholesterolemia) have been associated to ED. Patients affected by FCHL have evidence of ED [48].

FCHL and Inflammation

The growing evidence relating inflammation markers to the atherosclerotic process [49,50] could cast new light on the diagnostic profile of FCHL. The role of an acute-phase reactant like C-reactive protein (CRP) is now well established as a marker of CVD, particularly in patients with stable or unstable CHD. More uncertain is the role of CRP in primary prevention, although CRP levels are associated with elevated blood pressure, elevated body mass index (BMI) and low HDL/high triglycerides, all features of FCHL. Atherosclerotic process and CRP itself are associated with increased plasma levels of cell adhesion molecules (CAMs), which mediate rolling and then attachment of leucocytes along the endothelium. In particular, high levels of intercellular adhesion molecule-1 (ICAM-1) and of soluble e- and p-selectin were found in healthy individuals subsequently developing MI or other CVD events. High levels of vascular CAM (VCAM)-1 were found in CHD patients. It should be considered that among patients with FCHL, both categories of subjects with possibly high levels of CAMs (high-risk healthy subjects and CVD patients) are represented. In addition, the same clinical and biochemical charac-

teristics often found in FCHL and associated with high plasma levels of CRP (elevated blood pressure and BMI, as well as HDL, triglycerides, and blood glucose alterations) are associated with increased levels of CAMs.

Once attached—through the CAMs—to the endothelial cells, the leucocytes migrate into the subendothelial space where they contribute to the inflammatory process inducing production from macrophages and smooth muscle cells of proinflammatory cytokines. In particular, interleukin (IL)-6 is expressed in human atheromas, is a predictor of CVD events in healthy subjects and in acute coronary syndromes, and can induce a prothrombotic state [50].

TNF-α is another cytokine that is related to CVD events both in healthy individuals and in CVD patients [50]. IL-6 and TNF-α were found to be related—like CAMs—to the clinical features of FCHL, like obesity, low HDL, and hypertriglyceridemia, hypertension, hyperglycemia, and prothrombotic state. TNF-α is a cytokine that is secreted within the endothelial wall, but also in adipose tissue by adipose cells and macrophages. Among the inflammatory markers most commonly measured, only TNF-α was associated with FCHL independently of age, gender, BMI, and homeostatis model assessment (HOMA). The association of TNF-α with FCHL was also independent of the MetS [36].

Management, Diet

On the basis of the observation that abdominal obesity enhances the expression of FCHL [43], correction of overweight is the first-line intervention in nonpharmacological management of FCHL. Physical exercise might contribute to both weight control and correction of low HDL-C of FCHL (see Chapter 20).

A low-fat diet is recommended for FCHL. However, LDL responses depend on the type of hyperlipidemia (i.e., simple hypercholesterolemia or mixed hyperlipidemia). In mixed hyperlipidemia, LDL levels are only one-third as responsive to fat and cholesterol restriction as simple hypercholesterolemia.

FCHL is caused by heightened lipid secretion by the liver. A moderate-fat, moderate-carbohydrate diet employing allowable fats is expected to reduce endogenous lipoprotein production in combined hyperlipidemia. After such a diet, triglyceride, LDL, and sd-LDL levels should be lower, and high-density lipoprotein, ApoA-I, and buoyant LDL levels should be higher [51].

It has been suggested that the current dietary recommendations (low-fat, high-carbohydrate diet) may promote the intake of sugar and highly refined starches which could have adverse effects on the metabolic risk profile. The short-term nutritional and metabolic effects of an ad libitum low-glycemic index, low-fat, high-protein diet (prepared according to the Montignac method) was compared with the American Heart Association (AHA) phase I diet consumed ad libitum [52]. Favorable changes in the metabolic risk profile noted with the ad libitum consumption of the low-glycemic index, low-fat, high-protein diet (decreases in triacylglycerols, lack of increase in cholesterol:HDL-C ratio, increase in LDL particle size) were demonstrated in the comparison with the AHA phase I diet.

Management, Drugs

In FCHL the lipid abnormalities before treatment are different from patient to patient, by definition. In all cases, statin treatment reduces LDL-C, triglycerides (generally in direct proportion to baseline levels), with variable changes of HDL-C. The mechanism underlying the triglyceride-lowering effect has been documented for atorvastatin. The FCHL patients have an impaired catabolism of postprandial triglyceride (TG)-rich lipoproteins (TGRLs). Atorvastatin improves the delayed clearance of large TGRLs in FCHL (as evaluated by measuring the acute clearance of intravenous intralipid) and TGRLs after oral fat-loading tests. Atorvastatin significantly reduced fasting intermediate density lipoprotein (Svedberg flotation, 12-20)-ApoB100 concentrations. Investigated with oral fat-loading tests, the clearance of VLDL (Sf20-60)-ApoB100 was improved by 24%, without major changes in the other fractions. In FCHL, the effects of atorvastatin on postprandial lipemia were on hepatic TGRLs, without major improvements on intestinal TGRLs [53].

Among statins, rosuvastatin produces a more favorable response in terms of HDL-C [54,55]. Rosuvastatin and atorvastatin, given at their maximal doses, favorably alter the HDL subpopulation profile, but rosuvastatin is more effective in this regard than atorvastatin. In mixed dyslipidemia (simultaneous increase of LDL-C and triglycerides), different drug associations have been suggested, in order to reduce LDL-C and triglycerides and increase HDL-C, including fenofibrate + statin [56,57] or fenofibrate+ezetimibe [58]. In mixed dyslipidemia, it would be advisable to associate a statin with nicotinic acid to achieve an optimal lipid response, but the preparation of nicotinic acid so far available produce an unpleasant face flush, which is poorly tolerated by patients, especially long term.

Rosuvastatin and extended-release (ER) niacin alone and in combination [59] were assessed in patients with combined hyperlipidemia and low HDL-C levels. Daily doses of rosuvastatin 40 mg reduced LDL-C significantly more than either ER niacin 2 g or rosuvastatin 10 mg/ER niacin 2 g (−48% vs. −0.1% and −36%). Triglyceride reductions ranged from −21% (ER niacin monotherapy) to −39% (rosuvastatin 40 mg/ER niacin 1 g). Compared with rosuvastatin alone, rosuvastatin 10 mg/ER niacin 2 g produced significantly greater increases in HDL-C (11% vs. 24%, $p < .001$) and ApoA-I (5% vs. 11%, $p < .017$). Over 24 weeks, rosuvastatin alone was better tolerated than either ER niacin alone or the combinations of rosuvastatin and ER niacin.

It is well established that patients with combined hyperlipidemia, defined as elevated triglyceride levels between 200 and 500 mg/dl and elevated LDL-C > 130 mg/dl, are at increased risk for CAD. The optimal assessment of reaching lipid goals in patients with combined hyperlipidemia is still far from settled and has been an area of revision and modification in recent guidelines [17]. Although controversy remains as to the best single measurement to be used in treatment goals, current focus is on the use of LDL-C, non-HDL-C, and ApoB [60].

Type III HLP

Type III hyperlipoproteinemia (HLP) is a genetic disorder characterized by accumulation of remnant lipoproteins in the plasma and development of premature atherosclerosis. Defective forms of ApoE are the common denominator in this disorder, leading to impaired binding of remnant particles to a liver cell receptor and delayed removal from plasma [61–63].

In humans, ApoE is a polymorphic protein of which three common isoforms can be distinguished, designated ApoE2, ApoE3, and ApoE4. This genetic variation is associated with different plasma lipoprotein levels, different response to diet and lipid-lowering therapy, and a variable risk for CVD and Alzheimer's disease. Defective ApoE (commonly ApoE2) is essential but not sufficient to cause overt type III HLP. In fact, most ApoE2 homozygotes are hypolipidemic. Transgenic animal models [63] have demonstrated the impact of other genes or hormones in converting the hypolipidemia to hyperlipidemia.

Type III HLP or familial dysbetalipoproteinemia (FD) is an ApoE-mediated, autosomal recessive lipid disorder that is caused by mutations in the ApoE gene. Homozygosity for APOE2 (1 in 170 persons) causes FD or type III HLP in less than 20% of the adult APOE2 homozygotes. Less common, dominant negative mutations may also cause the disorder.

Additional gene and environmental factors are necessary for the expression of this hyperlipoproteinemia, including hyperinsulinemia and/or defects in other genes involved in the hydrolysis of triglycerides. The type III HLP phenotype is characterized by both hypercholesterolemia and hypertriglyceridemia. The hypercholesterolemia is caused by impaired receptor-mediated clearance of remnants by the liver, whereas the hypertriglyceridemia is caused primarily by impaired lipolytic processing of remnants and increased VLDL production associated with increased levels of ApoE.

The patients [61] may present with typical skin lesions and elevated plasma levels of cholesterol and triglycerides, mainly in VLDL remnants and intermediate-density lipoproteins. Estrogen affects both LDLR expression and lipolytic processing, explaining the resistance of women to this disorder until after menopause. The disorder is associated with frequent occurrence of premature peripheral and CAD. Diet and weight reduction are effective but usually not sufficient to normalize the lipid levels. Additional therapy with statins or fibrates is necessary and effective in most patients.

Familial Hypertriglyceridemia

In the paper first associating premature CVD with familial dyslipidemia, a distinct disorder, namely familial hypertriglyceridemia, was identified and described [64]. It is defined with the presence of a hypertriglyceridemic phenotype in all the affected members of the families and with a relatively high risk of eruptive cutaneous xanthomas and pancreatitis, especially in cases of severe hypertriglyceridemia, exceeding 1,000 mg/dl.

Several molecular abnormalities have been associated with genetic hypertriglyceridemia involving LPL and ApoC-II, or ApoA-V genes. Also, the loci identified for lipodystrophy syndromes have been associated with severe hypertriglyceridemia [31].

With regard to cardiovascular risk, it is suggested that familial hypertriglyceridemia is associated with risk increase, in the same order of magnitude of FCHL [46,64].

Chylomicronemia

Chylomicronemia [65] is present when triglyceride levels exceed 1,000 mg/dl. When accompanied by eruptive xanthoma, lipemia retinalis, or abdominal symptoms, chylomicronemia is referred to as the "chylomicronemia syndrome" and can cause acute pancreatitis.

Treatment aimed at reducing triglyceride levels includes lifestyle modifications to promote weight loss with diet and physical activity coupled with medications, including fibrates, n-3 polyunsaturated fatty acids, and nicotinic acid.

Familial chylomicronemia syndrome [66] is a rare disorder of lipoprotein metabolism due to familial LPL or ApoC-II deficiency or the presence of inhibitors to lipoprotein lipase. It manifests as eruptive xanthomas, acute pancreatitis, and lipemic plasma due to marked elevation of triglyceride and chylomicron levels. In many cases, patients with genetic lipodystrophies develop chylomicronemia and acute pancreatitis as well as cutaneous xanthomas [31].

Selected References

1. Bhatnagar D. Diagnosis and screening for familial hypercholesterolaemia: finding the patients, finding the genes. Ann Clin Biochem 2006;43:441–56.

29. Sniderman AD, Ribalta J, Castro Cabezas M. How should FCHL be defined and how should we think about its metabolic bases? Nutr Metab Cardiovasc Dis 2001;11:259–73.

41. Pauciullo P, Gentile M, Marotta G, Baiano A, Ubaldi S, Jossa F, Iannuzzo G, Faccenda F, Panico S, Rubba P. Small dense low-density lipoprotein in familial combined hyperlipidemia: independent of metabolic syndrome and related to history of cardiovascular events. Atherosclerosis 2009;2003(1):320–24.

42. Carr MC, Brunzell JD. Abdominal obesity and dyslipidemia in the metabolic syndrome: importance of type 2 diabetes and familial combined hyperlipidemia in coronary artery disease risk. J Clin Endocrinol Metab 2004;89:2601–7.

48. De Michele M, Iannuzzi A, Salvato A, Pauciullo P, Gentile M, Iannuzzo G, Panico S, Pujia A, Bond GM, Rubba P. Impaired endothelium-dependent vascular reactivity in patients with familial combined hyperlipidaemia. Heart 2007;93:78–81.

CHAPTER 20

HDL, Reverse Cholesterol Transport, and Atherosclerosis

Guido Franceschini, Monica Gomaraschi, & Laura Calabresi
University of Milano, Milan, Italy

High-Density Lipoproteins: Structure and Metabolism

Plasma high-density lipoproteins (HDLs) are a highly heterogeneous lipoprotein family consisting of several subspecies, with varying shape, density, size, and apolipoprotein composition. They sediment in the density region 1.063–1.210 g/ml, and range in diameter from 70 to 130 Å and in mass from 200,000 to 400,000 Daltons. When separated according to particle density, two major subfractions can be identified, called HDL$_2$ (1.063–1.125 g/ml) and HDL$_3$ (1.125–1.21 g/ml); HDL$_2$ particles are larger and relatively lipid rich and protein poor compared with HDL$_3$ particles. On average, HDLs contain 50% lipid and 50% protein. Most plasma HDLs have a spherical shape, with a central core of nonpolar lipids (triglycerides and cholesteryl esters) surrounded by a monolayer of polar lipids (phospholipids and unesterified cholesterol) and apolipoproteins; they migrate to α-position on agarose gel electrophoresis. A minor fraction of plasma HDLs have a disk-shaped structure with pre-beta mobility on electrophoresis; these particles, also called nascent HDLs (see below), lack the nonpolar core and are composed of a bilayer of polar lipids with apolipoproteins running around of the disk. Apolipoprotein A-I (ApoA-I) is the major protein component of HDL (about 70% of total proteins), followed by ApoA-II (about 20%). HDLs also contain other apolipoproteins (such as ApoA-IV, ApoCs, and ApoE) and a variety of enzymes and transfer proteins, including lecithin:cholesterol acyltransferase (LCAT), paraoxonase (PON), platelet-activating factor acetylhydrolase (PAF-AH), cholesteryl ester transfer protein (CETP), and phospholipid transfer protein (PLTP).

HDL metabolism is very complex, because HDL components are assembled after secretion, frequently exchanged among different HDL particles and between HDL and other lipoproteins, and mostly cleared independent from one another. Moreover, HDL particles are actively remodeled within the plasma compartment, through the combined action of enzymes and lipid transfer proteins. ApoA-I and ApoA-II are synthesized mainly by the liver and, to a lesser extent, by the small intestine and are secreted with very-low-density lipoproteins (VLDLs) and chylomicrons, respectively. During lipolysis of these triglyceride-rich lipoproteins, some surface components (phospholipids, cholesterol, and apolipoproteins) dissociate, generating preβ-HDLs or being incorporated into existing HDL particles, through the action of PLTP. Hepatocytes also secrete lipid-free ApoA-I, which then interacts with the ATP-binding cassette transporter A1 (ABCA1), acquiring phospholipids and cholesterol pericellularly and thereby forming preβ-HDLs [1]. In the circulation, preβ-HDLs are acted on by LCAT, which converts lecithin and cholesterol into lysolecithin and cholesteryl esters in a reaction that has ApoA-I as cofactor. The nonpolar cholesteryl esters split the bilayer and give rise to the mature spherical α-HDLs that

Nutritional and Metabolic Bases of Cardiovascular Disease, 1st edition.
Edited by Mario Mancini, José M. Ordovas, Gabriele Riccardi,
Paolo Rubba and Pasquale Strazzullo. © 2011 Blackwell Publishing Ltd.

predominate in plasma. The cholesteryl ester-rich mature α-HDLs follow a dual destiny. First, α-HDLs interact with CETP, which exchanges cholesteryl esters for triglycerides between HDLs and triglyceride-rich lipoproteins, generating large cholesteryl ester-poor and triglyceride-rich HDL particles. HDL triglycerides and phospholipids are then hydrolyzed by lipolytic enzymes (lipoprotein, hepatic, and endothelial lipases), converting spherical α-HDL back to discoidal preβ-HDL particles. During this process, some ApoA-I dissociates from HDLs and is cleared from the circulation, mainly through the kidney [2]. Second, mature α-HDLs are recognized by the scavenger receptor type BI (SR-BI), located on the surface of liver and adrenal cells, which mediates the selective uptake of cholesteryl esters from HDLs, without the internalization and degradation of the lipoprotein itself. The generated cholesteryl ester-depleted, small HDL particles are either remodeled into large HDLs by incorporation into preexisting HDLs, or are cleared through the kidney [2]. HDLs can be removed from the circulation through holoparticle endocytosis, following interaction with different "receptors," like the scavenger receptor class B type II (SR-BII) [3], the β-chain of ATP synthase [4], and others; however, this does not seem to be a major pathway for HDL catabolism. Rather HDL lipids and ApoA-I appear to be catabolized through distinct pathways, which require the dissociation of the apolipoprotein from its bound lipids. HDL lipid clearance occurs by the processes of cellular selective uptake through SR-BI, transfer to other lipoproteins by CETP and PLTP, and hydrolysis by lipolytic enzymes. The kidney is the principal site of ApoA-I degradation; cubilin, a multiligand receptor expressed in the apical membrane of various absorptive epithelia, including that of the kidney, binds ApoA-I with high affinity and mediates ApoA-I endocytosis. Whether the internalized ApoA-I may escape degradation and recycle back to the plasma is unknown.

HDL and Cardiovascular Disease

In the early 1950s, Barr et al. [5] were first to note that plasma concentrations of HDL-cholesterol (HDL-C) were lower in patients with coronary heart disease (CHD) than in healthy men. The Framingham Heart Study and other prospective studies during the 1980s confirmed the existence of a strong inverse association between HDL-C and cardiovascular risk. This inverse relation was observed at all levels of LDL-C, including concentrations well below the desirable level [6]. An aggregate analysis of four of the largest prospective U.S. studies indicated that for every 1-mg/dl increase in plasma HDL-C, the predicted incidence of coronary events decreases by 2% in men and 3% in women [7]. A low plasma HDL-C level is associated with not only an increased incidence of CHD but also with a greater risk for carotid atherosclerosis and ischemic stroke [8], for re-stenosis after coronary angioplasty [9], and for recurrent venous thromboembolism [10].

A low plasma HDL-C level is not simply a marker of cardiovascular risk, because several lines of evidence indicate a cause–effect relationship between low plasma HDL levels and cardiovascular disease. Studies in genetically modified animal models have established that interventions that raise the plasma HDL-C level, for example, by overexpression of ApoA-I, protect against the development of diet-induced and genetically determined atherosclerosis [11,12], while those that lower plasma HDL-C, for example, by deletion of the ApoA-I gene in an atherosclerosis-prone mouse, almost double lesion area [13]. Finally, *in vitro* and *in vivo* studies provide mechanistic explanations for the atheroprotective effects of HDL. The central role of HDL in reverse cholesterol transport (RCT), the process by which cholesterol within the arterial wall is routed to the liver for disposal (Figure 20.1), is widely considered the main mechanism responsible for HDL-mediated atheroprotection. However, it has been long recognized that apart from its role in RCT, HDL exert a series of non-lipid-related activities that may well contribute to HDL-mediated atheroprotection. In particular, HDLs have anti-inflammatory and antioxidant properties that cooperate in maintaining endothelium homeostasis, thus attenuating endothelial dysfunction, an hallmark of atherosclerosis [14]. It is not clear what the relative contribution of these non-lipid-related activities to human atheroprotection is, especially when compared with HDL function in RCT. However, recent work in mice lacking ApoA-I in the context of preserved plasma HDL-C levels provides some important clues to clarify this issue [15]. In these animals, a highly significant inverse

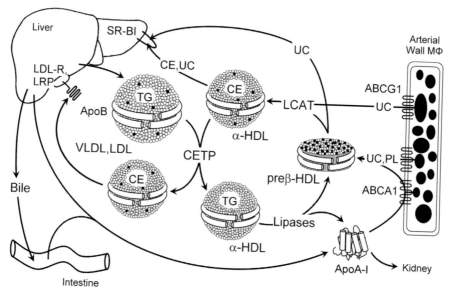

Figure 20.1 Schematic overview of HDL metabolism and reverse cholesterol transport. (ABCA1: ATP binding cassette transporter A1; ABCG1: ATP binding cassette transporter G1; ApoA-I: Apolipoprotein A-I; ApoB: apolipoprotein B; CE: cholesteryl ester; CETP: CE transfer protein; HDL: high-density lipoprotein; LCAT: lecithin:cholesterol acyltransferase; LDL: low-density lipoprotein; LDL-R: LDL-receptor; LRP: LDL-receptor related protein; Mɸ: macrophage; PL: phospholipid; SR-BI: scavenger receptor type BI; TG: triglyceride; UC: unesterified cholesterol; VLDL: very-low-density lipoprotein.)

relationship was observed between ApoA-I gene dose and the extent of atherosclerosis; the enhanced atherosclerosis in mice lacking ApoA-I was associated with defective RCT, increased vascular inflammation and greater oxidative stress, implying that all known HDL activities contribute to HDL-mediated atheroprotection.

The plasma HDL-C level quantifies the cholesterol content of HDL and is generally taken as a measure of the number of circulating HDL particles. Therefore, the consistent and highly significant inverse relationship between plasma HDL-C levels and cardiovascular risk found in many human population studies is assumed as an indication that the atheroprotective activity of HDL is closely linked to their concentration in plasma. Conversely, there is convincing evidence that at least some of the potentially atheroprotective functions of HDL relate to properties of specific HDL components or subpopulations, which concentration in plasma may be totally unrelated to the HDL-C level. So, small preβ-HDLs and large α-HDLs remove cell cholesterol through distinct pathways (see below); small

HDLs are also more efficient than larger particles in preventing endothelial dysfunction [14] and in protecting LDLs from oxidative stress[16]. Mechanistically, small HDLs, thus, appear as the most effective particles in arterial protection. Nevertheless, there is conflicting epidemiologic evidence on the relative atheroprotective potential of small HDL$_3$ versus large HDL$_2$, preβ-HDL versus α-HDL particles. In earlier prospective studies the plasma HDL$_3$-C level was a stronger predictor of coronary disease than was HDL$_2$-C [17]. Consistent with this finding, in the Veterans Affairs HDL Intervention Trial, plasma HDL$_3$-C, but not HDL$_2$-C levels at baseline, and as percentage change during treatment, were significantly related to the development of new coronary events [18]. However, when in the same trial HDL particles were separated by size and charge, case subjects had lower levels of large α-migrating HDL particles (mostly HDL$_2$) as compared to subjects without events [19]; this is in agreement with data from the Framingham Offspring Study, also showing that coronary patients have lower levels of large α-HDL than controls

[20]. Discordance in these epidemiological findings likely reflects complex relationships between HDL particles separated according to different chemicophysical properties. Indeed, which is the "good" HDL particle in arterial protection is largely indeterminate.

Genetic HDL Disorders

Up to 70% of the variation in plasma HDL-C levels is genetically determined. Familial hypo-alphalipoproteinemias and hyper-alphalipoproteinemias (FHALPs and FHrALPs) constitute a genetically heterogeneous group of inherited HDL disorders, defined by extremely low or high plasma HDL-C levels and caused by mutations in known candidate genes or in other genes yet to be identified. Some mutations are associated with unique HDL features and with paradoxical phenotypes, that is, low HDL-C but unaltered CHD risk, or high HDL-C with enhanced CHD risk.

FHALP is characterized by a plasma HDL-C level below the fifth percentile for the general population. Among the known causes of FHALP are mutations in major candidate genes, such as the *apoA-I*, *ABCA1*, and *LCAT* genes. Studies of American general populations revealed that mutations in these three genes account for 10%–16% of FHALP cases [21]. At least 70 different mutations in the *apoA-I* gene have been identified since the discovery of apoA-I$_{Milano}$ [22]. Only half of them cause FHALP [23]. While mutations that abolish ApoA-I synthesis are definitely associated with premature CHD, missense mutations that cause even marked reductions of plasma HDL-C do not necessarily lead to enhanced CHD risk [23]. So, carriers of the apoA-I$_{Milano}$ mutation, who do not show any structural and functional evidence of vascular disease [24,25], behave clearly distinct from carriers of the ApoA-I (L178P) mutation, who instead present with accelerated carotid arterial wall thickening and endothelial dysfunction, associated with premature CHD [26]. This dramatic difference in CHD risk may be due to remarkably distinct HDL features, as illustrated by the accumulation in ApoA-I$_{Milano}$ plasma of small HDL with improved cholesterol removal and vasculoprotective properties [25,27]. Familial HDL deficiency and Tangier disease are two FHALPs caused by the inheritance of either one or two mutant ABCA1 alleles, respectively.

Approximately 100 mutations distributed over the entire *ABCA1* gene have been described. These mutations may cause a variety of functional defects in the ABCA1 pathway, such as increased intracellular degradation, block of the intracellular transport, failure to act as phospholipid-cholesterol transporter, and increased degradation due to a defective interaction with ApoA-I [28]. The defective ABCA1 protein impairs the formation of preβ-HDL and the subsequent maturation to α-HDL. Homozygotes and heterozygotes for different ABCA1 mutations display a wide range of phenotypes at both the biochemical and cellular levels [29], which may translate into a variable CHD risk. Indeed, whether carriers of ABCA1 mutations are at increased CHD risk is not firmly established, although there is evidence of an enhanced preclinical atherosclerosis [30]. Mutations in the *LCAT* gene also cause two distinct FHALP syndromes: familial LCAT deficiency (FLD) and fish-eye disease (FED). FLD is characterized by a complete deficiency of LCAT activity, whereas in FED the enzyme does not esterifies cholesterol within HDL but retains its capacity to esterify cholesterol within other lipoproteins [31]. In recent years, 14 Italian families carrying 17 different LCAT mutations causing partial or complete LCAT deficiency have been identified [31]. Analysis of these families revealed a gene-dose-dependent effect of the mutations on various plasma lipid-lipoprotein parameters; however, the plasma lipoprotein profile, and in particular the HDL subspecies distribution, varied widely among families carrying different mutations. Despite the different functional defect of the LCAT enzyme in FLD and FED cases, resulting in clearly distinct cholesterol esterification profiles, the biochemical phenotype was quite similar, suggesting the possibility that FLD and FED are not two distinct syndromes, but the same disease at different levels of LCAT impairment. There was no evidence of premature CHD in these families [31]. Whether the HDL deficiency in carriers of *LCAT* gene mutations is associated with alterations in arterial structure and function is largely unknown [30]. In addition to the major candidate genes discussed above, mutations in other "minor" candidate genes, such as the *LPL*, *GBA*, *ABCG1*, *PLTP* and *ANGPTL-3* genes, have been found to be, or have the potential of being associated with FHALP.

FHrALP is characterized by a plasma HDL-C above the 95th percentile for the general population. The best known monogenic cause of FHrALP is a mutation in the *CETP* gene abolishing CETP activity. This disorder is relatively common in Japan, but is thought to be rare among Caucasians. CETP deficiency leads to the accumulation in plasma of cholesterol enriched, large α-HDL particles with either defective or normal capacity to promote cholesterol efflux from macrophages [32,33]. Its relationship to CHD risk is also debated [34,35].

Mutations in the *LIPG* gene, which encodes the endothelial lipase (EL), abolish the activity of this enzyme, and are associated with a substantial increase of plasma HDL-C in mice [36]. No EL deficiency has been detected so far in humans, but several potential functional polymorphisms of the *LIPG* gene were found in subjects with elevated HDL levels [37]. Similar considerations apply to the *SCARB1* gene, which encodes for SR-BI. Its deletion in mice leads to a marked increase of plasma HDL-C, with accumulation of large α-HDL [38]. Three common sequence variants in the human *SCARB1* gene have been found to be associated with variations in HDL-C [39], but no loss of function mutations causing FHrALP have been reported to date. Whether FHrALP due to molecular defects in the *LIPG* or *SCARB1* genes are protective against premature atherosclerosis and CHD is unknown.

Reverse Cholesterol Transport

Atherogenesis is a complex process characterized by a chronic inflammatory response to an excessive accumulation of cholesterol in the arterial wall. Early in the development of an atherosclerotic lesion, monocytes transmigrate through the endothelium into the intima layer, where they differentiate to macrophages; the excessive uptake of modified LDL or remnant lipoproteins by sub-endothelial macrophages gives rise to cholesterol-loaded cells known as "foam cells," which represent the major cell component of fatty streaks, the earliest grossly visible atherosclerotic lesions. By mediating cholesterol efflux from foam cells and its transport to the liver, the RCT represents a key process for the prevention and reversal of atherosclerosis. HDLs play

a pivotal role in RCT, being the main carriers of cholesterol in this process and different HDL subspecies are involved in different steps of RCT (Figure 20.1).

The efflux of unesterified cholesterol from cell plasma membranes to extracellular acceptors is the first and rate-limiting step of RCT. This movement can occur simply by aqueous diffusion according to the direction of cholesterol gradient. However, cell culture studies have clarified that cholesterol efflux is a highly regulated process and, to date, three distinct pathways other than passive diffusion have been identified [40,41]: 1) an ATP-dependent pathway mediated by ABCA1; 2) an ATP-dependent pathway mediated by the ABCG1 transporter; and 3) an ATP-independent pathway involving the SR-BI. Both ABCA1- and ABCG1-mediated pathways are energy-consuming processes that promote net cholesterol efflux from cells [40,41]. On the contrary, SR-BI mediates a bidirectional cholesterol exchange between cell membranes and extracellular acceptors; thus, like the passive diffusion, the net movement of cholesterol depends on the direction of the cholesterol gradient [40]. Lipid-free ApoA-I and preβ-HDL particles are the preferential acceptors for ABCA1-mediated efflux, whereas mature α-HDLs are the best acceptors for ABCG1- and SR-BI-mediated efflux [40–42]. ABCA1 and ABCG1 seem to act as a lipid translocase, increasing the availability of phospholipids and cholesterol at the cell surface, but while the binding of ApoA-I to ABCA1 is essential for ABCA1-mediated efflux, ABCG1-mediated efflux does not seem to require a direct interaction between the acceptors and the transporter. Therefore, cell cholesterol efflux is a complex and saturable process that critically depends on the availability of transporters on cell surface and of suitable cholesterol acceptors in the extracellular space.

Cholesterol carried by HDL is esterified within the plasma by the LCAT enzyme, and the synthesized cholesteryl esters are transported to the liver through two major routes: direct and indirect transport. During direct transport, HDLs deliver cholesteryl esters directly to hepatocytes, through SR-BI-mediated selective uptake; the cholesteryl esters are then hydrolyzed, and the unesterified cholesterol is excreted into the bile as it is, in a process that involves the ABCG5/ABCG8 transporters

[43], or in the form of bile acids. During indirect transport, a substantial part of HDL-cholesteryl esters is transferred by CETP to triglyceride-rich lipoproteins, which are metabolized into remnants and then removed by the liver either directly or after conversion into LDLs [44]. In addition to the two routes for HDL-cholesteryl esters transport to the liver, there is also an SR-BI-dependent pathway for the direct uptake of HDL unesterified cholesterol in the liver, with its subsequent excretion into bile [45] (Figure 20.1).

HDL as a Therapeutic Target for Cardiovascular Disease

The epidemiologic and experimental evidence of an atheroprotective function of HDL provides the background for the development of novel therapeutic interventions targeting HDL-C for the treatment of atherosclerotic cardiovascular disease. Plasma concentrations of HDL-C are the net result of a number of sources: 1) de novo production of HDL apolipoproteins by the liver and the intestine; 2) rates of ApoA-I lipidation in the liver and periphery by ABCA1; 3) remodeling of HDL particles through the action of multiple enzymes and lipid transfer proteins; and 4) fractional catabolic rates of HDL lipids, proteins and particles. A number of therapeutic approaches with the potential to raise plasma HDL-C levels and/or increase RCT rate are being pursued. Although these approaches appear all promising, doubts on the clinical benefit achievable with such interventions have been raised by the recent failure of torcetrapib, the most potent and furthest developed HDL-C raising compound to date.

Torcetrapib is a small lipophilic molecule that binds CETP to inhibit its lipid transfer activities. Clinical studies demonstrated that CETP inhibition by torcetrapib was effective in 1) increasing plasma HDL-C and decreasing LDL-C levels [46], 2) enhancing plasma α-HDL levels [47], and 3) increasing plasma concentrations of ApoA-I by delaying its catabolism [47]. Despite these impressive effects on lipid parameters long associated with cardiovascular risk, the ILLUMINATE study, a Phase III trial in more than 15,000 subjects comparing the combination of torcetrapib and atorvastatin versus atorvastatin alone, was prematurely halted because of an excess mortality in the combination

therapy arm. As a consequence, torcetrapib development was stopped. While the ILLUMINATE trial was ongoing, three imaging studies to investigate the effects of torcetrapib on atherosclerosis progression/regression in atorvastatin-treated patients were concluded. In all three studies, the torcetrapib-induced improvement in lipid/lipoprotein profiles did not translate in a reduced progression of atherosclerosis, as measured as percent atheroma volume by intravascular ultrasound, or carotid intima-media thickness by B-mode ultrasonography [48,49]. Although the imaging studies were not powered to evaluate cardiovascular outcomes, the number of severe adverse cardiovascular events was consistently greater in the groups treated with the combination of torcetrapib and atorvastatin than with atorvastatin alone. Theorized reasons for the unexpected results of the ILLUMINATE and imaging studies include 1) off-target effects of torcetrapib, as the increase in blood pressure; 2) a decrease in ABCA1-mediated macrophage cholesterol removal due to impaired recycling of mature α-HDL into preβ-HDL; and 3) accumulation in plasma of HDL particles that are dysfunctional in RCT or other atheroprotective mechanisms.

The failure of torcetrapib does not mean that the concept of targeting HDL-C to further reduce cardiovascular risk in the statin era is definitely dead. CETP inhibitors, which do not raise blood pressure, are under investigation by various companies; more research with these compounds is needed to answer the crucial question on whether the lack of clinical benefit with torcetrapib is a failure of CETP inhibition as a strategy for HDL-C raising or is due to a unique drug toxicity. The real beneficiaries of torcetrapib failure might be other HDL-C raising therapies, which act through disparate molecular mechanisms, and are in various stages of preclinical and clinical development. Nevertheless, further advancement in basic and translational research on the molecular mechanisms regulating HDL metabolism and mediating HDL atheroprotection is needed to define the best molecular targets for drug development. An important concept is that the plasma HDL-C level per se may not reflect the functionality of HDL; the function of HDL is likely more important than its concentration, at least as assessed by measuring plasma HDL-C concentration. Even if they do not increase plasma HDL-C levels, therapies that improve HDL function may have important antiatherogenic and vascular protective effects. There is a critical need for the development of HDL-related biomarkers that will allow the assessment of HDL function in a simple and reliable way, to determine whether a new HDL-targeted therapy indeed improves HDL function in preclinical models and early in clinical development before moving into a high-risk cardiovascular outcome trial.

The concept of providing patients directly with functional HDLs, instead of administering small compounds that enhance plasma HDL-C levels, is particularly attractive to overcome problems related to the still incomplete knowledge of factors regulating HDL metabolism and function. There is experimental and clinical evidence that such approach is feasible and likely successful. In a first clinical study in hypercholesterolemic patients, a single injection of synthetic HDL (sHDL) caused a rapid augmentation of plasma HDL levels followed by an increase of fecal sterol excretion, suggestive of an enhanced RCT [50]. In a second study in healthy males, all steps of RCT were stimulated by sHDL administration [51]. There was an increase in the cholesterol content of lymph lipoproteins, indicative of peripheral cholesterol mobilization; the plasma cholesterol esterification increased, indicating an enhanced flux of cholesteryl esters through plasma HDL; and there was a late increase in fecal bile acid excretion, indicating that the mobilized cholesterol had been indeed transported to the liver and utilized for bile acid synthesis [51]. In 2003, a small imaging study in coronary patients demonstrated that 5 weekly injections of sHDL containing a recombinant ApoA-I$_{Milano}$ variant (ETC-216, 15 or 45 mg/kg) provide a clear ben-

efit on atheroma regression, as assessed by IVUS [52]. More recently, a similar result, that is, a significant reduction of total atheroma volume versus baseline (but no difference vs. placebo), was achieved in a larger number of coronary patients receiving 4 weekly injections of sHDL containing wild-type ApoA-I (CSL-111, 40 mg/kg) [53]. sHDLs were generally well tolerated in both studies, although CSL-111 treatment at high dose (80 mg/kg) had to be discontinued because of a high incidence of liver function test abnormalities [53]. Therefore, there is mechanistic and imaging trial evidence that sHDL injections represent a viable treatment option for atherosclerosis regression, but only a clinical outcome study will allow us to quantify the risk/benefit ratio of such treatments and identify their place in the cardiovascular therapeutic arsenal.

Selected References

6. Barter PJ, Gotto AM, LaRosa JC, et al. HDL cholesterol, very low levels of LDL cholesterol, and cardiovascular events. N Engl J Med 2007;357:1301–10.
8. Sanossian N, Saver JL, Navab M, et al. High-density lipoprotein cholesterol: an emerging target for stroke treatment. Stroke 2007;38:1104–9.
14. Calabresi L, Gomaraschi M, Franceschini G. Endothelial protection by high-density lipoproteins: from bench to bedside. Arterioscler Thromb Vasc Biol 2003;23:1724–31.
29. Singaraja RR, Visscher H, James ER, et al. Specific mutations in ABCA1 have discrete effects on ABCA1 function and lipid phenotypes both in vivo and in vitro. Circ Res 2006;99:389–97.
44. Lewis GF, Rader DJ. New insights into the regulation of HDL metabolism and reverse cholesterol transport. Circ Res 2005;96:1221–32.

CHAPTER 21

Role of Polyunsaturated Omega-3 Fatty Acids and Micronutrient Intake on Atherosclerosis and Cardiovascular Disease

Francesco Visioli[1], Doriane Richard[1],
Pedro Bausero[1], & Claudio Galli[2]

[1] UPMC University, Paris, France
[2] University of Milan, Milan, Italy

Cardiovascular Disease, Diet, and Mortality in Contemporary Societies

Cardiovascular disease (CVD) is one of the major causes of mortality in developed countries (as reported in 2003 by the World Health Organization [WHO] [1]) and it will soon become a major cause also in countries undergoing rapid changes in their socioeconomic setup and, consequently, in their lifestyles. Indeed, it has been estimated that environmental changes and dietary habits will soon become the major factors responsible for most chronic diseases (namely, cardiovascular, metabolic, respiratory, and cancer) and related deaths. There is growing awareness that the profound changes in environment, diet, and lifestyle that began with the introduction of agriculture and animal husbandry 10,000 years ago occurred too recently and too rapidly on an evolutionary timescale for the human genome to adjust. In conjunction with this discordance between our ancient, genetically determined biology and the nutritional, cultural, and activity patterns of contemporary Western populations,

Nutritional and Metabolic Bases of Cardiovascular Disease, 1st edition.
Edited by Mario Mancini, José M. Ordovas, Gabriele Riccardi,
Paolo Rubba and Pasquale Strazzullo. © 2011 Blackwell Publishing Ltd.

many of the so-called diseases of civilization have emerged.

The large numbers of subjects affected by the disease for long periods pose the problem of a strictly pharmacological approach, that is, massive and prolonged drug treatments in large population groups, and underline the relevance of preventive approaches, based on lifestyle and especially dietary changes. This approach is very important from a public health point of view and has important economic connotations.

In this chapter, we focus on fatty acids (FAs) and micronutrients as examples of dietary approaches to CVD prevention/therapy.

Dietary Fats

Among dietary factors, fats, mainly represented by FAs esterified in triglycerides (TGs) are major determinants of the health status. In fact, their intakes are quantitatively relevant in the diet, due to several factors: high availability of fats derived from massive cultivation of plants for oil production, associated with low costs of energy-rich, fatty foods. On the other side, FAs play very relevant roles in the body, not only as energetic sources, but also in the case of selected types of FA—such as the long-chain, highly unsaturated FA (LC-HUFA) of the omega-6 and omega-3 series—as modulators of cell function. Under these conditions, the frequent excess of fat intake, mainly as saturated FAs, monounsaturated FAs (MUFAs), and polyunsaturated FAs (PUFAs) of the omega-6 series—such as linoleic acid (LA), present in high concentrations in most vegetable (seed) oils—leads to a "dilution" of the omega-3 FAs, poorly represented in most common foods. Omega-3 FAs, especially those that are most relevant in biological terms (i.e., the long-chain HU-FAs eicosapentaenoic [EPA] and docosahexaenoic [DHA]), have become analogous to micronutrients (intakes of a few hundreds of milligrams per day in most populations out of over 100 g/day of total fat).

The Omega-3 Fatty Acids

Their Origin in Biology and Shore-Based Foods in Human Diet

Omega-3 FAs are a family of compounds with a typical FA structure, that is, a carbon chain with a methyl group at one end and a carboxyl (acid) group at the other, acting as the esterification site into glycerolipids, with at least three double bonds (PUFA). They are characterized by their "essentiality," or the inability to be synthesized in animals; therefore, they need to be supplied by the diet and are endowed of properties that are essential for biological systems. While the reader is referred to specialized publications for details on the chemistry and the metabolism of these compounds, a few key relevant features are given here:

a The series is defined as omega-3 or *n*-3 because, in each component, three carbon atoms are interposed between the methyl end of the carbon chain and the closest double bond. This part of the molecule cannot be modified by the metabolic processes in the series, namely elongation and desaturation of precursors to products.

b They include precursors with 18 carbon atoms and 3 double bonds, that is, α-linolenic acid (ALA) (18:3 ω3) in positions Δ9,12,15 from the carboxyl end and, consequently, with 3 carbon atoms interposed between the double bond in position Δ15 and the methyl end. From ALA, a series of longer chain and more unsaturated FA is generated through subsequent elongation and desaturation reactions.

c Desaturases are critical in the conversion of shorter chain to longer chain PUFA (LC-PUFA) or HUFA and are modulated by a number of factors and conditions. In particular, they are activated by dietary factors (carbohydrate intakes, insulin, and low intakes of the 18 carbon precursors of both series), and by agents such as peroxisome proliferators and statins. In contrast they are inhibited by high fat diets, diets enriched in omega-3 FAs, and cholesterol, hormones (adrenaline, glucagon, and steroids), oxysterols, and cigarette smoke.

d The same desaturases function in both series, that is, in the omega-3 and in the omega-6. In the latter, they are involved in the conversion of LA (18:2 ω6), the most abundant PUFA in nature and in our diet, to the most abundant long-chain PUFA in biological systems arachidonic acid (AA) (20:4ω6). While the Δ6D is ubiquitously found in nature and operates also in plants, the Δ5D is exclusively found in animals (with exclusion of aquatic plants). The two pathways are completely independent, but since the same enzymes are involved in both series, competitions based on the relative abundance of substrates quantitatively affect the relative rates of conversion.

e Elongases are not rate limiting and do not appear to play major regulatory roles in the overall metabolic conversion in the two series.

f Relevant differences between the omega-6 and omega-3 series concern the major products of the series. In fact, while in the omega-6 series the metabolic pathway basically does not proceed beyond AA, the major LC-PUFA (DHA, 22:6 ω3) of the omega-3 series is produced through rather complex steps. In fact, the metabolic sequence after eicosapentaenoic acid (EPA) (20:5ω3) involves two elongation steps, leading to the formation of 24:5, followed by a Δ6D reaction producing 24:6. These steps take place in the endoplasmic reticulum and are kinetically rather efficient. However, the step yielding 22:6, that is, the retroconversion of 24:6 to 22:6, involves a peroxisomal β-oxidation. As a consequence, while AA is rather abundant in cells and tissues, due to the combined effect of high intakes of both its precursor LA with the diet and its biosynthetic pathway, omega-3 FA concentrations are, in general, low as a consequence of their lower levels in the diet and, in particular, of the fact that DHA is not very efficiently produced from its precursors.

Fish, Omega-3 Fatty Acids, and CVDs

The first observation that populations consuming high amounts of fish, namely the Greenland Eskimos, had a lower incidence of CVDs compared to populations on a typical Western diet dates back to the 1970s, after studies of Danish investigators [2]. Cardiovascular protection associated to fish consumption was soon attributed to the large intakes of the typical FA in fish, namely those of the *n*-3 series, accredited with protection of the Greenland population from ischemic processes [2].

The initial observations on the relationship between fish consumption and CVD were followed by several studies, which were recently reviewed [3] and which can be subdivided into (a) epidemio-

logic investigations (associations between fish consumption and clinical outcomes); (b) randomized controlled trials (RCTs) on the estimated intakes of fish or on controlled intakes of omega-3 FA; and (c) cohort studies. The effects on mortality and on various relevant parameters related to CV disease have been analyzed and the results are summarized in Table 21.1.

In synthesis, there is general consensus on the favorable effects of increased intakes of fish or omega-3 FA preparations on clinical cardiovascular outcomes, especially on sudden death, as well as on other cardiac events such as myocardial infarction [4]. However, the results, in terms of effectiveness, are variable, mainly due to the different designs of the studies. In fact, assessments of omega-3 FA consumption based on estimates of fish intake (with

Table 21.1   Major studies on the effects of fish or omega-3 fatty acid intakes on outcomes in cardiovascular pathologies.

A. Secondary prevention: RCT of the effects of a) dietary fish advice and b) long-chain omega 3 fatty acid supplements

No. of studies	n (intervention-control)	Omega-3 intakes (g/day)	All-cause mortality	Cardiac death	Sudden death	Myocardial infarction	Stroke
					Favorable effects on		
a) 2	~1,500-~1,100	0.9–1.1	1/2	1/2	1	1	–
b) 7	30-5,665		3/5	4/5	3	6/7 (1/7*)	1/4 (3/4*)

B. Case-control studies of the association of estimated of a) omega-3 fatty acids or b) fish consumption with clinical outcomes in the general population

No. of studies	n (min-max)	Sudden death	Myocardial infarction	Stroke
		Favorable effects on		
a) 3	827-975	1/3	1/3	Nd
b) 7	234-1,846	1/7	4/7	1/7

C. Cohort studies of the association of estimates of a) long-chain omega-3 fatty acids and b) fish consumption with clinical outcomes in the general population

No. of studies	n (min-max)	Duration (yr; min-max)	All-cause mortality	Cardiac death	Sudden death	Myocardial infarction	Stroke
					Favorable effects on		
a) 12	2,283-79,839	4-15.5	3/12	1/12	1/12	3/12	3/12
b) 27	603-223,170	4-30	3/27	11/27	2/27	5/27	6/27

*Relative number of adverse events concerning the specific outcomes. RCT: randomized clinical trials.
Adapted from Wang et al. [34], with permission.

rather different omega-3 FA contents and subjected to different cooking procedures) and on food composition tables, are often unreliable. The same applies to studies based on recommendations to increase fish consumption. On the other hand, RCTs based on the controlled administration of pharmaceutical preparations of omega-3 FA, that is, when intakes are more accurately defined, provide more reliable results. It is important to mention that the effects, especially those on sudden death and cardiovascular mortality, are reached more rapidly than the ones obtained through changes in the intakes of major dietary FA, for example, reduction of saturated FAs, increase of MUFA and especially PUFA of the omega-6 series, mainly LA. As pointed out in a meta-analysis by Hooper et al. [3], this is due to the fact that the favorable effects of modifications of major dietary FA on CVD are mainly dependent upon changes of lipid/lipoprotein profiles (especially reduction of low-density lipoprotein [LDL]-cholesterol [LDL-C]). These parameters are very slowly modified by dietary modifications.

Fish consumption may have several advantages over formulations:

A) In addition to providing omega-3 FAs, fish meat is a good source of other valuable nutrients such as A, B, and D vitamins. As for minerals, fish meat is regarded as a valuable source of calcium and phosphorus in particular, but also of iron, copper, and selenium. Finally, saltwater fish has a high content of iodine.

B) The resistance toward oxidation of omega-3 FA in extracted and purified preparations is lower than that of omega-3 FA in fish (where they are protected by various stabilizing agents), unless adequate amounts of antioxidants are incorporated in the preparations.

C) The bioavailability of omega-3 FA might be higher when they are ingested as components of fish, or of foods in general [5,6].

One relevant feature of LC-omega-3 PUFA is that they are present in very low amounts in conventional diets; yet, compared to that of total fat, relatively small intakes are able to effectively modulate key biological functions. Alas, reliable information on the concentrations of these FAs in the body, that is, their status in populations and population groups, is rather limited, and data on their dietary intakes extrapolated from food composition might

not be very reliable because of methodological limitations. Finally, recommendations on their optimal intakes should take into consideration, as previously mentioned, that their bioavailability appears to depend upon the matrix or the formulation, a parameter that so far has not been adequately assessed.

Mechanisms of Cardioprotection by Omega-3 Fatty Acids

Over the years, research has been extensively devoted to investigate, from *in vitro* to animal to human studies, the mechanisms underlying the effects of omega-3 FAs on the cardiovascular system.

Due to their involvement in the control of various metabolic and functional processes taking place in the cardiovascular system through multiple interactions, a number of mechanisms have been identified and proposed. Such mechanisms can be classified as follows:

A) Metabolic, namely effects on lipid metabolism. Relatively large intakes of omega-3 FA ($\geq$2 g/day) have been shown to effectively reduce plasma triacylglycerol (TG) concentrations. This is the major effect of omega-3 FA on circulating lipids and is likely consequent to i) lower TG synthesis due to reduced substrate (i.e., FA) availability, secondary to increase in β-oxidation; ii) decreased delivery of free FA to the liver; and iii) redirection of lipid synthesis vs. phospholipids rather than TG. An additional, less relevant effect of omega-3 FA on lipid parameters is their elevation of HDL cholesterolemia. The effects on LDL-C are, conversely, rather complex. In fact, plasma total and LDL-C may be increased by omega-3 FA supplementation, but the LDL particles that are formed are of larger volumes (with a consequently lower surface/volume ratio) and in lower concentrations. These particles are considered to be less atherogenic, as arterial lesions induced by LDL are related to surface-surface interactions: These processes are lessened in the case of particles with lower surface/volume ratios. In addition, it has been shown that omega-3 FAs are readily incorporated in atherosclerotic plaques where they induce changes that can enhance their stability [7].

B) Modulation of cell functions, namely reduced platelets aggregability, resulting in antithrombotic activity, and reduced proinflammatory activity of leukocytes. Major mechanisms are the competitive interactions with the production of bioactive metabolites (eicosanoids) generated from arachidonic acid. In particular, reduced production of pro-thrombotic thromboxanes (TxA_2) generated by platelets and of proinflammatory leukotrienes (LTB_4 and LTC_4), generated by leukocytes, both derived from AA, and production of less active metabolites derived from EPA, that is, TxA_3 and LTB_5 and LTC_5, appear responsible for these effects. More recently, the activities of anti-inflammatory protective compounds from DHA (resolvins and neuroprotectins) have also been described [8]. Finally, mounting evidence points to the antioxidant activities of omega-3 FAs [9].

C) Reduced production of proinflammatory cytokines (interleukin [IL]-1β, IL-6, IL-8, tumor necrosis factor [TNF]-α) by altered expression of inflammatory genes, through effects on transcription factors activation [10].

D) Antiarrhythmic myocardial activity, as tested *in vitro* by the exposure of cardiomyocytes to arrhythmogenic compounds, and in animal models of fatal arrhythmias related to myocardial infarction. These activities appear to be mediated by the inhibition of the fast, voltage-dependent sodium current and the L-type calcium currents, and to be responsible of the reduction of sudden death in human studies [11].

Concerning omega 3 FAs and CVD, the following general conclusions can be drawn: Enhanced intakes of omega-3 FA are cardioprotective via modulation of various parameters. The effects are obtained with relatively low amounts of omega-3 FA, on the order of approximately 1 g/day, which is a small fraction of total fat ingested daily (at least 100 g in most countries). The effects on plasma TG, the major modification of lipid parameters induced by omega 3 FAs, are usually obtained with high doses. Rather scarce in our diets, omega-3 FAs are selectively and specifically incorporated in cellular lipid pools, mainly in glycero-phospholipids, where they exert their modulatory roles. One feature of omega-3 FA treatment is, in fact, that their increments in plasma and cell lipids are relevant, even at relatively low levels of intakes. Also, these compounds accumulate mainly in rather stable lipid pools and are retained even after long washout periods. This implies that preservation

Table 21.2 Recommendations on fish and omega-3 fatty acids intake.

A. General population	
Fish: consumption of (fatty) fish at least twice /week	
omega-3:	
EPA+DHA	at least 0.65 g/day
EPA	*Minimum* 0.22 g/day
DHA	*Minimum* 0.22 g/day
B. Patients with documented cardiovascular disease	
EPA+DHA	At least 1 g/day
C. Patients with hypertriglyceridemia	At least 2 g/day

EPA: eicosapentaenoic acid; DHA: docosahexaenoic acid.

of body levels does not require daily administration, but just a maintenance schedule. In particular, fish consumption provides adequate intakes of omega-3 and exerts cardioprotective effects with consumption levels of two servings of fatty fish per week.

Recommendations on appropriate intakes of omega-3 FA and of fish are summarized in Table 21.2 and are further discussed in the authoritative International Society for the Study of Fatty Acids and Lipids (ISSFAL) website (www.issfal.co.uk).

In synthesis, there is solid and convincing evidence that increased consumption of fish, providing long-chain omega-3 FA on the order of 1 g/day results in cardioprotective effects (and activities on other major systems such as the nervous, respiratory, and immune systems) [34]. Development of appropriate public health strategies might lead to improvement of the health status of populations from pregnancy to the elderly.

Micronutrients and Cardiovascular Disease

The traditional dietary habits of the Mediterranean area have been consistently associated with lower incidence of CVD (coronary heart disease [CHD]) and cancer [12]. Although the healthful properties of Mediterranean diets as a whole have gained recognition, basic researchers are nowadays concentrating their efforts on individual food items, such as cereals, fruits, vegetable, olive oil, and their components, such as fibers, vitamins, polyphenols [12]. By singling out the contribution of micronutrients to the protective activities, one can better focus dietary guidelines and, possibly, formulate appropriate functional foods or nutraceuticals [13]. One approach is based on *in vitro* observations of potentially healthful properties of plant extracts or their isolated components. There is indeed extensive literature that reports on the antioxidant and enzyme-modulating activities of numerous herbs and their extracts. However, the transposition of these basic observations into claims of human effects is, at present, not entirely backed by solid evidence. Human studies are difficult to perform because of ethical and practical reasons. Hence, even though *in vitro* studies abound, human (and even animal) intervention studies are scant. Thus, it is mandatory to confirm *in vitro* observations in *in vitro* studies before definitive claims can be made.

In this chapter, we use olive oil and tomato, whose consumption has been linked to CHD- and chemoprotection, as examples of the epidemiology-to-trial approach to food minor components. In this respect, we pioneered research on the biological properties of olive oil polyphenols, whose wide range of pharmacological activities might provide a partial explanation for the high longevity and low incidence of degenerative diseases observed in the Mediterranean area, where olive oil is the predominant source of fat. Moreover, we investigated the effects of tomato supplementation, by providing healthy volunteers with purified tomato extracts in an attempt to identify the contribution of individual tomato components, for example, carotenoids such as lycopene. Finally, we more recently followed an *in vitro*-to-*in vivo* approach to test and validate the vasomodulatory properties of plant food extracts, selected within a European Union (EU)-funded project on Local Food Nutraceuticals (www.biozentrum.uni-frankfurt.de/Pharmakologie/EU-Web/index.html).

Plant-Derived Phenols

Phenolics are derivatives of benzene with one or more hydroxyl groups associated with their ring and they can be conveniently classified into at least ten different classes according to their chemical structure. Such compounds are important to plant physiology, contributing to resistance to microorganisms and insects, pigmentation and organoleptic characteristics (odor and flavor).

It is noteworthy that fruits and vegetables require a variety of antioxidant compounds of different origin that may protect plants from environmental stress, including ultraviolet (UV) light radiation, and relatively high temperatures. Accordingly, phenolics-rich crops such as grapes, olives, and heavily pigmented vegetables are particularly abundant in the Mediterranean area, where the combination of heat and light radiation stimulates plant antioxidant defenses. In addition to phenolic compounds, legumes (soybeans, peanuts, beans, and peas) contain flavanoids, isoflavanoids, isoflavones, coumestans, lignans, and other molecules, some of which also act as estrogenic agonist/antagonist; such compounds have bee suggested to contribute to reducing risk of atherosclerosis.

Extra Virgin Olive Oil: Human Evidence

Olive oil is the most typical source of visible fat of the Mediterranean diets. The healthful properties of olive oil have been often attributed to its high MUFA content, namely in the form of oleic acid (18:1n-9). However, there is currently no consensus on the effects of MUFA on circulating lipids and lipoproteins. The effects of high MUFA intakes on serum cholesterol might be indirect and due to the associated replacement of saturated FAs. Yet, some studies attributed a direct, although modest, cholesterol-lowering effect to MFA alone, when they equicalorically replace carbohydrates [14,15]. It should also be underlined that oleic acid is one of the predominant FA in worldwide largely consumed animal foods, such as poultry and pork; thus, the percentage of oleic acid in the Mediterranean diet is only slightly higher than that of other kinds of Western diets, such as the North American one. It is therefore unlikely that oleic acid is exclusively accountable for the healthful properties of olive oil. In turn, even though the salubrious effects of a high proportion of oleic acid intake—including reduced endothelial activation and lower susceptibility of LDL to oxidation—should not be overlooked, what really sets extra virgin olive oil apart from other vegetable oils is its content in phenolic compounds. From a public health viewpoint, it needs to be underlined that only extra virgin olive oil, as opposed to that labeled as "olive oil" contains polyphenols and confusion should be avoided.

Olives are rich in phenolic components. Approximately 15 years ago, we started our investigations on the antioxidant properties of olive oil phenolics and, subsequently our and others' groups followed up on this. In synthesis, hydroxytyrosol and oleuropein have been shown to be potent scavengers of superoxide anion and other reactive species (peroxynitrite, hypochlorous acid) possibly implicated in the onset of CHD and mutagenesis. Moreover, hydroxytyrosol and oleuropein are also capable to modulate enzymatic processes, some of which might be relevant to CHD. As an example, hydroxytyrosol has been shown to inhibit platelet aggregation, suggestive of an antithrombotic potential [16].

Human absorption and metabolism of olive oil phenolics have been well documented, and *in vivo* studies of antioxidant potential and biological activity have been the subject of approximately 15 trials. Indeed, research in this field is rapidly progressing and data proving in vivo activities of olive oil polyphenols accumulate relatively rapidly [17,18].

One of the interesting aspects of the latest studies performed with extra virgin olive oil is that they have been obtained by providing doses of phenolic compounds comparable to those currently consumed by many population groups in the Mediterranean area [18].

Tomato

Tomato was imported in the Mediterranean area from South America at the beginning of the eighteenth century and is now an important component of the Mediterranean diet. Among the minor components of tomato, carotenoids such as beta-carotene, lycopene, lutein, and zeaxanthin have been extensively investigated because of their relative abundance in human plasma and their antioxidant properties [19]. Accordingly, both basic research and epidemiologic studies concur to suggest the cardioprotective and chemopreventive activities of carotenoids, in particular of beta-carotene and lycopene. However, it should be noted that the results of the ATBC and CARET trials [20,21]

conducted among smokers (who are exposed to enhanced oxidative stress) supplemented with β-carotene demonstrated excess risk for cancer and cardiovascular endpoints. In addition, other clinical trials did not demonstrate any effect of β-carotene supplementation on cancer. The major conundrum in carotenoid research now is, Why is it that consumption of tomato and tomato products is associated with lower cancer and cardiovascular risks, whereas supplementation with β-carotene is yet to be proven beneficial? Suggestions include the co-carcinogenic and pro-oxidant potential of beta-carotene under certain conditions, the presence of concomitant liver disease in ATBC and CARET patients, and the confounding interference by smoking habits and alcohol consumption on overall outcomes. As a final point, the healthful effects of tomato consumption might not be limited to its carotenoid content, as suggested by some experimental data.

In an attempt to discern the contribution of tomato components to human health, some intervention studies with carefully standardized diets, added with well-defined amounts of carotenoids, were undertaken. Porrini et al. verified if regular consumption of tomato products could protect lymphocytes and plasma from oxidative stress [22]. Lycopene concentrations increased significantly after tomato intervention both in plasma (+53%) and in lymphocytes (+72%), confirming data in the literature. Conversely, limited literature exists on the intracellular concentrations of lycopene, although this is very important for understanding the role of this antioxidant on tissue activity.

For this reason, research focused on lycopene and its biological effects [23]. The purpose was to verify that the daily intake of a beverage containing a natural tomato extract (Lyc-o-mato® oleoresin 6%), was able to modified plasma carotenoids concentration and that this intake could protect DNA in lymphocytes from oxidative stress. Lycopene, phytoene, phytofluene and beta-carotene concentrations increased significantly by about 68%, 92%, 61%, and 28%, respectively, after 26 days of Lyc-o-mato® drinking, but not after placebo intake. Conversely, the consumption of Lyc-o-mato® did not affect the plasma concentrations of lutein, zeaxanthin, β-cryptoxanthin and

α-carotene, which were not present in the drink; plasma concentrations of α-tocopherol also did not change throughout the intervention, possibly due to the relatively low amount of this vitamin present in the Lyc-o-mato® drink. In brief, it is possible to increase carotenoid plasma and cellular concentrations by providing adequate amounts of tomato, its products, or supplements. One of the most interesting aspects of the potentially cardioprotective and chemopreventive properties of carotenoids is that lycopene is more bioavailable from tomato products, such as paste, puree, and sauce, than from raw tomatoes [24]. Also, addition of olive oil and cooking further promotes absorption. In addition to raw tomatoes, which are important constituents of salads, consumption of processed, cooked tomato products might provide additional benefits deriving from lycopene.

The second aim of these studies was to verify if the increased of carotenoids concentration was able to increase cellular defenses against the oxidative stress. The percentage of DNA in the tail of lymphocytes subjected to the comet assay decreased by about 42% ($p < .0001$), as calculated by considering the variation between the percentage of DNA in the tail registered before and after Lyc-o-mato® intake with respect to the value recorded before Lyc-o-mato®. In addition, a decrease in 8-OHdG/dG was observed in the prostate tissue. Also, Rao et al. found that one week of supplementation with lycopene or tomato products let to a fall in leukocyte 8-OHdG/dG level [19].

Wild Plants and Cardiovascular Health

Endothelial dysfunction is a major complication of atherosclerosis and accumulating evidence suggests that oxidative stress plays a major role in its onset and maintenance. Reduced production/availability of the vasorelaxant factor nitric oxide (NO) plays a major role in the oxidative stress-related development of endothelial dysfunction [25]. Indeed, administration of some antioxidants, such as lipoic acid, vitamin C, and flavonoids from tea and wine, has been shown to ameliorate endothelial function and vasomotion [26] and increasing evidence over the past decade shows that several dietary factors may partly modulate nitric oxide synthase (NOS) activity. The project "Local Food Nutraceuticals" was undertaken to investigate the effects of extracts obtained from selected, phenol-rich wild plants traditionally eaten in the Mediterranean area on the production of NO and prostacyclin by cultured aortic endothelial cells.

Supplementation of porcine aortic endothelial cells (PAEC) with *Cynara cardunculus* or *Thymus pulegioides* extracts increases NO production. Moreover, enhanced secretion into the medium of prostacyclin, another important vasorelaxant factor, further confirms the vasomodulatory potential of these wild plants [27]. Recently, we further tested a *Cynara cardunculus* extract on isolated aortic rings and after supplementation to aged rats. The results confirm that the vasorelaxant properties of *Cynara cardunculus* are maintained *in vivo* (Figure 21.1),

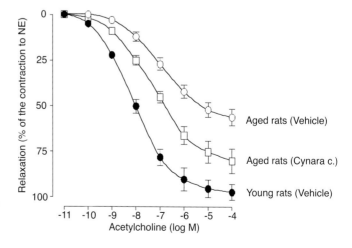

Figure 21.1 Wild artichoke (*Cynara cardunculus*) ameliorates the age-associated decline in vasomotion, as shown by cumulative concentration-response curves of acetylcholine in norepinephrine (NE)-precontracted aortic rings prepared from vehicle-treated young and aged rats or from *Cynara c.*-treated aged rats. (Reproduced from Rossoni et al. [27], with permission.)

suggesting that part of the lower incidence of endothelial dysfunction and the higher vascular health observed in the Mediterranean area are to be attributed to the consumption of wild plants [27].

Finally, wild artichoke has been shown to inhibit metalloproteinase 9 and hypochlorous acid–induced protein modification, hence further contributing to the reduction of noxious events in vascular cells.

Vitamin E

Vitamin E is the most widely studied antioxidant in the cardiovascular area. The involvement of lipid, namely LDL, peroxidation in the initiation of atherosclerosis led to several studies aimed at finding cardioprotective actions of vitamin E. In brief, epidemiological as well as animal and clinical studies are inconsistent as to whether vitamin E lowers the risk for atherosclerosis and CHD: whereas some studies show an association between high dietary vitamin E intake and/or its high serum concentrations and lower rates of CHD, other controlled trials examining vitamin E intake in populations with different risks for CHD did not confirm such observations. Supplementation studies also did not show cardioprotective activities of vitamin E [28], with the exception of a paper published in 2005, which reported cardioprotective effects of vitamin E in women older than 45 years [29]. The causes for these discrepancies are not clear but might be due to subject compliance, study design, dosage regime, timing of therapy, and the isoform of vitamin E used, that is, natural versus synthetic. Moreover, there is currently no clear evidence that vitamin E exerts antioxidant activities *in vivo*. In turn, administration of vitamin E to cardiovascular patients is, at the moment, unjustified.

Vitamin C

The results of most prospective studies indicate that low or deficient intakes of vitamin C are associated with an increased risk of CVDs. However, several studies had failed to find significant reductions in the risk of CHD among vitamin C supplement users in well-nourished populations, with the exception of the First National Health and Nutrition Examination Survey (NHANES-I) Epidemiologic Follow-up Study and the Nurses' Health Study. More recently, a pooled analysis of nine prospective cohort studies,

including more than 290,000 adults who were free of CHD at baseline and followed for an average of 10 years, found that those who took more than 700 mg/day of supplemental vitamin C had a 25% lower risk of CHD than those who did not take vitamin C supplements [30]. This suggests that reduction of CHD risk may require vitamin C intakes high enough to saturate plasma and circulating cells, that is, the use of supplements or a well-balanced diet.

In terms of cardiovascular therapy, it is noteworthy that treatment with vitamin C has consistently resulted in improved dilation of blood vessels in individuals with atherosclerosis as well as those with angina pectoris, congestive heart failure, high cholesterol, and high blood pressure. Improved blood vessel dilation has been demonstrated at a dose of 500 mg of vitamin C daily [31].

Moreover, several studies have demonstrated a blood pressure–lowering effect of vitamin C supplementation, again in the range of 500 mg/day in addition to antihypertensive medications.

In turn, there is enough scientific evidence to encourage the use of vitamin C supplements (500 mg/day) in cardiovascular patients with vascular complications, namely hypertension and endothelial dysfunction.

Why This Emphasis on Micronutrients?

Micronutrient intakes less than the estimated average requirement (EAR), that is, more than 2 standard deviations below the recommended dietary allowance (RDA), are considered inadequate, and by this definition, inadequacy is widespread in the United States and Western populations, especially in the lower socioeconomic class, children, adolescents, the obese, and the elderly. A number of these micronutrient inadequacies affect more than half the U.S. population (e.g., for Mg^{2+}, 56% of the U.S. population is below EAR; for vitamin D, African Americans as a group are below EAR). These findings are likely extendable to other areas of the world, where diets are becoming calorie rich and nutrient poor. Medical concern is currently low because no overt pathology has been associated with these levels of deficiency beyond doubt.

A new theory about homeostasis during micronutrient shortage has been proposed by

Dr. Bruce Ames [32]. His *triage hypothesis* posits that the risk of degenerative diseases associated with aging, including cancer, cognitive decline, and immune dysfunction, can be decreased by ensuring adequate intake of micronutrients (the 40 essential vitamins, minerals, amino acids, and FAs) earlier in life. According to this hypothesis, during evolution one homeostatic mechanism that developed during shortage of any micronutrient involves protein triage, such that metabolism essential for short-term survival is maintained at the expense of metabolism that only impacts years later. A possible mechanism is that enzymes required for short-term survival have tighter binding constants for micronutrient cofactors than enzymes involved in functions whose loss has less immediate adverse impacts. A corollary of the triage hypothesis is that micronutrient deficiencies would accelerate late-onset diseases causally linked to these earlier subclinical insults, including cancer, cognitive decline, and vulnerability to infection. Thus, the triage hypothesis predicts a rebalancing of metabolism during micronutrient shortage that eventually results in late-onset disease but has insidious but detectable immediate effects in areas of metabolism not essential for short-term survival. In turn, the role of micronutrients in human health might be subtle in the short term, with no apparent clinical manifestations, but bears important consequences in the development of degenerative disease such as atherosclerosis [33]. Regardless of whether this hypothesis will be confirmed or disputed, the modern-day diet favors the diffusion of micronutrient deficiencies, which in the absence of overt clinical symptoms are often dismissed by general practitioners.

Conclusions

The link between diet and CVD is now undisputable: adherence to a healthful diet affords protection from CVD and cancer. Currently, researchers are concentrating their efforts on the identification of novel biological activities of food components, such as omega-3 FAs, vitamins, and plant metabolites, which are many. *In vitro* studies abound and human trials (which provide the most useful information) are in progress, despite the current scarcity of appropriate biomarkers and difficulties inherent to diet modification and related compliance. However, future availability of appropriate techniques to evaluate the *in vivo* activities of food items or of their isolated components will likely resolve this issue. For the time being, the advice to incorporate proper quantities of plant foods and omega 3-FAs in the diet has strong epidemiologic grounds and increasing clinical justification. From a public health viewpoint, and in light of the current escalating cost of healthcare, it appears appropriate for physicians to pay particular attention to the diets of their patients, not only in terms of calories, but also by discussing the nutritional profile of their dietary habits.

Selected References

10. Leaf A, Kang JX, Xiao YF. Fish oil Fatty acids as cardiovascular drugs. Curr Vasc Pharmacol 2008 Jan;6(1):1–12.

12. Visioli F, Bogani P, Grande S, et al. Mediterranean food and health: building human evidence. J Physiol Pharmacol 2005 Mar;56(Suppl 1):37–49.

30. Knekt P, Ritz J, Pereira MA, et al. Antioxidant vitamins and coronary heart disease risk: a pooled analysis of 9 cohorts. Am J Clin Nutr 2004 Dec;80(6):1508–20.

33. Visioli F, Hagen TM. Nutritional strategies for healthy cardiovascular aging: Focus on micronutrients. Pharmacol Res 2007 Mar;55(3):199–206.

34. Wang C, Harris WS, Chung M, et al. n-3 Fatty acids from fish or fish-oil supplements, but not alpha-linolenic acid, benefit cardiovascular disease outcomes in primary- and secondary-prevention studies: a systematic review. Am J Clin Nutr 2006 Jul;84(1):5–17.

CHAPTER 22

Alcohol Intake, Dyslipidemia, and CVD

Saverio Stranges[1,2] *& Maurizio Trevisan*[2]

[1] University of Warwick Medical School, Coventry, UK
[2] University of Nevada Health Sciences System, Nevada System of Higher Education, Las Vegas, NV, USA

Introduction

The association between alcohol consumption and coronary heart disease (CHD) has been the focus of intensive investigation over the past 3 decades. A number of ecological, case-control, and cohort studies have addressed this complex relationship, in both men and women, across diverse populations throughout the world, showing a tendency for light or moderate drinkers to exhibit lower rates of mortality and morbidity from CHD than non-drinkers or heavy drinkers [1–4]. This association also explains the beneficial effects of moderate alcohol consumption on total mortality observed in both men and women of middle-aged populations [5]. The epidemiologic evidence is corroborated by laboratory and physiologic studies supporting the existence of plausible biologic pathways underlying the cardiovascular benefits of moderate drinking. Some of these biologic mechanisms include favorable effects on metabolic pathways such as an improvement of the lipid profile, especially high-density lipoprotein (HDL)-cholesterol (HDL-C) [6], and enhanced insulin sensitivity [7].

However, important questions about the effects of alcohol consumption on CHD still need to be addressed. First, although recent evidence indicates that drinking pattern may modify the underlying association between moderate alcohol consumption and CHD, information regarding the cardio-

Nutritional and Metabolic Bases of Cardiovascular Disease, 1st edition.
Edited by Mario Mancini, José M. Ordovas, Gabriele Riccardi,
Paolo Rubba and Pasquale Strazzullo. © 2011 Blackwell Publishing Ltd.

vascular effects of the various aspects of drinking pattern (i.e., frequency and intensity of consumption, beverage preference, drinking with/without meals) is still limited and poorly understood. Second, the potential biological mechanisms underlying the beneficial and detrimental effects of alcohol consumption and drinking pattern on cardiovascular risk have not been definitively established. Third, the majority of studies evaluating the effects of alcohol consumption on CHD risk have focused on a single-point assessment of alcohol exposure, mostly focusing on current assessment at the time of the examination. However, many vitally important effects of alcohol consumption on health and well-being, including cardiovascular disease (CVD), are likely to be the result of long-term drinking habits. Moreover, the impact of variability in drinking patterns over the lifetime is unknown. Finally, there is relatively little epidemiologic data on the effects of alcohol consumption on prognosis among individuals with established CHD.

We evaluate the existing evidence in relation to the outlined issues, with a specific focus on recent studies supporting the important role of drinking patterns in the association between alcohol consumption and CHD.

Biologic Pathways

The mechanisms to explain the beneficial effect of alcohol consumption on CVD risk are not completely understood, although several biological pathways have been suggested. For some of them, such as increases in HDL-C and inhibition of thrombogenesis, the experimental and epidemiologic evidence is substantial, whereas for other potential biologic mechanisms (e.g., favorable effects on insulin resistance, anti-inflammatory action, and influence on body fat distribution) the evidence is still limited or less consistent. Conversely, increased blood pressure observed with larger amounts of alcohol consumption is one potential mechanism suggested to contribute, in large part, to the increased risk observed in heavy drinkers.

Lipids

One of the most frequently studied mechanisms for the beneficial effect of moderate alcohol consumption on CHD concerns alcohol and lipid profiles. Moderate alcohol intake has been clearly linked to favorable lipid profiles, especially an increase in HDL-C [8–9]. It has been estimated that at least 50% of the protective effect of moderate alcohol consumption on CHD may be attributable to alcohol-induced elevation of HDL-C [6]. On the other hand, moderate to heavy drinking raises serum triglyceride levels [6]. However, the measures of alcohol consumption utilized in these studies have been restricted to daily or weekly averages of quantity of alcohol, with little regard to alcohol drinking pattern. The potential exists for various patterns of alcohol consumption to have different effects on lipid profiles, with high-intensity drinking possibly attenuating the relationship between alcohol and HDL-C. This possibility was first raised by Gruchow et al. who noted a significantly greater HDL-C component of total cholesterol in regular drinkers compared to drinkers with a more variable drinking pattern [10]. Likewise, Taskinen et al. reported that large doses of alcohol administered to healthy males over a weekend failed to raise HDL-C [11]. Conversely, a controlled trial in moderate to heavy drinkers did not confirm a more atherogenic lipid profile associated with weekend drinking as opposed to daily regular drinking [12]. Little information is available regarding the effects of lifetime drinking on lipid profiles. A recently published analysis from the Western New York Health Study (WNYHS) suggests that a pattern of high intensity and low frequency of drinking may counteract the cardiometabolic benefits of alcohol consump-

tion [13]. Specifically, lifetime average intensity of drinking was directly related to high triglycerides, whereas lifetime drinking frequency was inversely related to low HDL-C. These preliminary results indicate the need for further research to examine the association between patterns of alcohol consumption and lipoprotein levels.

Thrombogenic Factors

Another mechanism whereby alcohol may affect the risk of CHD is through an inhibitory effect on thrombogenesis, in particular through its effects on platelet aggregation and fibrinolysis. A meta-analysis confirmed the favorable effect of moderate alcohol intake on coagulation profiles and attributed to this mechanism a further 20%–30% of the overall protective effect of moderate alcohol consumption on CHD [6]. Alcohol can inhibit platelet production, activation and aggregation. An inverse relationship between plasma fibrinogen concentration and alcohol intake has been demonstrated in several cross-sectional studies [14–15]. Other effects of alcohol on the fibrinolytic pathway include modulation of the activity of plasminogen activator inhibitor-1 (PAI-1) and of tissue-plasminogen activator (t-PA), with alcohol initially decreasing but in the long-term possibly promoting fibrinolysis [16]. In a study examining the effect of drinking pattern in relation to food consumption on fibrinolysis, alcohol ingestion with a meal was associated with anti-fibrinolytic activity [17].

Insulin Resistance

Several studies have shown that moderate alcohol consumption is associated with a reduced incidence of type 2 diabetes mellitus (DM). A recent meta-analysis pooling 15 cohort studies on the relationship between alcohol consumption and risk of type 2 diabetes showed a U-shaped relationship with a 30% reduced risk of type 2 DM in alcohol consumers of 6–48 g/day compared with heavier consumers or abstainers [18]. Enhanced insulin sensitivity with lower plasma insulin concentrations is the plausible mechanism for this association because inverse and U-shaped relationships between alcohol consumption and insulin levels and other indicators of insulin sensitivity/resistance have been reported in several cross-sectional studies among both young and elderly individuals [19–20]. These findings have been corroborated by two controlled trials examining the effect of alcohol use on insulin sensitivity [21,22]. Little is known, however, on the possible influence of alcohol drinking patterns as well as of lifetime drinking on the glucose-insulin axis. A recently published analysis from the WNYHS indicated that lifetime average intensity of drinking was directly related to impaired fasting glucose and the metabolic syndrome overall [13].

Inflammation

With the emergence of the crucial role of inflammation in both initiation and progression of atherosclerosis as well as in mediating atherosclerotic plaque stability, some studies have begun to look at the association between alcohol intake and inflammation as a further mechanism for the beneficial effect of moderate alcohol consumption on CHD. From the available population-based data, there is some indication of an anti-inflammatory effect of moderate amounts of alcohol. For example, in a West German cohort of 2,006 men and women, moderate male drinkers had lower levels of C-reactive protein (CRP), a systemic marker of inflammation, than either abstainers or heavier drinkers. However, the association was less strong among women [23]. In a further cross-sectional investigation among 1,732 men and 1,101 women participating in the Pravastatin Inflammation/CRP Evaluation Study, moderate alcohol consumption was again associated with lower CRP concentrations than occasional or no alcohol intake in both men and women, as well as in participants with or without a history of CVD [24]. These results were further corroborated by findings of the Health, Aging, and Body Composition Study, which reported similar associations of moderate alcohol consumption with lower concentrations of both CRP and interleukin-6 (IL-6) [25].

Body Fat Distribution

The effect of alcohol on body fat distribution has received increasing consideration because abdominal obesity is an important risk factor for CVD morbidity and mortality. Alcohol ingestion suppresses the oxidation of fat, favoring fat storage, and can serve as a precursor for fat synthesis [26]. However, epidemiologic research in this area re-

mains inconsistent, with some studies showing positive associations between volume of alcohol consumption and body weight and abdominal obesity, other showing no or inverse association [27–29]. Differential effects have also been reported among various race-gender groups, and for different beverage types. Little is known, however, about the association of body fat distribution with patterns of alcohol use. A cross-sectional analysis from the WNYHS examined some aspects of current drinking pattern in relation to central adiposity [28]. In this study, drinking frequency was inversely associated, whereas drinking intensity (i.e., number of drinks per drinking day) was positively associated with central adiposity in women and men, even when total volume of alcohol was included in multivariate analyses. When frequency and intensity were considered together, daily drinkers of less than one drink per drinking day had the smallest mean abdominal height measures, whereas the largest measures were observed among less than weekly drinkers who consumed four or more drinks per drinking day. These results support the hypothesis that aspects of drinking pattern such as frequency and high intensity may have important implications for the distribution of body fat, an important CHD risk factor.

Moreover, in a cross-sectional analysis from the British Regional Heart Study on a large sample of men 60–79 years of age, higher alcohol consumption (i.e., ≥21 standard drinks/wk) was positively associated with central adiposity, irrespective of the type of beverage or time in relation to meals [29]. Finally, a further analysis from the WNYHS indicated that, among women only, lifetime average intensity of drinking was directly related to abdominal obesity, whereas lifetime drinking frequency was inversely related to abdominal obesity [13]. No association was found among men.

Effects of Alcohol Drinking Patterns

Numerous scientific studies have investigated the relation between average volume of alcohol consumption and risk of CHD morbidity and mortality. Despite its known adverse health and social effects, a substantial amount of evidence exists indicating that light to moderate drinking is associated with lower risk for CHD incidence and mortality compared to abstention or heavy consumption in men and women [1–4]. The J-shape relationship has been supported by findings of a meta-analysis [5]. However, important questions about this association, mainly concerning the role of drinking patterns as well as the possible influence of long-term exposure and variability in drinking pattern over time, remain unanswered and are outlined below.

Frequency and Intensity

Much of what is known about the role of alcohol in the etiology of CHD comes from observational epidemiologic studies in which a variety of methods have been used to measure alcohol. In many studies, ascertainment of alcohol consumption has been limited, often focusing only on volume, without considering different components of consumption, particularly drinking pattern [3]. The majority of studies have used an average index of drinks consumed within a given time period, monthly, weekly, or daily, and have not addressed specific questions regarding the frequency and intensity of consumption. Consequently, certain categories of drinking have included individuals with widely differing drinking patterns. The speculation that light to moderate drinking (i.e., one to two drinks per day) is related to a reduced CHD risk is often based upon information from studies that report average drinks per day. However, evidence exists that average drinks per day does not adequately represent the actual drinking practices. For example, in the United States, the pattern of light, daily drinking has been reported by only 2% of the population; in addition, most daily drinkers are not light drinkers and most light drinkers do not drink every day. Therefore, it may be misleading to attribute putative health benefits associated with low average drinks per day to light, daily drinking. A number of studies suggest that a binge pattern of drinking may counteract the cardioprotective effects of alcohol consumption [30]. For example, in a large case-control study from Australia, there were no protective effects for major coronary events in binge drinkers of both sexes, who experienced higher CHD risk compared to abstainers [31]. This elevated risk was

present even in individuals with low overall volume of drinking. Likewise, findings from a longitudinal, population-based study from Canada showed that binge drinking increased the risk of CHD in men and women compared to regular drinking [32]. These findings emphasizing the frequency/intensity of alcohol consumption as the primary determinant of its association with CHD risk were further corroborated by findings from a population-based case-control study on male participants in the WNYHS [33]. In this analysis, among current drinkers, men who reported drinking only on weekends had a nearly twofold significant increased risk of myocardial infarction (MI) compared to men who drank less than once a week. These results were independent from the effects of differences in the amount of alcohol consumed among individuals of different drinking pattern categories. These findings further suggest that consuming alcoholic beverages in a concentrated fashion (weekend only) and without food may counteract any potential benefit associated with moderate alcohol consumption on the cardiovascular system. In a further analysis from the WNYHS, based on female participants, women who reported being intoxicated at least once a month in the past 12–24 months had a nearly threefold significant increased risk of MI than lifetime abstainers [34].

Consistent with these epidemiologic reports, angiographic findings showed that the inverse association between amount of alcohol consumed and the level of occlusion of coronary vessels can be reversed in individuals with variable or sporadic patterns of alcohol intake [10]. These findings are also supported by the physiological mechanisms of increased clotting, unfavorable lipid profile and reduced threshold for ventricular fibrillation associated with irregular heavy drinking occasions [3].

Beverage Preference

Another important component of the pattern of alcohol use is beverage preference. A number of observational studies supported similar benefits on CHD risk for wine, beer, or liquor. In a review of the literature on beverage-specific effects on CHD, no systematic effect was found, and the authors raised the hypothesis that the beverage most widely consumed by a given population is the one most likely to be inversely associated with CHD risk in that population [35]. In addition, beverage preferences in most cultures are linked with other variables. Therefore, studies may have been confounded by sociocultural factors such as socioeconomic status, diet, and other lifestyle habits. In fact, there is ample evidence suggesting that uncontrolled confounding may explain the greater benefits attributed to wine in some studies, because wine drinkers have been found to have healthier lifestyles and better sociodemographic characteristics than drinkers of other beverages and, in some cases, even than nondrinkers [3]. For example, data from the WNYHS showed that diet of wine drinkers was, on average, healthier than diet of drinkers of other beverages and nondrinkers. Specifically, among drinkers, consumers of wine ate more fruits and vegetables, fewer desserts, and less meat than drinkers of other beverages [36].

Drinking in Relation to Food Consumption

A further aspect of the multidimensional pattern of alcohol consumption pertains to the proportion consumed in conjunction with meals. For example, in a 7-year follow-up analysis of the Risk Factor and Life Expectancy Study, wine drinking outside meals was associated with higher rates of all-cause, CVD, CHD, non-CVD, and cancer mortality compared with wine drinking with meals among male participants, independent of average volume [37]. These findings were corroborated by results of a population-based case-control study on participants in the WNYHS, where men who drank mostly without food had an increased risk of MI compared to those who drank mostly with food [33].

The potential mechanisms linking consumption of alcohol with a meal to a lower CHD risk compared with drinking outside meals are still unclear; however, a few plausible physiological pathways have been suggested. Drinking with meals has been shown to exert beneficial effects on fibrinolysis [17] and lipids [38]. A potential explanation may reside as well in the effect of food on absorption and intragastric metabolism of ethanol leading to a slower increase and lower peak of blood alcohol concentration, and increased alcohol elimination rates [39]. Furthermore, two cross-sectional studies conducted in two different populations from Italy

and the United States showed that drinking outside meals was associated with a higher prevalence of hypertension compared to drinking in conjunction with meals, even after adjustment for volume of alcohol [40–41]. Finally, drinking alcohol with or without food may represent a marker of lifestyle profile and health-related behaviors, which may itself be the link to protective and detrimental health effects, such as different dietary habits [3].

Variability of Lifetime Drinking Habits

Most previous epidemiologic studies on the effects of alcohol consumption and drinking pattern on CHD morbidity and mortality have based their exposure assessment on a single measurement of current alcohol consumption at the time of the examination under the assumption that drinking patterns are fairly stable over the lifetime. In cases in which this assumption is met, current and past drinking patterns are very similar, making it difficult, if not impossible, to disaggregate acute and chronic effects of alcohol on health. It has been suggested, however, that alcohol consumption varies considerably over the course of a lifetime, but the relation of this variability to health is still poorly understood [42].

Only a few prospective studies have assessed alcohol intake at two or more points in time. For example, Sesso et al. reported a reduction in CVD risk from increasing alcohol intake among men with initially low alcohol consumption (≤ 1 drink/wk) but not among men initially consuming more than 1 drink/wk [43]. Moreover, findings from the British Regional Heart Study showed that nondrinkers and occasional drinkers who took up regular drinking in middle age subsequently experienced reduced risk of CHD morbidity compared with those who remained nondrinkers or occasional drinkers, but did not report benefit for mortality from CHD or CVD [44]. In a later analysis from the British Regional Heart Study, based on five measurements of alcohol intake over 20 years of follow-up, the baseline U-shaped relations of alcohol intake with CVD and all-cause mortality changed after taking into account variation in alcohol intake. Specifically, risks associated with non-drinking were reduced, while risks associated with moderate and heavy drinking increased [45]. These findings suggest that previous prospective studies may have overestimated the benefits on CVD risk from moderate alcohol consumption and underestimated the risks associated with heavy drinking.

A recently published analysis from the WNYHS attempted to examine the impact of lifetime drinking trajectories on the cardiovascular risk factors included in the cluster of the metabolic syndrome, in the attempt to account for the effects of variability of drinking habits over time [46]. In this specific study, participants were lifetime regular drinkers selected from healthy controls for the WNYHS in which lifetime lifestyle was ascertained retrospectively. Trajectory analyses were based on estimates of standardized total adjusted ounces of ethanol for each decade between 10 and 59 years. Two groups with distinct lifetime drinking trajectories were obtained, an early peak and a stable trajectory group. Compared to stable trajectory drinkers, early peak drinkers had earlier onset of regular drinking, drank heavily in late adolescence and early adulthood tapering off in middle age, averaged more drinks per drinking day, drank less frequently, preferred beer or liquor to wine, were more likely to drink without food, drank fewer years, had lower lifetime alcohol intakes, and were more likely to abstain when interviewed. After controlling for potential confounders, early peak trajectories were associated with an unfavorable cardiometabolic profile. Specifically, they exhibited higher likelihoods of low HDL-C, abdominal obesity, overweight, and the metabolic syndrome overall as compared to stable drinkers. These findings further emphasize that a binge pattern of drinking, especially when initiated at younger ages, may produce long-term detrimental effects on cardiovascular and metabolic health. Binge drinking is likely to be associated with other unhealthy lifestyle habits and drinking patterns (e.g., drinking without meals), as well as with a higher likelihood of alcoholism. This is an issue of considerable public health significance given the increasing trends in the prevalence of binge drinking among both adolescents and young adults in many western countries [47]. Further studies are needed to clarify the impact of variability of drinking patterns over time on cardiovascular and metabolic health in order to better inform public health guidelines.

Alcohol Intake and Prognosis in Patients with Established CHD

A few epidemiologic studies have specifically examined the long-term effects of alcohol consumption in individuals with established CHD. These studies have generally confirmed protective effect of light to moderate alcohol intake among these individuals [48]. For example, Thun et al. found that, in 490,000 middle-aged and elderly U.S. adults, the adjusted death rates from CHD were 30%–40% lower among regular drinkers with preexisting CHD than among nondrinkers [49]. Likewise, in the Physicians' Health Study, there was a reduction of total and CVD mortality associated with moderate alcohol consumption among middle-aged men with a history of previous MI, the maximum apparent benefit (a 24% reduction of CVD mortality) coming from 2 to 6 drinks/wk [50]. However, these earlier reports were limited by their restriction to individuals with a remote history of previous CHD and use of self-reported diagnoses. Findings from the Onset Study examining the effect of alcohol consumption on mortality among early survivors of a first acute MI showed that moderate alcohol consumption in the year prior to the first clinical event was associated with lower subsequent mortality [51]. This association was present in both men and women, was similar for cardiovascular and all-cause mortality and among different types of alcoholic beverages. Moreover, in a French study examining the role of alcohol consumption subsequent to an acute MI in the secondary prevention of several cardiovascular complications, among 437 middle-aged male survivors of a recent acute MI, moderate wine drinking was associated with a significant reduction in the risk of cardiovascular complications [52]. Finally, in a further analysis from the Onset Study, binge drinkers (i.e., ≥3 drinks within 1–2 hours) experienced a twofold higher risk of total mortality, after a first acute MI, than drinkers who did not binge in the year preceding the first clinical event, independently of the average amount of alcohol consumed [53].

Conclusions

CHD remains one of the leading causes of death and a major health concern in women and men. Alcohol is one of the lifestyle behaviors frequently considered in both primary and secondary prevention of CHD. While the epidemiologic evidence, with reasonable biologic plausibility, indicates that moderate drinking is likely to confer cardiometabolic benefits, some methodological limitations in the studies conducted thus far raise uncertainties on a number of unresolved issues. For example, the magnitude of these benefits may be biased by the choice of reference categories, because it has been argued persuasively that quitters may well be less healthy for reasons unrelated to the fact that they are not currently drinking [54]. Therefore, studies that fail to distinguish former drinkers from lifetime abstainers may overestimate the health benefits of moderate alcohol consumption.

A further issue resides in the role of drinking pattern. In fact, a number of the studies conducted thus far were not originally designed to examine the effects of alcohol consumption on health and did not employ standard quantity-frequency questions to assess intake. Moreover, most of these studies did not adequately measure drinking pattern, and that is a problem, not only because it renders uncertain the actual volume of alcohol consumed, but because the pattern of drinking is likely to influence the effect of alcohol consumption on health. Clearly, the effect on health of having seven drinks on a Saturday night are likely to differ from that of having a glass of wine with dinner every evening of the week. Yet the volume measures employed in many of the studies define both as one drink a day, moderate drinking. Substantial evidence from studies designed to look specifically at drinking pattern now verifies that the way alcohol is consumed (i.e., frequency and intensity of consumption, binge drinking, drinking with/without meals) may modify the underlying association between alcohol consumption and both total mortality and cardiometabolic risk [3]. In particular, a number of recent studies suggest that a binge pattern of drinking or heavy episodic drinking may counteract the cardiometabolic benefits of alcohol consumption. Moreover, it has been shown that consuming alcohol in a concentrated fashion (weekend only) and without food may counteract any potential benefit associated with moderate alcohol consumption on the cardiovascular system. Together, these findings emphasize the importance of the frequency and intensity of alcohol consumption as the primary determinants of its association with the cardiometabolic risk. Thus, a recommendation that moderate drinking confers cardiovascular benefits, without considering the risks associated with "unhealthy" patterns of drinking, could potentially lead to unbalanced advice given to individuals and the population at large with regard to drinking habits.

Selected References

5. Di Castelnuovo A, Costanzo S, Bagnardi V, et al. Alcohol dosing and total mortality in men and women: an updated meta-analysis of 34 prospective studies. Arch Intern Med 2006;166:2437–45.
18. Koppes LL, Dekker JM, Hendriks HF, et al. Moderate alcohol consumption lowers the risk of type 2 diabetes: a meta-analysis of prospective observational studies. Diabetes Care 2005;28:719–25.
19. Dal Maso L, La Vecchia C, Augustin LS, et al. Relationship between a wide range of alcohol consumptions, components of the insulin-like growth factor system and adiponectin. Eur J Clin Nutr 2007;61:221–5.
41. Stranges S, Wu T, Dorn JM, et al. Relationship of alcohol drinking pattern to the risk of hypertension: a population-based study. Hypertension 2004;44:813–9.
42. Fillmore KM, Kerr W, Stockwell T, et al. Moderate alcohol use and reduced mortality risk: Systematic error in prospective studies and new hypotheses. Addiction Res Theory 2006;14:101–32.

CHAPTER 23

Dyslipidemia in Chronic Renal Disease

Carmine Zoccali

Nephrology, Hypertension and Renal Transplantation Unit, and National Research Council-IBIM Clinical Epidemiology of Renal Diseases and Hypertension, Reggio Calabria, Italy

Introduction

Chronic kidney disease (CKD) is now recognized as a major public health problem [1]. In the perspective of systemic epidemiology, this disease is part of the current epidemic of chronic diseases that followed the decline of infectious diseases [2]. This disease is formally defined as a glomerular filtration rate < 60 ml/min/1.73 m² and/or evidence of kidney damage as identified by biochemical, histopathology, or imaging studies. It is now solidly established that in the majority of economically developed Western countries, CKD has a population prevalence ranging from 6% to 10%. Concerns related to CKD derive more from the cardiovascular rather than from the renal sequelae of this condition [3]. Indeed, patients with CKD are more likely to die of cardiovascular complications than to progress to end-stage renal disease (ESRD). Even though the magnitude of the cardiovascular risk excess associated with moderate CKD (i.e., with a GFR in the 60- to 30-ml/min/1.73 m² range) is less than that of diabetes or of a previous myocardial infarction (MI) episode [4] the Kidney Disease Outcomes Quality Initiative (K/DOQI) guidelines formally consider CKD a cardiovascular disease (CVD) risk equivalent [5]. Furthermore CKD patients frequently display a number of nontraditional risk factors including proteinuria, inflammation, increased oxidative stress, and altered nitric oxide (NO) synthesis [6].

Altered lipid metabolism was one of the first biochemical corollaries of advanced renal dysfunction to be identified. The founding father of nephrology, Richard Bright, is being credited as the first to report such an alteration in patients with renal diseases [7]. Apart from Bright, dyslipidemia was recognized as a common sequela of chronic renal insufficiency by clinicians in the early twentieth century, but interest on this disturbance as a risk factor for cardiovascular complication and renal damage is relatively recent and dates to the 1970s when analyses of the first case-series of long-term dialysis patients by Scribner group disclosed the dim cardiovascular prognosis of ESRD [8].

In the eighties Moorhead [9] hypothesized that renal diseases may be mediated by abnormalities of lipid metabolism. This author envisaged that a loss of lipoprotein lipase activators brought about by defective glomerular membrane barrier may result in hyperlipidemia and that high circulating low-density lipoprotein (LDL) by binding glycosaminoglycans in the glomerular basement membrane may increase membrane permeability thereby perpetuating a vicious cycle. In keeping with this hypothesis, it is now well established that in diverse models of renal damage, high-lipid diets or other experimental interventions that produce hyperlipidemia aggravate glomerular damage and renal dysfunction and that oxidized lipids are particularly noxious in this context.

Nutritional and Metabolic Bases of Cardiovascular Disease, 1st edition.
Edited by Mario Mancini, José M. Ordovas, Gabriele Riccardi,
Paolo Rubba and Pasquale Strazzullo. © 2011 Blackwell Publishing Ltd.

Biochemistry

In routine clinical practice, the physician observes just two lipid abnormalities in CKD patients: low high-density lipoprotein (HDL)-cholesterol (HDL-C) and high triglycerides. On average, low-density lipoprotein (LDL)-cholesterol (LDL-C), a highly atherogenic lipoprotein, is indeed normal in these patients. However, detailed analyses by high-performance liquid chromatography (HPLC) and other techniques applied in clinical research unveil a much more complex scenario (Table 23.1). Very LDLs (VLDLs) as well as VLDL remnants and intermediate-density lipoproteins are substantially increased in patients with renal insufficiency [10–12]. Furthermore, it is well documented that clearance of chylomicron remnants is impaired in these patients [13], a process going along with accumulation of small dense LDLs. The atherogenic potential of lipoproteins is increased by secondary structural modification of these molecules. Glycation, oxidation, and carbamoylation all amplify the proinflammatory effect of these compounds [14]. On the other hand, increased lipoprotein(a) [Lp(a)] levels [15] and accumulation of acute-phase HDLs, that is, an HDL subclass that may have noxious rather than protective effects on the cardiovascular system [16], further aggravate the atherogenic risk profile of CKD. As intermediate-density lipoproteins signal a high risk for atherosclerosis [17], estimation of non-HDL-C levels (which can be easily calculated by summing up LDL-D and VLDL-C) has been proposed as a practical means for evaluating the lipid-dependent atherogenic potential of CKD.

Serum Cholesterol and Lp(a) in CKD

The first large-scale epidemiologic study [18] investigating the relationship between dyslipidemia and survival in ESRD was published about 8 years after the seminal study by Scribner group that highlighted the high risk for atherosclerotic complications of ESRD [19]. Surprisingly, the Degoulet study showed that hypocholesterolemia rather than hypercholesterolemia is associated with death in this population. Since then, this observation was confirmed in a large series of surveys and in cohort studies [20]. This apparently counterintuitive finding was initially considered as prima facie evidence that dyslipidemia is not harmful in ESRD patients. In interpreting this observation, one should consider that in clinical and experimental medicine, effects observed in a given clinical or experimental context are not necessarily observed in other contexts [21]. For example, studies in experimental models and in humans have consistently shown that chronic exposure to high levels of angiotensin II produces extensive renal damage. On the other hand, high levels of angiotensin II are fundamental for maintaining the GFR in situations of sodium deprivation and low extracellular volume, as is exemplified by the fact that angiotensin II antagonism precipitates acute renal failure in volume-depleted patients. Similarly, in epidemiologic studies, a given relationship between a predictor variable and an outcome variable may be very consistently found in some clinical contexts but not in other situations. The relationship between cholesterol and cardiovascular events is indeed a case in point. Compelling evidence has been gathered that in the general population the relationship between cholesterol and cardiovascular risk is linear without evidence of any threshold [22]. This relationship is coherent with physiological and pathophysiological studies in experimental models, as well as with intervention studies showing that reducing the level of cholesterol lowers the risk

Table 23.1 Lipid abnormalities in CKD: The individual alterations are commented in the main text.

Alterations detected in routine clinical practice

Low HDL-C
High triglyceride
Low total and LDL-C

Alterations emerging in sophisticated studies

High lipoprotein(a)
VLDL remnants/IDL
Chylomicron remnants
Glycated, oxidized, and carbamylated small dense LDL
Advanced glycosylation of ApoB
Acute-phase HDL

CKD: chronic kidney disease; HDL-C: high-density lipoprotein-cholesterol; LDL-C: low-density lipoprotein-cholesterol; IDL: intermediate-density lipoprotein; VLDL: very-low-density lipoprotein.

of disease. Because of these large, coherent series of observations, we believe that hypercholesterolemia should be regarded as a "risk factor" of primary importance. However, coherent with experimental evidence and with intervention studies, the continuous relationship between cholesterol and cardiovascular events observed in the general population may not apply to different populations, such as high-risk populations and populations with a heavy burden of comorbidities. In other words, the linear relationship between cholesterol and cardiovascular events only applies to the population wherefrom it was derived and not to the universe of disease and pathophysiological conditions. In different populations, and in different conditions, the association between cholesterol and risk may even take an opposite direction. While obesity and hypercholesterolemia in otherwise healthy individuals predict adverse outcomes in the long term, these risk factors are associated with decreased rather than increased risk of death in patients with heart failure [23,24]. This "inverse epidemiology" does not negate that obesity and hypercholesterolemia are dangerous to our health in the long term. Centuries ago, when famine was a major cause of death and the average lifespan was 40 years or less, obesity was undoubtedly a survival advantage for our ancestors. As the lifespan became longer and access to food virtually unlimited, obesity was no longer a protective factor in long-term survivors. Indeed, in the long term, the metabolic alterations associated with obesity, particularly hypercholesterolemia, determine atherosclerotic complications. Life expectancy in patients with ESRD is considerably shorter than in the general population. Obesity and high cholesterol in patients with severe CKD and ESRD may appear protective because low body weight and hypocholesterolemia in these conditions denote a situation of particular frailty rather than because obesity and hypercholesterolemia per se are protective. Well beyond serum cholesterol, ESRD is a situation where inverse epidemiology is truly pervasive [25]. In this condition, various risk factors, from blood pressure to serum cholesterol, body weight, homocysteine, and other factors, are inversely related to death and cardiovascular complications. That low cholesterol in ESRD is an indicator of frailty and high risk is supported by the observation that in analyses stratified according to nutritional

status cholesterol maintains the expected direct link with mortality in ESRD patients without malnutrition [26]. Thus, malnutrition (i.e., a condition determining a reduction in plasma cholesterol) is a confounder for the interpretation of the association between this factor and clinical outcomes.

Prospective studies in the general population in the 1990s described Lp(a) as an independent risk factor for coronary artery disease [27], a finding that contrasts with the observation that the plasma concentration of this lipoprotein is high in centenarians [28]. In healthy individuals, plasma Lp(a) is almost exclusively controlled by the apolipoprotein A ApoA gene locus on chromosome 6q2.6-q2.7. More than 30 alleles at this highly polymorphic gene locus determine a size polymorphism of ApoA and an inverse correlation exists between the size (molecular weight) of ApoA isoforms and Lp(a) plasma concentrations [29]. Therefore, Individuals with low molecular weight ApoA isoforms are expected to have the highest serum Lp(a) levels. More recent studies testing the prognostic value of this protein in patients with coronary heart disease (CHD) reported that the association between Lp(a) and cardiovascular risk is in fact confined only to some genotypes and that it is critically dependent on levels of ApoA isoforms [30]. In patients with renal diseases, the average Lp(a) concentration is substantially increased, but a it was observed in patients with CHD, the predictive power of Lp(a) for cardiovascular events appears dictated by the particular type of ApoA isoform rather than by the magnitude of plasma Lp(a) increase. Indeed, rather than Lp(a) plasma concentration, it is the level of the low molecular weight ApoA isoform that determines the risk for coronary artery disease events in ESRD patients [31].

Atherosclerosis in CKD and in ESRD Patients

Autopsy studies coherently showed that no vascular territory is spared by atherosclerosis in patients with renal insufficiency and that, in particular, advanced coronary atherosclerosis is a prominent problem in these patients [32]. *In vivo*, imaging studies by ultrasound clearly documented that atherosclerosis is exceedingly frequent in the carotid arteries in patients with CKD [33] and in patients with ESRD [34]. The high frequency of CHD in this condition has been confirmed by angiography [35] and electron beam computed tomography [36] studies. Coronary calcification is common in CKD patients, and as hypothesized by Lindner in the 1970s, this process appears to be not only much accelerated as compared to that in patients without renal insufficiency, but also much precocious, being evident in the early phases of renal disease [37].

The accelerated nature of atherosclerosis in renal insufficiency is epitomized by observations in the experimental model of ApoE knockout mouse [38]. In this model, a 50% renal mass ablation (uninephrectomy) is sufficient to trigger the atherosclerosis process. Remarkably angiotensin receptor blockers [39], a class of drugs that favorably affect the course of renal disease, also limit atherosclerosis in this model.

Lipids and the Evolution of CKD

As alluded to in the introductory paragraph, the Moorhead hypothesis has now convincing experimental underpinnings. In animal models, high-cholesterol diets worsen renal injury, and conversely, lipid-lowering interventions limit renal injury [40–44]. Virtually all cell species represented in the kidney are prone to lipid-mediated damage, endothelial and mesangial cells, podocytes as well as tubular cells (Figure 23.1). Mesangial cells express receptors for LDL and oxidized LDL, which when activated by the key ligand trigger mesangial cell proliferation, mesangial matrix deposition, and production of a variety of inflammatory proteins including macrophage chemoattractant protein-1 (MCP-1), IL-6, and other proinflammatory proteins and growth factors. MCP-1 elicits the recruitment of macrophages, which infiltrate the

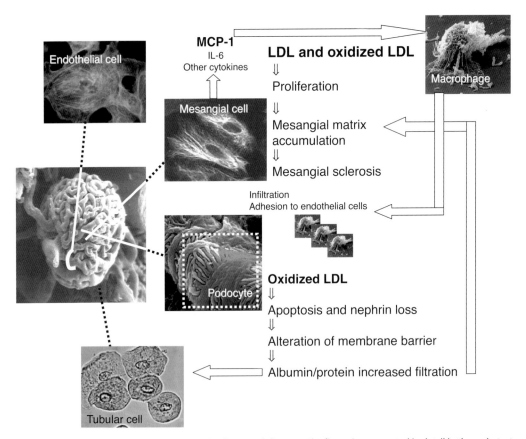

Figure 23.1 Mechanisms whereby dyslipidemia leads to renal damage. The figure is commented in detail in the main text. (MCP-1: monocyte chemoattractant protein-1.)

glomerulus to become foam cells, the prototypical cells species of atherosclerotic/inflammatory damage. On the other hand, oxidized LDL also prompts the adhesion of monocytes to glomerular endothelial cells, thereby initiating infiltration of the renal parenchyma by these cells. As previously mentioned, lipid-mediated renal damage is extended to tubular cells, which undergo regressive changes [45]. Hypercholesterolemia and hypertriglyceridemia are noxious also to podocytes. Oxidized LDL causes apoptosis and nephrin loss (a protein of fundamental importance for the functionality of the glomerular filtration barrier), thereby increasing transcapillary albumin diffusion and, by this mechanism, eventually determines mesangial sclerosis [46].

Although observational studies have shown that ApoB-containing lipoproteins are associated with a more rapid loss of renal function in humans [47], the effect of statins on progression to ESRD still remains intensely debated. Two meta-analyses concluded that renal outcomes are improved by statins in the predialysis phase [48,49] depending on proteinuria. Indeed, in patients with protein excretion >300 mg/day, a beneficial effect was apparent, whereas no influence on progression of renal disease was seen in those with microalbuminuria or normoalbuminuria [50]. By the same token, a reduction in progression rate of renal insufficiency and a concomitant decrease in cardiovascular complications was reported with improvement in proteinuria in the other meta-analysis [51]. A most recent meta-analysis that evaluated the efficacy and safety of statins for renal and cardiovascular outcomes at the various stages of CKD (predialysis, dialysis, and transplantation) [52] came to the conclusion that the purported renoprotective effect of statins remains unproven because of relatively sparse data and possible outcomes reporting bias. In reality, this meta-analysis, which considered randomized and quasi-randomized studies did not include a solid secondary analysis of three pravastatin studies (PPP) by Tonelli, which was based on GFR changes over time [53]. In this study, which gathered 18,569 subjects at risk for cardiovascular disease, pravastatin reduced the adjusted rate of kidney function loss by 8% (0.08 ml/min.1.73 m^2/yr by MDRD-GFR; 95% confidence interval [CI], 0.01–0.15) and the risk of acute renal failure as well (relative risk

[RR], 0.60; 95% CI, 0.41–0.86). On the other hand, a nephroprotective effect by another statin was ascertained in another very recent subanalysis of the Treating to New Targets study [54]. In this study, treatment with 80 mg of atorvastatin resulted not only in a significant reduction in major cardiovascular events compared with 10 mg/day atorvastatin but also in a better evolution of renal function. Indeed, in the 80-mg arm, estimated GFR improved to >60 ml/min/1.73 m^2 in significantly more patients and declined to <60 ml/min/1.73 m^2 in significantly fewer patients than in the 10-mg arm. Overall, the sparing effect of statins on the GFR in patients at high risk for cardiovascular events appears quantitatively modest. However, in a public health perspective, given the high prevalence of cardiovascular and CKD at population level, even modest effects on the GFR by statins may be of relevance.

Efficacy of Statins in Cardiovascular Prevention in CKD Patients

No specifically designed major trial (i.e., a well-powered, randomized study based on clinical endpoints) has been performed in patients with CKD in the predialysis phase. Such specific information is important because renal dysfunction may alter the pathophysiology of CVD [55], and therefore, therapies that reduce cardiovascular risk in the general population may not be equally effective in CKD patients. Risk factors related to CKD, such as malnutrition, chronic inflammation, anemia, and abnormal calcium and phosphate metabolism, represent potential risk factors for CVD, which are overrepresented among people with renal insufficiency. Renal dysfunction has a 10% prevalence in the adult population, and it is even more common among patients with established coronary artery disease. Thus, information on the effect of statins in the prevention of cardiovascular complications in CKD can be derived from secondary analyses of major randomized clinical trials performed so far.

West of Scotland Coronary Prevention Study (WOSCOPS), Cholesterol and Recurrent Events (CARE), and Long-Term Intervention with Pravastatin in Ischemic Disease (LIPID) are three major randomized, double-blinded studies comparing pravastatin 40 mg daily with placebo over a long (5 years) follow-up. WOSCOPS studied high-risk individuals who had not previously experienced a MI. CARE and LIPID were trials of subjects with previous acute coronary syndromes and average cholesterol levels. The maximum baseline serum creatinine values for subjects included in WOSCOPS, CARE, and LIPID were 1.7, 2.5, and 4.5 mg/dl, respectively. In 2004, Tonelli et al., [56] published a combined analysis of individual patient data of these three studies, which constitutes the most solid information available about cardiovascular prevention by statins in CKD. As expected, CKD was quite common in the high-risk patients enrolled in these trials. Of 19,700 participants, about 23% had moderate CKD as defined by a GFR of 30.00–59.99 ml/min/1.73 m^2. In keeping with previous knowledge, also in this combined analysis, kidney function was a strong and independent predictor of cardiovascular complications. When the primary outcome of coronary death, nonfatal MI, or the need for coronary revascularization was considered, a 20-ml/min/1.73 m^2 decrease in GFR was independently associated with a 9% increase in risk. Overall, pravastatin reduced LDL-C levels by 48 mg/dl and triglyceride levels by 17 mg/dl and raised HDL-C by 2.3 mg/dl at 12 months, compared with baseline. LDL was reduced by a significantly greater extent in subjects with more severe renal insufficiency. Of note, such changes went along with a significant (−23%) reduction of the primary outcome and this risk reduction was almost identical to that registered in patients without renal impairment (−22%). Thus, because of the higher rate of cardiovascular events in CKD patients, the absolute risk reduction in these patients was even greater than that observed in patients with normal GFR. In the aggregate, this elegant analysis of three large trials of similar design, including use of pravastatin at the same dose (40 mg), leaves little doubt that this statin in CKD is at least as efficacious as it is in patients without renal disease. This analysis by Tonelli was apparently in contrast with the above mentioned meta-analysis by Strippoli [57], which negated a protective effect on all-cause and cardiovascular death and nonfatal cardiovascular events in CKD patients as a whole. Such a combined analysis was apparently justified by the lack of heterogeneity between studies in predialysis, dialysis, and transplant patients. In fact, a tendency toward heterogeneity did exist ($p = .12$). Furthermore the subanalysis of patients in the predialysis phase, which was dominated by the three pravastatin studies (16,824 patients, 93% of all patients included in this subanalysis), was still highly significant, confirming the benefit of statins at this CKD stage.

In the sole large trial performed so far in ESRD the Die Deutsche Diabetes Dialyse (4D) study, which tested the effect of 20 mg/day atorvastatin [58] in more than 1,000 diabetic patients on chronic dialysis, LDL-C was lowered as effectively as it was in previous studies with the same drug. However, the risk reduction in the primary composite end-point (cardiac death, fatal MI, stroke) was relatively small (−8%) and failed to reach statistical significance. Yet, a preplanned secondary analysis restricted to a cardiac end-point showed a risk reduction (-18%) similar to that which was expected on the basis of previous trials of statins in high-risk patients. It was noted that death in 4D patients was mainly due to noncoronary causes, such as sudden death and heart failure, and that the study power was inadequate. The question of whether statins afford cardiovascular protection in hemodialysis patients is also being tested in the AURORA study (Assessment of Survival and Cardiovascular Events Trial) [59], a trial focusing on the effects of rosuvastatin on cardiovascular morbidity and mortality in about 2,700 ESRD patients. The final, much awaited, answer on whether statins are cardiovasculoprotective in moderate to advanced CKD and ESRD will be given in the Study of Heart and Renal Protection (SHARP) [60] and Heart and Renal Protection (HARP) Study [61]. This is a quite large study that tests the effect of simvastatin (20 mg/day) combined to ezetimibe (10 mg/day), which enrolled 3,000 patients on dialysis and 6,000 patients with moderate to severe CKD.

Conclusion

Patients with CKD are at high cardiovascular risk. Such a risk excess appears in the early stages of CKD. In mild and mild to moderate CKD (i.e., when the GFR ranges from 90 to 45 ml/min/1.73 m^2, particularly in the absence of proteinuria), Framingham risk factors still represent the main cause of cardio-vascular complications in patients with renal diseases, and therefore, treatment with statins appears warranted. For more severe degrees of renal function loss, no definitive recommendations can be made. Even though we have no evidence to support the use of statins in patients with advanced renal insufficiency, awaiting the results of well-powered definitive trials such as AURORA and SHARP, there is no convincing rationale for denying the use of these drugs to patients with established coronary artery disease and moderate to severe CKD and to dialysis patients. Such a provisional recommendation rests on two arguments: 1) In the 4D study, a beneficial effect of atorvastatin was evident for the cardiac end-point (a secondary end-point) and 2) neither atorvastatin in the 4D study nor cerivastatin in the CHORUS study (Cerivastatin in Heart Outcomes in Renal Disease: Understanding Survival) [62] produced an excessive number of adverse effects in comparison to the adverse-event rate observed in other patient populations.

Selected References

6. Zoccali C. Traditional and emerging cardiovascular and renal risk factors: an epidemiologic perspective. Kidney Int 2006;70:26–33.

CHAPTER 24

Subclinical Hypothyroidism, Dyslipidemia, and Cardiovascular Risk

Jan Kvetny[1] & Jørgen Gram[2]

[1] Endocrinological Clinic, University of Copenhagen, Naestved Hospital, Naestved, Denmark
[2] University of Southern Denmark, Esbjerg, Denmark

Thyroid Physiology

The thyroid gland efficiently concentrates iodine and couples it to tyrosine residues from thyroglobulin protein, forming monoiodothyrosines and diiodothyrosines. These are in turn condensed to produce iodothyronines, and hence thyroid hormone (TH). The thyroid gland produces two main iodothyronines: $3,5,3',5'$-tetraiodothyronine (T_4) and $3,5,3'$-triiodo-l-thyronine (T_3), as well as small amounts of other iodothyronines. The control of TH secretion is exerted by a negative feedback loop: Thyrotropin-releasing hormone (TRH), produced in the hypothalamus, stimulates the release of thyrotropin-stimulating hormone (TSH) from the pituitary, and this in turns stimulates TH synthesis and release. The increase in blood concentration of TH inhibits the production of both TSH and TRH, leading to a down-regulation of thyrocyte function [1].

Until a few years ago, it was a common assumption in the literature that T_4 was a precursor and that T_3 was the only active TH, but a growing body of evidence seems to suggest that other iodothyronines (such as T_4 itself, and $3,5$-T_2) could be of biological relevance [2,3]. These other iodothyronines including T_3 are not produced centrally by the thyroid but by the action of the deiodinase enzymes present in various tissues.

TH is circulating bound to thyroxin-binding globulin (TBG), prealbumin, and albumin. However, while it was previously anticipated that the lipophilic TH passively diffused into the cell, TH transporters located in the plasma membrane and able to regulate TH uptake into cells have been described [4].

Thyroid Hormone Receptor Binding and Extranuclear Activation Sites

TH is expressed both by transcriptional pathways and by non-transcriptional pathways.

For almost 30 years, high-affinity nuclear-binding sites (TH receptor [TR]) for TH have been known [5,6]. TRs act as ligand-adjustable transcription factors because they bind both TH and TH-response elements (TREs) that are typically located in the promoters of target genes.

It is known that TR alters the level of gene transcription both in the absence and in the presence of TH, so the unliganded receptors repress expression. Microarray studies have led to the identification of novel target genes (both positively and negatively regulated) that are involved in a wide range of cellular pathways and functions, including gluconeogenesis, lipogenesis, insulin signaling, adenylate cyclase signaling, cell proliferation, and apoptosis [7].

Nutritional and Metabolic Bases of Cardiovascular Disease, 1st edition.
Edited by Mario Mancini, José M. Ordovas, Gabriele Riccardi,
Paolo Rubba and Pasquale Strazzullo. © 2011 Blackwell Publishing Ltd.

However, non-transcriptional pathways are also regulated by TH. At the plasma membrane, TH stimulates glucose uptake [8], and mitochondrial biogenesis and activity are regulated by TH both by a direct pathway of TH binding to mitochondrial TR isoforms and by an indirect pathway via intermediate factors [9].

Subclinical Hypothyroidism

Subclinical hypothyroidism (subhypo) is defined as a biochemical condition where serum free T_4 and total or free T_3 are within the respective reference limits and serum TSH is above the respective reference limits, as there are often only subtle clinical signs [10].

The prevalence of this condition in women ranges from 4% at age 20 years to 17% at age 65 years and in men from 2% at age 20 years to 7% at age 65 years [10]. Because subclinical thyroid disease is only detected as a TSH abnormality, the definition of the TSH reference range is crucial. Thus, the variation in the reference intervals obtained with different methods reflects differences in epitope recognition of different TSH isoforms. These differences make it difficult to establish a universal upper TSH reference limit, more so as the clinical state of test persons and the conditions in which the blood samples for establishment of the reference limits are seldom reported.

TSH reference interval should, therefore, be established using blood sampled in the morning from fasting euthyroid subjects in whom basal oxygen consumption (VO_2) is normal [11]. Furthermore, a recent study has demonstrated that test results within laboratory reference limits are not necessarily normal for an individual, due to individual reference range [12].

Thyroid Hormone Effect on Lipids

Although a number of alterations induced by lack of TH may contribute to the development of cardiovascular disease (CVD) (left ventricular dysfunction, endothelial dysfunction, alteration of coagulation parameters, low-grade inflammation), we focus on the significance of lipid disturbances.

It has long been known that hypothyroidism alters serum levels of lipids [13]. A recent review summarized alterations in lipids in overt hypothyroidism [14]: elevated levels of total cholesterol, low-density lipoprotein (LDL)-cholesterol (LDL-C), and apolipoprotein B (ApoB), increased levels of lipoprotein(a) [Lp(a)], a reversible reduction in clearance of chylomicron remnants, reduced activity of cholesteryl ester transfer protein, and decreased activity of hepatic lipase and lipoprotein lipase (LPL). All these alterations are attributed basically to the lack of TH effect [15].

When the serum TSH level remains elevated, as in subhypo, the TH levels are not truly normal for that individual. Because the half-life of T_4 is 7 days and that of T_3 is 1 day, the serum TSH, which has a half-life of less than 1 hour, would be expected to return to normal if TH levels were normal for that individual. Thus, an elevated TSH in subhypo means that the circulating TH concentrations are insufficient, and the above-described alterations in lipids would be liable in this condition also.

The effect of subhypo on plasma lipids has been evaluated either by direct observations in patients with subhypo or by observation of the effect of T_4 treatment on plasma lipids in patients with subhypo.

In studies on patients with subhypo, a small increase in LDL-C and a decrease in high-density lipoprotein (HDL)-cholesterol (HDL-C) were reported; changes that enhance the risk of development of atherosclerosis and coronary artery disease [16]. Furthermore, subhypo has been reported to be associated with a higher concentration of triglycerides (TGs) [17], and it is also noteworthy that the increased cardiovascular risk associated with subhypo seems to extend into the normal range of thyroid function [18].

A review of thyroxin treatment in subhypo has shown that treatment with T_4 lowers mean serum total cholesterol and LDL-C concentrations [19].

What then appears to be the relation between lipid metabolism and thyroid hormones? Peroxisome-proliferator-activated receptors (PPARs) are intimately involved in nutrient sensing and the regulation of carbohydrate and lipid metabolism. PPARα and PPARδ appear primarily to stimulate oxidative lipid metabolism, while PPARγ is principally involved in the cellular assimilation of lipids via anabolic pathways (fatty acid β-oxidation, lipoprotein synthesis). Activation of PPARγ induces the expression of genes controlling adipocyte fatty acid (FA) metabolism, including those that encode

LPL and FA transport proteins, thus leading to lipolysis of plasma TGs, uptake of FAs, and storage of TGs in adipocytes. It has also been shown that subjects with PPARγ ligand resistance have marked dyslipidemia, characterized by high TG and low HDL-C levels and impaired mitochondrial function [20].

TR interacts with PPAR by sharing binding sites and heterodimeric partners (retinoid X receptors [RXRs]), and it is known that variable cross-talk patterns between TRs and PPARs exist [21,22] and that TH modulates mitochondrial maturation partly through posttranscriptional control of PPAR coactivator-1 (PGC-1) [23,24].

Macrophages play a pivotal role in the development of atherosclerosis. Monocytes, well-known target cells for TH [25], differentiate into macrophages and accumulate lipids, thus forming foam cells. Research over the last few years has revealed important roles for PPARs and LXRs in macrophage inflammation and cholesterol homoeostasis with consequences in atherosclerosis development [26]. It is feasible that intracellular lack of THs interacts with PPARs leading into altered lipid profiles and finally to development of atherosclerosis.

Dyslipidemia and Cardiovascular Disease

CVD (e.g., coronary heart disease [CHD]) is a major threat to the population in Western societies affecting a larger number of persons older than 60 years [27]. CVD represents a systemic disorder, as it has been reported that the presence of noncoronary atherosclerotic disease carries the same risk of future cardiac events as CHD [28]. A number of risk factors, often acting in synergy, are associated with evolution of CHD [29]. Some of the most prevailing of these risk factors are associated with abnormalities of lipid metabolism. Obviously, the prevalence of dyslipidemia depends on definitions and the populations studied. However, the incidence is highest in patients with premature CHD and in patients with clinically overt disease at younger than 55 years, the prevalence of dyslipidemia is as high as 48% compared with age-matched controls [30].

Since screening tests for dyslipidemia are widely available, it is possible to identify high-risk groups, and since several factors of the lipid system are mod-

ifiable, there has been a huge interest in studying the association between lipids and CHD. Thus, it is well established that there are associations between CHD and high levels of total cholesterol, high levels of LDL-C, low levels of HDL-C and high levels of TGs [31]. In addition, it has been indicated that excess of Lp(a), excess of small LDL particle size, and excess of ApoB and low ApoA-1 are associated with evolution of CHD [32].

Evidence accumulated during the last decade has revealed that the presence of a low-grade chronic inflammation in subjects with dyslipidemia causes a deterioration of prognosis with respect to evolution of CHD [33,34]. The presence of low-grade inflammation in such patients may increase vulnerability of atherosclerotic plaques, thereby increasing the risk of myocardial infarction. Also noteworthy is that cholesterol-lowering therapy with statins has a much more pronounced effect on subjects with an ongoing chronic low-grade inflammation [35] compared with subjects with no signs of inflammation. Thus, an increasing body of evidence suggests a link between dyslipidemia and inflammation. Therefore, it is of particular interest to note that subjects with subhypo are characterized by both dyslipidemia and low-grade inflammation [17]. This raises the question of whether medical normalization of subhypo per se normalizes markers of inflammation and lipid abnormalities.

Subclinical Hypothyroidism as a Risk Factor for Cardiovascular Disease

Although a number of studies have addressed the subject, it is still uncertain whether subclinical hypothyroidism is associated with increased cardiovascular risk. In 2000, it was demonstrated that subhypo is a strong indicator of risk of atherosclerosis and myocardial infarction in elderly women [36], an observation that was in conflict with the Wickham Survey in which subhypo was not related to ischemic heart disease [37]. However, in this latter study, separation between subhypo and autoimmune thyroid disease was not distinct and subjects treated for myxedema were included.

Subsequent studies demonstrated that subjects with subhypo have increased levels of TGs and signs of low-grade inflammation (raised C-reactive protein [CRP] levels) associated with an increased risk of developing CVD in younger men [17], and that subjects with subhypo had a significantly higher prevalence of CHD than euthyroid subjects, indicating that subhypo may be an independent risk factor of CHD [38].

In a population-based study of mortality in a cohort of 1,191 individuals 60 years or older, comparison of mortality in those with high serum thyrotropin and normal serum thyrotropin revealed no significant difference, although subhypo was not separated from overt hypothyroidism [39].

Subhypo (TSH > 5.0 mU/L) was associated with ischemic heart disease independent of a number of predictors for CVD in 257 subjects compared to 2,293 control subjects [40], and in a 10-year follow-up study, increased mortalities from all causes in years 3–6 after baseline measurement were apparent in men with subhypo, but not in women [40].

In a prospective, observational, population-based follow-up study within the Leiden 85-Plus Study of a 2-year birth cohort (1912–1914), a total of 599 participants were followed from age 85 through 89 years. Increasing levels of thyrotropin were surprisingly associated with a lower mortality rate, which remained after adjustments for baseline disability and health status [41].

Subhypo in persons aged 70–79 years was associated with an increased risk of CHF (congestive heart failure) among older adults with a TSH level of 7.0 mU/L or greater, but not with other cardiovascular events and mortality [42].

In a study of 3,233 U.S. community-dwelling individuals 65 years or older, 15% had subhypo (TSH > 4.5 mU/L), but there were no differences between the subclinical hypothyroidism group and the euthyroid group for cardiovascular outcomes or mortality [43].

Although CVD was not examined, subhypo in middle-aged women was reported to be associated with hypertension, hypertriglyceridemia, and elevated total cholesterol/HDL-C ratio, thus increasing the risk of accelerated atherosclerosis and coronary artery disease in some patients [44].

In a recent review, it was stated that subhypo was associated with raised serum levels of total colesterol and LDL-C and, therefore, an increased risk of the development of atherosclerosis existed [45].

In another review, based on all case-control and cohort studies published in peer-reviewed journals, it was concluded that it is somewhat biologically

plausible to assume a causal relation of thyroid dysfunction with all-cause and circulatory mortality [46]. In another extensive review, it was similarly concluded that the influence of subhypo on lipids was directly proportional to the degree of TSH elevation [47].

There are several reasons for the conflicting results on an association between subhypo and CVD. The study populations differ regarding age, sex, and the TSH range that defines subhypo and methods of evaluation of CVD. However, it appears that association between subhypo and CVD primarily is present in the younger populations (younger than 70 years) and in populations consisting predominantly of males, suggesting that older age and inclusion of females introduce significant confounders (Table 24.1). It has recently been stressed that reference intervals for older persons should be higher than for younger [48]. Therefore, subhypo may have been overdiagnosed in a number of studies including older persons and underdiagnosed in groups of younger persons, which again may explain the difference of the reported prevalence of subhypo, from 20% [17] to 9% and 1% [49,50]. Another point of caution is the fact that the association between subhypo and CVD is often evaluated on basis of the effect of treatment with thyroxin. However, this approach is uncertain for a number of reasons. For example, to which level should TSH be titrated? It is also questionable to assume that euthyroidism is equivalent to a TSH level within reference limits. Additionally, it is currently discussed whether T_3 (or other intracellular iodothyronines) may have separate effects. This would imply that a simple substitution with T_4, though a decrease of TSH is achieved, does not restore intracellular mitochondrial function based on activation of TRs and PPARs.

Relevance to the Public Health: Necessity for Screening for Subclinical Hypothyroidism?

Although subhypo is a condition that occurs frequently in the general population, it is still uncertain whether screening strategies should be recommended as part of screening for CVD. If screening should be advisable, there is a need to know

Table 24.1 Lipid status, frequency of cardiovascular disease, and prevalence of subclinical hypothyroidism reported in the literature.

	Male/female (%)	Age (median + range)	Lipid changes	Increased frequency of CVD	Prevalence of subclinical hypothyroidism
Vanderpump 1996	47/53	44+15	?	No	8.1%
Hak et al. 2000	0/100	69+7.5	Chol, HDL	Yes	10.8%
Parle et al. 2001	43/57	70+7	?	No	
Kvetny et al. 2004	42/58	42+13	TG	Yes, males	19.7%
Imaizumi et al. 2004	39/61	57+11	?	Yes, males	10.2%
Gussekloo et al. 2004	34/66	85+	Chol, TG	No	5%
Rodondi et al. 2005	45/55	74+3	Chol	No	12.4%
Walsch et al. 2005	50/50	58+14	Chol, TG	Yes	5.6%
Cappola et al. 2006	41/59	73+6	Chol? Statin treated?	No	15%

Chol: cholesterol; HDL: high-density lipoprotein; TG: triglyceride; CVD: cardiovascular disease.

whether medical treatment of subhypo reduces future events of subjects with CVD. It has been reported that medical treatment of subhypo causes a moderate decrease in concentrations of cholesterol and LDL-C, but it remains unknown whether treatment affects, for example, inflammation caused by intracellular malfunction of organelles involved in lipid metabolism. Importantly, no studies have been reported on a possible favorable effect of treatment of subhypo on cardiovascular death or myocardial infarction. It is, therefore, questionable to recommend routine population screening, as there is no convincing evidence of an effective treatment. For the present, further studies on different treatment regimens in selected population groups are needed before screening can be recommended.

Acknowledgment

The authors want to thank Maria Kvetny, MA, scientific linguistic consultant, Institute of Odontology, Faculty of Health Sciences, University of Copenhagen, for linguistic support.

Selected References

10. Biondi B, Cooper D. The clinical significance of subclinical thyroid dysfunction. Endocrine Reviews 2007;10:1–236.

17. Kvetny J, Heldgaard PE, Bladbjerg E-M, Gram J. Subclinical hypothyroidism is associated with a lowgrade inflammation, increased triglyceride levels and predicts cardiovascular disease in males below 50 years. Clin Endocrinol 2004; 61:232–8.

38. Walsh J, Brenner A, Bulsara M, et al. Subclinical thyroid dysfunction as a risk factor for cardiovascular disease. Arch Intern Med 2005;165:2467–72.

43. Cappola AR, Fried L, Arnold A, et al. Thyroid status, cardiovascular risk, and mortality in older adults. JAMA 2006;295:1033–41.

46. Völzke H, Schwahn C, Wallaschofski H, Dörr M. REVIEW: the association of thyroid dysfunction with all-cause and circulatory mortality: is there a causal relationship? J Clin Endocrinol Metab 2007;92: 2421–9.

CHAPTER 25

Genetic Influences on Blood Lipids and Cardiovascular Disease Risk

Jose M. Ordovas & Mireia Junyent

Tufts University, Boston, MA, USA

Introduction

Cardiovascular disease (CVD) is the major cause of morbidity and mortality in developed countries. As a multifactorial disease, its manifestation is determined by interactions among genes, environmental factors, as well as gene–environment interactions [1]. Major risk factors for CVD are blood lipids, particularly increased serum low-density lipoprotein (LDL)-cholesterol (LDL-C) and triglyceride (TG) levels, as well as reduced high-density lipoprotein (HDL)-cholesterol (HDL-C) levels. It has been clearly demonstrated that variation at several candidate genes has significant effects on blood lipids, and these effects are also modulated by nonmodifiable factors such as gender and age, and modifiable factors, including diet, smoking, alcohol intake, obesity, and physical activity, among many others.

Although most of the beneficial evidence from lowering LDL-C values in reducing CVD morbidity and mortality comes from pharmacological interventions, the National Cholesterol Education Program (NCEP) has continuously emphasized that therapeutic lifestyle changes (TLCs) should be the primary treatment for lowering cholesterol values, reserving drug therapies for cases in which TLCs are ineffective [2]. These TLCs advocate dietary changes, increased physical activity, and weight management. However, it is not known how many individuals can achieve the recommended levels of

Nutritional and Metabolic Bases of Cardiovascular Disease, 1st edition.
Edited by Mario Mancini, José M. Ordovas, Gabriele Riccardi,
Paolo Rubba and Pasquale Strazzullo. © 2011 Blackwell Publishing Ltd.

lipids using this approach, and this is a major reason for the inability to predict individual plasma lipid responses to dietary changes [1].

We have traditionally measured the success of CVD risk-reducing strategies on the basis of their effect on lipids. Lipid metabolism can be viewed as a complex biological pathway containing multiple steps. Indeed, lipid homeostasis is achieved by the coordinated action of a large number of nuclear factors, binding proteins, apolipoproteins, enzymes, and receptors involving hundreds of previously known candidate genes and many others recently identified [3]. Lipoprotein metabolism is commonly subdivided into three components: the exogenous pathway, the endogenous pathway, and the reverse cholesterol transport (RCT) (Figure 25.1).

Exogenous Lipoprotein Pathway

The exogenous lipoprotein pathway has its origin in the enterocyte with the synthesis of chylomicron particles. Dietary fats absorbed in the intestine are packaged into large, TG-rich chylomicrons. During their transit to the liver, these particles interact with lipoprotein lipase (LPL) and undergo partial lipolysis to form chylomicron remnants. These chylomicron remnants pick up apolipoprotein E (ApoE) and cholesteryl esters from HDL particles and are taken up by the liver. The most relevant candidate genes involved in this metabolic pathway and their known associations with lipids and dietary response are described below.

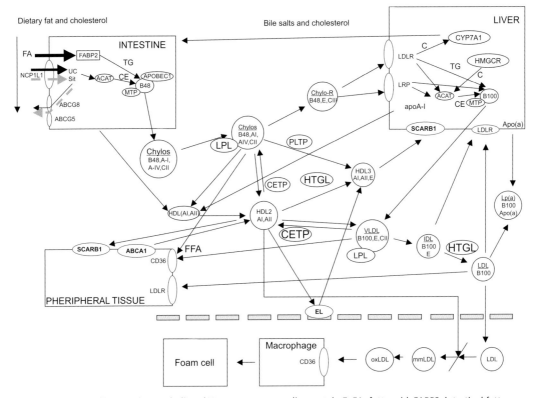

Figure 25.1 Human lipoprotein metabolism. (AI: apolipoprotein A-I; AII: apolipoprotein A-II; AIV: apolipoprotein A-IV; AV: apolipoprotein A-V; ABCA1: ATP-binding cassette, subfamily A, member 1; ABCG5: ATP-binding cassette, subfamily G, member 5; ABCG8: ATP-binding cassette, subfamily G, member 8; ACAT2: cytosolic acetoacetyl-CoA thiolase; apo: apolipoprotein; APOBEC1: apolipoprotein B mRNA editing enzyme; B48: apolipoprotein B-48; B100: apolipoprotein B-100; CII: apolipoprotein C-II; CIII: apolipoprotein C-III; CD36: CD36 antigen; CE: cholesteryl esters; CETP: cholesteryl ester transfer protein; chylos: chylomicron; chylo-R: chylomicron remnants; CYP7A1: cholesterol-7-alpha-hydroxylase; E: apolipoprotein E; FA: fatty acid; FABP2: intestinal fatty acid–binding protein; FFA: free fatty acid; HDL: high-density lipoprotein; HMGCR: 3-hydroxy-3-methylglutaryl-CoA reductase; HTGL: hepatic triglyceride lipase; IDL: intermediate-density lipoprotein; LDL: low-density lipoprotein; LDLR: LDL receptor; Lp(a): lipoprotein a; LPL: lipoprotein lipase; mmLDL: minimally modified LDL; MTP: microsomal triglyceride transfer protein; NPC1L1: Niemann-Pick C1-like 1; oxLDL: oxidized LDL; PLTP: phospholipid transfer protein; SCARB1: scavenger receptor type I B; Sit: sitosterol; TG: triglyceride; UC: unesterified cholesterol; VLDL: very-low-density lipoprotein.

Apolipoprotein B

ApoB is the major protein of chylomicrons, LDL, and very low-density lipoprotein (VLDL) particles, by which genetic variation at this locus can influence cholesterol and TG levels. Although several ApoB polymorphisms have been correlated with lipids and CVD risk, the outcomes of these studies have not been unanimous [4].

A silent mutation causing a cytosine to thymidine (C→T) change characterizes the well-studied *ApoB XbaI* restriction fragment length polymorphism (RFLP). The association between this polymorphism and variability in dietary response has

been studied with controversial results. Some reports shown that the response to a low-fat, low-cholesterol diet was influenced by the *ApoB XbaI* genotype [5,6], by which subject carriers of the X+ allele displayed greater reductions of plasma LDL-C, ApoB, and HDL-C levels compared to X−X− genotype [5]. However, a meta-analysis suggested that this polymorphism played a minor role in determining individual variability in response to dietary intervention [7]. Another interesting polymorphism is the three-codon (Leu-Ala-Leu) insertion (I)/deletion (D) polymorphism in the signal peptide region of the *ApoB* gene [8].

Xu et al. [9] reported that I/I subjects displayed higher TG levels than D/D subjects after a high-fat, high-cholesterol diet. Importantly, this effect disappeared when subjects were switched from a high-fat, high-cholesterol diet to a low-fat, low-cholesterol diet. However, these results were not confirmed by Boerwinkle et al. [10] in which this gene locus did not have a major effect on the response of lipids to increased dietary cholesterol.

The *Msp*I polymorphism in exon 26 causes an adenine to guanosine change (Arg^{3611}→Glu). We found a significant association between the minor allele of this variant and the presence of CVD [11].

Apolipoprotein A-IV

In humans, apolipoprotein A-IV (ApoA4) plays a key role in dietary fat absorption and chylomicron synthesis. Multiple genetic variants have been examined in *ApoA4* locus in order to determine their associations with lipids and CVD risk. However, these studies have been complicated by the close proximity of other candidate genes such as *ApoA1*, *ApoC3*, and *ApoA5* [12]. In whites, the most common isoforms are *ApoA4*-1 and *ApoA4*–2, with allele frequencies around 88%–95% and 5%–12%, respectively. The *ApoA4*-2 allele has been associated with higher levels of HDL-C and/or lower TGs [13–15], whereas no lipid associations have been reported in other studies [15–17].

The effect of *ApoA4* genetic variation on dietary response of plasma lipids has been examined previously [18–20]. Our own data [19] show that the *ApoA4*-2 (Gln^{360}→His) isoform was associated with hyporesponsiveness of LDL-C to dietary therapy consisting of reduction in total fat and cholesterol intakes. McCombs et al. [20] demonstrated that the *ApoA4*-2 allele attenuated the hypercholesterolemic response to the ingestion of a very-high-cholesterol diet. We also observed that subjects with the *ApoA4*-2 allele tended to have greater decreases in HDL-C after a low-fat, low-cholesterol diet. We next examined the effect of this polymorphism on HDL-C response in 41 healthy males [18] after feeding with three consecutive diets (high-saturated, low-fat, and high-monounsaturated fat [MUFA] diets) during diet phases of 4 weeks each. After consuming the high-saturated fat diet, carriers of the *ApoA4*-2 allele displayed decreased HDL-C and ApoA1 levels. In these subjects, replacement of a

high-carbohydrate diet by a diet rich in MUFAs, resulted in a higher increase in HDL-C and ApoA1 levels compared to homozygotes for the *ApoA4*-2 allele. We also examined the association between the *ApoA4* (Thr^{347}→Ser) variant observed within the *ApoA4*-1 allele and the LDL-C response to dietary intervention [18]. Our data show that carriers of the less common Ser^{347} allele displayed lower LDL-C and APOB concentrations when they were switched from a low-fat, cholesterol diet to a high-MUFA diet as compared with homozygous carriers of the Thr^{347} allele.

Apolipoprotein E

Apolipoprotein E (ApoE) in serum is associated with chylomicrons, VLDL, and HDL and serves as a ligand for the LDL receptor (LDLR). When ApoE deficiency is present, there is a marked accumulation of cholesterol-enriched lipoproteins [21]. Population studies have shown that plasma LDL-C, and ApoB levels are highest in subjects carrying the *ApoE4* isoform, intermediate in those with the *ApoE3* isoform and lowest in those with the *ApoE2* isoform [22]. In the general population, *ApoE* allelic variation may account for up to 7% of the variation in LDL-C levels [23], and this effect is modulated by environmental factors such as diet. Therefore, it appears that the association of the *ApoE4* isoform with elevated cholesterol levels is greater in populations consuming diets rich in saturated fat and cholesterol than in others. Although some investigators reported greater lipid responses in subjects carrying the *ApoE4* allele, others failed to find significant associations between *ApoE* genotypes and plasma lipid responses [1,24]. Differences in age, gender, and lipids may explain these discrepancies.

Apolipoprotein C-III

Apolipoprotein C-III (APOC3) is a component of chylomicrons, VLDL, and HDL particles. The S2 allele of the SstI SNP (C3238G) has been associated with hypertriglyceridemia and increased CVD risk [12]. A PvuII RFLP located in the first intron of the *ApoC3* gene has also been associated with HDL-C levels. In addition, several polymorphisms have been identified in the promoter region of the gene (C^{-641}→A, G^{630}→A, T^{-625} → deletion, C^{-482} → T, and T^{-455} → C) [25]. Our own studies show that after a diet rich in MUFAs, S1S1 subjects displayed increased LDL-C levels, whereas LDL-C decreased in S1S2 subjects [26], suggesting that *ApoC3* locus was involved in LDL-C responsiveness to dietary fat.

Apolipoprotein A5

Apolipoprotein A5 (*ApoA5*) and its genetic variability have a great impact on TG-rich lipoprotein (TRL) metabolism. Five common *ApoA5* polymorphisms have been reported in several populations: −1131T>C, −3A>G, 56C>G IVS3+476G>A, and 1259T>C. These variants have been associated with increased TG concentrations [27–30]. However, the association between *ApoA5* polymorphisms and CVD risk remains still controversial [30–34].

In the Framingham Heart Study (FHS), we reported a gene–diet interaction between *ApoA5* gene variation and polyunsaturated fatty acids (PUFAs) in relation to plasma lipid concentrations and lipoprotein particle size [35]. More recently, we found a gene–diet interaction between *ApoA5* and total fat intake in relation to obesity risk [36]. The −1131C allele was associated with higher TGs only in subjects consuming a high n-6 PUFA diet, suggesting that n-6 PUFA-rich diets were related to a more atherogenic lipid profile.

Lipoprotein Lipase

LPL is an enzyme that plays a key role in lipoprotein metabolism by the hydrolysis of the TGs of chylomicrons and VLDL particles. Hundreds of polymorphisms have been reported at this locus, some of them with a loss of enzymatic function. Conversely, the S447X variant has been associated with an increased lipolytic function considered as a gain-of-function mutation. Consistenly, 447X carriers displayed lower TG levels and increased HDL-C levels with a lower incidence of CVD risk compared to noncarriers.

The Asn291Ser is the most common mutation that reduces LPL activity with a frequency of 2%–5% in the white population. Less common mutations are Asp9Asn (1.5%) and Gly188Glu (0.06%). The French Canadian population has a high rate of LPL mutations, up to 17% (Pro207Leu, Gly188Glu, and Asp250Asn), whereas in the Japanese population, the frameshift mutation G916 deletion is the most common. On the other hand, the promoter variant T-93G was found in 76.4% of South African blacks and in only 1.7% of whites.

A systematic review [37] reported that the T-93G polymorphism was a risk factor for hypertriglyceridemia and low HDL-C levels. Moreover, this gene variant may predispose to coronary heart disease (CHD).

In addition to the LPL polymorphisms described above, some other less frequent mutations have been associated with LPL deficiency and with atherogenic lipid profiles. When these mutations are gathered with other risk factors, a significant increase in CVD risk is observed.

Intestinal Fatty Acid-Binding Protein

Intestinal FA-binding protein (IFABP) is a member of a family of cytoplasmic hydrophobic ligand-binding proteins. IFABP is involved in several steps of fat absorption and transport, and its expression is under nutritional control.

Baier et al. [38] initially reported a G→A mutation, which results in an amino acid substitution in IFABP at residue 54, alanine54 (wild-type) →threonine (mutant type). Associations of this polymorphism with elevated insulin levels and insulin resistance have been investigated in Pima Indians, Japanese, Mexican Americans, Native Americans, and white populations [38,39]. Conversely, a study of Keewatin Inuit (Eskimos) found that the Thr54 allele was associated with lower glucose concentrations [40]. These phenotypic differences may be explained by the high content in PUFA omega-3 from Eskimo diets. Other studies have found an association between the presence of the Thr54 mutation and a higher fat oxidation rate [38], greater fasting plasma TG [41], and internal carotid artery (ICA) stenosis [42].

Regarding differences in dietary response, Hegele et al. [40] found that the Ala54Thr mutation was associated with variation in the response of plasma lipoproteins to dietary fiber. Compared to those homozygous for the ala54 allele, subjects with the mutant Thr54 allele had greater decreases in LDL-C and ApoB after consuming a high-soluble-fiber diet.

Endogenous Lipoprotein Metabolism

The hepatocyte synthesizes and secretes VLDL-TGs, which are converted first to intermediate-density lipoproteins (IDLs) and then to LDLs through lipolysis by LPL enzyme. The excess of surface components is usually transferred to HDLs. Some of these remnants are taken up by the liver, whereas others are further lipolyzed and converted into LDL particles. This pathway shares many of the genes described already for the exogenous pathway. This section describes briefly some of the studies related to the *LDLR* gene, which has a major responsibility for the catabolism of LDL particles, and the 3-hydroxy–3-methylglutaryl coenzyme A (HMG-CoA) reductase gene, coding for a key enzyme in the synthesis *de novo* of cholesterol.

LDL Receptor

Mutations at the *LDLR* are responsible for familial hypercholesterolemia (FH), an autosomal dominant disorder characterized by elevation of LDL-C levels and premature CVD. In addition to those rare mutations associated with FH, several common polymorphisms have also been associated with lipids in the general population.

The role of common genetic variations in the 3'UTR of the LDLR in relation to plasma cholesterol has been recently examined [43]. Six polymorphisms, G44243A, G44332A, C44506G, G44695A, C44857T, and A44964G, within the 5' region of the 3'UTR fall into three common haplotypes, GGCGCA, AGCACG, and GGCGTA, occurring at frequencies of 0.45, 0.31, 0.17 and 0.13, 0.13, 0.38 in whites and African Americans, respectively. Genotyping of two "haplotype tagging" polymorphisms, C44857T and A44964G, in the Atherosclerosis Risk in Communities (ARIC) study population showed that in whites, but not in African Americans, the inferred TA haplotype had a significant LDL-C–lowering effect. White men homozygous for CA, in contrast, showed significantly higher LDL-C and lower HDL-C. These data show that 3'UTR sequences that cause higher gene expression *in vitro* are associated in whites with atherogenic plasma lipid profiles. Some investigators found an association between the polymorphism (A370T) and stroke, independently of lipids [44], whereas no associations with lipids were reported by Vieira et al. [45]. So far, no gene–diet interactions have been reported for this locus.

3-Hydroxy–3-Methylglutaryl-Coenzyme A Reductase

Similar to the LDLR locus, and despite its important biological role as a drug target in the form of HMG-CoA reductase inhibitors, this gene has been barely examined in terms of association with lipids and related phenotypes. Some studies have investigated this locus regarding its potential pharmacogenetic value [46,47].

Reverse Cholesterol Transport

HDL is synthesized by the liver and the intestine. The HDL precursor form has a discoidal shape and matures in circulation through picking up unesterified cholesterol from cell membranes, other lipids (phospholipids and TG), and proteins from TRL. The cholesterol is esterified by the action of lecithin cholesterol acyltransferase (LCAT), and thereby, small HDL_3 particles are converted into large HDL_2 particles. The esterified cholesterol is either delivered to the liver or transferred by the action of the cholesterol ester transfer protein (CETP) to TRL in exchange for TG. The liver may take up this cholesterol via specific receptors for these lipoproteins, or can be delivered to peripheral tissues. TGs received by the HDL_2 are hydrolysed by hepatic lipase enzyme (LIPC) and particles are converted to HDL_3. In the liver, cholesterol can be excreted directly into bile, converted to bile acids, or reutilized in lipoprotein production.

The study of genetics of the RCT has been restricted mainly driven by the complexity of the several pathways involved in this process. The understanding of the molecular basis for HDL deficiency is crucial to target this information for CVD prevention. This section provides an overview of the current status of common polymorphisms related to RCT and their potential interactions with diet.

Apolipoprotein A-I

ApoA1 is the most abundant protein of HDL. The common variant most intensively studied is the resulting from an adenine (A) to guanine (G) transition (G/A), 75-bp upstream from the *ApoA1* transcription start. Several studies have reported that carriers of the A allele display higher HDL-C levels than subjects homozygous for the G allele. Our own data [48] supported that the A allele was associated with hyperresponse to changes in the dietary saturated fat. In addition, different rare genetic abnormalities have been reported within this locus and some of them have been associated with severe HDL deficiency and premature coronary atherosclerosis. However, other studies have not found an association with CVD risk, and at least one of these mutations has shown a protective effect despite its association with low HDL-C [49].

Apolipoprotein A-II

ApoA2 as the second most abundant protein of HDL constitutes a candidate gene for the study of the RCT. Although some initial studies reported an inverse relationship between plasma ApoA2 concentrations and CVD risk [50,51], subsequent studies did not find significant associations or even suggested a proatherogenic role [52]. Few studies have examined the association between *ApoA2* polymorphisms and phenotypic traits [53,54]. We studied the association between a functional *ApoA2* promoter polymorphism (−265T>C) and lipids, anthropometric variables, and food intake in subjects who participated in the Genetics of Lipid Lowering Drugs and Diet Network (GOLDN) study [55]. We observed that individuals homozygous for the −265C allele displayed more obesity than T allele carriers. Interestingly, total energy, total fat, and protein intakes were higher in CC individuals than T allele carriers, suggesting a new role for *ApoA2* in the regulation of dietary intake.

Cholesteryl Ester Transfer Protein

CETP facilitates the exchange of cholesteryl esters from HDL or LDL into TRLs and, thereby, stimulates the RCT. The most studied polymorphism in the *CETP* gene has been the variant TaqIB, characterized by a silent base change affecting the 277th nucleotide in the first intron of the *CETP* gene, with a restriction site for the endonuclease TaqI. The B2 allele (absence of the TaqI restriction site) at this polymorphic site has been firmly associated with increased HDL-C levels [56]. In addition, significant interactions have been reported between *CETP* variants and diet [57]. Given the consistent association between *CETP* polymorphisms and CVD risk factors, mainly HDL-C concentrations, several studies have reported significant associations with CVD risk [58].

Hepatic Lipase (LIPC)

LIPC is a lipolytic enzyme involved in the catabolism of plasma lipoproteins and an important determinant of HDL concentrations. The lipid profile of individuals with complete LIPC deficiency is characterized by elevated cholesterol and TG levels, as well as an impaired metabolism of TG-enriched particles [59].

Four LIPC polymorphisms located in the 780-bp region upstream of the transcription start (−250 G to A, −514 C to T, −710 T to C, and −763 A to G) are in complete LD. The −514T allele has been associated with increased HDL-C and ApoA1 concentrations [60]. Indeed, Tahvanainen et al. [61] reported an association between the −514T allele and TG content of LDL, IDL, and HDL particles in male Finnish patients with CHD. Our own data from the FHS have showed a gender-specific association with HDL-C levels that became stronger after examining more specific markers of HDL metabolism such as HDL subfractions and HDL size [62]. In addition to those polymorphisms presented in several ethnic groups, other common polymorphisms have been shown in Chinese populations with significant associations with HDL-C concentrations and CVD risk [63].

Cholesterol-7-Alpha-Hydroxylase (CYP7A1)

Cholesterol-7-alpha-hydroxylas (CYP7A1) is a rate-limiting enzyme in bile acid synthesis and plays an important role in cholesterol homeostasis. A common A-to-C substitution at position −204 of the promoter of the *CYP7A1* gene has been associated with plasma LDL-C levels [64]. The effect of the A278-C promoter polymorphism on plasma lipid responses to an increased intake in dietary cholesterol, saturated fat and trans-fat has been investigated in normolipidemic subjects [65]. AA subjects who consumed a cholesterol-rich diet had a significantly smaller increase in HDL-C levels than CC subjects. No effects were seen in saturated and trans fat interventions. Another study [66] measured LDL-C levels in healthy men who were homozygous for either the −204A or −204C allele, after 3 weeks on a low-fat (LF) diet and 3 weeks on a high-fat (HF) diet. In subjects homozygous for the −204C allele, the concentrations of LDL-C were significantly higher in subjects with HF diet than LF diet, whereas no significant changes were observed in subjects homozygous for the −204A allele.

Scavenger Receptor B Type I

Although scavenger receptor B type I (SCARB1) was the first HDL transmembrane receptor identified, it is a multilipoprotein receptor involved in the selective uptake of cholesteryl esters from HDL, LDL, and VLDL particles. Preliminary evidence from our studies indicated that the SCARB1 gene played a significant role in determining lipids and body mass index [67]. Moreover, we found that lipid response was modified by one common polymorphism located in exon 1 at SCARB1 gene [68].

ATP-Binding Cassette Transporters (ABCA1, ABCG5, ABCG8)

For several decades, the elucidation of the RCT involving the cholesterol efflux from cells and its transport and internalization by the liver has been intensively studied. Mutations in the ABCA1 gene are responsible for the Tangier phenotype characterized by the almost complete absence of HDL and the accumulation of cholesteryl esters in tissues. Patients with Tangier disease tend to develop premature CVD, despite low levels of LDL-C. Since the initial discovery of the ABCA1 gene as a key player in lipoprotein metabolism, other members of the ATP-binding cassette (ABC) transporter family have been shown to play similar roles [69]. In this regard, ABCG5 and ABCG8 form heterodimers that limit absorption of dietary sterols in the intestine and promote cholesterol elimination from the body through the RCT. Recently, we demonstrated that HDL-C levels were determined by the interaction between several common ABCG5/G8 variants and smoking [70]. ABCA1 has not been properly investigated in terms of dietary response; however, several ABCG5 polymorphisms have been examined regarding the variability in dietary response [71].

Conclusions

In summary, gene–diet interactions modulate plasma lipids and potentially CVD risk. However, the application of these findings to the clinical environment is not ready for prime time. Current and future findings need to be replicated using experimental approaches providing the highest level of scientific evidence. To assess the modulation by specific polymorphisms of the effects of dietary interventions on lipids, there is a need for well-designed, adequately powered, and appropriate studies to increase the consistency of the reported results. Overall, future large genetic epidemiologic studies and intervention studies involving groups of individuals selected for specific genotype combinations and phenotypic characteristics are required.

Acknowledgments

This work was supported by National Institutes of Health (NIH) grants HL54776 and DK75030 and contract 58-1950-9-001 from the U.S. Department of Agriculture Research Service. M.J is supported by a grant from the Fulbright-Spanish Ministry of Education and Science (reference 2007-1086).

Selected References

3. Kathiresan S, Manning AK, Demissie S, , et al. A genome-wide association study for blood lipid phenotypes in the Framingham Heart Study. BMC Med Genet 2007; 8(Suppl 1): S17.

24. Masson LF, McNeill G. The effect of genetic variation on the lipid response to dietary change: recent findings. Curr Opin Lipidol 2005;16:61–7.

58. Barter PJ, Brewer HB Jr, Chapman MJ, et al. Cholesteryl ester transfer protein: a novel target for raising HDL and inhibiting atherosclerosis. Arterioscler Thromb Vasc Biol 2003;23:160–7.

69. Ordovas JM, Tai ES. The babel of the ABCs: novel transporters involved in the regulation of sterol absorption and excretion. Nutr Rev 2002;60:30–3.

71. Herron KL, McGrane MM, Waters D,et al. The ABCG5 polymorphism contributes to individual responses to dietary cholesterol and carotenoids in eggs. J Nutr 2006; 136:1161–5.

CHAPTER 26

The Relationship between Dyslipidemia and Inflammation

Branislav Vohnout[1], Giovanni de Gaetano[2],
Maria Benedetta Donati[2] & Licia Iacoviello[2]
[1] Slovak Medical University, Bratislava, Slovakia
[2] John Paul II Center for High Technology Research and Education in Biomedical Sciences,
Catholic University, Campobasso, Italy

Introduction

Atherosclerosis is a chronic and progressive disease morphologically characterized as asymmetric focal thickenings of the intima in primarily large and medium-sized elastic and muscular arteries, such as aorta, coronary, carotid, and femoral arteries [1,2]. A wide range of clinical manifestations are related to atherosclerosis. It can be presented chronically, such as stable angina pectoris, or can manifest suddenly with myocardial infarction (MI) or stroke with or without preceding clinical symptoms. However, some individuals can live without any clinical consequence despite the evidence of extensive atherosclerosis found postmortem.

Critical Steps for Development of Atherosclerosis

Endothelial Dysfunction

Endothelium, the continuous single-cell lining covering the inner surface of blood vessels, plays a crucial role in regulating vascular tone, growth, vascular inflammation, coagulation, and thrombosis. Endothelial dysfunction can be induced by elevated and modified low-density lipoprotein (LDL), smoking, hypertension, diabetes mellitus, genetic alterations, and combinations of these or other factors [1]. As a consequence of endothelium activation by atherogenic and proinflammatory stimuli, the expression of adhesion molecules is upregulated and monocytes and T cells are recruited. Moreover, at the site of defective endothelium, plasma molecules and lipoprotein particles enter into the subendothelial space, where lipoproteins can be trapped and modified and manifest proinflammatory, chemotaxic, and cytotoxic activities. LDL, which can be modified by oxidation, glycation, aggregation, association with proteoglycans, or incorporation into immune complexes, is a major cause of injury to the endothelium and the underlying smooth muscle [1]. Finally, reduced endothelial availability of nitric oxide (NO), in part due to oxidative stress, has been shown to promote a proinflammatory and prothrombotic phenotype of endothelium.

Although the entire vascular system is exposed to the effects of the risk factors, atherosclerotic lesions are not equally distributed over the arterial system. Atherosclerotic lesions form at specific arterial sites, such as bifurcations, at or near side branches, at the inner wall of curvatures, or where low and oscillatory endothelial shear stress (ESS) occur [3]. Endothelial cells (ECs) detect and respond to ESS by activating numerous mechanoreceptors at the EC surfaces with a trigger of several intracellular pathways in a process known as mechanotransduction. Low ESS modulates endothelial gene expression by suppressing atheroprotective and up-regulating

Nutritional and Metabolic Bases of Cardiovascular Disease, 1st edition.
Edited by Mario Mancini, José M. Ordovas, Gabriele Riccardi,
Paolo Rubba and Pasquale Strazzullo. © 2011 Blackwell Publishing Ltd.

pro-atherogenic genes and induces an atherogenic endothelial phenotype. It impairs flow dependent vasodilation through down-regulation of NO and prostacyclin and up-regulation of endothelin-1 and promotes LDL uptake, synthesis, permeability, and subendothelial accumulation of LDL [3]. Moreover, it induces production of reactive oxygen species (ROS) in the intima and down-regulates intracellular ROS scavengers. Oxidative stress represents a common feature of all known cardiovascular risk factors and leads to the formation of oxidized LDL (oxLDL), one of the key mediators of atherosclerosis. ECs at low shear regions show high levels of nuclear factor-κB (NF-κB) molecules and elevated NF-κB transcriptional activity [4]. NF-κB activation induces downstream up-regulation of various endothelial genes, including genes encoding adhesion molecules (such as vascular cell adhesion molecule [VCAM]-1, E-selectin), monocyte chemoattractant protein (MCP)-1, and proinflammatory cytokines (tumor necrosis factor [TNF]-α, interleukin 1 [IL-1], and interferon [IFN]-γ).

Monocyte Recruitment, Macrophages, and Foam Cell Formation, and T Cell Recruitment and Activation

The recruitment of circulating inflammatory cells into the intima to scavenge oxidized LDL constitutes a major pathogenic concept of atherosclerosis. Lesion initiation is caused by infiltration of monocytes into the subendothelial space and subsequent accumulation of lipid-loaded macrophages. Recruitment of monocytes in lesion-prone sites is regulated by endothelial adhesion molecules and their corresponding monocyte ligands, such as VCAM-1, selectins (E, P), and intracellular adhesion molecule-1 (ICAM-1). Monocytes (with their ligands) initially interact with selectins on ECs in a low-affinity interaction that permits leukocyte tethering and rolling. This initial interaction is followed by firmer attachment, mediated by VCAM-1, ICAM-1, and integrins. Once adherent to endothelium, monocytes migrate by diapedesis into the intima under the influence of modified LDL and chemoattractant molecules, particularly MCP-1 that attracts leukocytes carrying its receptor CCR-2. The expression of these adhesion molecules and chemokines is under control of inflammatory cytokines (e.g., interleukin [IL]-6, IL-10, and TNF-α).

In the intima, infiltrated monocytes in response to monocyte colony-stimulating factor (M-CSF) further differentiate into macrophages. The macrophages express scavenger receptors (such as scavenger receptor A and CD36) that internalize modified lipoprotein particles (such as oxLDL) and extracellular debris, accumulate cholesteryl esters in the cytoplasm, and thus become foam cells. Macrophage-derived foam cells in turn lead to production of ROS, growth factors, and proinflammatory cytokines, including TNF-α and IL-1, and amplify the local inflammatory response. Activated macrophages present antigens, and by triggering activation of antigen-specific T cells macrophages also participate in the adaptive immune response. In addition to their inflammatory attributes, foamy macrophages also have active lipid metabolism (taking up, building, and exporting lipids). The development of lipid-loaded macrophages containing massive amounts of cholesteryl esters is a hallmark of both early and late atherosclerosis.

Lymphocytes enter into the endothelial space of the developing lesion by adhesion molecules and a chemokine-guided process similar to that of recruitment of monocytes. Once present in the intima, T cells may encounter antigens (e.g., oxLDL, heat shock protein [HSP] 60, and microbial antigens) bound to major histocompatibility complex molecules on the surface of antigen-presenting cells (such as macrophages and dendritic cells). Upon activation, several types of effector responses occur in atheroma, with predominant T helper-1 response. This leads to production of several proinflammatory cytokines (e.g., IFN-γ, TNF, and CD40 ligand), mononuclear cells recruitment, macrophage activation, and promotes lesion formation and plaque vulnerability. Regulatory T cells inhibit this process, although the role of Th$_2$ cells remains controversial [5].

Accumulation of lipid-laden macrophages, together with some T cells, dendritic cells, and mast cells, is a hallmark of fatty streaks. Even if not clinically important, fatty streaks can evolve into more complex atheroma lesions or eventually disappear.

Advanced Lesions and Plaque Disruption

In the disease progression, the immuno-inflammatory response is joined by a fibro-proliferative response mediated by intimal smooth muscle cells (SMCs). The process involves migration of SMCs from media into the intima with subsequent proliferation, cholesterol accumulation, and SMC-derived foam cells formation and synthesis of extracellular matrix proteins (such as collagen and elastin) leading to the development of the fibrous cap [6]. Migration of SMC is directed by chemoattractants such as platelet-derived growth factor, produced by activated leukocytes or by SMCs themselves when appropriately stimulated. Secretion of extracellular matrix proteins is stimulated by TGF-β, which is a product mainly of regulatory T cells.

During the progression of atherosclerosis, foam cells die by apoptosis or necrosis which leads to the formation of a necrotic, cholesterol-rich core. This core region consisting of foam cells, dead cells, and extracellular accumulation of lipids is covered by the fibrous cap of SMCs and a collagen-rich matrix. Its formation is important in maintaining plaque stability by isolating the lipid core and inflammatory cells from circulating blood.

Plaque growth may result in luminal narrowing that can lead to clinical consequences of atherosclerosis, such as stable angina pectoris, or intermittent claudication, although even large plaques may be asymptomatic. Indeed, the vascular wall can enlarge and compensate for the developing plaque via outward remodeling ("positive remodeling"), so that the lumen is not significantly narrowed and blood flow is preserved.

Although advanced lesions can lead to clinical symptoms, the majority of acute events such as MI or stroke are due to plaque rupture or superficial endothelial erosion and thrombosis. Plaque rupture is responsible for approximately three out of four fatal heart attacks caused by coronary thrombosis, while the remaining one is caused by plaque erosion and other less known mechanisms.

Plaque ruptures generally occur at the shoulder region of the plaque and more likely occur in lesions with thin fibrous caps, a relatively high concentration of lipid-filled macrophages within the shoulder region or large necrotic cores. As the lesion grows, increased modified lipid content and activation of macrophages around the necrotic core and in shoulders area results in secretion of proinflammatory cytokines, synthesis of tissue factor, and production of matrix metalloproteinases (MMPs) and other proteolytic enzymes, which in turn cause collagen and matrix degradation. In addition, loss of SMCs occurs in the fibrous cap as a result of SMC apoptosis induced by activated macrophages and reduced collagen synthesis. These changes can make the fibrous cap thinner and render it weak and rupture prone. With plaque progression, vasa vasorum invade the medial wall and the intima, where proangiogenic factors stimulate their further growth. Local hemorrhage, due to fragility of the neovascularization, promotes expansion of the necrotic core, stimulates inflammation, and contributes to weakening of the fibrous plaque.

Under hemodynamic forces, the weakened cap can fissure and rupture and, thus, allow contact of blood with thrombogenic plaque material with subsequent initialization of coagulation, recruitment of platelets, and the formation of a thrombus, which causes most acute coronary syndromes.

Dyslipidemia

A causal relationship between plasma lipoproteins (mainly LDL) and development of atherosclerosis and cardiovascular disease (CVD) has been confirmed and accepted for many years. Although the relationship of increased concentration of LDL and the catabolic remnants of triglyceride-rich lipoproteins (chylomicrons and very LDLs [VLDLs]) as well as inverse correlation of high-density lipoprotein (HDL) with atherosclerosis are widely accepted, there is still continuous uncertainty about the precise mechanism of the effects of different lipoproteins in the process of atherosclerosis.

In a very simple concept of atherosclerosis, LDL carries cholesterol into the intima and HDL removes it from there. However, the roles of lipids and lipoproteins in atherogenesis are more complex.

Low-Density Lipoprotein-Cholesterol

The atherosclerotic lesion begins with the entry of LDL-cholesterol (LDL-C) into the vascular intima. It has been shown both in animal and human studies that lipid deposition can precede macrophage infiltration in the arterial wall [7]. Maternal hypercholesterolemia in pregnancy is associated with increased fatty streak formation in human fetal arteries and accelerated progression of atherosclerosis in normocholesterolemic children [8]. The hypothesis of inflammation as a consequence of lipoprotein retention (that is the basis for the so-called response-to-retention model) is supported by findings, that NF-κB is activated in mice models only in the setting of hypercholesterolemia [9]. NF-κB is a transcription factor that plays a major role in the regulation of inflammatory gene expression.

However, to trigger inflammation, LDL must be modified, progressing from minimally modified LDL (mmLDL) to extensively oxidized LDL (oxLDL). So far, oxidative changes have been the most *in vivo* and *in vitro* studied modifications. Modified lipoproteins play a crucial role in the recruitment of monocytes (and T lymphocytes) and in their migration and differentiation in the intima. In ECs, modified LDL induces expression of adhesion molecules (such as VCAM-1, ICAM-1), chemokines (MCP-1, IL-8) and growth factors (M-CSF) [10]. Oxidized LDL is also itself a potent chemoattractant with direct effect on monocytes and T cells [10]. Monocyte expression of MCP-1 receptor CCR2 is stimulated and increased in hypercholesterolemia and increased chemotactic response to MCP-1 has been shown in hypercholesterolemic patients [6]. OxLDL has been shown to specifically induce differentiation of human monocytes to macrophages in vitro and it has been demonstrated in vivo that oxLDL triggers monocyte-to-macrophage differentiation through the activation of the macrophage colony stimulating factor receptor [11]. OxLDL also induce several chemokines, chemokine receptors and adhesion molecules in monocytes and macrophages. Uptake of modified lipoproteins by scavenger receptors can lead to MHC class II–restricted antigen presentation and activation of T-lymphocytes and thereby links innate and adaptive immunity [5]. In addition to the effect on ECs and monocytes and macrophages, oxLDL also promotes platelet interaction with monocytes and ECs that, in turn, induces monocyte adherence to the endothelium [10].

In mice models of atherosclerosis cholesterol feeding induces a rapid inflammatory response in the liver, including serum amyloid A (SAA), various cytokines (IL-1, vascular endothelial growth factor, granulocyte macrophage colony-stimulating factor), transcription factors (NF-κB), and proteases expression. The hepatic response precedes the development of atherosclerotic lesions in the vessel wall and the development of first atherosclerotic lesions in the aortic root [12]. Cholesterol feeding was also associated with significant increases in both CRP and SAA in lean insulin sensitive healthy human subjects [13]. In patients with familial hypercholesterolemia (FH) peripheral blood mononuclear cells have enhanced spontaneous release of different chemokines and this release correlated with plasma concentration of total and LDL-C [14]. FH heterozygotes are born with increased LDL levels due to mutations in LDL receptor gene and suffer of premature atherosclerosis. Heterozygous FH children are characterized by an enhanced systemic inflammation involving a selective up-regulation of the CC-chemokine RANTES (regulated on activation normally T-cell expressed and secreted) in circulating monocytes, as well as raised levels of neopterin, a marker of monocyte/macrophage activation [15].

High-Density Lipoprotein-Cholesterol

HDL is involved in pathophysiology of atherosclerosis by several complex mechanisms that are not yet clearly understood [16]. Antiatherogenic properties of HDL are mainly attributed to its role in reverse cholesterol transport, a pathway in which peripheral cellular cholesterol is transported to the liver (see corresponding chapter). Beyond lipid transport function, HDL has additional but not well-characterized antiatherogenic functions, including antioxidative, antithrombotic, and anti-inflammatory effects.

HDL inhibits oxidative modification of LDL through the activity of its associated enzymes and apolipoproteins, such as ApoA1, ApoE, paraoxonase 1 (PON1), platelet-activating factor acetylhydrolase (PAF-AH), and glutathione peroxidase. *In vitro* HDL antagonizes the proinflammatory effect of oxLDL by inhibiting the ROS/NF-κB signaling pathway, through preventing the ROS rise at the cellular level [17]. Inhibition of ROS by HDL has also been shown *in vivo* in a rabbit model of acute arterial inflammation [18].

In addition to its antioxidative activity, HDL possesses important anti-inflammatory properties. *In vitro*, HDL has been shown to inhibit cytokine-induced expression of VCAM-1, ICAM-1, and E-selectin and the binding of monocytes and neutrophils to cultured ECs. *In vivo*, in a normocholesterolemic rabbit model of acute arterial inflammation, induced by a periarterial collar. Infusion of reconstituted HDL (rHDL) and ApoA1 inhibited endothelial expression of VCAM-1, ICAM-1, and MCP-1 and polymorphonuclear leukocytes infiltration [18]. A similar effect was seen with intravenous infusion of rHDL in ApoE-knockout mice studies. In humans, subjects with low HDL levels showed elevated plasma levels of soluble ICAM-1 and soluble E-selectin, whose concentrations were inversely correlated with HDL concentration. In contrast, such correlation was not evident in subjects with normal or elevated HDL levels [19]. In a subsequent placebo-controlled double-blind crossover study, treating 20 subjects with low HDL with fenofibrate raised plasma HDL-C levels by 21%. This rise was inversely correlated with significant reductions of plasma soluble ICAM-1 and E-selectin. Finally, a significant increase in TNF-α, IL-1β, IL-6, IL-8, MCP-1, and hsCRP was observed after endotoxin challenge in healthy men with genetically determined isolated low HDL-C [20].

Several rare genetic causes of low HDL-C have been described, but not all of them are associated with an increased risk of coronary disease. The well-known variant ApoA1 Milano is associated with very low levels of HDL, without any increase in the risk of premature CHD. On the contrary, increased coronary risk has been reported in the presence of increased HDL levels. More recently, inhibition of one of the key enzymes of HDL metabolism cholesterol ester transfer protein (CETP) despite an impressive effect in increasing HDL and decreasing LDL, resulted in disappointing clinical results: increase in mortality/CVD incidence in the group of patients treated with torcetrapib plus atorvastatin as compared to atorvastatin alone. This suggests that rather than quantitative evaluation of HDL, HDL composition is important. HDL particles are highly heterogeneous and vary substantially in size, composition and functionality. In some circumstances abnormal HDL particles can be created with proinflammatory and proatherogenic properties [21]. Acute or chronic inflammation can neg-atively influence the original protective properties of HDL resulting in the so-called "dysfunctional HDL." Such proinflammatory form is an HDL that accumulated oxidants derived from an inflammatory reaction, which inhibit the HDL-associated antioxidant enzymes and render ApoA1 unable to promote ABCA-1–mediated cholesterol efflux [21]. During inflammation levels of HDL and related apolipoproteins are altered. Synthesis of ApoA1 in liver is decreased and ApoA1 in HDL is replaced by SAA. Like CRP, SAA is produced by the liver in response to systemic inflammation. Apart from its replacement by SAA, ApoA1 in the circulation and in atherosclerotic lesions is selectively nitrated or chlorinated by myeloperoxidase, which leads to reduced ability of ApoA1 to promote cholesterol efflux from macrophages via the ATP-binding cassette transporter A-I (ABCA-1) pathway [21]. Increased proinflammatory HDL, expressed as "HDL inflammatory index" was seen in patients with CHD or CHD equivalents and also in patients with CHD and elevated HDL levels [22]. It thus seems that HDL in the presence of systemic inflammation can become proinflammatory due to inactivation of HDL related antioxidant enzymes and modification of ApoA1. Qualitative measures of HDL and related apolipoproteins rather than quantitative estimate of HDL can be potentially useful in determining individual risk prediction and in pharmacological treatment targeting.

Biomarkers of Inflammation in the Disease Risk Prediction

In general, traditional risk factors (such as lipid levels, diabetes, hypertension, obesity, and smoking) are used for determination of cardiovascular risk. However, these factors do not identify a considerable number of patients at risk and this leads to attempts to improve cardiovascular risk prediction by introducing several biomarkers related to different pathways involved in the process of atherothrombosis. As atherosclerosis is considered an inflammatory disease, research and clinical interest has focused on whether markers of inflammation can add some predictive value over the traditional risk factors.

C-Reactive Protein

Among proposed new biomarkers, CRP is the most extensively studied marker of inflammation and emerges as the most powerful inflammatory predictor of future cardiovascular risk. CRP is an acute phase protein involved in the systemic response to inflammation. It is mainly synthesized in the liver under the regulation of IL-6, which is up-regulated by other cytokines such as IL-1 and TNF-α. However, it can also be produced locally by lymphocytes, alveolar macrophages, and by SMCs and monocytic cells in atherosclerotic lesions.

CRP has been suggested to be involved in several mechanisms of atherosclerosis. It reduces NO production, causes the expression of adhesion molecules ICAM-1 and VCAM-1 by ECs, induces MCP-1, binds oxidized LDL, enhances cholesterol uptake by macrophages, can stimulate monocytes to secrete tissue factor and proinflammatory cytokines through the up-regulation of NF-κ, and stimulates vascular smooth muscle migration, proliferation, neointimal formation, and ROS production [23]. However, most of these data are extrapolated from studies of cultured cells and it has been suggested that some of the biological effects observed with CRP *in vitro* can be caused by contamination of the commercial CRP preparation used by azide or bacterial lipopolysaccharides. CRP can activate complement factors and thus increases the inflammatory activity in the entire body and in the atheromatous plaques too. The complement activation in fact has been suggested to explain the relation between CRP and CVD [24]. In both familial hypercholesterolemic and normocholesterolemic human subjects, high purity recombinant human CRP infusion has been shown to increase plasma levels of MCP-1, IL-8, and soluble E-selectin [25]. In contrast to normocholesterolemic subjects, stimulation of thrombin generation and PAI-1 by the CRP in the study was more pronounced in FH patients and CRP infusion caused marked deterioration of endothelium-dependent vasodilation in FH patients only.

CRP levels are strongly associated with several cardiovascular risk factors, such as increased triglycerides, low HDL, hypertension, increased blood glucose, metabolic syndrome, age, smoking, and some other clinical and environmental risk factors. In particular, abdominal obesity and adiposity are strong correlates of CRP levels [26]. Genetic variation has been suggested to importantly influence CRP levels. Heritability estimates of CRP range from 27% to 40% and several single nucleotide polymorphisms (SNPs) are associated with CRP levels. Evidence of a common association between individual SNPs or common haplotypes, CRP levels, and risk of CVD, however, remains controversial, and even reports have suggested an inverse relation between genetic regulation, CRP levels, and the cardiovascular risk [27].

CRP has been shown to independently predict risk of future cardiovascular events, both in primary and in secondary risk. However, in light of more recent studies, the magnitude of this risk seems to be lower than suggested by older studies published before 2000. A meta-analysis of 22 prospective studies reported a multivariable adjusted odds ratio for coronary heart disease (CHD) of 1.58 (95% confidence interval [CI], 1.48–1.68) in a comparison of subjects in the top third of the baseline CRP values with those in the bottom third [28]. When only studies involving more than 500 subjects were considered, the combined odds ratio was 1.49 (95% CI, 1.37–1.62). The authors of the meta-analysis consider CRP as a relatively moderate predictor of CHD.

In clinical practice, high-sensitivity assays of CRP measurement have been standardized, are broadly available, and show sufficient precision. A recent American Heart Association/Centers for Disease Control and Prevention consensus report has recommended the CRP measurement in asymptomatic subjects at intermediate risk for future coronary events. Several different statistical approaches have been proposed to evaluate risk calculation; however, whether measurement of CRP adds additional predictive value beyond major risk factors is still widely discussed [29].

It is also important to distinguish whether CRP is a marker or a causal factor of atherosclerosis, as this can answer the question whether CRP is a potential target for therapy. It has been suggested in individual primary and secondary clinical trials that statins lower plasma levels of hs-CRP in a manner largely independent of LDL cholesterol lowering. In primary prevention benefit from statin therapy has been shown in individuals with elevated hs-CRP but not elevated LDL, and in a secondary prevention trial, post-MI patients with elevated hs-CRP had a greater relative clinical benefit from statin therapy than those with lower levels [30]. However, meta-analysis of randomized placebo-controlled studies on the effects of cholesterol-lowering interventions on LDL and CRP in healthy and clinically stable subjects revealed that in the range of LDL reduction typically seen with statin therapy 90% or more of the changes in CRP was related to LDL reduction and only 10% or less to non-LDL effects of statins [31]. Moreover, lack of direct evidence that treatment solely on the basis of CRP levels decreases cardiovascular events, still makes causality of CRP in CVD controversial.

The exact role of CRP still needs to be more investigated to be accepted as a standard cardiovascular risk factor or even considered as a therapeutic target.

Lipoprotein-Associated Phospholipase A₂ (Lp-PLA₂)

Lp-PLA2, also known as platelet-activating factor acetylhydrolase, is an enzyme involved in lipid metabolism and inflammatory pathways that belongs to the phospholipase A_2 superfamily. The enzyme is produced mainly by monocytes, macrophages, T lymphocytes and mast cells. It circulates in the blood bound to LDL (approximately 80%) and HDL and VLDL (remaining 20%). Levels of Lp-PLA2 have been reported to be elevated in hypercholesterolemia and there is a strong correlation between Lp-PLA2 and LDL levels. It is present in the media of normal and diseased arteries and increase of Lp-PLA2 mRNA expression has been shown in atherosclerotic lesions both in humans and rabbits [32]. Similarly, increased Lp-PLA2 mRNA was associated with accelerated atherogenesis in mice models. Circulating levels of Lp-PLA2 increase after inflammatory stimuli and during infection. However, the exact role of Lp-PLA2 is not clear. Both atherogenic and antiatherogenic functions have been suggested. Lp-PLA2 hydrolyzes oxidized phospholipids within modified LDL and thus generates proinflammatory and proatherogenic lysophosphatidylcholine and oxidized free fatty acids which lead to recruitment and activa-

tion of monocyte/macrophages and T cells, migration of VSMC and to increased expression of adhesion molecules and cytokines [32]. Inhibition of Lp-PLA2 in severely hypercholesterolemic rabbits resulted in downregulation of the atherosclerotic process. It has been suggested that Lp-PLA2 may be independently regulated in LDL and HDL and the enzyme in HDL may have an atheroprotective role by hydrolyzing oxidized phospholipids in HDL [33]. Moreover, it could also play an antithrombotic and anti-inflammatory role through hydrolysis of platelet-activating factor. In humans, epidemiologic studies favor a proatherogenic role for the Lp-PLA2; an adjusted odds ratio of 1.6 (95% CI, 1.36–1.89) has been reported in a recent meta-analysis of prospective and case-control studies and the unadjusted risk estimate appears to be relatively unaffected by conventional risk factors [32]. However, considering the relatively weak strength of association it remains questionable, whether its incorporation into current risk assessment algorithms can add additional predictive power over the traditional risk factors.

Serum Amyloid A

SAA is an acute-phase protein that had been shown to reflect systemic inflammation, and as with CRP, its levels can increase by several hundred-fold in response to an acute inflammation. In the circulation, SAA is transported primarily in association with HDL, but also with VLDL particles, particularly in inflammatory states [34]. In acute inflammation, SAA (mainly its isoforms SAA1 and 2) is produced principally by liver upon induction of IL-1β, IL-6, and TNF-α. It was, however, recently suggested that in humans, particularly in obese, SAA1 and SAA2 are predominantly expressed in adipocytes [35]. During the acute phase, SAA is able to replace ApoA1 from the surface of HDL (particularly in small dense HDL3) and alter HDL-mediated cholesterol delivery to cells, enhances HDL binding to proteoglycans, promotes HDL immobilization in the arterial wall, and accelerates HDL clearance from the circulation [16]. In addition to its role in formation of functionally deficient HDL, SAA can also act as a chemoattractant for inflammatory cells and stimulate expression and release of IL-1β, IL-8, and TNF-α in neutrophils, stimulate the production of inflammatory cytokines in coronary ECs and monocytes and by adipose tissue stromal-vascular cells [35]. SAA mRNA has been present in all of the major cell types in human atherosclerotic lesions [34].

Elevated levels of SAA are associated with obesity, insulin resistance, metabolic syndrome, and diabetes [34,35]. Interventions, such as weight loss and rosiglitazone, have been shown to decrease adipose SAA secretion and circulating levels. Several epidemiological studies confirmed that the risk for CVD related to SAA runs parallel to that with CRP [34]. However, whether SAA is simply a marker, or mediator or causal factor in atherogenesis has still to be explored.

Interleukin-6

IL-6 is an immune-modulating pleiotropic cytokine and a proximal mediator that propagates the inflammatory cascade. IL-6 is the major initiator of acute phase response in liver and a primary determinant of acute phase proteins production. It can be produced during infection, trauma and immunological challenge by several immune system cells, ECs, SMCs, adipocytes, hepatocytes, and islet β-cells [36]. Besides affecting the immune system, IL-6 also acts in other biological systems. Even if considered to be proinflammatory, IL-6 can also elicit anti-inflammatory effects, depending on the *in vivo* environmental circumstances and different transcriptional regulation by different cells. A key feature in the regulation of IL-6 responses is a soluble IL-6 receptor (sIL-6R), which forms a ligand-receptor complex with IL-6 that is capable of stimulating a variety of cellular responses including proliferation, differentiation and activation of inflammatory processes, regulation of leukocyte recruitment and the complex may serve a positive role in the prothrombotic/proinflammatory activation of ECs [37]. In the atherosclerotic lesion, IL-6 is secreted by macrophages and SMCs and IL-6 gene transcripts are expressed in the lesions [38].

IL-6 levels have been shown to be moderately associated with smoking, diabetes and dyslipidemia, and consistent with its central role in the inflammatory cascade with several inflammatory factors [39]. Given the role of IL-6 in chronic inflammation, the role of IL-6 in CVD prediction has been extensively evaluated in epidemiological studies. Recent meta-analysis of such studies revealed a combined odds ratio of 1.61 (95% CI 1.42–1.83) per 2 standard deviation (SD) increase in baseline IL-6 and 3.34 (95% CI 2.45–4.56) per 2-SD increase in long-term average IL-6 levels for MI or coronary death [39]. However, the latter authors suggest the need of further studies to answer whether this association with CHD is importantly modified by lipid concentrations. The role of the genetic modulation of IL-6 has been recently studied in the postoperative systemic inflammatory reaction following revascularization procedures in atherosclerotic patients [40]. As in the case of other inflammatory factors, a possible causal link between IL-6 and CHD remains uncertain.

Interleukin-1

IL-1 family consists of three structurally related cytokines; isoforms IL-1α, IL-1β, and an IL-1 receptor antagonist (IL-1 RA) [41]. IL-1 is produced by monocytes, macrophages, ECs, vascular SMCs, and hepatocytes. Although IL-1α and IL-1β are products of distinct genes, they share various biological activities, cell surface receptors and agonistic effects. IL-1 RA is a naturally occurring antagonist of IL-1 activity and enacts an important role in determination of IL-1β's inflammatory activity *in vivo*. IL-1 as a proinflammatory cytokine may contribute to the pathogenesis of arteriosclerosis by different pathways including the stimulation of vascular SMCs by TGF-β, the suppression of EC proliferation, the expression of adhesion molecules by ECs and the modification of endothelium to favor coagulation and thrombosis [42]. Moreover, IL-1β stimulates the synthesis of IL-6, fibrinogen, CRP and other inflammatory mediators involved in coronary syndromes. Detection of increased levels of IL-1β mRNA in human arteriosclerotic plaque suggests that the protein synthesized locally may activate or enhance the synthesis of growth factors and other cytokines, leading to local inflammatory cascades, and is involved in the proliferation or differentiation of monocyte-derived cells and increased vascular permeability.

The role of IL-1 in atherosclerosis and lipid metabolism has been examined by using several mice models. After atherogenic diet, higher total cholesterol, due to higher VLDL and LDL cholesterol and lower SAA levels were observed in the IL-1α knock-out mice compared to IL-1β knock-out mice and wild-type mice. Nevertheless, both IL-1α and IL-1β knock-out mice showed in the same study a lower atherosclerotic lesion area at the aortic sinus compared to wild-type mice [43]. Lack of IL-1β has been shown to decrease the severity of atherosclerosis in apoE deficient mice, and to down regulate VCAM-1 and MCP-1 at both the mRNA and protein level in the aorta [44]. In agreement with this data, deletion of IL-1 RA in ApoE-deficient mice increased the mRNA expression of VCAM-1, ICAM-1, and IL-1β, enhanced mRNA levels of MCP-1, and increased the size of atherosclerotic lesions in the aorta of mice on a normal chow diet [45]. Furthermore, total cholesterol levels of IL-1 RA$^{-/-}$/ApoE$^{-/-}$ mice were significantly elevated and HDL-C levels lower compared to IL-1 RA$^{+/+}$/ApoE$^{-/-}$ mice [45]. Another study demonstrated that upon atherogenic diet in IL-1 RA–deficient mice, the levels of total cholesterol and VLDL and LDL fractions were significantly increased and HDL was significantly lower when compared with wild type mice. On atherogenic diet, increased cholesterol levels in the VLDL and LDL fractions, earlier start of lipid accumulation in liver, failure to induce mRNA expression of cholesterol 7α-hydroxylase and decreased bile acid excretion was shown in IL-1 RA–deficient mice compared to wild-type mice [46]. This data suggests that IL-1 and IL-1 RA play an important role not only in the regulation of vascular cell functions, but also in cholesterol homeostasis.

We have shown that genetic variations within the IL-1 gene cluster have been associated with inflammatory responses and levels of IL-1β *in vivo* and *in vitro* after inflammatory stimulation [47,48]. Moreover, the cluster is suggested to affect also the risk of MI and ischemic stroke at young age [47]. However, studies evaluating the association between polymorphisms in the IL-1 gene cluster and coronary artery disease have reported contrasting results [42].

Conclusion

Atherosclerosis is still the leading health-related problem worldwide. Both lipid accumulation and inflammation have been recognized as key players in atherogenesis. Therefore, atherosclerosis can be considered to be a lipid-driven inflammatory disease. However, the chicken-versus-egg problem of whether inflammation or dyslipidemia alone can initiate atherosclerosis or who comes first remains unclear. Current knowledge confirms an active interplay between inflammation and lipids and inflammation leads to changes in lipid metabolism aimed at responding to injury in the vessel wall and decreasing the toxic effect of harmful agents. However, the protective mechanism of inflammation with time and continuing damage may become overwhelming, so lipid changes will manifest chronic and such excess may represent the disease itself.

Our understanding of the relationship between inflammation and lipid metabolism has advanced greatly, however a coordinated effort is needed to use this knowledge to develop new preventive and treatment tools.

Acknowledgment

This study was partially supported by Italian Ministry of University and Research (MIUR, Decreto n. 1588 Rome, Italy) *Programma Triennale di Ricerca.*

Selected References

2. Hansson G. Inflammation, atherosclerosis, and coronary artery disease. N Engl J Med 2005;352:1685–95.

9. Tabas I, Williams KJ, Borén J. Subendothelial lipoprotein retention as the initiating process in atherosclerosis: update and therapeutic implications. Circulation 2007; 116:1832–44.

30. Ridker PM. C-reactive protein and the prediction of cardiovascular events among those at intermediate risk: moving an inflammatory hypothesis toward consensus. J Am Coll Cardiol 2007;49(21):2129–38.

39. Danesh J, Kaptoge S, Mann AG, et al. Long-term interleukin-6 levels and subsequent risk of coronary heart disease: two new prospective studies and a systematic review. PLoS Med 2008;5(4): e78.

47. Iacoviello L, Di Castelnuovo A, Gattone M, et al. Polymorphisms of the interleukin-1beta gene affect the risk of myocardial infarction and ischemic stroke at young age and the response of mononuclear cells to stimulation in vitro. Arterioscler Thromb Vasc Biol 2005;25(1): 222–7.

CHAPTER 27

Dyslipidemia in Children: Diagnosis and Management

Leiv Ose

Oslo University Hospital, Rikshospitalet, Oslo, Norway

Introduction

Familial hypercholesterolemia (FH) is the most frequent diagnose of dyslipidemia in children with marked elevation of low-density lipoprotein (LDL)-cholesterol (LDL-C). Other dyslipidemias such as combined dyslipidemia and polygenic hyperlipidemia are not well studied in the pediatric population. Studies in FH in this age-group are well suited for investigations of the various aspects of dyslipidemia such as diagnosis, genetic testing, and dietary and pharmaceutical treatment. Currently, we have the diagnostic tools for FH in children. We have safe dietary recommendations and pharmaceutical treatments. Statins and resins are available for treatment of these high-risk children with FH.

Clinical Diagnosis

The clinical diagnosis of FH in children is based on family history and laboratory findings. Because of its autosomal dominant inheritance mode, each child with heterozygous FH consequently has one affected parent and often a positive family history for premature cardiovascular disease (CVD). With a prevalence of 0.2%–1.0%, FH is a common autosomal dominant disorder of lipoprotein metabolism. The hallmark of the disease is a severely elevated total cholesterol (TC) and LDL-C level, which predisposes to premature CVD [1]. The molecular basis of FH is a vast array of more than 1,000 mutations

in the LDL receptor (LDLR) gene. Each country seems to have its own specific mutations, but many mutations are shared by different countries, an observation that can be explained in some cases by historical or demographic conditions. The LDLR locus is located on the distal part of the short arm of chromosome 19, on band p13.1 to p13.3. The locus stretches over 45,000 base pairs or 45 kilobases and comprises 18 exons and 17 intervening introns [2].

Clinical symptoms of the disease found frequently in adult patients with FH such as arcus lipoidus, xanthelasmas, and xanthomas are rarely seen in heterozygous children with FH. Less than 10% of heterozygous FH children have tendon xanthomas and these are primarily found in the second decade of life [3]. Some children may complain of tenderness and pain in the Achilles tendons. However, the disease is mostly asymptomatic in children. Children with homozygous FH have frequent xanthomas on the Achilles tendons and xanthelasmas when diagnosed before puberty.

In children, plasma levels of TC and LDL-C above the 95th percentile for age and gender with high-density lipoprotein (HDL)-cholesterol (HDL-C) characterize the disease. Triglycerides are in the normal range, although HDL-C plasma levels are usually slightly decreased in children and in adult FH patients [4]. Thus, the diagnosis of FH in children is usually based on elevated levels of LDL-C. In 1992, an expert panel of the National Cholesterol Education Program (NCEP) recommended screening guidelines to identify these children and recommended a lipid profile to be obtained in the

Nutritional and Metabolic Bases of Cardiovascular Disease, 1st edition.
Edited by Mario Mancini, José M. Ordovas, Gabriele Riccardi,
Paolo Rubba and Pasquale Strazzullo. © 2011 Blackwell Publishing Ltd.

following children: 1) those whose parents and grandparents who have undergone coronary arteriography at younger than 55 years and found to have coronary atherosclerosis, 2) whose parents or grandparents had a previously documented myocardial infarction, angina pectoris, peripheral vascular disease, cerebral vascular disease, or sudden cardiac death at an age younger than 55 years, 3) those who have a parent who has been found to have high blood cholesterol (TC $\geq$ 6.2 mmol/L), and 4) those whose parental or grandparental history is unobtainable and the children have two or more other cardiovascular risk factors [5]. The recommendations of the European Atherosclerosis Society (EAS) concerning whom to screen included children of a parent who has familial hyperlipidemia or a cholesterol $\geq$7.8 mmol/L.

The best available LDL-C value for diagnosis of FH in children is $\geq$3.50 mmol/L [6]. Levels below this concentration were found in only 4.3% of those with a mutation the LDLR gene. In contrast, children with LDL-C $\geq$3.50 mmol/L had 0.98 posttest probability of FH. It is important to realize that these results were valid only against the background of a family investigation with a definitive diagnosis of FH established. These data do not apply to the general population or to other children with dyslipidemia. When LDLR gene identification has not been performed in the family or is not available, the cutoff value for the LDL-C should be increased. In 742 FH children with a mean age of 11.0 years (2.0–18.7), LDL-C was 5.62 ± 0.06 mmol/L in comparison to their unaffected siblings 2.55 ± 0.05 mmol/L.

The lipoprotein levels have been analyzed according to family history of premature CVD in relatives in 408 index FH children with the FH mutation. The LDL-C in children with first-degree relatives with premature CVD was 5.90 ± 0.13 mmol/L, second-degree relative with premature CVD was 5.67 ± 0.09 mmol/L, and 5.09 ± 0.18 mmol/L with no such relatives. The p for trend was .001. The LDL-C and HDL-C of an index child have indicated length of event-free survival among their FH parents. The event-free survival was significantly better in the parents of children who had LDL-C levels below 6.23 mmol/L, and if the FH child have HDL-C $\geq$ 1.00 mmol/L, the event-free survival was significantly better in their parents [6].

The family history, sex, and TC of the FH child have been proposed to be included in the classification of a risk category for children and adolescents with FH [7]. As this classification was not based on epidemiologic studies at that time, these guidelines should be revised based on LDL-C, HDL-C, sex, flow-mediated dilatation (FMD), IMT, family history of CVD, and other risk factors [8–10]. Although the documentation of an LDL receptor gene mutation is important for the diagnosis of FH, significant variation of LDL-C and null alleles were associated with more severe elevated LDL-C, whereas the frequent Dutch N53H/2393del9 mutation (19.0% of the Dutch FH mutations) had less elevated LDL-C [11]. The risk of CVD was demonstrated to be lower. When excluding this specific founder mutation, no difference was found between the mutations, LDL-C, and CVD risk. Other not-lipid risk factors may be important for the development of early CVD in FH patients. An association of specific LDLR gene mutations with differential plasma lipoprotein response has been observed in children [12]. The patients were grouped according to known LDLR genotype and treated with 20 mg/day of simvastatin. The mean reduction in plasma LDL-C in patients with the W66G mutation was 31%, whereas the deletion >15 kb and C646Y mutation groups was 38% and 42%, respectively. Multiple regression analysis suggested that 42% of the variation of the LDL-C response to simvastatin can be attributed to variation in the LDLR locus, ApoE genotype, and body mass index, while the observed increase in HDL-C was explained by sex and baseline HDL-C. Molecular assays can assist in establishing the diagnosis. In a Dutch population, the molecular basis was established in more than 80% of FH cases investigated. In the other remaining 20% of patients with a definitive clinical diagnosis of FH, no detectable mutations were found after complete analysis of the LDLR gene and the ApoB gene, which indicated that other genes may be involved in inherited hypercholesterolemia. A study of Southeast Asian patients demonstrated that a portion of the patients had a slightly milder FH phenotype. This is in keeping with recent evidence that besides the LDLR gene (FH1) and the ApoB gene (FH2), a third gene located on the short arm of chromosome 1 can produce a somewhat milder but definitive FH-like phenotype. By evidence of this so-called FH3 gene, the heterogeneity of FH is further enlarged [13].

In contrast to most genetic diseases, efficient therapy is now available for FH in the form of (lifestyle changes) and lipid-lowering drugs for children, adolescents, and adults. A study from 14 Western countries revealed that only 20% of FH heterozygotes had been diagnosed and only 7% were being adequately treated. These observations reflect the situation in the adult FH population. In the younger FH population (children and adolescents), no data is available. The most cost-effective strategy to diagnose both adult and adolescent FH patients is to screen first-degree relatives already diagnosed as having FH. In Norway, we evaluated the cascade genetic screening of 1,805 relatives, of which 390 were 17 years or younger [14]. A total of 2,272 first-degree relatives of 440 index patients had initially consented to genetic testing. Some concern has been raised that cascade genetic screening for FH might cause adverse psychological effects. However, no clinically relevant adverse psychological affects have been observed. Tension may also develop between an individual's right of confidentiality and the rights of family members to be informed of potential harms. However, in the study of Bhatnager et al., 99% of the index patients gave consent that first-degree relatives could be contacted for cascade genetic screening [15]. A population-based survey in Norway has shown that 77% of the responders would enter a cascade screening program for FH if they had a family member with FH [16]. Moreover, the findings that 72%–90% of first-degree relatives who are being offered cascade genetic screening actually undergo genetic screening support the notion that genetic screening is well accepted [17].

Screening for genetic diseases in children has been debated and is subject to specific regulations in different countries. However, there is no data to suggest that children diagnosed with FH differ in psychological function compared to children without FH. The legislation on genetic screening in Norway allows screening for children younger than 16 years if the test result might have therapeutic consequences. A positive attitude of parents with FH to have their children screened for FH has been demonstrated by Umans-Eckenhausen et al. [18]. In their study, 87% of the parents wanted their children 16 years or younger to undergo genetic screen-

ing for FH. When FH is diagnosed by measurements of serum lipids, the American Academy of Pediatrics recommends screening children 2 years and older. When FH is diagnosed by the use of molecular gene tic testing, diagnosis can be performed at an age younger than 2 years, even the cord blood.

The diagnosis of FH in unselected children is difficult because of the overlap of cholesterol values in affected and nonaffected and paucity of physical signs. Campagna et al. carried out a combination of family study and molecular analyses of the LDLR gene [19]. They estimated that LDL-C >3.9 mmol/L was the best cutoff for diagnosing FH in these children, showing 79% sensitivity and 71.0% specificity. They proposed the use of LDL-C cutoff level associated with a family study to identify FH among hypercholesterolemic children. Widhalm et al. [20] demonstrated that the diagnosis of FH can be improved by using genetic testing. When the MEDPED limits were adopted with LDL-C < 3.5 mmol/L, they showed that at least 21% of the FH children were missed by conventional laboratory methods.

Wald et al. [21] performed a meta-analysis of published data on TC and LDL-C in people with and without FH according to age. They reported 13 studies on 1,907 cases and 16,221 controls. They concluded that screening by measurements of serum cholesterol is most effective done in early childhood after the first year of life; between ages 1 and 9 years, an estimated 88% of affected children would be identified with a positive rate of 0.1%. Screening newborns was much less effective. Once an affected child is identified, measurements of cholesterol would detect about 96% of parents with FH using the simple rule that the parent with higher serum cholesterol is the affected parent. This proposed child–parent screening population strategy needs to be tested but has the potential to prevent the medical consequences of this disorder in two generations simultaneously [21].

As the FH gene mutation is only found in 85% of the FH families, it will always be important to use the combination of LDL-C and family history to make the FH diagnosis in a child. Cholesterol levels decrease at puberty, but the difference between the pubertal stages was greater than expected [17,22]. Although secondary hyperlipidemia is rare in childhood, in healthy children we recommend testing TSH, blood sugar, creatine, and liver enzymes as part of the initial diagnostic workup of every child and adolescent screened for FH.

Therapeutic Aspects

In children, the disease is mostly asymptomatic. However, even in the general population, autopsy reports of healthy children and adolescents show atherosclerotic lesions at young age. Morphological and functional changes of the arteries have been shown to be predictive of future CVD and have been documented in young children with FH. The data emphasize the importance of considering aggressive and early treatment of dyslipidemia to prevent premature atherosclerotic events. Endothelial function can be assessed by testing the FMD in the brachial artery. deJongh et al. evaluated weather FH children with a positive family history of premature CVD have more pronounced endothelial dysfunction compared to children with a negative family history 50 children 10–18 years of age [23]. In FH, FMD was significantly impaired to compared to matched controls. In addition, FMD was significantly more impaired in FH children with a positive family history of premature CVD.

Wiegman et al. [24] demonstrated that 2-year treatment with pravastatin in a placebo-controlled trial reduced atherosclerosis progression, as measured by IMT. Since longer term studies in children are lacking, it is unknown at which age statin treatment should be initiated in terms of safety and CHD risk reduction. The group (Academic Medical Center in Amsterdam), therefore, continued to follow the 214 subjects of the previous study [25]. Pravastatin was given in a dose of 20 or 40 mg dependant on their age (<14 years 20 mg; >14 years 40 mg). The subjects on placebo in the original study were treated with statins for at least 2 years and subjects on statin treatment for at least 4 years. Follow-up data of the 187 children revealed that age of statin initiation was an independent predictor for carotid IMT after follow-up, when adjusted for carotid IMT at initiation of statin treatment, gender, and duration of treatment. Early initiation of statin treatment was associated with subsequent smaller IMT. Furthermore, no serious laboratory adverse events were reported during follow-up, and statin treatment had no untoward effects on sexual maturation. Even in the apparently healthy non-FH population, the initial stages of atherogenesis are already clearly present at young age [26,27]. The Muscatine study measured carotid IMT in healthy young and middle-aged individuals over a period of 25 years to determine the relationship between IMT and risk factors for CVD. This study demonstrated that the main predictors of an increase of IMT were age and LDL-C in adulthood and interestingly TC levels during childhood [28]. Consequently, as in FH children both LDL-C and TC levels are severely elevated, they are also characterized by an increased IMT in these children [9,29]. FH children were found to have an IMT of 0.50 mm versus 0.47 mm in healthy controls [30]. Mabuchi et al. [31] have demonstrated that in heterozygous FH patients older than 18 years, significant stenosis was already visible on their coronary arteries, as seen on coronary angiograms.

The sequence of events in the atherogenesis of FH children, therefore, seems to proceed from endothelial dysfunction to increased arterial stiffness and subsequently to increased arterial wall thickness and finally to coronary stenosis in the time span of 2 decades. Thus, this process develops three times more rapidly than in healthy individuals, which exposes FH patients to very early and life-threatening coronary disease. Conversely, it provides us with a plethora of intermediate end-points for the prevention of clinical sequelae.

Although dietary treatments always are implemented in the treatment of FH, very few randomized controlled trials have been performed. A recent Cochrane Review stated that no conclusion can be made about the effectiveness of the cholesterol-lowering diet or any other dietary intervention suggested for FH, because of lack of adequate data [32]. A cholesterol-lowering diet based on the following principles is recommended: 1) a reduction of total fat intake, 2) a reduction in the intake of saturated fatty acids, 3) a reduction in dietary cholesterol intake, and 4) manipulation of carbohydrate intake to replace the energy deficit of the low-fat diet. The currently prescribed diet should not be considered to be monotonous and will seldom lead to problems with compliance.

In view of this, a number of other dietary therapies have been considered for treatment of FH including 1) the manipulation of different types of fatty acids while maintaining normal total fat intake, 2) increasing dietary intake of soluble fiber, 3) increasing the dietary intake of antioxidants, and 4) increasing the intake of certain dietary components, such as garlic, onions, soy protein, plant sterols, and stanols. Only five studies met the strict criteria for inclusion in the Cochrane Review. They were randomized controlled crossover trials [33]. All were short-term studies with each arm of the trial lasting between 1 and 3 months. However, information on long-term compliance is lacking [34]. We will, therefore, always recommend a low-fat diet as a first step in treatment of FH children irrespective of age. Gylling et al. demonstrated an 11% reduction of TC and 15% reduction of LDL-C in a small crossover study including 14 FH children [35]. We have recently studied the effect of 18.2 ± 1.5 g/day spread/day corresponding to 1.60 ± 0.13 g plant sterol esters in 41 FH children aged 7–12 years [36]. Plasma LDL-C decreased by 10.2% during the plant sterol period. TC and ApoB were reduced by 7.4% during the plant sterol period. No changes were observed in HDL-C, triglycerides, or ApoA1. In 26 weeks, an open-label follow-up study of children who had previously been studied in the controlled crossover design [37], their parents were also included in the open-label arm of the study. Thirty-seven children (7–13 years) and 20 parents diagnosed with "definite" or "possible" heterozygous FH. Nineteen of the parents used statins. The subjects were recommended to eat 20 g/day of plant sterol spread (1.76 g plant sterols) as part of their lipid-lowering diet. Plasma TC decreased significantly by 8.5% and 8.1% in the children and parents, respectively. The corresponding decreases in LDL-C were 10.5% and 8.4%.

Long-term compliance of plant sterol consumption and sustained efficacy of cholesterol reduction was demonstrated in this study. In a short-term study, 2.3 g/day plant sterol decreased TC with 11% and LDL-C with 14%. Endothelial function was assessed as FMD of the brachial artery. However, although a clear reduction of the LDL-C by plant sterol therapy, this did not improve the impaired endothelial function in FH children. The difference in potency between statins and sterols is the most likely to explain the difference in vascular effects in FH children [38].

Untreated FH carry a substantial burden of morbidity and mortality if left untreated or inadequately treated. The NCEP guidelines from 1992 suggested that drug treatment be considered from the age of 10 years and older if LDL-C levels are ≥ 4.9 mmol/L or ≥ 4.1 mmol/L in the presence of other cardiovascular risk factors, including a positive family history of premature CVD [39]. Applying these guidelines to FH means that most children with FH would be eligible for treatment. While bile acid sequestrants (resins) have long been considered the drug of choice in children, they have actually never been approved for the pediatric use by the Food and Drug Administration (FDA), are poorly tolerated, marginally effective at lowering LDL-C, and have few well-controlled studies in children upon which to adequately asses safety. We attempted to determine the efficacy and safety of cholestyramine therapy in children with FH [40]. Ninety-eight FH children 6–11 years were included. During dietary therapy alone, LDL-C levels were reduced by 5.5%. With the addition of cholestyramine, in an ingested dose of about 6 gm daily, LDL-C levels were reduced by 17%–19% and ApoB levels about 13%. The long-term compliance was not satisfactory. A study with colestipol tables was also disappointing [41]. Recently, a prospective study (DISC) found a similar growth rate in children with elevated LDL-C levels randomly assigned to a low-fat diet compared with control subjects [42].

However, the compliance is too low to recommend the use of resin as a drug for treatment of FH children. A new resin, colesevelam, now available in the United States and Europe has not yet been approved for the use in children and adolescents [43]. However, the size of the tablets is smaller and the compliance in adults is better as observed for the "old" resins. In adults 3.8 g/day will reduce LDL-C with 16% [44].

Over the last decade, statins have been studied extensively in children and adolescents. Although many of these studies have been poorly controlled, of short duration, too small and lacking detailed assessment, several well-controlled studies with pravastatin, simvastatin, and atorvastatin have recently been published [45–47]. It is opportune to evaluate the current treatment guidelines in FH children and adolescents. Stein et al. [48] were the first to show a 40% reduction of LDL-C in FH children treated with lovastatin, but this study was not controlled and only involved a small group of boys [49]. Later, three other statin studies in children and adolescents were reported. In the first study, 72 FH children (66% girls), age 10–16 years, were randomized to placebo or pravastatin 5, 10, or 20 mg [50]. After 12 weeks, LDL-C was reduced by 23%, 24%, and 33% in the groups receiving pravastatin 5, 10, and 20 mg, respectively. Short-term safety and tolerability were excellent. The second study reported an uncontrolled study in which boys were randomized to lovastatin 10, 20, 30, and 40 mg/day for 12 weeks [51]. LDL-C was reduced by 21%–36% and lovastatin was again well tolerated with no serious adverse events. In the last study, 132 boys, between 10 and 17 years of age, were randomized to either lovastatin or placebo. Lovastatin was started at 10 mg/day and the dosage was doubled every 8 weeks to a maximum of 40 mg/day. Mean LDL-C levels decreased significantly relative to placebo in all active groups [52].

In an international multicenter, double-blind, randomized, parallel designed study of 175 FH children, 99 boys and 76 girls were randomized, 69 were randomized to placebo, and 106 to simvastatin [46]. The mean age for the boys was 13.2 ± 2.3 years and the girls 14.5 ±1.6 years. TC level was 6.78 ± 1.03 mmol/L in the boys and 7.44 ± 1.35 mmol/L in the girls. Simvastatin was gradually increased over a period of 24 weeks to 10, 20, and 40 mg/day reducing the LDL-C to 31.4%, 34.7%, and 38.4%, respectively. The study was continued 48 weeks and LDL-C was reduced 40.7%, ApoB levels down 34.2% ± 14.0%, and ApoA1 up 10.4% ± 13.9%. There were no serious adverse events and the only discontinuation was a child on simvastatin who developed infectious mononucleosis. No serious laboratory adverse events and none of the children discontinued the study due to laboratory adverse events. No significant differences were observed between the simvastatin or placebo groups with regard to height, BMI, and cortisol (boys and girls), testicle size and testosterone levels (boys), and menstrual cycle and estradiol levels (girls). An analysis of the Tanner stage from baseline showed that there was a similar progression of the Tanner stages for both boys and girls on simvastatin and placebo.

To examine the safety and efficacy of atorvastatin 10–20 mg in children and adolescents subjects with FH and/or severe hypercholesterolemia ($n = 187$) were randomized to 26 weeks of treatment with atorvastatin 10 mg or placebo [46]. Atorvastatin was titrated to 20 mg in subjects with LDL-C levels >3.4 mmol/L at week 4. At week 26, subjects received 10 mg atorvastatin for an additional 26 weeks. Percent changes at week 26 also significantly favored atorvastatin for TC (−32% vs. −2%; $p < .001$), TG (−12% vs. +1%; $p = .03$), and ApoB (−32% vs. +2%; $p < .001$). Atorvastatin was as well tolerated as placebo, and administration of atorvastatin for 12 months was effective and safe for the treatment of pediatric subjects with known FH or severe hypercholesterolemia.

Avis et al. [53] performed a review and meta-analysis of randomized, double-blind, placebo-controlled trials evaluating statin therapy in children aged 8–18 years with heterozygous FH. Of the 537 publications on the topic, only 10 were randomized placebo-controlled trials that evaluated statin treatment in patients with heterozygous FH less than 18 years of age. Analyses of the pooled data of these studies showed an LDL-C reduction of 30%.

Four of the included studies reported on adverse events. Analysis of the pooled data revealed no increased risk of adverse events when receiving statin therapy. With respect to growth, four studies reported data on height of the participants. The analysis of the pooled data revealed a minimally but statistically significant change in height favoring the treatment group. None of the three studies that evaluated sexual development reported a difference between statin and placebo-treated children. All studies reported data on ASAT, ALAT, and CK. However, due to the sample size studies, definitive conclusions with respect of liver and muscle-related adverse events cannot be drawn. Thus, even though statins seem safe, long-term muscle and liver safety in children and adolescents should still be monitored. No consistent changes were found for hormone levels in these studies. In 2007, the American Heart Association (AHA) presented its scientific statement whose purposes were 1) to examine the atherosclerosis process in children and its relationship to lipid abnormalities, 2) to review and discuss existing screening and management guidelines and their limitations, 3) to highlight therapy in children and current knowledge specific to drug, and 4) to provide general recommendations for pharmacological management of high-risk lipid abnormalities in children and adolescents [54]. No change is made in the NCEP criteria for drug therapy, only in children older than 10 years after 6–12 months of diet intervention. In general, treatment do not start before 10 years of age in boys and preferable after onset of menses in girls. Patients should ideally be at Tanner stage II or higher. The therapy may be influenced by the presence and number of other cardiovascular risk factors. Important is to include the preferences of patients and family in the decision making. Based on this statement, at our Lipid Clinic we currently follow the recommended patient's selection for drug treatment. In addition, the choice of the particular statin is a matter of preference; we prefer to start with the statin, which is prescribed to the parent. We start with a dose given in the placebo-controlled such as pravastatin 20 or 40 mg day, simvastatin 40 mg, or atorvastatin 10 or 20 mg day. We measure the fasting lipid profile after 4–6 weeks with ALT, AST, and CK. The target levels for LDL is by the AHA statement set to a minimum for LDL-C < 3.35 mmol/L, with the ideal being <2.85 mmol/L. The target levels are not based on evidence from placebo-controlled studies and must be individualized based on the cardiovascular risk factors present as risk scores predicting atherosclerotic lesion in young FH patients have not been developed, as has been for young people with no genetic disorder [55]. On the other hand, the risk score developed based on the Pathological Determinants of Atherosclerosis in Youth (PDAY) research group may represent the findings in adolescents with no genetic lipid disorder and may serve as a minimal estimation of the process [56].

We prefer to see the young patient back for a clinic visit after 6 months; the first adjustment of the medication is made at this visit. An increase of the statin dose is made in some patients, but adding colesevelam can be an alternative when the target level is not reached. We then monitor growth, including height, and weight (BMI) related to normal growth charts, and sexual maturation. We monitor and encourage compliance with lipid-lowering dietary and the drug therapy every 12 months thereafter. Serial assessment and council are given for other risk factors, such as weight gain, smoking,

and physical inactivity. In the beginning, the children are seen with their parents, but from the age of 13–14 years, the consultations are individualized as accepted and preferred by the patient and parent. A consultation with a clinical nutritionist is mandatory in our clinic for the children and adolescents and throughout the teenage period. If FH diagnosis has been established, we prefer to have the first clinical consultation at the age of 6–8 years. The genetic DNA and laboratory diagnosis with a lipid profile may be performed earlier based on the request of the parents.

It has been suggested that identification of children who are at risk for CVD is unnecessary and might be harmful [57,58]. One important issue in diagnosing and treating FH children, therefore, is to be aware of the data available on the psychosocial function of children treated for FH. Awareness of sharing an inherited trait with a family member who has died or who has serious disease may predispose the child to anxiety or mood disorders and have a detrimental impact on the child's self-image. The diet could contribute to social isolation and eating disorders or would exacerbate family conflicts. The availability of frequent medical checkups and access to medical care could lead to somatization and unnecessary intervention. Tonstad et al. studied 86 boys and 66 girls, 7–16 years of age attending a lipid clinic [58]. They were all screened and instructed to follow a diet low in saturated fat and cholesterol 1–9 years earlier (mean: 4 years). One-fourth had lost a parent or had a parent who had CVD due to FH. Psychosocial scores were similar in children with FH and the population sample. Tests showed that children with FH did not have increased symptoms in any area of function, and scores for family, mood, and expression of anger were lower (less symptomatic). The prevalence of a psychiatric diagnosis was 10%, which was not greater than expected. However, within the group with FH, those who had a parent who died or had disease had somewhat poorer psychological function, beyond the acute bereavement or event. A recent study assessed the influence of statin therapy on quality of life, anxiety, and concerns of children with FH and their parents. A total of 69 FH children on statin therapy and 87 parents participated in this study [59]. FH children and their parents report no problems with regard to quality of life and anxiety.

However, a specific FH survey with question on 1) knowledge of FH, 2) experience of the disease, 3) family communication, 4) screening, 5) diet, and 6) experience of medication therapy did show that one-third of the children thinks FH can be cured, 43.4% of the children suffer from the fact they have FH, but taking medication (statin) makes them feel safer (62.3%). Almost 38% of the parents experience FH as a burden to their family and 79.3% suffer because they have a child with FH. To improve the knowledge of FH and family communication, the families would benefit from additional information focusing on the various aspects of living with FH. Improvement and help to the FH families will improve family communication and might lead to better compliance of both the diet and medication in the future. A prospective registry study from the Simon Broome Register in statin-treated patients with FH demonstrated a 48% reduction of CHD mortality, with a smaller reduction of nearly 25% in patients with established disease. The results in the follow-up of 3,382 patients followed between 1980 and 2006 emphasized the importance of early identification of FH and treatment of statins [60].

Selected References

53. Avis HJ, Vissers MN, Stein EA, et al. Systematic review and meta-analysis of statin therapy in children with familial hypercholesterolemia. Arteriocler Trombo Vasc Biol 2007;27:1803.

54. McCrindle BW, Urbina EM, Dennison BA, et al. Drug therapy of high-risk lipid abnormalities in children and adolescents. A scientific statement of the American Heart Association atherosclerosis, hypertension, and obesity in youth committee, council of cardiovascular disease in the young, with the Council on Cardiovascular Nursing. Circulation 2007;115:1948–67.

55. McGill HC, McMahan CA, Gidding SS. Preventing heart disease in the 21st century. Implications of the pathological determinants of the atherosclerosis in youth (PDAY) study Circulation 2008;117:1216–27.

59. De Jongh S, Kerckhoffs MC, Grootenhuis MA, et al. The influence of statin therapy on quality of life, anxiety and concerns in children with familial hypercholesterolemia and their parents. Acta Paediatr 2003;92:1096–1101.

60. Neil A, Cooper J, Betteridge J, et al. Reductions in all-course, cancer, and coronary mortality in statin-treated patients with heterozygous familial hypercholesterolemia: A prospective registry study. Eur Heart J 2008; 29:2624–33.

CHAPTER 28

Early Atherosclerotic Lesions in Childhood and Adolescence

Paolo Rubba[1], Gabriella Iannuzzo[1], Fabrizio Jossa[1], Gennaro Marotta[1], & Arcangelo Iannuzzi[2]

[1] Federico II University, Naples, Italy
[2] A. Cardarelli Hospital, Naples, Italy

Atherogenesis in Children

When atherosclerosis develops in adults, advanced lesions form first in well-known arterial regions with adaptive intimal thickening, which is present at constant locations and represents arterial wall adaptation to local mechanical forces [1]. Differently from many animals, whose intima is represented by a single layer of endothelial cells separated from underlying media by a thin basement membrane and rare smooth muscle cells (SMCs), in humans a thickened intimal layer can be observed in almost 30% of newborns.

This intimal layer is exposed to blood-borne components and hemodynamically active forces that could influence the development of atherosclerosis. The earliest atherosclerotic events involve both cellular elements and extracellular matrix (ECM) proteins. Consequently, diffuse intimal thickenings are characterized by SMCs, ECM, and small groups of a few macrophages in the superficial layer. Macrophages are present both without and with intracellular accumulated lipid (referred to as *foam cells*). SMCs are present in the intima and especially in areas of intimal thickening, even though the majority of SMCs are contained in the medial layer.

Eccentric intimal thickenings tend to be focal and are found in specific locations, especially areas of turbulent blood flow and branch points. In humans, areas of advanced atherosclerotic lesions and of intimal thickening share the same topographic distribution: coronary arteries, renal arteries, carotid arteries, and the aorta [2–4]. Areas of arteries in which intimal thickening and, subsequently, advanced atherosclerotic lesions most frequently develop are referred to as atherosclerotic-prone regions. It should be remembered that in 45% of infants, in their first 8 months of life, it is possible to find macrophage foam cells in the coronary arteries [5].

Frequently, we use the term "early atherosclerotic lesions" (i.e., lesions that appear early in life and that could proceed to advanced atherosclerotic lesions) to indicate intimal thickening and fatty streaks. These types of lesions are generally the only lesions present in children. In these lesions, often there is an abnormal accumulation of lipoproteins and cholesteryl esters. At these stages, usually there is no disruption of the intimal architecture, no alterations in media and adventitia [1]. Fatty streaks macroscopically present as yellow streaks, patches, or spots on the intimal surface of arteries and are constituted mostly of foam cells, whereas extracellular lipids are present in small quantities in the extracellular space and are visible only by electronic microscopy as lipid droplets or vesicular particles. These extracellular lipids derive mostly from disrupted foam cells.

The development of these early abnormalities into advanced atherosclerotic lesions mostly

Nutritional and Metabolic Bases of Cardiovascular Disease, 1st edition.
Edited by Mario Mancini, José M. Ordovas, Gabriele Riccardi,
Paolo Rubba and Pasquale Strazzullo. © 2011 Blackwell Publishing Ltd.

depends on mechanical forces that permit an increased influx, stay, and early accumulation of lipids in hypercholesterolemic children. In particular, low shear stress increases the interaction time between low-density lipoprotein (LDL) and the arterial wall and promotes trans-endothelial diffusion [6]. The preferred location of fatty streaks in the aorta is the posterolateral walls between the origin of the inferior mesenteric artery and the bifurcation of the common iliac arteries. This site is available for ultrasound studies in children. In coronary arteries, fatty streaks usually appear around puberty and are rarely seen before the age of 9 years [7]. In an autopsy study, 65% of adolescents (12–14 years of age) had microscopically visible early atherosclerotic lesions in their coronary arteries, and an additional 8% had more advanced lesions. We do not know the precise factors that play a role in the development of fatty streaks around puberty. What we know is that hypercholesterolemic adolescents more frequently have atherosclerotic lesions in their arteries, even if in this case puberty is not associated with higher cholesterol levels [8,9]. A possible mechanism could be an increase of blood pressure during puberty [10].

The morphological bridge between early atherosclerotic lesions and more advanced lesions could be represented by progression-prone regions of arteries (i.e., locations with focal adaptive thickening). Preatheroma lesions are microscopically visible as extracellular lipid droplets and particles. Pools of this material form among the layers of SMCs in the arterial sites, where adaptive intimal thickening develops. The lipid accumulation occurs just below the layers of macrophages and macrophage foam cells, replace intercellular matrix proteoglycans and fibers, and drive SMCs apart [11]. Intimal SMCs may contain lipid droplets. Multiple separate extracellular lipid pools that disrupt the coherence of intimal SMCs represent progression beyond fatty streaks. At this lesion stage, a massive, confluent, well-delineated accumulation of extracellular lipid (a lipid core) has not yet developed. Early in life, progression-prone locations shelter fatty streaks; later, in young adults, preatheroma and the first atheroma-type lesions are found in the same locations. Fatty streaks and preatheroma lesions in these locations are morphologically similar to atheroma.

The term "*pathologic intimal thickening*" (PIT) was recently proposed to define an early stage of atherosclerosis found in human coronary lesions at autopsies of sudden death victims [12]. This term refers to preatheroma or "intermediate" lesion, and it has been suggested as the morphological and chemical bridge to more advanced plaques. PIT identifies a lesion with an extracellular lipid pool with intimal SMC loss typically adjacent to the medial wall in addition to varying degrees of macrophage infiltration near the lumen. These morphological features indicate a progressive lesion in the earlier stages of atherosclerosis, while a necrotic core is not yet present [13]. Macrophages, macrophage-derived foam cells, and SMCs are the cellular components of early histological damage of the human intima. In fatty streaks and preatheroma lesions, intimal SMCs and to lesser extent lymphocytes, plasma cells, and mast cells are also involved. SMCs are responsible for the production of most of the ECM within the vessel wall. Increases in collagen types may be a result of SMC hyperplasia in developing atherosclerotic lesions. Under the influence of atherogenic stimuli, SMCs can also modify the type of matrix proteins produced. Whereas most of the ECM within a healthy artery is type I and type III fibrillar collagen, atherosclerotic lesions tend to contain mostly proteoglycans with scattered type I collagen fibrils and fibronectin [14].

This transition can not only alter the architecture of the vessel, but also influence the lipid content and the proliferative index. During the progression of atherosclerosis from the initial through the intermediate lesion, a significant increase in dermatan sulfate proteoglycan of the ECM occurs [15]. On the other hand, heparan sulfate is reduced in human lesions when atherosclerosis severity increases. The lipid accumulation in the deep intimal layer in the earliest stage of lesion growth is associated with the expression of proteoglycans, biglycan, and decorin [16].

Transforming growth factor (TGF) plays an important role in the production of proteoglycans and, hence, derives its importance in early lesion development. Elastin content is decreased in advanced atherosclerotic lesions. In initial and fatty streak lesions, only few changes in elastin content are reported, while significant consequences may be due to damage of the elastic fibers in early lesions. An interesting observation is the absence of the elastin barrier and the exposure of a dense collagen/proteoglycan network at arterial branch points in animal models [17]. Furthermore, binding of lipids to elastic fibers may change elasticity of tissue, through changes in the conformation of the elastin.

Early Atherosclerotic Lesions in Childhood and Adolescence: Noninvasive *In Vivo* Evaluation

In the previous section, we have considered that atherosclerosis is preceded by a phase of changes in the arterial wall that could have functional consequences even before the appearance of atheromatous changes. It is, therefore, possible that early alterations of the mechanical properties of the arterial wall could precede clinical and echographic anatomical modifications. These preclinical alterations include pathologic intima-media thickening (IMT), increased collagen fibrosis, and foam cell infiltration.

By using noninvasive ultrasound for testing endothelial function, we can gain considerable information on the early stages of atherosclerosis and on the effects of cardiovascular risk factors on vasculature in childhood. The physiological atheroprotective function of the endothelium is attenuated in the presence of atherosclerotic risk factors such as hyperlipidemia. In addition, a partial loss of this endothelial function may be a key event in atherogenesis and may precede the development of structural and clinical atherosclerosis.

Endothelial function can be assessed by measuring the vascular response to infused acetylcholine, which increases nitric oxide production. However, this approach is invasive and not considered ethically appropriate for use in children. Therefore, other methods were developed to noninvasively test endothelial function and the most popular is ultrasound-measured flow-mediated dilation (FMD). FMD is obtained by inducing a hyperemic response after release of a cuff inflated above the systolic pressure to induce ischemia in the forearm: The artery dilates as a result of nitric oxide release produced by shear stress. The amount of dilation represents an index of endothelial func-

tion and can be accurately measured using high-resolution ultrasound. In order to obtain reproducible and reliable results, it is necessary to follow a strict and standardized exam protocol [18], but it should be acknowledged that there is a wide day-to-day variability of endothelial function.

Keeping these limitations in mind, the measurement of FMD might be a useful test, as arterial endothelial function reflects the proneness of the vascular tree to develop early atherosclerosis. For example, in the early phases of hyperlipidemia, the function of endothelium is modified with impairment in endothelium-dependent relaxation, which has been recognized as a very precocious abnormality. In children (6–7 years) with heterozygous familial hypercholesterolemia (FH), an impaired FMD was demonstrated even in the absence of visible atherosclerotic lesions [19]; moreover, a positive family history for cardiovascular disease was shown to carry additional risk in young patients with FH [20]. Children with familial combined hyperlipidemia also exhibited an impaired FMD [21].

Moreover, FMD might be a valuable tool in determining the benefits of early risk factor therapy in dyslipidemic children. In 9- to 18-year-old children with heterozygous FH, endothelial dysfunction has been shown to be potentially reversible by the use of statins [22] as well as, in another group of hypercholesterolemic children, by use of combined tocopherol and ascorbic acid antioxidant therapy [21]. Ultrasonic assessment of arterial endothelial function is a safe and widely available procedure, but no data are yet available on the predictive value of childhood endothelial function on cardiovascular prognosis in adults.

Another way of studying arterial response to vasodilating stimuli is by means of plethysmographic measurements during a reactive hyperemia test. An early impairment of vasodilating response to reactive hyperemia in lower limb arterial district, and its correction after LDL-apheresis has been demonstrated in young familial hypercholesterolemic patients [23]. Plethysmographic determination of blood flow is easier to perform than ultrasound measurements of FMD and has the advantage that gives a quantitative estimate of blood flow. However, the principal limitation of this technique is a wide coefficient of variation for repeated measurements.

Another noninvasive indicator of atherosclerosis, especially in the early phases of the disease, is arterial stiffness measurements. Stiffening of large arteries could anticipate increased IMT and the appearance of echographic plaques. Carotid arteries and aorta are the most extensively studied vessels, for the determination of ultrasound calculated arterial stiffness. Common carotid artery is relatively close to the heart, rich in elastic fibers, and easily available by ultrasound methodology.

Arterial stiffness can be assessed noninvasively using B- or M-mode imaging by measuring change in lumen diameter from systole to diastole, coupled with the measure of the logarithmically transformed pulse pressure normalized for diastolic pressure. A more accurate way to monitor changes in vessel diameters from diastole to systole and calculate carotid stiffness is by means of echotracking techniques which use radiofrequency signals coupled with B-mode ultrasonic images. In a recent study, children with hypercholesterolemia had a stiffer carotid arterial wall than the healthy control population [24]. The young age of these FH subjects is not compatible with an advanced sclerosis of the arterial wall. Foam cells are likely to be present in the early atherosclerotic alterations and are known to be mainly composed of soft material. Thus, it is difficult to attribute the arterial stiffening to accumulation of foam cells in the arterial wall. The increased stiffness of carotid arteries in young FH patients could rather be attributed to an altered ECM. SMCs are the major producers of ECM within the vessel wall and in response to atherogenic stimuli can modify the type of matrix proteins produced. Increases in collagen types may be a result of SMC hyperplasia, in developing atherosclerotic lesions, and might modify arterial rigidity. However, one endothelium function is the control of both smooth muscle tone and vascular wall remodeling. We do not know the precise molecular mechanisms by which the endothelium controls vascular remodeling. It is possible that nitric oxide, vasoactive molecules, and growth factors play an important role. In particular, nitric oxide inhibits the turnover of ECM and could modify the mechanical properties of the arterial wall.

The metabolic syndrome is the clustering of many cardiovascular risk factors: dyslipidemia, obesity, high blood pressure, and glucose metabolism abnormalities. First described in adults, it is reported to occur also in children. In a recent study, it was demonstrated that carotid stiffness was higher in children with metabolic syndrome compared to obese children (with a similar BMI) without metabolic syndrome, suggesting that the coexistence of multiple cardiovascular risk factors in pediatric age could further deteriorate arterial function compared to obesity alone [25]. The Bogalusa Heart Study performed on 10- to 17-year-old adolescents demonstrated stiffer carotid arteries in adolescents whose serum total cholesterol and systolic blood pressure was in the upper tertile [26]. Taken together, all these observations in pediatric populations indicate that increased arterial stiffness in conditions predisposing to atherosclerosis may be present at a young age. These alterations of the mechanical properties of the arterial wall in dyslipidemic high-risk children could be useful markers of preclinical vascular disease and could allow identification of children who would benefit most from intensive therapy.

High-resolution B-mode ultrasound measurement of carotid IMT is the most widely accepted marker of early atherosclerosis and in adults correlates with coronary artery disease and is associated with myocardial infarction and stroke. There are also clear indications that carotid IMT is a marker of the increased atherosclerotic burden in childhood. Carotid IMT has been used as an index of generalized atherosclerotic vascular process that can be used to study subclinical atherosclerosis *in vivo* in children.

There is evidence in hypercholesterolemic children of an increased carotid IMT, which is detectable after the age of 6 years [27]. In another study, the presence of plaque, found in 10% of children with FH, was associated with higher lifetime levels of total cholesterol and LDL-C and ApoB and cholesterol-years score [28]. Carotid IMT was also used to evaluate the relationship between LDL receptor genotype and response to pravastatin treatment in children with FH [29].

Several studies investigated the tracking of cardiovascular risk factors determined in childhood and their effects on atherosclerosis in adult age: most of these studies used IMT as a measure of subclinical atherosclerosis [30,31]. In particular, in the

Bogalusa Heart Study, childhood measures of LDL-C levels predict carotid IMT in young adults [32].

In another study, children with metabolic syndrome had not only greater IMT, but also a greater cross-sectional area of the intima-media complex compared to healthy control children [33]. The significance of childhood IMT and the long-term consequences remain unknown. In fact, carotid IMT differences between normal and high-risk pediatric populations are very small and their clinical or functional relevance is, therefore, questionable.

Lifestyle interventions and pharmacologic therapies have been successful in improving arterial health and have led to a speculation that these interventions in childhood may lead to improved arterial health in adulthood. However, the question is whether reducing the risk factors in childhood, leading to improvement in arterial structure and function, will truly affect the risk for cardiovascular events in adulthood.

Selected References

13. Kolodgie FD, Burke AP, Nakazawa G, et al. Is pathologic intimal thickening the key to understanding early plaque progression in human atherosclerotic disease? Arterioscler Thromb Vasc Biol 2007;27: 986–9.
14. Doran AC, Meller N, McNamara CA. Role of smooth muscle cells in the initiation and early progression of atherosclerosis. Arterioscler Thromb Vasc Biol 2008;28:812–9.
30. Raitakari OT, Juonala M, Kähönen M, et al. Cardiovascular risk factors in childhood and carotid artery intima-media thickness in adulthood: the Cardiovascular Risk in Young Finns Study. JAMA 2003;290:2277–83.
31. Johnson HM, Douglas PS, Srinivasan SR, et al. Predictors of carotid intima-media thickness progression in young adults. The Bogalusa Heart Study. Stroke 2007;38: 900–5.
33. Iannuzzi A, Licenziati MR, Acampora C, et al. Carotid artery wall hypertrophy in children with metabolic syndrome. J Hum Hypertens 2008;22:83–8.

CHAPTER 29

Phytosterols, Plasma Lipids and CVD Risk

Gerd Assmann[1] *& Udo Seedorf*[2]

[1]Assmann-Stiftung für Prävention, Münster, Germany
[2]University of Münster, Münster, Germany

Introduction

In many countries of the world, more than 20% of all adult men and women are either at risk for or affected by cardiovascular disease (CVD). Despite notable progress in primary, secondary, and tertiary prevention of CVD over the past 10 years, CVD prevention remains an exceedingly important public health challenge because of demographic changes and obesity-related morbidities. The benefits that have occurred because of the widespread introduction of effective cholesterol-lowering drugs (i.e., statins) and an improved awareness concerning a healthy lifestyle in parts of the population are counteracted by steeply increasing rates of overweight and obesity in many populations worldwide [1]. Overweight and obesity are well-established risk factors of the metabolic syndrome (also called syndrome X), which is an expanding health threat due to its tight association with diabetes, hypertension, hyperlipidemia, and atherosclerosis [2,3]. The metabolic syndrome is associated with approximately a twofold increased risk of myocardial infarction [4], and it was predicted that life expectancy will plateau or even decline in the United States and other Western societies within the first half of this century as a consequence of rising incidence rates of the metabolic syndrome [5].

Phytosterols and their ester derivatives have been introduced as food supplements by the food industry as part of a population-targeted strategy to reduce CVD risk because these natural compounds reduce the absorption of both dietary and biliary cholesterol from the intestinal tract, thereby lowering low-density lipoprotein (LDL)-cholesterol (LDL-C) levels. The primary aim of this chapter is to discuss potential benefits and risks that may be associated with this approach.

Relation between Phytosterols and the Metabolic Syndrome

One important reason for the growing interest in phytosterols relates to the fact that their serum levels and ratios to serum cholesterol were shown to be influenced by the metabolic syndrome. It was shown that sitosterol-to-cholesterol ratios (reflecting intestinal absorption of dietary and biliary cholesterol [6]) were inversely related to body mass index (BMI) values in male and female participants of the Prospective Cardiovascular Munster (PROCAM) Study, a large prospective epidemiologic study on risk factors for CVD performed in the northwestern part of Germany [7].

Conversely, another sterol ratio, lathosterol to cholesterol (reflecting *de novo* synthesis of body cholesterol [6]), was positively related to BMI [7]. Moreover, these sterol ratios followed a graded trend for the severity of individual components of the syndrome and for an index of the severity of the metabolic syndrome, which was based on the number of metabolic syndrome components present in the study participants [7]. Interestingly,

Nutritional and Metabolic Bases of Cardiovascular Disease, 1st edition.
Edited by Mario Mancini, José M. Ordovas, Gabriele Riccardi,
Paolo Rubba and Pasquale Strazzullo. © 2011 Blackwell Publishing Ltd.

high-density lipoprotein (HDL)-cholesterol (HDL-C) was negatively related with the lathosterol-to-cholesterol ratio (indicating the rate of cholesterol synthesis), whereas triglyceride levels showed a negative relationship with the sitosterol-to-cholesterol ratio (indicating the rate of cholesterol absorption) [7].Thus, these PROCAM study data support the notion that increased cholesterol synthesis and reduced cholesterol absorption may be seen in a context with the pathogenesis of the metabolic syndrome, and that plasma phytosterol levels and their ratios to plasma cholesterol may serve as novel biomarkers in CVD risk assessment by virtue of their association with the metabolic syndrome.

Phytosterols as Biomarkers to Identify Cholesterol Hyperabsorbers

A potential relationship existing between phytosterol levels and coronary risk was disclosed by Miettinen et al. who showed that coronary patients with low baseline ratios of serum phytosterols to cholesterol (indicating low cholesterol absorption) but not those with high ratios (indicating high cholesterol absorption) experienced reduced recurrences of coronary events during simvastatin treatment in the Scandinavian Simvastatin Survival Study [8]. Miettinen et al. also demonstrated that patients requiring large statin doses to normalize their cholesterol levels (poor statin responders) had higher baseline ratios of serum phytosterols to cholesterol than good statin responders (reaching target cholesterol levels at lower statin doses). Moreover, the good statin responders had higher ratios of cholesterol precursor sterols to cholesterol than the poor statin responders [9].

These findings led to the concept that poor responders to statin monotherapy would profit from a therapy that combines a statin with a cholesterol absorption inhibitor, such as ezetimibe. It could meanwhile be demonstrated that such combinations result in highly effective LDL-C lowering and that ezetimibe monotherapy reduces serum phytosterol concentrations significantly from baseline compared with placebo. Conversely, statin therapy profoundly lowers the levels of cholesterol synthesis precursor sterols, such as desmosterol and lathosterol, whereas a combination therapy with ezetim-

ibe and statin decreases serum levels of all of these sterols together [10].

Several trials have been initiated with the aim to evaluate whether combining a statin with ezetimibe is not only effective to lower LDL-C and plasma phytosterol levels but would also improve well-established surrogate markers of vascular disease. Results of the first trial, the Ezetimibe and Simvastatin in Hypercholesterolemia Enhances Atherosclerosis Regression (ENHANCE) trial, were published recently [11]. The ENHANCE trial compared 2-year daily therapy with 80 mg of simvastatin plus either placebo or 10 mg of ezetimibe on the average change in LDL-C and carotid intima—media thickness (IMT) in patients with familial hypercholesterolemia. Unexpectedly, no difference between the simvastatin monotherapy and the simvastatin-ezetimibe combined therapy groups with respect to IMT (a commonly used risk surrogate for vascular disease) or any other studied clinical end-point could be demonstrated, despite the substantial additional lowering of LDL-C resulting from ezetimibe, which exceeded 50 mg/dl (1.3 mmol/L) in the combined therapy group at the end of the study [11].

The outcome of the ENHANCE trial profoundly contradicted previous expectations. It used to be a widely accepted assumption that "lower is better" with respect to LDL-C. Essentially all previous controlled trials of statins, resins, or partial ileal bypass had shown rather convincing benefits on several CVD-related outcome measures, which seemed to correlate with the corresponding reductions in LDL-C [12,13]. What may be the reason for the limited effect of ezetimibe on IMT in the ENHANCE trial? The preclinical studies have shown that neither ezetimibe nor its glucoronidated metabolites affect drug-metabolizing enzymes or interact with cytochrome P450 (CYP450) substrates, thus excluding a negative impact of ezetimibe on statin drug availability. However, as noted by the U.S. National Lipid Association [14], more than 80% of the trial participants had been treated with statins prior to their recruitment into the ENHANCE study, many as part of a previous statin trial [13]. Thus, previous plaque lipid depletion may provide an explanation for the results of the ENHANCE study. Further clarification of these questions is expected from the results of the ongoing Improved Reduction of Outcomes: Vytorin Efficacy International Trial (IMPROVE IT) [15], which are due sometime around 2011.

Ezetimibe is highly effectively conjugated to a phenolic glucuronide, which is readily absorbed, pharmacologically active, and reaches fairly high systemic concentrations (~70 ng/ml at a dose of 10 mg) [16,17]. Moreover, since the glucuronide is transported in lipoproteins, one may expect it to accumulate considerably locally within the lipid core of the atherosclerotic plaque. Thus far, however, only a few publications have addressed potential consequences of the presence of the glucuronide outside the intestine. Seedorf et al. have shown that non-glucuronidated ezetimibe is bound to specific cell surface receptors followed by endocytosis via the classical endocytic pathway in human monocyte-derived macrophages [18]. The non-glucuronidated drug had no effect on uptake and/or processing of acetylated LDL, but it inhibited uptake of oxidized LDL by approximately 50% in a dose-dependent manner. Sehayek and Hazen reported that treatment of mice with ezetimibe resulted in increased cholesterol efflux from peripheral tissue macrophages [19], and Davis et al. demonstrated that ezetimibe inhibited development of atherosclerosis in apolipoprotein E (ApoE)-deficient mice [20]. All these results suggest potentially beneficial pleiotropic effects besides LDL-C lowering, which would promote rather than inhibit plaque regression. Nevertheless, further studies are warranted to definitively exclude the possibility that negative effects may result from the direct interaction of glucoronidated ezetimibe with cells at the arterial wall.

Are Phytosterols Biomarkers Predicting the Risk of Cardiovascular Disease?

To date, several studies have dealt with the question of whether baseline phytosterol levels are associated with altered risk of CVD. High dietary intake of phytosterols reduces LDL-C, and thus, a diet rich in phytosterols may theoretically be considered beneficial (see following section). On the other hand, individuals who are carriers for mutated forms of ABCG5 and/or ABCG8 (encoding ABC transporters, which limit intestinal absorption of plant sterols) develop sitosterolemia, a rare in-

born error of metabolism that is associated with elevated phytosterol concentrations along with highly elevated risk for coronary heart disease (CHD) and myocardial infarction [21].

Based on data from a prospective nested study derived from the PROCAM study, our laboratory found that high phytosterol level or a high phytosterol-to-cholesterol ratio was a risk factor of major coronary events [22]. The relative hazard ratios obtained upon univariate analysis for high phytosterol levels were similar to those of other well-established risk factors (i.e., hypertension, diabetes, the metabolic syndrome, or family history for myocardial infarction). The most pronounced relative risk increase with elevated sitosterol-to-cholesterol ratios was observed in male study participants who were at high global risk for myocardial infarction (risk of >20% in 10 years according to the PROCAM risk algorithm). As shown in Figure 29.1, these individuals had approximately a three-fold higher relative hazard ratio for the development of a major coronary event compared with corresponding study participants who had low sitosterol-to-cholesterol ratios [22].

The hypothesis that plasma phytosterol levels may be associated with increased coronary risk in non-sitosterolemic individuals has also been supported by findings in the Framingham Offspring Study, showing a significant association between phytosterol to cholesterol ratios and coronary artery disease [23]. Moreover, Glueck et al. reported that phytosterol levels were associated with a personal or family history of coronary artery disease in hypercholesterolemic individuals who were younger than 55 years [24]. In line with these epidemiologic findings, Weingartner et al. could demonstrate recently that dietary phytosterol ester supplementation in mice may lead to impairment of endothelium-dependent vasorelaxation, increased cerebral lesion size after middle cerebral artery occlusion and increased atherosclerotic lesion formation in apolipoprotein E deficient mice [25]. Moreover, patients with aortic stenosis who were receiving phytosterol supplemented margarine showed fivefold higher sterol concentrations in aortic valve tissue compared with corresponding control patients [25].

On the other hand, mice with inactivated forms of ABCG5 and ABCG8, leading to >20-fold higher

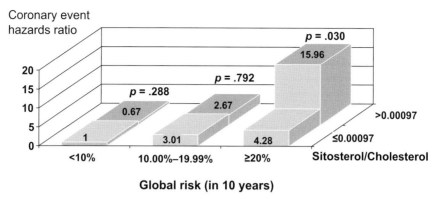

Global risk (in 10 years)

Figure 29.1 Hazard ratios for major coronary events according to sitosterol/cholesterol ratios and global risk. Study participants with high global risk (≥20% within 10 years of follow-up according to the PROCAM risk algorithm) and sitosterol/cholesterol ratios >0.00097 had an approximate threefold elevated hazards ratio compared with those having ratios ≤0.00097. Note that this difference was not present in the probands with lower global risk. The shown results are from a PROCAM nested study comprising 177 cases and 354 controls (see [22] for details).

plasma levels of phytosterols, showed no significant increase of aortic lesion area compared with controls [26]. Moreover, plasma levels of phytosterols were not associated with elevated coronary calcium scores (detected by electron beam computer tomography) in 2,542 subjects aged 30–67 years [26]. In another study, the Longitudinal Aging Study Amsterdam (LASA), high plasma concentrations of sitosterol were associated with a markedly reduced risk for CHD in a cohort of 1,242 subjects older than 65 years [27]. Conversely, no association between plasma phytosterol levels and risk of coronary artery disease could be detected in a prospective nested case-control study derived from the EPIC-Norfolk study, consisting of 373 cases and 758 controls [28].

In discussing these apparently conflicting results, it is important to consider that all studies differ with respect to study design, inclusion and exclusion criteria for study participants, regional differences with respect to the study population, and the analytical methods used to measure phytosterol levels. The last point may be of particular importance because accurate quantitation of phytosterols in nonsitosterolemic individuals is not trivial.

Phytosterols as Food Supplements to Lower LDL-C

Phytosterols, phytostanols, and their ester derivatives have been introduced as food supplements by the food industry because these natural compounds reduce the absorption of both dietary and biliary cholesterol from the intestinal tract by 30%–50% [29]. Although the exact mechanism is not entirely clear, it is generally assumed that increased concentrations of phytosterols in the gut interfere with the micellar solubility of cholesterol, thus lowering the amount of cholesterol available for absorption by the intestine [29]. Recent advancements in food technology have led to a number of food products, including margarine, milk, yogurt, and cereal products, which are enriched for plant sterols or their stanol derivatives. These products are extensively promoted by the food industry to lower serum cholesterol levels.

The Adult Treatment Panel (ATPIII) of the U.S. National Cholesterol Education Program (NCEP) has issued a number of dietary recommendations as part of therapeutic lifestyle changes to reduce the risk of CVD. In response to the growing amount of evidence showing significant cholesterol-lowering resulting from phytosterol/phytostanol-enriched margarines, these recommendations have recently been extended by giving the advice to include 2 g/ day of phytosterols or their stanol derivatives into the diet for those individuals who have elevated serum LDL-C levels [30]. Similar recommendations have also been issued by the International Atherosclerosis Society [31] and the National Heart Foundation of Australia [32].

The most common unsaturated phytosterols are β-sitosterol, campesterol, and stigmasterol, whereas the most common saturated phytostanols are sitostanol and campestanol [33]. Research over the past decade has focused primarily on the esterified forms of phytosterols, which result in superior product stability if used in food products, although free forms of phytosterols have also been employed, primarily in yogurt [34].

The evidence that dietary phytosterols lower total plasma cholesterol and LDL-C levels is well documented. The efficacy of phytosterol and phytostanol esters to reduce total cholesterol and LDL-C was studied in normocholesterolemic, hypercholesterolemic, and diabetic individuals in at least 57 trials [35]. When phytosterols or phytostanols were added to foods such as margarine with an average dose of about 2 g/day, LDL-C was lowered approximately 10% [35]. The efficacy between phytosterols and stanols in the esterified form, which was used in most studies, was essentially identical [36]. With respect to different food vehicles, there seemed to be a relative advantage for enrichment of milk or yogurt compared with bread or cereal [37].

Some concerns have been raised with respect to reductions of absorption of fat-soluble vitamins resulting from functional food enriched for phytosterols. High levels of phytosterols and stanols (>5 g/day) have been shown to reduce β-carotene, α-carotene, and vitamin E levels by approximately 25%, 10%, and 8%, respectively [38,39]. Moreover, currently only very few trial results are available that deal with the question of whether phytosterol-enriched foods are effective to improve well-established surrogate markers of atherosclerosis in humans or reduce the number of real clinical CVD end-points such as stroke, CHD, or myocardial infarction. Very recently, Weingartner et al. published an interesting study on the effects of dietary phytosterol ester supplementation on endothelial function, cerebral lesion size, and atherosclerosis in mice [25]. The data provided evidence for impairment of endothelium-dependent vasorelaxation and increased cerebral lesion size after middle cerebral artery occlusion resulting from dietary phytosterol supplementation. In addition, plant sterol plasma concentration strongly correlated with increased atherosclerotic lesion formation in ApoE-deficient mice and patients with aortic stenosis who were receiving phytosterol supplemented margarine showed fivefold higher sterol concentrations in aortic valve tissue compared with corresponding control patients [25]. Thus, food supplementation with phytosterol esters may not be as beneficial as originally assumed. Therefore, additional intervention trials and prospective studies that evaluate effects of phytosterols not only on LDL-C concentrations but also on well-established surrogate CVD markers and/or real clinical end-points are highly warranted in order to prove the safety of these extensively promoted and widely used functional food products.

Selected References

7. Assmann G, Cullen P, Kannenberg F, Schulte H. Relationship between phytosterol levels and components of the metabolic syndrome in the PROCAM study. Eur J Cardiovasc Prev Rehabil 2007;14:208–14.

19. Sehayek E, Hazen SL. Cholesterol absorption from the intestine is a major determinant of reverse cholesterol transport from peripheral tissue macrophages. Arterioscler Thromb Vasc Biol 2008 Apr 17.

25. Weingartner O, Lütjohann D, Ji S, et al. Vascular effects of diet supplementation with plant sterols. J Am Coll Cardiol 2008;51:1553–61.

27. Fassbender K, Lütjohann D, Dik MG, et al. Moderately elevated plant sterol levels are associated with reduced cardiovascular risk—the LASA study. Atherosclerosis 2008;196:283–8.

28. Pinedo S, Vissers MN, von Bergmann K, et al. Plasma levels of plant sterols and the risk of coronary artery disease: the prospective EPIC-Norfolk Population Study. J Lipid Res 2007;48:139–44.

CHAPTER 30

Nitric Oxide in the Development of Vascular Diseases and Regenerative Angiogenesis

Claudio Napoli[1] *& Louis J. Ignarro*[2]

[1] 1st School of Medicine, II University of Naples, Naples, Italy; *and* Boston University, Boston, MA, USA

[2] David Geffen School of Medicine, University of California, Los Angeles, CA, USA

Nitric Oxide Signaling

Nitric oxide (NO) acts as a key signaling messenger in the cardiovascular system [1]. NO participates in well-established regulatory functions including control of hemostasis, fibrinolysis, proliferation of vascular smooth muscle cells (VSMCs), and homeostasis of blood pressure [2–4].

Disturbances in NO bioavailability have been linked to cause endothelial dysfunction, leading to increased susceptibility to atherothrombosis, hypertension, hypercholesterolemia, diabetes mellitus, congestive heart failure, and stroke [2,3]. However, it is unclear whether this is a cause of or result of endothelial dysfunction or, more likely, both events. NO is produced by a family of NO synthase (NOS) enzymes of which there are three main isoforms, encoded on separate chromosomes by separate genes [2,3]: neuronal NOS (nNOS) predominantly expressed in certain neurons and in skeletal muscle, endothelial NOS (eNOS) predominantly expressed in endothelial cells, and inducible NOS (iNOS) expressed by macrophage/monocyte lineage cells. nNOS, also known as NOS-1, and eNOS (or NOS-3) are constitutively expressed and regulated by calcium and calmodulin and by post-translational modifications of the enzymes. The

Nutritional and Metabolic Bases of Cardiovascular Disease, 1st edition.
Edited by Mario Mancini, José M. Ordovas, Gabriele Riccardi,
Paolo Rubba and Pasquale Strazzullo. © 2011 Blackwell Publishing Ltd.

third isoform, iNOS (or NOS-2) is regulated by cytokines and produces quantities of NO far exceeding those produced by the other two isoforms. The three NOS isoforms have similar enzymatic mechanisms that involve electron transfer for oxidation of the terminal guanidin nitrogen of L-arginine. These enzymes all require several cofactors, including tetrahydrobiopterin (BH4), nicotinamide-adenine-dinucleotide phosphate (NADPH), flavin adenine dinucleotide (FAD), and flavin mononucleotide (FMN). Each isoform of NOS has been genetically disrupted in mice providing useful tools to complement other approaches investigating the multiple roles of NO in the cardiovascular system. Mice lacking the endothelial isoform are hypertensive, have endothelial dysfunction and show a more severe outcome in response to vascular injury, to cerebral ischemia, and to diet-induced atherosclerosis [5]. Mice lacking the neuronal isoform show a less severe outcome in response to cerebral ischemia but have increased diet-induced atherosclerosis, and, mice lacking the inducible isoform show reduced hypotension to septic shock [5,6].

The physiologic target of NO is soluble guanylate cyclase [2,3,6]. NO activates guanylate cyclase by binding to its heme moiety, resulting in increased cyclic guanosine monophosphate (cGMP) levels. In the vasculature, cGMP mediates NO-dependent relaxation of VSMCs, resulting in vasodilation. Similarly, NO produced as a neurotransmitter in the gastrointestinal, urinary, and the respiratory tract mediates smooth muscle relaxation by increasing cGMP production. These effects are mediated by the phosphorylation of downstream proteins by cGMP-dependent protein kinases, including myosin light chain [2,3]. Another target for NO is sulfhydryl groups on proteins to form nitrosothiol (SNOs) compounds.

Alterations in endogenous S-nitrosylated proteins that include eNOS, β-actin, vinculin, diacylglycerol kinase-alpha, GRP78, extracellular signal-regulated kinase 1, and transcription factor nuclear factor-κB (NF-κB) may underlie the adverse effect of hyperglycemia on the vasculature and the development of vascular complications [6,7]. Interestingly, studies indicate that these changes can be completely reversed by inhibition of superoxide production, suggesting a key role for oxidative stress in the regulation of S-nitrosylation under hyperglycemic conditions [7]. NO and/or SNOs can prevent the loss of β adrenergic receptor signaling *in vivo* and regulation occurs through modulation of G-protein–coupled receptor kinase 2 (GRK2) [8]. Indeed, in both cells and tissues, GRK2 resulted to be S-nitrosylated by SNOs, and Cys340 of GRK2 has been identified as a principal locus of inhibition by S-nitrosylation [8]. Moreover, regulation of cytokine-induced S-nitrosylation of p65 by NOS-2 delineates a novel mechanism by which NOS-2 modulates NF-κB activity and regulates gene expression in inflammation [9].

Hemoglobin (Hb), which may serve as a natural carrier for SNO derivative of Hb (SNO-Hb), is formed *in vivo* and circulating concentrations are capable of dilating blood vessels. A number of novel reactions of NO, nitrite, and SNO that produce SNO-Hb *in situ* [10] and result in release of NO bioactivity under hypoxic conditions [4,5] have been described. Levels of SNO-Hb are altered in disorders in tissue oxygenation [11] and NO bioactivity is depleted in banked blood, impairing the vasodilatory response to hypoxia raising the hypothesis that pathogenic microbes and viruses may induce S-nitrosylation of dynamin to facilitate cellular entry [12].

Pharmacological modulation of NO and combined therapy with antioxidant and L-arginine may restore endothelial dysfunction, inhibit oxidation-sensitive mechanisms, reduce atherogenesis, and improve bone marrow cell (BMC)–mediated vascular repair and regeneration [3,13,14]. Some pharmacological agents exert direct beneficial effects on endothelium [15,16], while others elicit their actions by improving the deleterious oxidation-sensitive mechanisms leading to vascular dysfunction and atherosclerosis [17].

NO in Cascular Dysfunction

An early event in the pathophysiology of atherosclerosis is the impairment of endothelial function before structural changes such as intimal hyperplasia or lipid deposition occurs. Diminished levels of bioavailable NO occur through several potential mechanisms, such as reduced eNOS expression levels, reduced eNOS enzymatic activity, and reduced NO bioavailability [2,3,5]. Endothelial dysfunction is associated with an increase in reactive oxygen species (ROS) production in the bloodstream, which occurs via activation of the NADPH oxidase(s) in endothelial cells, VSMCs, or adventitial cells or via the enzyme xanthine oxidase [3,18]. Activation of the endothelial cell NADPH oxidase and formation of peroxynitrite during angiotensin II–induced mitochondrial dysfunction modulates endothelial NO and superoxide generation, which in turn has ramifications for the development of endothelial dysfunction.

Despite the transient compensatory increase in iNOS and nNOS expression, NO bioavailability is reduced because of increased reaction rates with superoxide, yielding as byproducts reactive nitrogen/oxygen species that induce protein nitration [2,3]. Indeed, superoxide radical reacts with NO to form peroxynitrite, which at very low concentrations possesses the same biologic activity as NO. It is only at higher levels that peroxynitrite exerts its toxic effects by forming the cytotoxic peroxynitrous acid, as well as resulting in protein modification by nitration of amino acids [2,3].

Besides the key role of the decreased NO bioactivity in endothelial dysfunction and vascular damage, NOS itself is capable of producing ROS in the absence of substrate, L-arginine, or BH_4 [2,3]. BH_4, whose synthesis is rate limited by GTP cyclohydrolase, is an important cofactor, because in its absence, electron transport through eNOS can become "uncoupled," resulting in generation of superoxide anion.

Thus, coronary heart disease (CHD) risk factors that deplete levels of L-arginine or BH_4 may promote NOS-mediated ROS formation and, in turn, increase peroxynitrite generation [19].

Clinical Measurements of Endothelial Function

Assessment of endothelial function is a useful diagnostic and prognostic tool [20]. The pathophysiology of endothelial dysfunction includes abnormal vasomotor function, proinflammatory, and prothrombotic state. Some laboratory markers have been used as indicators of abnormal function of the endothelium, such as E-selectin, intercellular adhesion molecule (ICAM)-1, vascular cell adhesion molecule (VCAM)-1, CD40L, C-reactive protein (CRP), interleukin (IL)-1, tumor necrosis factor (TNF)-α interferon (IFN)-γ, monocyte chemotactic protein (MCP)-1, von Willebrand factor, tissue plasminogen activator (tPA), plasminogen activator inhibitor (PAI)-1, microalbuminuria, and tests of apoptosis [21]. Although cinical utility of these measurements is limited due to their non-specific character, they represent good complement to imaging assessment of endothelial function.

Quantitative coronary angiography after intraarterial infusion of acetylcholine is a clinical gold standard for the assessment of coronary endothelial function. Vasoconstriction or even no arterial diameter change after acetylcholine stimulation disclose endothelial dysfunction and indicate "hot" places, at risk of atherosclerosis. Assessment of coronary vasoreactivity using acetylcholine, cold pressor testing, and increased blood flow in 147 patients (57% with angiographic evidence of atherosclerosis) showed that responses to each of these tests independently predicted cardiovascular events [22].

Angiographically smooth epicardial coronary arteries can be associated with endothelial dysfunction and a worse long-term outcome in low-risk population [22]. A high-resolution ultrasound imaging of brachial artery flow-mediated dilation (FMD) is a noninvasive, sensitive, and re-producible ultrasonic measurement of endothelial function [23], which has been shown to correlate with invasive testing of coronary endothelial function [23]. FMD has been most commonly studied in the brachial artery [23,24]. FMD can be conducted among children and young adults, especially if repeated measurements are required [24]. The occlusion-induced production of reactive hyperemia to promote endothelial NO-dependent vasodilation evaluates the shear stress. Subjects with small sized brachial arteries may have normal arterial dilation, even in the presence of endothelial dysfunction. Mean FMD values can vary considerably across studies in similar populations: in CHD ranging from −1.3% to 14%, in diabetes mellitus from 0.75% to 12%, and in healthy volunteers from 0.2% to 19.2% [25]. Endothelial function is reduced in the early morning, around the time of waking (6 AM), compared with measurements obtained before sleep (9 PM) and later in the day (11 AM) in healthy humans [23–25]. FMD at 6 AM (4.4%) was markedly decreased, compared with the measurements at 9 PM (7.5%) and 11 AM (7.7%).

Reduced brachial artery vasoreactivity was demonstrated as an independent predictor for increased cardiovascular risk in patients with peripheral arterial disease (PAD) [3,23]. Median FMD was significantly lower in patients with an event (5.8%) than in those without (7.6%). More importantly, measurement of FMD improved the prognostic value of ankle-brachial pressure index, which is the powerful prognostic indicator in PAD.

There is substantial evidence suggesting an improvement in FMD following exercise training in general population [26] with the subsequent reduction of cardiovascular risk. Furthermore, 45 minutes of moderate-intensity (acute) exercise has been shown to improve FMD and other parameters of endothelial function [27].

Another clinical tool for measurement of endothelial function is the reactive-hyperemia peripheral arterial tonometry (RH-PAT), a noninvasive and operator-independent technique used to assess peripheral microvascular endothelial function by measuring changes in digital pulse volume during reactive hyperemia [28]. Digital hyperemic response is attenuated in patients with established coronary endothelial dysfunction.

NOS Competitive Inhibitors

Abnormalities in the coagulation system take part to the setting of established atherosclerosis (reviewed in [3,19]). Analogues of L-arginine such as NG-monomethyl-L-arginine (L-NMMA) and asymmetric dimethylarginine (ADMA), an endgenous competitive inhibitor of NOS, have been used to inhibit NOS. Plasma levels of ADMA are elevated in hypercholesterolemic and atherosclerotic patients and have been correlated with the severity of risk factors and endothelial dysfunction [29]. The inhibitory effect of ADMA on endothelial function has been shown not only to involve NO-mediated endothelium-dependent vasodilatation but also the endothelium-derived hyperpolarizing factor mediated pathways in hypertensive individuals [30]. In healthy subjects without symptomatic coronary arterial disease or PAD, the plasma ADMA level varied with age, blood pressure, glucose tolerance, and carotid IMT [3]. An acute infusion of ADMA (2.0–10.0 μmol/L) given to healthy subjects caused a significant decrease in plasma cGMP concentration, the main second messenger of NO inducing a significant decrease in cardiac output [31]. Cardounel et al. [32] provided some insight into the open question of whether the small change in the plasma level of ADMA in patients with CHD is sufficient to alter significantly NO production and contribute to the development of CHD. Indeed, ADMA is preferentially taken up by endothelial cells and the intracellular level of ADMA is five to tem times that of the extracellular level. Therefore, a small change in the plasma level of ADMA would presumably have a large effect on the intracellular level of ADMA and on NO production.

Finally, advanced glycation end-products, senescent macroprotein derivatives closely linked to the development of diabetic atherosclerosis [31,33], accelerate the development of diabetic atherosclerosis via iNOS and heme oxygenase induction.

NOS Knockout Mice

Ex vivo gene transfer of eNOS to atherosclerotic rabbit aortic rings improves relaxations to acetylcholine [34], suggesting that reduced NO bioavailability observed in cholesterol-induced vascular

dysfunction can be partially overcome by eNOS gene transfer. NOS gene therapy also rapidly reduces inflammatory cell infiltration in carotids of cholesterol-fed rabbits [35]. Gene transfer of eNOS, but not eNOS plus iNOS, regressed atherosclerosis in rabbits [36].

A complementary approach is to manipulate the genes that encode the NOS enzymes to generate knockout mice [5]. Results from eNOS knockout (eNOS$^{-/-}$) mice confirm results using pharmacological agents. Indeed, eNOS$^{-/-}$ mice show significantly greater neointima formation after cuff injury than wild-type mice [5]. ApoE/eNOS double knockout mice (ApoE$^{-/-}$/eNOS$^{-/-}$) on a Western diet develop atherosclerosis significantly faster than ApoE$^{-/-}$ and have almost twice as many lesions [5].

After a Western-type diet, ApoE$^{-/-}$/eNOS$^{-/-}$ males and females showed significant increases in lesions compared with ApoE$^{-/-}$ mice, respectively [5]. They also show evidence of CHD, left ventricular dysfunction, aortic aneurysm, and aortic dissection, and the phenotype more closely resembles the spectrum of cardiovascular complications seen in humans. ApoE$^{-/-}$/eNOS$^{-/-}$ mice are hypertensive, but pharmacological control of blood pressure still leads to accelerated atherosclerosis and development of aortic aneurysms [5]. Several studies have implicated dysfunctional eNOS as a common pathogenic pathway in diabetic complications [37]. Diabetic eNOS$^{-/-}$ mice developed hypertension, albuminuria, and renal insufficiency with arteriolar hyalinosis, mesangial matrix expansion, mesangiolysis with microaneurysms, gracilis muscle arterioles, and Kimmelstiel–Wilson nodules [38].

Contractions to endothelin-1 (ET-1) may be enhanced during chronic deficiency in expression or activity of NOS. Vasoconstriction to ET-1 is enhanced under conditions of chronic deficiency in eNOS$^{-/-}$ mice [5]. ET-1–induced contraction of aorta from wild-type mice increases twofold following acute inhibition of all NOS isoforms with N(G)-nitro-l-arginine (l-NNA). Arterioles of eNOS$^{-/-}$ mice express high levels of cyclooxygenase-2 (COX-2) protein, together with an upregulation of COX-2 gene expression [5].

In contrast, ApoE$^{-/-}$/iNOS$^{-/-}$ mice show significantly smaller lesions compared to ApoE$^{-/-}$ mice [5]. The reduction in atherosclerosis in double knockout animals is associated with decreased plasma levels of lipoperoxides, suggesting that reduction in iNOS-mediated oxidative stress may explain the protection from lesion formation in double knockout animals [5]. The critical role of the endogenous NOS system in maintaining cardiometabolic homeostasis has been demonstrated using a mice model deficient in all 3 NOS isoforms (triply n/i/eNOS$^{-/-}$ mice). Indeed, genetic disruption of the whole NOS system causes spontaneous mouse infarction associated with risk factors of metabolic origin [5]. Importantly, activation of the renin-angiotensin system was noted in the triply n/i/eNOS$^{-/-}$ mice, and long-term oral treatment with an angiotensin II type 1 receptor blocker significantly suppressed coronary lesions and the occurrence of spontaneous myocardial infarction (MI) and improved the prognosis, along with ameliorating the metabolic abnormalities [5].

NO and Oxidation-Sensitive Mechanisms

An extensive exploration of the oxidation-dependent mechanisms has been described elsewhere [2,17,19]. Atherogenic lipids, particularly oxidized low-density lipoproteins (oxLDLs), are responsible for a wide range of cellular dysfunctions within the vessel wall, playing a pivotal role in human early atherogenesis [2,17,19]. Indeed, oxidized LDL induces monocyte adhesion to the endothelium, migration and proliferation of smooth muscle cells, injures cells, interferes with NO release, and promotes procoagulant properties of vascular cells. Native and oxLDL can uncouple eNOS and may also induce a decreased uptake of L-arginine. The local depletion of the L-arginine substrate may derange the eNOS, leading to overproduction of superoxide radical from oxygen, the co-substrate of eNOS [2,17,19]. Moreover, oxLDL increases the availability and activity of arginase II (at both transcriptional and posttranslational levels), reciprocally decreases NOx production, and contributes to impaired vascular NO signaling.

Superoxide can also be formed from all NOS isoforms under specific conditions, for example, lack of essential cofactors. Identification of LOX-1 as the major receptor for oxLDL in endothelial cells has provided a new clue to the mechanisms involved in oxLDL accumulation in the arteries. This receptor, by facilitating the uptake of oxLDL, induces endothelial dysfunction and mediates numerous oxLDL-induced proatherogenic effects [39]. Besides endothelial cells, LOX-1 is also expressed by VSMC and macrophages. Here, LOX-1 may function as a scavenger receptor and promote foam cell formation. Another mechanism, also at least partly involving the LOX-1 receptor, is the impact of OxLDL on ADMA. OxLDL can acutely increase ADMA concentration in endothelial cells, and leads to overexpression of protein arginine N-methyltransferases, the enzymes that generate ADMA [40]. In endothelium, ADMA increases oxidative stress, and in activated macrophages it upregulates the expression of LOX-1, thus causing a vicious circle.

Interestingly, physiological differences can affect arterial segments from different regions [41–43]. For example, oxLDL impairs contraction and endothelium-dependent relaxation in carotid but not in basilar artery [43], indicating that intracranial arteries are relatively protected from atherosclerosis via resistance to oxidative injury. Finally, a multitude of oxidation-sensitive apoptotic signaling can interact with NO in the vessel wall [17,44]. This concept demonstrates that L-arginine hypothesis and the increased oxidative stress may actually fit together and are not two concepts which exclude each other.

eNOS Polymorphisms

Some studies demonstrate that eNOS gene polymorphism can be considered an additional risk factor contributing to atherosclerosis [3]. The two polymorphisms located in the exon 7 (894 G→T which encodes a Glu298→Asp amino acid substitution in eNOS gene) and in the promoter region (T-786→C) of the eNOS gene are associated with functional changes in the endothelium and carotid IMT, mild modulation of the predisposition abdominal aortic aneurysm (reviewed in [3,45]) and could be a risk factor for angiographic CHD and recent MI (3).

However, data about the association between polymorphisms in heart disease–related genes and the early onset of a first MI are limited. Multivariate regression analysis evaluates age at onset of a first MI in relationship to individual single-nucleotide polymorphisms in a cohort of patients enrolled in the Thrombogenic Factors and Recurrent Coronary Events (THROMBO) [46]. Patients who had the high-risk genotype eNOS E298D showed ages at onset of a first MI of 3.5 years ($p = .02$) earlier than in noncarriers of the genotype. Consistently, high-risk genotypes of the eNOS E298D polymorphisms were significantly associated with onset of a first MI at younger than 50 years (adjusted odds ratio 1.70, $p = .005$, adjusted odds ratio 2.15, $p = .01$, respectively) [46].

Analysis of the GluAsp or AspAsp genotype of the Glu298Asp polymorphism in 337 Japanese patients with diabetes indicates that this polymorphism is significantly associated with CHD [47]. Of the 337 subjects analysed for polymorphisms of the eNOS gene, 45 with the GluAsp and 5 with the AspAsp genotype were combined into one group (GluAsp or AspAsp group). Among these 50 subjects, 16 (32%) have shown CHD, and among 287 subjects with the GluGlu genotype, 38 (13.2%) have shown CHD. The number of subjects with CHD was significantly greater in the GluAsp or AspAsp group than in the GluGlu group ($p = .0006$) [70].

Several studies evaluate the relationship between common variants of eNOS gene and the risk of CHD [47–49]. In the evaluation of the association between presence of CHD documented by angiography and the -786T>C polymorphism of the eNOS gene in Chilean patient with CHD and controls, the frequency of CC homozygous genotype for -786T>C polymorphism is 6% in CAD patients and 4% in the control group [48]. However, the genotype distribution and allele frequencies are not significantly different between CHD patients and control subjects. Moreover, the odds ratio for CHD associated with the C variant failed to reach statistical significance, suggesting that the -786T>C polymorphism of the eNOS gene is not associated with CHD [48].

In a case-control study performed to evaluate the association between the eNOS -786T>C, 4a4b, or 894G>T polymorphism and CHD in Koreans patients and healthy controls, the eNOS-786T>C, 894G>T and 4a4b polymorphisms were not an independent predisposition factor to CHD [49]. However, a subgroup analysis adjusted with various risk factors confirmed positive association of the -786T>C polymorphism in CHD patients with hypertension and a smoking history and also a significant association of the intron 4 genotypes with a smoking history, but no significance has been found in the eNOS polymorphisms of 894G>T upon any risk adjustment. Distribution of heterozygotes (-786TC, 894GT, and 4a4b) and variant homozygotes for the -786C, 894T, and intron 4a alleles of eNOS in Koreans resulted also significantly lower than in white populations [49].

A systematic examination of the associations of eight variants of the eNOS gene [-786T>C and Glu298Asp] and six tagging single nucleotide polymorphisms with CHD risk in a cohort of diabetics suggests that -786T>C, Glu298Asp, and an intron 8 polymorphism of the eNOS gene are potentially involved in the atherogenic pathway among U.S. diabetic men [50]. Indeed, among 861 diabetic men (>97% white), 220 developed CHD. Genotype distributions of -786T>C and Glu298Asp polymorphisms were not significantly different between case and control subjects, and CHD risk was significantly higher among men with the variant allele at the rs1541861 locus (intron 8 A/C) than men without it. The Asp298 allele of the eNOS gene is significantly associated with impaired coronary collateral development, especially in diabetic patients [51].

The T(-786)C single-nucleotide polymorphism of eNOS gene implies a blunted endothelium-dependent vasodilation in hypertensive patients and is associated with multivessel CHD in cross-sectional studies. This polymorphism is associated with changes in markers of oxidant stress in high-risk white patients referred for coronary angiography [52]. In white patients of the GENICA (Genetic and Environmental Factors in Coronary Atherosclerosis) study, who underwent coronary angiography, the eNOS T(-786)C was determined by melting curve analysis of amplicons from allele-specific fluorescence resonance energy transfer probes. After a median follow-up of 1,296 days, 85 (8.2%) deaths are reported with a significant impact of the T(-786)C eNOS genotype on cardiovascular death-free ($p = .01$) survival [52].

NO and Vascular Regeneration

Preclinical Studies

Administration of L-arginine to hypercholesterolemic rabbits increases the number of apoptotic macrophages in lesions and results in a regression of the atherosclerotic plaque [2,3]. This suggested that intervention of the NOS pathway may represent a therapeutic approach to resolving the inflammatory response in the artery [2,3]. In a murine model of hindlimb ischemia, autologous Bone Marrow Cell (BMC) together with metabolic intervention significantly ameliorated ischemia-induced angiogenesis in C57BL/6J [53] and hypercholesterolemic mice [54] by modulation of cellular oxidation-selective mechanisms and augmentation of NO production. This was amplified by metabolic treatment (vitamins C/E, and L-arginine), which induced vascular protection, at least in part, through the NO pathway, and reduced systemic oxidative stress.

Moreover, a long-term combined beneficial effect of L-arginine treatment is also observed on atherosclerosis in hypercholesterolemic mice during graduated physical training [55]. BMC therapy alone and, more consistently, in combination with metabolic treatment, ameliorated bone marrow-derived endothelial progenitor cells (BM-EPC) functional activity via decreased cellular senescence and improved homing capacity by increasing CXCR4-expression levels [56]. L-arginine potentiates the effects of moderate physical exercise by increasing EPCs number and VEGF serum levels supporting the evidence that L-arginine positively modulates EPC levels [57].

Combined antioxidant and gene therapy is also shown on middle-cerebral artery occlusion (MCAO) in the rat [58]. Rats that 3 days before MCAO received a pretreatment with L-arginine, vitamin E, and gene therapy with virus-mediated overexpression of tissue inhibitors of matrix metalloproteinases (TIMPs) showed a smaller brain lesions than control rats or those treated with single treatment. The combined treatment of BMC with TIMPs and metabolic supplementation added further beneficial neuroprotective effects improving histological and functional outcome in brain ischemia [58].

Clinical Studies

Early clinical studies describing the effect of L-arginine supplementation [3,15,16] indicate its clinical beneficial effects in patients with CVD. Some clinical studies on NO and vascular regeneration are shown in Table 30.1. L-arginine administration partially restores endothelium-dependent vasodilation in hypercholesterolemia [59,60], dilates coronary stenoses in patients with CHD [61], and improves coronary small-vessel function in patients with endothelial dysfunction and non-obstructive CHD [62]. Oral treatment with L-arginine (5.6–12.6 g/day) in patients with heart failure caused a drop in arterial blood pressure whereas the administration L-arginine (21 g for 3 days) to young men with CHD determined no changes in arterial pressure, despite the fact that the brachial artery was dilated [63]. Intracoronary infusion of L-arginine in patients with hyperlipidemia, CHD, or cardiac transplant recipients induced attenuation of serotonin-induced constriction, dilatation of coronary segments and stenoses, and improvement of abnormal microvascular responses to sympathetic activation [64,65].

L-arginine administered intravenously is somewhat effective in patients with PAD. Clinical improvement was manifested in the extension of painless intermittent claudication distance, shortening of pain regression after walking, improvement of lower limb blood supply and increase in ankle-arm pressure ratio [66].

In the Nitric Oxide in Peripheral Arterial Insufficiency (NO-PAIN) randomized trial, subjects with intermittent claudication due to PAD received oral L-arginine (3 g/day) [67]. The primary endpoint was the change at 6 months in the absolute claudication distance. Although absolute claudication distance improved in both L-arginine- and placebo-treated patients, the improvement in the L-arginine–treated group was significantly lesser than that in the placebo group [67]. A study conducted to establish the lowest effective oral dose of L-arginine in patients with PAD and intermittent claudication demonstrated a trend of a greater increase in walking distance and walking speed in the

Table 30.1 Published clinical studies on L-arginine and vascular function.

Condition	Intervention	Clinical outcome
Hypercolesterolemia	*i.v.* administration of L-arginine	Improvement of endothelium-dependent vasodilation
	L-arginine infusion	Improvement of coronary microcirculation
	Intra-coronary infusion of L-arginine	Improvement of abnormal microvascular function
CHD	L-arginine infusion	Dilatation of coronary stenoses
	Oral supplementation of L-arginine	Reduced arterial blood pressure
	Intra-coronary infusion of L-arginine	Dilatation of coronary segments
	Oral supplementation of L-arginine	Ineffective in influencing endothelial function
	Oral supplementation of L-arginine	Improvement of small-vessel coronary endothelial function
Gestational hypertension	Oral supplementation of L-arginine	Reduced blood pressure, improved endothelial function
Type 2 diabes	Oral supplementation of L-arginine	Improved endothelial function, oxidative stress, and adipokine release
Congestive heart failure	Oral supplementation of L-arginine	Ineffective in influencing endothelial function
Cardiac transplant	Intra-coronary infusion of L-arginine	Attenuation of serotonin-induced constriction
Myocardial infarction	Oral supplementation of L-arginine	No improvements of vascular stiffness measurements or ejection fraction
	Oral supplementation of L-arginine	Beneficial not-significant trend towards reduction of major clinical events
	Oral supplementation of L-arginine	Ineffective in influencing endothelial function
PAD	*i.v.* administration of L-arginine	Extension of painless intermittent claudication distance, improvement of lower limb blood supply
	Oral supplementation of L-arginine	No significant improvements of claudication distance
	Oral supplementation of L-arginine	Increased in walking distance

Reviewed in references [16,59–68]. i.v.: intravenous; CHD: coronary heart disease; PAD: peripheral arterial disease.

group treated with L-arginine [68]. Recently, we have established that the neovascularization capacity of autologous BMC transplantation is effective during cotreatment with vitamin C, vitamin E, and L-arginine in severe PAD [69].

Finally, nitrite functions as a physiological regulator of vascular function and NO homeostasis,

suggesting that it is an active metabolite of the organic nitrates that can be used therapeutically to bypass enzymatic tolerance in healthy human volunteers [70]. Sodium nitrite, along with saline to maintain a total infusion volume of 120 ml/hr, was infused at doses from 0, 7, 14, 28, and 55 to 110 $\mu g \times kg^{-1} \times min^{-1}$ (Figure 30.1). Results

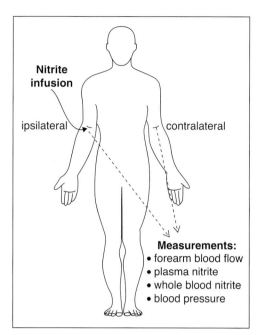

Figure 30.1 Nitrite infusion in humans. Schematic protocol of nitrite infusion performed at doses from 0, 7, 14, 28, and 55–110 μg × kg^{-1} × min^{-1}, as described by Dejam et al. [70]. After each dose was infused, blood was drawn from both veins to measure plasma and whole blood nitrite, blood pressure, and heart rate. Forearm blood flow was measured in the opposite arms. (Adapted from Dejam et al. [70], with permission.)

revealed that nitrite is a potent and rapid regional and systemic vasodilator, an effect slightly potentiated by systemic reductants and inhibition of xanthine oxidase [70].

Acknowledgments

We apologize to colleagues of many original articles that were not quoted due to strict limitation of space allowed. Moreover, we thank our colleague Joseph Loscalzo for helpful discussions in the field and our colleague Mario Mancini for his fascinating mentorship in the field of atherosclerosis.

Selected References

32. Cardounel AJ, Cui H, Samouilov A, et al. Evidence for the pathophysiological role of endogenous methylarginines in regulation of endothelial no production and vascular function. J Biol Chem 2007;282:879–87.
45. Napoli C, Ignarro LJ. Polymorphisms in endothelial nitric oxide synthase and carotid artery atherosclerosis. J Clin Pathol 2007;60:341–4.
46. Morray B, Goldenberg I, Moss AJ, et al. Polymorphisms in the paraoxonase and endothelial nitric oxide synthase genes and the risk of early-onset myocardial infarction. Am J Cardiol 2007;99:1100–5.
69. Napoli C, Farzati B, Sica V, et al. Beneficial effects of autologous bone marrow cell infusion and antioxidants/L-arginine in patients with chronic critical limb ischemia. Eur J Cardiovasc Prev Rehabil 2008;15:709–18.
70. Dejam A, Hunter CJ, Tremonti C, et al. Nitrite infusion in humans and nonhuman primates: endocrine effects, pharmacokinetics, and tolerance formation. Circulation 2007;116:1821–31.

CHAPTER 31

Impact of Treating Dyslipidemia on Cardiovascular Events

Željko Reiner & Diana Muačević-Katanec
University Hospital Center Zagreb, Zagreb, Croatia

Introduction

A large body of evidence indicates a direct association between dyslipidemia and the development of cardiovascular diseases (CVDs) (coronary heart diseases [CHD], myocardial infarction [MI], stroke, and peripheral arterial disease [PAD]) [1–5]. Dyslipidemias, particularly hyperlipoproteinemias are at the same time the most in-depth studied risk factor for CVD [6–8]. Results of numerous large studies illustrate the importance of hyperlipoproteinemia treatment aimed at preventing atherosclerosis and CVD [9–11]. It is certain that reduction of low-density lipoprotein (LDL)-cholesterol (LDL-C) concentration in plasma significantly reduces cardiovascular morbidity and mortality [4,11,12]. Clinical trials testing the "lipid hypothesis," based on the view that lowering plasma total and LDL-C leads to decreased risk of CHD, were first conducted in the 1970s and 1980s. Results were generally positive and led to the conclusion that MI could be prevented by lipid-lowering therapy. However, definitive proof that such treatment could reduce cardiovascular mortality and improve overall survival was not available until the publication of landmark studies in primary and secondary prevention using 3-hydroxy-3-methylglutaryl-coenzyme A (HMG-CoA) reductase inhibitors, statins, that were published in the 1990s and more recently [4,6,12].

In addition to decreasing elevated LDL-C levels to prevent or delay the development of atherosclerosis, in the past decades elevated triglyceride levels and decreased protective high-density lipoprotein (HDL)-cholesterol (HDL-C) have also become recognized as important and worth intervention [10,13–20].

The effectiveness in reducing morbidity and mortality from CHD was demonstrated by many studies. The most significant primary and secondary prevention studies are discussed.

Studies on Treatment of Hypercholesterolemia

Scandinavian Study of Survival with Simvastatin

The Scandinavian Study of Survival with Simvastatin (4S) study, which recruited patients from throughout the Scandinavian countries, was the first large clinical trial to have shown positive clinical outcomes (reduced risk of mortality and vascular events) due to lowering cholesterol with simvastatin, an HMG-CoA reductase inhibitor [12]. After a 5.4-year follow-up, 182 (8%) fatalities occurred in patients on simvastatin, and 256 (12%) in those on placebo, respectively. Reduction in the relative risk of death due to any cause amounted to 30% (p = 0.0003) in the group receiving simvastatin. Simvastatin also reduced risks of major coronary events (death from coronary disease, nonfatal definite or probable myocardial infarction (MI), silent myocardial infarction or recurrent cardiac arrest) by 34% (353 − 16%) vs. 502 − 23%; p < 0.00001) [12].

Nutritional and Metabolic Bases of Cardiovascular Disease, 1st edition.
Edited by Mario Mancini, José M. Ordovas, Gabriele Riccardi,
Paolo Rubba and Pasquale Strazzullo. © 2011 Blackwell Publishing Ltd.

West of Scotland Coronary Prevention Study

West of Scotland Coronary Prevention Study (WOSCOPS) was a primary prevention trial that demonstrated the effectiveness of pravastatin (40 mg/day) in reducing morbidity and mortality from CHD in moderately hypercholesterolemic men [4,21].

Long-term follow-up results of WOSCOPS have been published. The results show that men to whom statin therapy was prescribed for 5 years during the clinical trial period had fewer cardiovascular events a decade later, although a large majority of those included in the study cohort had stopped taking their cholesterol-lowering medication. About 10 years after trial end, the risk for death from CHD or nonfatal MI was 10.3% in the placebo group and 8.6% in the pravastatin group ($p = .02$). During the entire follow-up period, this rate was 15.5% versus 11.8% ($p < .001$). According to the investigators, the results are presumably due to the stabilization of existing plaques [22].

Air Force Texas Coronary Atherosclerosis Prevention Study

Air Force Texas Coronary Atherosclerosis Prevention Study (AFCAPS/TexCAPS) was a primary prevention, placebo-controlled randomized trial demonstrating that reduction of LDL-C is an appropriate treatment also for persons with "average" LDL-C levels and with the additional risk of below-average HDL levels [23,24].

The number needed to treat over 5 years to prevent one event was 46 among men. AFCAPS/TexCAPS emphasizes the point that in primary prevention, targeting patients at higher risk will produce a bigger impact at relatively lower cost [23,24].

LIPID

The LIPID study emphasized the importance of hypolipemic therapy in the secondary prevention setting [25]. Patients included in the study had a history of MI or unstable angina with a very broad range of initial total cholesterol levels varying from 4.0 to 7.0 mmol/L. The incidence of the primary end point which was death from CHD was 6.4% in the pravastatin group, as compared to 8.3% in the placebo group (reduction in RR with pravastatin 24%; 95%, CI, 12 to 35% ; P < 0.001). The overall

mortality was 22% lower (95% CI, 13 to 31%) in the pravastatin group (11.0%) than in the placebo group (14.1%, P < 0.001). Mortality from all cardiovascular causes was 25% lower (7.3% vs. 9.6%, P < 0.001).

Cholesterol and Recurrent Events

The Cholesterol And Recurrent Events (CARE) trial, a 5-year trial that compared the effect of pravastatin and placebo, included 586 patients (14.1%) with clinical diagnosis of diabetes. The participants with diabetes were older, more obese, and more hypertensive. The mean baseline lipid concentrations in the group with diabetes –136 mg/dL LDL cholesterol, 38 mg/dL HDL cholesterol, and 164 mg/dL triglycerides – were similar to those in the nondiabetic group. Pravastatin treatment reduced the absolute risk of coronary events for the diabetic and nondiabetic patients by 8.1% and 5.2% and the relative risk by 25% (P = 0.05) and 23% (P < 0.001), respectively [26,27].

Heart Protection Study

The Heart Protection Study (HPS) was carried out to investigate the long-term benefit of simvastatin and/or antioxidant therapy with vitamins on the incidence of coronary disease in a large number of patients at a high risk of CHD, independently of cholesterol level, including those with diabetes with or without CHD [13]. The study included men and women from 40 to 80 years of age with an increased 5-year risk of death from CHD ($n = 20{,}536$; 15,454 men and 5,082 women) in Great Britain. Based on age and medical history, patients who were at a high risk from CHD were divided into four major risk groups: 1) patients with coronary artery disease, 2) patients with occlusive disease of the noncoronary arteries, 3) diabetic patients, and 4) those treated for hypertension. Baseline total cholesterol in randomized patients was ≥135 mg/dl (≥3.5 mmol/L); the upper limit had not been defined by the inclusion criteria. Patients with normal or below-normal 100 mg/dl (<2.6 mmol/L) baseline LDL-C levels were included, in order to evaluate if a reduction of LDL-C to a level below that of 3.2 mmol/L (125 mg/dl) was able to reduce the risk of CHD. Previous statin or other lipid-lowering therapy was not a criterion for excluding patients from the study.

Simvastatin therapy significantly reduced the risk of major vascular events, including nonfatal MI, coronary death, revascularization, and cerebral infarction. The incidence of any of the major vascular events was 19.8% ($n = 2,033$) among the 10,269 patients who received simvastatin and 25.2% ($n = 2,585$) among the 10,267 patients on placebo.

In the HPS, 40 mg of simvastatin per day significantly reduced the relative risk (RR) of major vascular events, independently of baseline LDL-C or total cholesterol levels (RR = 24%, $p < .0001$). Patients with a low baseline LDL-C benefited from simvastatin treatment equally to those with intermediate or high levels of LDL-C. In patients with baseline LDL-C <3.0 mmol/L, simvastatin therapy reduced the 5-year absolute risk of major vascular events by 4.6%, from 27.6% to 22.2%. A 40 mg/day simvastatin therapy reduced the risk of major vascular events regardless of whether the patients had a history of CHD at the beginning of the study. Among the patients without previous CHD, major vascular events occurred in 574 out of 3,575 patients (16.1%) treated with simvastatin and 744 out of 3,575 patients (20.8%) treated with placebo.

In patients with diabetes without a previous CHD, major vascular events were recorded in 276 out of 2,006 patients (13.8%) treated with simvastatin as compared to the 367 out of 1,976 patients (18.6%) on placebo therapy.

Anglo-Scandinavian Cardiac Outcomes Trial Lipid Lowering Arm (ASCOT-LLA)

The Anglo-Scandinavian Cardiac Outcomes Trial—Lipid Lowering Arm (ASCOT-LLA) study investigated the effect of atorvastatin on clinical events in high-risk patients (hypertension plus at least three other cardiovascular risk factors) and total cholesterol <250 mg/dl (6.5 mmol/L). In this study, 10,305 patients were randomized to atorvastatin 10 mg or placebo. Although the planned follow-up was 5 years, the trial was stopped at 3 years because of clear benefit of the statin therapy. In atorvastatin patients, the primary end-point of nonfatal MI or CHD death was significantly reduced by 36%.

Patients studied in ASCOT-LLA were at increased risk because of hypertension and other cardiovascular risk factors such as age, diabetes, or other

vascular disease, although they did not have known CHD or substantially elevated LDL-C. The clinical interpretation of these data suggests that high-risk patients with low or normal levels of LDL-C benefit from intensive reductions of LDL-C and non-HDL-C with statin therapy [28].

Greek Atorvastatin and Coronary Heart Disease Evaluation

The Greek Atorvastatin and Coronary Heart Disease Evaluation (GREACE) study was an independent, prospective, randomized, open-label study designed to compare two standards of treatment and management in hypercholesterolemic patients with CHD. This study enrolled 1,600 hypercholesterolemic patients with CHD and LDL-C levels >100 mg/dl (> 2.6 mmol/L) after a 6-week period of lipid-lowering diet. CHD was documented by a coronary angiogram. Patients were randomized into one of two treatment groups. Atorvastatin was initiated at a dosage of 10 mg/day. If the National Cholesterol Educational Program (NCEP) Adult Treatment Panel (ATP) III LDL-C goal of <100 mg/dl (2.6 mmol/L) was not reached within 6 weeks, the dose of atorvastatin was increased to 20 mg/day. With evaluations every 6 weeks, the dose of atorvastatin was titrated up to a maximum of 80 mg/day depending on patient response. The GREACE study demonstrated significant reductions in morbidity and mortality associated with active dose titration of atorvastatin and structured management of dyslipidemia. Higher levels of LDL-C at baseline were associated with a greater risk of subsequent events among patients randomized to usual care. This study demonstrated significant reductions in morbidity and mortality associated with active dose titration of atorvastatin and structured management of dyslipidemia. Reducing the LDL-C and the non-HDL-C level to the NCEP ATP-III goals required greater doses of atorvastatin for the higher baseline quartile of LDL-C, after achieving the LDL-C treatment goal [29].

Myocardial Ischemia Reduction with Aggressive Cholesterol Lowering

The Myocardial Ischemia Reduction with Aggressive Cholesterol Lowering (MIRACL) study was a randomized, double-blind trial that demonstrated the effectiveness of atorvastatin therapy

(80 mg/day) initiated 24–96 hours after an acute coronary syndrome (ACS) in reducing death and nonfatal ischemic events. Atorvastatin and placebo were compared in 3,086 adults 18 years or older with unstable angina or non-Q-wave acute MI with a follow-up through 16 weeks at 122 clinical centers in Europe, North America, South Africa, and Australasia. The primary end-point event was defined as death, nonfatal acute MI, cardiac arrest with resuscitation, or recurrent symptomatic myocardial ischemia with objective evidence and requiring emergency rehospitalization. It occurred in 228 patients (14.8%) in the atorvastatin group and 269 patients (17.4%) in the placebo group (RR 0.84; 95% confidence interval [CI], 0.70–1.00; $p =$ .048). There were no significant differences in risk of death, nonfatal MI, or cardiac arrest between the atorvastatin group and the placebo group, although the atorvastatin group had a lower risk of symptomatic ischemia with objective evidence and requiring emergency rehospitalization (6.2% vs. 8.4%; RR, 0.74; 95% CI, 0.57–0.95; $p = .02$). The MIRACL study clearly emphasized the importance of beginning with hypolipemic therapy within the first days after an ACS to reduce recurrent ischemic events requiring rehospitalization [30,31].

Pravastatin or Atorvastatin Evaluation and Infection Therapy – Thrombolysis in Myocardial Infarction 22

The Pravastatin or Atorvastatin Evaluation and Infection Therapy—Thrombolysis in Myocardial Infarction 22 (PROVE IT-TIMI 22) study compared the clinical efficacy of reduction in LDL-C to approximately 100 mg/dl (2.6 mmol/L) with pravastatin 40 mg/ day (the dose being increased to 80 mg/day if the LDL-C level was greater than 125 mg/dl (3.2 mmol/L) on two consecutive visits) with a more intensive one to approximately 70 mg/dl (1.8 mmol/L) with 80 mg/day of atorvastatin. The study included 4,162 patients hospitalized for ACS within the previous 10 days. Mean follow-up was 2 years.

Primary end-point events included fatal outcome, MI, unstable angina requiring hospitalization, revascularization at least 30 days after randomization, and stroke. They occurred in 26% of pravastatin-treated patients and 22% of atorvastatin-treated subjects, showing a 16% reduction in the hazard ratio with atorvastatin, which has

also been found to be significantly more beneficial with respect to secondary end-points.

Although the study was designed to produce evidence that therapy with 40 mg of pravastatin was not inferior to that with 80 mg of atorvastatin after ACS, it has revealed that a more intensive therapy reduced primary end-point clinical events by 16%. Earlier studies, which have shown that more intensive lipid-modifying therapy was more efficient in stopping the development of atherosclerosis or reversing it based on carotid or coronary artery ultrasonographic measurements, have used surrogate end-points. This study, however, was the first to corroborate that "lower was better" using clinical end-points [32].

The PROVE IT-TIMI 22 trial has achieved an approximate 50% reduction in LDL-C, reducing it to 62 mg/dl (1.6 mmol/L), a level substantially lower than the current target one (100 mg/dl, or 2.6 mmol/L). This has indicated that individuals with ACS benefit significantly from intensive lipid-lowering therapy as first suggested by the REVERSAL trial, using intravascular ultrasound and the same statin regimens, although not aimed at identifying differences in clinical outcomes [33].

Treatment to New Targets

In the Treatment to New Targets (TNT) study, patients with CHD and LDL-C levels <130 mg/dl (3.4 mmol/L) were randomized to atorvastatin 10 mg/day (5,006 patients) or 80 mg/day (4,995 patients). A highly significant reduction of cardiovascular events with lower levels of LDL-C achieved with atorvastatin 80 mg/day was found ($p < .0001$), without increasing the rate of serious adverse effects thus proving once more "the lower the better" concept [34].

Collaborative Atorvastatin Diabetes Study

Diabetes mellitus is associated with a twofold to fourfold increased risk of CHD and death after MI in comparison with patients without diabetes. The Collaborative Atorvastatin Diabetes Study (CARDS) was a 4-year multicenter, randomized, placebo-controlled, double-blind trial of atorvastatin administered in a dose of 10 mg/day. It was the first study set to prospectively evaluate statin therapy specifically in patients with type 2 diabetes.

The patients included in the study, aged 40–75 years, had type 2 diabetes, LDL-C concentration of 160 mg/dl (4,1 mmol/L) or less, fasting triglycerides of 600 mg/dl (6.6 mmol/L) or less, at least one additional risk factor (hypertension, retinopathy, microalbuminuria or macroalbuminuria, or current smoking), and no history of CHD, cerebrovascular accident, or severe peripheral vascular disease.

Patients treated with 10 mg/day of atorvastatin showed a 26% (54 mg/dl, or 1.4 mmol/L) reduction in total cholesterol and a 40% (46 mg/dl, or 1.l7 mmol/L) reduction in LDL-C on the average. Mean reduction in triglycerides was 19%, with a 1% increase in HDL-C levels as compared with placebo.

The RR in the primary end-point of first acute CHD event (MI including silent infarction, unstable angina, acute CHD death, resuscitated cardiac arrest), coronary revascularization procedures, or fatal or nonfatal stroke was significantly reduced by 37% with 10 mg/day of atorvastatin as compared to placebo ($p = .001$). A significant reduction (by 48%; $p = .016$) was achieved for stroke and all-cause mortality (27%; $p = .059$). The CARDS results have pointed to a need to consider patients with type 2 diabetes as candidates for statin treatment even at a lower LDL-C level goal, as has been recommended by the American Diabetes Association [35].

REVERSing Atherosclerosis with Aggressive Lipid Lowering (REVERSAL)

The REVERSAL study measured changes in atheroma burden as assessed by intravascular ultrasound. It included 654 patients from 35 to 78 years of age with symptomatic coronary artery disease and a $\geq 20\%$ stenosis as determined by coronary angiography. After 8 weeks of washout period LDL-C ranged between 125 mg/dl (3.2 mmol/L) and 210 mg/dl (5.4 mmol/L) in all patients, randomly assigned to either moderate lipid-lowering therapy with 40 mg of pravastatin or to intensive lipid-lowering therapy with 80 mg of atorvastatin administered for 18 months. There was no progression of atherosclerosis in the intensive treatment group (−0.4%, CI, −2.4%, $p = .98$) as compared with the baseline, which was different from the pravastatin group in which progression of coronary atherosclerosis did occur in spite of treatment [33].

Aggressive statin therapy, which achieved LDL levels below those targeted by the NCEP, has been found to be clearly associated with clinical benefit in a wide range of primary and secondary prevention clinical studies of atorvastatin in patients with all levels of disease severity. The reduction in CRP and in other anti-inflammatory markers from other studies has been found to be an important pleiotropic effect [33,36].

ASTEROID

The ASTEROID study has shown that by using intravascular ultrasound (IVUS) a significant delay in the progression of atherosclerosis during statin treatment, as well as the regression in atheroma volume percentage. The study was carried out in 53 centers in the United States, Canada, Europe, and Australia. The size of coronary atheromas was compared in 349 patients treated with rosuvastatin in a single daily dose of 40 mg at the beginning of the study and after 24 months of treatment.

This study has shown a significantly greater reduction in LDL-C concentration using 40 mg of rosuvastatin in comparison to treatment with other statins, as well as an increase in HDL-C level by 14.7%. A resulting atheroma regression was significant.

The results of this study support the recommendation for treating CHD patients with higher doses of statins [37].

METEOR

A double-blind, placebo-controlled METEOR study, which included 984 patients with different 10-year risk factors for the development of CHD (age, mildly marked carotid intima-media thickness [IMT], elevated LDL-C concentration), was carried out in 60 primary care centers from the United States and Europe. The study was designed to investigate the effect of rosuvastatin on IMT during a 2-year period in middle-aged individuals with low Framingham risk scores, but with subclinical atherosclerosis, in comparison to the placebo. Of 984 patients enrolled, 702 were assigned to rosuvastatin and 282 were assigned placebo. At 2 years, rosuvastatin treatment was associated with a significant reduction in the rate of IMT progression, overall (0.0014 mm/yr decrease vs. progression of

0.0131 mm/yr on placebo, $p < .0001$), as well as for the individual carotid sites.

This study has shown that treatment with rosuvastatin in middle-aged persons with a Framingham 10-year risk of the development of atherosclerosis of less than 10% and with signs of subclinical atherosclerosis leads to a statistically significant delay in the progression in carotid IMT over a 2-year period in comparison to placebo [38].

JUPITER

In this study 11 001 men and 6801 women who had hsCRP levels >2 mg/L (median, 4.2 mg/L) and LDL-C levels <130 mg/dL or 4.4 mmol/L (median, 108 mg/dL) were randomized to either rosuvastatin 20 mg or to placebo. The best clinical outcomes (prevention of MI, stroke, hospitalization for unstable angina, arterial revascularization, or cardiovascular death) were observed among those receiving rosuvastatin who achieved low levels of both hsCRP and LDL-C (<70 mg/dL or 1.8 mmol/L)[39].

ENHANCE

In ENHANCE trial 720 patients with familial hypercholesterolemia were treated with 80 mg of simvastatin combined either with placebo or with 10 mg of ezetimibe. The primary outcome measure was the change in the mean carotid-artery IMT. Combined therapy with ezetimibe and simvastatin did not result in a significant difference in changes in intima-media thickness, as compared with simvastatin alone, despite stronger decreases in levels of LDL-C and hsCRP [40].

Studies on Treatment of Hypertriglyceridemia and Low HDL-Cholesterol

Although the role of high serum triglyceride levels in CHD has been debated for many years, evidence suggests that elevated serum triglyceride levels, especially in patients with additional lipoprotein abnormalities, predict an increased risk of CVD [41–46].

The Helsinki Heart Study

This study found a threefold increased risk of cardiac events in subjects with a high LDL-C/HDL-C ratio and triglyceride levels >200 mg/dl

(2.3 mmol/L) [47]. This 5-year, double-blind, placebo-controlled trial on 4,081 men without CHD showed that gemfibrozil 1,200 mg/day increased HDL-C by 11% and decreased triglycerides by 35% while decreasing total cholesterol by 10% and LDL-C by 11%. These effects were associated with a significant 34% reduction of total coronary events (nonfatal and fatal MI, sudden cardiac death).

Bezafibrate Infarction Prevention

The Bezafibrate Infarction Prevention (BIP) study [48] on 3,090 subjects aged 74 years showed a small, independent risk of increased mortality with elevated triglyceride levels in men and women with established CHD, especially in those with elevated LDL-C levels. Although the treatment with bezafibrate 400 mg/day showed no significant effect on the combined incidence of nonfatal MI or death from CHD in the total study population, there was a significant reduction in a subgroup of patients whose triglycerides were elevated at the beginning of the study. In this subgroup, the event rate was reduced by 39% from 19.7% in the placebo group to 12.0% in the bezafibrate group ($p = .02$).

In this study, 52% of the patients with total cholesterol <200 mg/dl (5.2 mmol/L) had HDL-C levels consistent with the accepted "high-risk" range of <35 mg/dl (0.9 mmol/L), whereas an increasing percentage of desirable HDL-C level was found with increasing levels of total cholesterol (14% with HDL-C). The number of previous infarctions, severity of congestive heart failure, and severity of angina was negatively correlated with mean HDL-C in a dose-response manner, whereas the association with mean triglycerides was inverted, creating a mirror image of that observed with HDL-C. These results also strongly establish the necessity for obtaining all three standard blood lipid determinations (total and HDL-C and triglycerides) and to adjust treatment modalities not only in patients with CHD but also in individuals at high risk for CHD [48].

Veterans Affairs High-Density Lipoprotein Cholesterol Intervention Trial

The Veterans Affairs High-Density Lipoprotein Cholesterol Intervention Trial (VA-HIT) was a five-year, multicenter, randomized, double-blind, placebo-controlled secondary prevention trial that was designed to test the hypothesis that decreasing triglycerides and/or raising HDL-C protects against CHD events [49]. In this study, 2,531 men with CHD and HDL-C of 40 mg/dl (1 mmol/L) or less and LDL-C of 140 mg/dl (3.6 mmol/L) or less were treated with 1,200 mg/day of gemfibrozil or placebo. Gemfibrozil treatment increased HDL by 6% and decreased triglycerides by 31%. Concentrations of HDL-C were inversely related to CHD events. CHD events were reduced by 11% with gemfibrozil for every 5 mg/dl (0.13 mmol/L) increase in HDL-C ($p =$ .02). LDL-C levels remained unchanged. There was a 22% reduction in RR of a major cardiac event (MI or death due to CHD) in the treated group, which was attributed to the significant increase in HDL-C. During gemfibrozil treatment, only the increase in HDL-C significantly predicted a lower risk of CHD events—neither triglycerides nor LDL-C levels at baseline or during the trial did it [48]. A significant reduction in stroke was also demonstrated in the group treated with gemfibrozil (RR reduction of 31%).

This study suggests that patients with low HDL-C, high triglyceride, and low LDL-C levels can benefit from therapy with fibrates [50].

Diabetes Atherosclerosis Intervention Study

The Diabetes Atherosclerosis Intervention Study (DAIS) was a 3-year angiographic trial performed to investigate whether the decrease of plasma triglycerides concentration with a consecutive shift toward larger, more buoyant LDL particles caused by fenofibrate was associated with significantly less progression of focal CHD. In this study, 418 patients with diabetes type 2 were randomized to receive 200 mg/day of micronized fenofibrate or placebo. Fenofibrate treatment significantly increased LDL particle size as well as HDL-C concentration and decreased plasma triglycerides. Fenofibrate treatment was associated with 40% less progression of minimum lumen diameter versus placebo treatment ($P = .029$).

The DAIS study has demonstrated that not only plasma lipoprotein concentrations, but also LDL size show statistically significant correlation with the progression of CHD [51].

The Fenofibrate Intervention and Event Lowering in Diabetes

The Fenofibrate Intervention and Event Lowering in Diabetes (FIELD) study was designed to assess the effect of fenofibrate on CVD events in diabetic patients. It was a randomized controlled trial with 9,795 participants aged 50–75 years, with type 2 diabetes. In the three countries, 14,247 patients were registered, of whom 4,900 were randomized to placebo and 4,895 to fenofibrate. The two treatment groups were well matched for baseline characteristics, including use of cardiovascular and glucose-lowering therapies. A total of 5,820 patients (59%) met the prespecified definition of low HDL-C (40 mg/dl (<1.03 mmol/L) in men, 50 mg/dl (<1.29 mmol/L) in women) and 5,093 (52%) had high triglyceride concentrations (>1.7 mmol/L). A total of 3,710 patients (38%) had both of these features, to meet the definition of dyslipidemia. Fenofibrate was associated with a nonsignificant 11% relative reduction in the primary outcome of first MI or CHD, but for the secondary outcome of total CVD events (the death of CVD, MI, stroke, coronary and carotid revascularization), there was a significant 11% reduction in patients receiving fenofibrate. The results are of particular importance suggesting the need to treat diabetic patients without previous CVD [52,53].

ACCORD

In this trial 5518 patients with type 2 diabetes who were being treated with open-label simvastatin were randomized to receive either additional fenofibrate or placebo. The primary outcome was the first occurrence of nonfatal MI, nonfatal stroke, or death from cardiovascular causes and the mean follow-up was 4.7 years. The combination treatment did not reduce the primary outcomes, as compared with simvastatin alone [54]. These results do not support the routine use of such a combination therapy to reduce cardiovascular risk in the majority of high-risk patients with type 2 diabetes but the subgroup analysis indicates that the patients with high TG (204 mg/dL or above) and low HDL-C (34 mg/dL 0.9 mmol/L or below) will benefit by adding fenofibrate due to additional decrease of TG and increase of HDL-C.

Studies on Treatment of Low HDL-Cholesterol

Reduction of atherogenic LDL-C has for years been considered the main therapeutic goal, while increasing low HDL-C has remained somehow neglected. It has been shown, nevertheless, that 40% of adult men who had MI had normal values of total cholesterol and LDL-C, but decreased HDL-C. On the other hand, it has been observed that the development of CVD in persons between 49 and 82 years of age was significantly delayed if their levels of protective HDL-C were elevated [55,56]. Today it is accepted that a 1% increase in HDL-C level reduces the risk of the development of CVD by 2% [55,57]. Increase in HDL-C can be influenced by physical activity, diet, fibrates, and nicotinic acid (niacin). Nicotinic acid is most effective in HDL-C elevation, particularly affecting HDL2 particles, which are responsible for the transport of esterified cholesterol from the periphery into the liver during the process of reverse cholesterol transport. Therefore, most studies used nicotinic acid to increase HDL-C levels. It has been shown that it also lowers elevated lipoprotein(a), an independent risk factor (at least in some studies) for the development of atherosclerosis [58]. Nicotinic acid has been shown to have the whole range of antiatherogenic effects independent of its beneficial effect on lipid profile. It has antioxidant properties [59], significantly reduces inflammation markers, especially phospholipase A2 and CRP [60], and lowers the concentration of prothrombotic factors such as fibrinogen and cellular adhesion molecules [61]. During treatment with nicotinic acid a rise in adiponectin, an important antiatherogenic substance, which is reduced in patients with diabetes and the metabolic syndrome, has also been observed [62].

Studies have demonstrated a benefit from niacin treatment in inhibiting or delaying the progression of CVD, which is explained by its efficacy in elevating HDL-C. This is considered important because of the growing body of evidence showing that mere reduction of atherogenic LDL-C is insufficient prevention if HDL-C is low, or even, additionally reduced during statin treatment.

Coronary Drug Project

The Coronary Drug Project is one of the most significant studies on the effect of niacin on the progression of atherosclerosis. It was a placebo-controlled secondary prevention study that included 1,119 men who were treated with niacin and 2,789 men who received placebo. The group treated with 2,000 mg/day of niacin for 6 years revealed a 26% reduction in the incidence of nonfatal MI and a 24% decrease in cerebrovascular events in comparison with the placebo group ($p < .05$) [63].

Nine years after the completion of the study, total mortality was 11% lower in the niacin-treated group as compared to that receiving placebo ($p = .0004$) [64].

Cholesterol-Lowering Atherosclerosis Study and Familial Atherosclerosis Treatment Study

Using quantitative coronary angiography, the Cholesterol-Lowering Atherosclerosis Study and Familial Atherosclerosis Treatment Study showed that niacin in a combination with cholestipol reduced the progression of atherosclerosis and increased coronary plaque regression [65].

HDL Atherosclerosis Treatment Study

The HDL Atherosclerosis Treatment Study (HATS) was a double-blind, placebo-controlled, 3-year angiographic trial on 160 patients with CHD and low HDL-C. Patients were assigned to four treatment groups: simvastatin plus niacin, antioxidants, simvastatin plus niacin plus antioxidants, and placebo. After 3 years of placebo therapy, the mean percent stenosis in proximal arteries increased on average by 3.9%, it increased by 1.8% (Bonferroni-adjusted $p = .16$ for the comparison with the placebo group) after antioxidant therapy, but regressed by 0.4% ($p < .001$) after simvastatin–niacin therapy. With simvastatin–niacin plus antioxidants, proximal stenosis increased by 0.7% ($p = .004$) [66].

Arterial Biology for the Investigation of the Treatment Effects of Reducing Cholesterol

The second and third Arterial Biology for the Investigation of the Treatment Effects of Reducing Cholesterol (ARBITER 2 and 3) studies investigated the beneficial effects of niacin in addition to statin treatment by measuring carotid IMT after 1 and 2 years of treatment [67,68]. Carotid IMT significantly increased in patients receiving placebo, while remaining unchanged in those treated with niacin. Regression by 0.027 mm was observed after 12 months of niacin treatment, and after 24 months, IMT was reduced by 0.041 mm. Results of this study have demonstrated that niacin has a significant effect on the regression of atherosclerosis, possibly due to raising HDL-C.

Conclusion

Evidence from large, randomized trials clearly demonstrates that total cholesterol and LDL-C lowering for 25%–45% achieved with statins reduces the risk of coronary events by 20%–40% over a period of 3–6 years. Larger reductions in LDL-C are associated with greater improvements in CVD morbidity and mortality [69]. Although the issue of very low cholesterol levels and mental disorders is still controversial, the rates of serious mental disorders and suicide seem to be unaffected by statin therapy [70]. However, factors other than total cholesterol and LDL-C levels such as increasing low HDL-C or reducing the proportion of small dense LDL particles, which are highly atherogenic, may provide an additional therapeutic approach to decrease significant residual CVD risk in patients treated with statins.

Despite the clear evidence of the benefits of lipid-lowering treatment in both primary and particularly secondary prevention a large majority of CVD patients with dyslipidemia is still inadequately treated and a significant number of patients on lipid-lowering therapy are still not reaching the treatment goals [71]. This is despite much better lipid control and the increase in the use of lipid-lowering therapy, particularly statins, over the past decade [72]. Economic constrains within certain healthcare systems could partly explain why the pharmacological treatment of dyslipidemia is not more effective and the treatment goals are not achieved, especially in low- and middle-income countries [73,74]. Although according to the guidelines [1] and based upon clear evidence statins should be initiated while patients are in hospital with an acute coronary event, this is not universally followed [75]. Therefore, a considerable potential still exists to reduce CVD mortality and morbidity rates as well as cardiovascular events through better treatment of dyslipidemia [73].

Selected References

13. Heart Protection Study Collaborative Group. MRC/BHF Heart Protection Study of cholesterol lowering with simvastatin in 20, 536 high-risk individuals: a randomised placebo-controlled trial. Lancet 2002;360:7–22.

34. La Rosa JC, Grundy SM, Kastelein JJ, et al. Treating to New Targets (TNT) Steering Committee and Investigators. Safety and efficacy of atorvastatin-induced very low density lipoprotein cholestrol levels in patients with coronary heart disease (a post hoc analysis of the Treating to New Targets (TNT) Study). Am J Cardiol 2007;100:747–52.

38. Crouse JR, Raichlen JS, Riley WA et al. Effect of Rosuvastatin on progression of carotid intima-media thickness in low-risk individuals with subclinical atherosclerosis. The METEOR Trial. JAMA 2007;297:1344–53.

71. Reiner Ž., Tedeschi-Reiner E. Atherosclerosis – A paradox of Eastern European countries. Atherosclerosis 2006;7(Suppl 3): 461.

73. Fruchart J-C, Sacks F, Hermans MP, et al. The Residual Risk Reduction Initiative: A call to action to reduce residual vascular risk in dyslipidemic patients. A position paper by the Residual Risk Reduction Initiative (R3I). Diabetes Vasc Dis Res 2008;4:319–35.

CHAPTER 32

Evolution of the Lipid Clinic, 1968–2008

Barry Lewis

University of Sydney, Sydney, NSW, Australia

Summary

This chapter outlines the evolution, during the past four decades, of the management of the hyperlipidemias as a clinical discipline. The development of this specialty paralleled the accumulating evidence that hypercholesterolemia is causally related to cardiovascular disease; the establishment of this relationship underlies the need to recognize and to achieve optimal control of lipid disorders. The discipline lies at the interface of internal medicine, clinical nutrition, and public health. Some unresolved complexities are reviewed, including the choice of target levels for lipid-lowering therapy, the indications for lipid-lowering drug treatment, and the need for noninvasive plaque imaging as an arbiter of cardiovascular risk.

Introduction

As the evidence base for treating hyperlipidemia becomes ever more compelling and as the effectiveness of therapy advances, clinical practice in centers for managing lipid disorders has evolved in several ways. One of the first lipid clinics, at the Hammersmith Hospital, London, was opened in 1968 by the author jointly with our Editor, Professor Mario Mancini. Its function was therapeutic as well as providing a research base, but the range of treatment was limited to diet, early bile acid

Nutritional and Metabolic Bases of Cardiovascular Disease, 1st edition.
Edited by Mario Mancini, José M. Ordovas, Gabriele Riccardi,
Paolo Rubba and Pasquale Strazzullo. © 2011 Blackwell Publishing Ltd.

sequestrants, nicotinic acid, and clofibrate; these were neither remarkably effective nor conducive to good compliance. The evidence base for treatment was underwhelming: Epidemiologic data on serum cholesterol from the Seven Country Study [1] and from Framingham [2] were already highly suggestive, but the few completed clinical trials were underpowered and based on low-fat or modified-fat diets of limited effectiveness [3,4], and a further study was uncontrolled [5]. Not surprisingly some failed to provide evidence of benefit, and it was said at the time that the lipid hypothesis could not survive many more negative results. Fortunately the Oslo Heart Study [6], a secondary prevention trial, yielded moderately significant evidence of reduction in coronary heart disease (CHD) events from dietary intervention; taken together with the epidemiology, such information at least justified nutritional management of hypercholesterolemia.

Climate of Opinion

In the 1960s, it was a tenable position to regard the lipid hypothesis of CHD as unproven, but during the 1970s and 1980s, the power of newer epidemiologic data [7] and the growing number of prestatin trials [8–11] made it increasingly anachronistic to hold such a view. Some elements within the food industry devoted their resources to undermining the role of diet, though others saw commercial opportunities. Much senior medical opinion remained unconvinced [12], although the reasons offered varied with the passage of time, as certain earlier objections were invalidated by new knowledge [13]. However opinions polarized and the public was often confused by competing polemics.

Later, the concerns that inhibited appropriate management of hyperlipidemia were that cholesterol lowering (or existing low serum cholesterol) led to increased risk of cancer, depression, and non-medical deaths [14]. Such concerns were shown to be baseless [15,16] even before the statin trials of the 1990s offered full reassurance. It was not until 1994 that a convincing meta-analysis of earlier trials confirmed, beyond reasonable doubt, both the effectiveness [17] and the safety [16] of lipid lowering. A large number of CHD deaths worldwide would have been averted by earlier acceptance of the favorable effects of lipid-lowering treatment. Schopenhauer has told us how the truth is first ridiculed, then opposed, and finally regarded as self-evident.

Despite these factors, the workload at the Hammersmith Hospital lipid clinic was substantial from the start and it, with other clinics that soon opened in all CHD-prone communities, rapidly experienced overwhelming numbers of referrals. Clearly a considerable number of practicing primary care doctors, cardiologists, and vascular surgeons were satisfied by the evidence.

The Patient Profile

Widespread screening for hyperlipidemia and inclusion of cholesterol and triglyceride measurements in biochemical profiles are comparatively recent developments. Initially the common reasons for referral to lipid clinics were early onset cardiovascular disease (CVD) and such clinical manifestations of severe hyperlipidemia as cutaneous and tendon xanthomas, recurrent pancreatitis, and visibly lipemic blood samples. It became good practice to measure plasma lipids in diabetics. Interestingly, referrals from occupational health physicians soon became an important source of patients, a consequence of the longstanding interest of this specialty in preventive care.

Thereafter, as lipid testing became more general, less-severe hyperlipidemias outnumbered the major lipid disorders at lipid clinics. This was a reflection, firstly, of the understandable reluctance

of many nonspecialists to prescribe lipid-lowering drugs, and secondly of lack of time and skill in establishing effective dietary management. Currently the latter remains a serious deficiency and is a source of inappropriate use of lipid-lowering drugs.

At the present time, statins are widely prescribed by primary care doctors and cardiologists, analogous to the transfer of most antihypertensive care from hypertension clinics to these areas of practice. Without doubt, it is highly desirable that statins should be extensively and appropriately used in primary and cardiological settings. This trend has influenced the type of problems addressed by lipid specialists.

Side Effects of Lipid-Active Drugs

In current hyperlipidemia practice, a large number of patients are referred to lipid specialists for untoward effects caused by or arising during lipid-lowering medication. By far the most widely prescribed group of drugs is the statins, and their untoward effects have been well documented and excellently reviewed [18], providing considerable reassurance. Among these, the most common statin side-effect is musculoskeletal pain, usually distinguishable on clinical grounds from the far rarer classical statin myopathy, and accompanied by normal or insignificantly raised creatine kinase levels; all too frequently therapy is withdrawn from patients in whom statins are strongly indicated by virtue of existing CVD or high-risk status. Often treatment is withdrawn without creatine kinase measurement. Hence, the lipid specialist must distinguish, by careful history taking and examination, and on occasion by cautious rechallenge with a statin and frequent creatine kinase testing, between true statin myopathy and the real, far commoner and apparently benign entity of nonspecific pain in muscles or joints also related to statin treatment.

Options include continuing treatment with firm reassurance or the reintroduction of statin treatment with a lower dose of a more potent member of this class. Low-dose statin may valuably be combined with a nonstatin "assist" drug, but the potential for additional side-effects must be considered. Whichever course is adopted, close clinical and biochemical monitoring is required.

Inadequate Response to Treatment

The other frequent reason for referral to lipid specialists is an inadequate lipid response to treatment. Compliance requires careful evaluation and is addressed with varying success. Even with consistent compliance, there is remarkable individual variation in the lipid response both to diet and to medication. Inflexible algorithms do not take this into account, and it would also limit the usefulness of "polypill" formulations.

Variation in the effect of saturated fats on serum cholesterol level has long been recognized [19,20] and women respond somewhat less well to diet than men [21]. Differing responsiveness to dietary cholesterol has been studied extensively [22,23]. Variability in response to diet is one reason for the occasional disenchantment expressed concerning nutritional management of hyperlipidemia, and another likely reason is insufficient skill in dietary counseling. This is highly unfortunate, given that nutrition is a fundamental etiological factor in atherosclerotic CVD.

Having dealt with any compliance problems, the lipid specialist has several options. In diet-treated patients, a lipid-lowering drug is introduced if further reduction of lipid levels is indicated. Patients receiving one of the earlier statins benefit from substitution of a more efficacious member of this class of drugs, sometimes even at reduced dosage. This is more effective than increasing the statin dose, both because of the flat dose-response curve of these drugs, and because most statin side-effects are dose related. A further step is to introduce a drug combination, for example, adding to statin treatment ezetimibe or a nicotinic acid preparation or a fibrate.

Major Hyperlipidemias

The management of familial hypercholesterolemia (FH), remnant (type III) hyperlipidemia, and familial combined hyperlipidemia falls within the province of the lipid specialist, exclusively so in the author's opinion. This is necessary for a number of reasons. These disorders confer very high risk of early onset CVD. In FH, more than 50% of heterozygous men develop CHD by age 50 years [24] and young men have a 100-fold excess risk of CHD

[25]; hence, it is imperative to ensure maximum control of lipid levels by appropriate use of one or more drugs, together with dietary care. Severe hypertriglyceridemic states also require specialist care, in view of the high risk of acute pancreatitis.

In order to minimize risk, it is also essential to identify (clinically and biochemically) and to manage accompanying cardiovascular risk factors effectively. Health-related behavior needs ongoing supervision and competent guidance regarding exercise, diet, weight control, and smoking cessation.

Further, patients at high vascular risk require regular review to identify early clinical and subclinical CVD; for this purpose, detailed history taking and examination are supplemented by regular noninvasive investigations that may entail exercise stress electrocardiography, carotid ultrasound by a standardized protocol, lower-limb Doppler studies, myocardial perfusion scanning, and possibly 64-slice computed tomographic (CT) coronary angiography pending the advent of improved vascular imaging methods.

Case Finding of Major Hyperlipidemias

An extensive untapped opportunity exists to practice highly effective CVD prevention. At present the majority of persons in the population with FH remain undiagnosed, at least until they present with CHD [26]. The disease is usually transmitted as an autosomal dominant trait. The prevalence of other major lipid disorders such as remnant hyperlipidemia is lower, but affected individuals are also at high cardiovascular risk. There is good evidence that cascade screening of relatives of patients with definite and probable FH will identify many such persons [27]. There is also evidence that effective treatment of FH substantially reduces risk [28] and favorably affects coronary atherosclerosis [29]. Lipid clinics are well placed to undertake formal cascade screening; clearly the wider the scope of such case detection the better, and formal screening of relatives needs to be based also in cardiology centers and general practices [26]. Cascade screening for FH is a service that should be mandatory in every lipid clinic.

Therapeutic Goals

Therapeutic target levels of plasma lipids are cited in guidelines for cardiovascular risk reduction. These are based on placebo-controlled trials, but a few recent secondary prevention trials have been designed to compare different degrees of lipid lowering. The latter trial design will in due course provide a clearer idea of optimal lipid lowering. There is a comparative dearth of primary prevention trials on which to base the inadequately studied issue of lipid goals in primary prevention.

Until 1990, it was widely believed that secondary prevention by lipid lowering was implausible or impossible [30]. Atherosclerosis was assumed to be irreversible. Like so many myths, this was dispelled, first, by the demonstration that cholesterol lowering induced regression of atherosclerosis in laboratory animals [31], and in the 1980s and 1990s by comparable findings in human coronary arteries [32,33]. A meta-analysis of prestatin secondary prevention trials showed significant benefit from even limited lipid lowering [34]; this put secondary prevention on a firm footing and helped to place lipid lowering in the care of patients with clinically evident CVD at the forefront of preventive efforts. Historically, it was appropriate at that time to concentrate on secondary prevention, as was well recognized by manufacturers of lipid-lowering drugs. The relatively small cost of secondary prevention trials helped to generate more such trials than those of primary prevention. Nevertheless the larger goal is prevention of CVD in the population; and to achieve this a renewed effort is now required to address primary prevention, both at a clinical level and in the population.

Risk Estimation and the Decision to Medicate

All sets of guidelines have taken into account that a number of risk factors contribute to global CVD risk. Hence, lipid-lowering targets and indications for the use of lipid-lowering medication necessarily vary according to estimated global risk. Target values for lipid levels are reasonably consistent among current guidelines. However, the level of risk regarded as justifying drug treatment has varied considerably between guidelines. These in-

consistencies reflect the essentially arbitrary choice of levels of risk considered to merit drug treatment. Lipid targets and the risk threshold for using medication have also varied over the past 25 years, being revised downward to conform with the results of successive trials. Unfortunately, there is no objective way of identifying a risk threshold that quantitatively reflects a balance between the benefits of treatment, the risks of drug side-effects, and the cost of medication. Among current lipid-lowering drugs, the statins have an impressive safety record, but with vast and increasing numbers of people on treatment, a significant absolute number of serious side-effects must occur. Less-serious untoward effects sufficient to lead to withdrawal of treatment are common (nonspecific musculoskeletal pain, sleep disturbance, constipation, indigestion, depression, elevation of hepatocellular enzymes [18]); hence, every decision to prescribe long-term lipid-lowering drugs requires weighty consideration, and treatment entails ongoing supervision. When a statin is clearly indicated, efforts should be made to persevere with treatment while assisting the patient to cope with non-serious subjective untoward effects.

Guidelines, Treatment Algorithms, and Clinical Judgment

There is no easy way out of this impasse. Risk estimation is a necessary and valuable part of clinical decision making, but the experienced lipid specialist will also be guided by clinical judgment in making therapeutic decisions as to risk level and management. The ability of the patient to comply with treatment, factors such as business travel that limit dietary compliance, and biological (as opposed to chronological) aging are examples of nonquantifiable variables that cannot be built into treatment algorithms. The attitude of the patient to long-term preventive medication must be considered, as must his or her ability to understand the attendant risk/benefit considerations. Family history is a cogent risk factor and clinical experience shows that it is an overriding risk determinant in some patients in whom other risk factors are unremarkable. The severity of family history is not readily quantifiable. Fewer individuals at low-to-moderate risk will present clinically once more- effective efforts are made to address the societal causes of CVD by modifying health-related behavior to avoid overweight, restrict saturated fat consumption, increase soluble fiber use, and to instill suitable regular exercise habits. Numerous studies in controlled circumstances [35] and in free-living populations [8,32,36] have attested the considerable effect of such measures on lipid and lipoprotein levels; dietary measures, resembling these in part, can also substantially lower blood pressure [37]. Educational and legislative measures to enhance the fuller adoption of these approaches are urgently needed. These measures would lessen the inappropriate use of long-term medication. Regrettably the success of the statins has lessened interest in such means.

Having said this, it must be emphasized that statin-induced reduction in low-density lipoprotein (LDL)-cholesterol (LDL-C) is one of the most salient advances in modern medicine. A recent meta-analysis of over 90,000 participants in 14 statin trials confirms both the safety and the consistent substantial reduction in major cardiovascular events by lowering LDL-C, and the relation between the extent of LDL-C lowering and reduction in events [38].

Target levels are useful for didactic purposes and have been utilized in setting official constraints on lipid-lowering drug use, but they draw attention away from the fact that the relation between lipid levels (such as blood pressure) and cardiovascular risk is continuous and graded. To the uninitiated, they imply that lipid levels can be dichotomized into "normal" and "abnormal" ranges. Thus, the concepts of target levels, action limits, and normal ranges are potentially misleading to the nonexpert, for whom they are designed to offer guidance or algorithms to achieve correct treatment decisions. Although there is no credible way of teaching good practice without some recourse to such numbers, it is essential that these be offered explicitly to provide only a general indication. Both at the national level and in primary care practices, for example, cost-containing policies have sometimes been adopted that depend on a rigid protocol for treatment choices and can lead to injudicious treatment decisions. This applies equally to lipid or lipoprotein levels and to estimated global cardiovascular risk.

Risk estimates based on the epidemiology of the major risk factors will remain a valuable guide to management. For many years, it has been common practice to supplement this information by quantitative carotid ultrasound, which adds a measure of independent coronary event risk prediction. When noninvasive imaging of coronary and carotid atherosclerosis achieves sufficient resolving power, the detailed assessment of plaque morphology will become possible. Data may become available on plaque burden, lipid content, fibrous cap thickness, and inflammatory cell activity. Depending on evidence that such information improves outcome and on cost-effectiveness such data may strikingly improve our ability to allocate appropriate intervention.

Successive generations of guidelines have played important roles in helping the nonspecialist to manage hyperlipidemic patients with confidence. In specialist practice, however, clinical judgment reinforces decision making; realistically there is no other way to factor in some of the nonquantitative variables noted above, and no alternative when taking into account the continuous, graded nature of the lipid level–cardiovascular risk relationship. Errors of judgment can and will occur, but this approach permits the specialist is to treat the "whole patient." Imparting experience-based clinical acumen to the nonspecialist is a further responsibility of the expert in the lipid clinic (see the section "Medical Education," later in this chapter).

"Normal," "Optimal," "Desirable," and Physiological Lipid Levels

Based on the population mean plus two standard deviations, pathology reports 50 years ago often cited an upper limit for serum cholesterol level of 7.8 mmol/L (300 mg/dl). By the 1970s, the limit had been revised to 6.5 mmol/L (250 mg/dl), and in the guidelines of the late 1970s [39], the cholesterol limit had fallen to 5.2 mmol/L (200 mg/dl) in subjects at high risk. Even at that time, it was clear from Framingham data and case-control studies that a many CHD patients had levels below this value before the cardiac event.

With the advent of the statin trials therapeutic targets for LDL-C and total cholesterol have decreased progressively. Data is now available from end-point trials comparing different degrees of LDL-C reduction [40,41] and from imaging trials using intensive lipid-lowering regimens [42]. Currently many lipid specialists and cardiologists aim to lower the LDL-C of patients with overt CVD to no higher than about 1.5 mmol/L (60 mg/dl). With currently available drugs, such levels are achievable in most patients, if necessary using drug combinations.

It is highly likely that the downward trend in recommended goals for lipid-lowering therapy will continue further. A recent analysis [43] of the results of the Treating New Targets (TNT) secondary prevention trial found that the incidence of CVD events increased directly with in-trial LDL cholesterol from the lowest quintile to the highest; mean LDL cholesterol in the lowest quintile was only 53.9 mg/dl (1.39 mmol/L). Confirmation of this finding in further trials of intensive lipid-lowering treatment will justify yet another downward revision of target levels in secondary prevention. Pending solid data for determining goals for primary prevention, it will be a reasonable implication that current primary prevention targets also need to be lowered.

It has been plausibly proposed that future target levels for LDL-C may approximate to putative human physiological concentrations [44]. Mean non-high-density lipoprotein (HDL)-cholesterol (HDL-C) in rural Chinese cantons is as low as 1.04 mmol/L (40.1 mg/dl) [45] and levels of LDL-C in human neonates are similar or even lower.

Regrettably the evidence on which to base recommendations for primary prevention is comparatively sparse. Despite the historical reasons for focusing on secondary prevention, primary prevention of CVD is self-evidently the goal of paramount importance. It is usually held that less rigorous targets are acceptable, and in most guidelines these are graded according to the number of non-lipid risk factors or, more recently, on estimates of CVD risk. Such recommendations may be appropriate but are insufficiently supported by solid evidence. The introduction of genetic markers of risk such as the 9p21.3 mutation [46] will inevitably sharpen risk prediction and allocation of appropriate therapy. Undeniably, the fractional reduction in CVD events achieved by lipid lowering is small in patients at low-to-moderate absolute global risk. However,

there are large numbers of such persons in the CVD-prone community, and a small percentage reduction translates into many preventable events [47]. A significant element in the prevailing threshold to drug treatment is concerns for side effects. However cogent the cost implications are to health administrators, Hippocratic considerations are a higher priority.

Cardiovascular Disease Prevention

The foregoing account of the development of the lipid clinic traces the initiation and growth of a novel and valuable area of clinical practice, specialization in lipid disorders. Expertise in other cardiovascular risk factors, particularly in hypertension and diabetes, has a longer history. In this section. the future of the lipid physician is discussed, and the prospect will be addressed that the lipid clinic, as a specific entity directed to one single risk factor, may now change direction.

The preceding sections are intended to document the scope of and demanding nature of practice in lipid disorders. Yet it is abundantly evident that the causation of cardiovascular diseases is multifactorial [7]; hence, a case can be made for subsuming selective attention to one risk factor into a multidisciplinary CVD prevention service. It goes without saying that lipid physicians are fully aware of the need to deal with all modifiable risk factors and many may be competent in several areas. The patient presenting with a single risk factor is frequently found to have other sources of risk or may develop other risk factors during treatment of the presenting abnormality. The case in favor of a multidisciplinary service is that this setting will ensure access by such a patient to the maximum level of expertise within a single clinic or institution, and preferably during a single visit. Additionally, the range of expertise ensures that advances in each discipline are promptly translated into patient care. A further efficiency is that some ancillary services and staff are common to the management of several risk factors, including dietetics, vascular imaging and other cardiovascular investigations, and nursing and reception personnel.

A design for a cardiovascular prevention service of this type was developed jointly by the author and Associate Professor DR Sullivan at Sydney University from 2005 to 2006 and a pilot service was inaugurated by the latter at the Royal Prince Alfred Hospital in 2007.

The requisite range of areas of expertise includes hypertension and hyperlipidemia management, smoking cessation/prevention, glucose intolerance/diabetes, and nutritional counseling. A cascade screening facility is essential. Many patients referred to such a service will have or be suspected of having overt end-organ CVD. Where possible, therefore, hypertension care should be provided by a cardiologist, in order to provide ready access to this specialty within the auspices of the same service and to focus requests for cardiovascular investigations.

In such a context, the lipid specialist continues to practice within his or her area and enjoys prompt and free recourse to related areas of specialization. The scope for clinical research in the area of lipid disorders remains, and the opportunity for multidisciplinary research is enhanced.

Medical Education

Many areas of clinical medicine have a role to play in prevention of CVD. Among these, primary care occupies a central position, in part because of the opportunity provided by frequent contact with patients. Among the elderly and middle-aged, a majority consult their primary care doctor at least once a year for routine attention or intercurrent problems. This affords a valuable opportunity to obtain information on personal history, family history, smoking, diet, exercise, blood pressure, body weight, and lipid and HDL-C levels. No other medical practitioner has a greater chance of assessing and managing risk factors than the primary care physician.

Undergraduate teaching and continuing medical education need to provide adequate attention to and interest in this aspect of preventive care. The CVD prevention center and the lipid clinic can and should provide such teaching at its most sophisticated level. The work of the lipid clinic was in the past regarded as somewhat esoteric, and in many countries, expertise in lipid disorders is not yet registerable as an area of specialization. The

educational role of lipid clinics and cardiovascular prevention services needs to be emphasized, and teaching by physicians working in this area is often an untapped resource in imparting clinical skills and judgment. A necessary component of a strategy for reducing the burden of cardiovascular disease is to extend training in the skills required to detect and manage lipid and other risk factors competently.

Risk Reduction in the Community

An extension of the role of lipid specialists and other physicians involved in cardiovascular disease prevention is to influence public policy. They are well placed to offer guidance as to the wise allocation of limited resources, the most burdensome problem faced by health administrators. The cost effectiveness of preventive measures, including statin therapy, is increasingly appreciated by such officials, but there is much scope for improvement in preventive care at the population level. The dramatic decline in CHD deaths that occurred in the 1970s and 1980s in Australia, the United States, Finland, and some other countries has slowed in many places. While great progress has been achieved in reducing the number of cigarette smokers in men (though not in women) intake of saturated fat by most populations has fallen to a less impressive extent. It is widely anticipated that the burgeoning epidemic of obesity and overweight may reverse the downward trend in cardiovascular deaths.

Thus, innovative measures are required in the areas of public education and in controls on the food and tobacco industries if public health policy is to resume the progress made 20–40 years ago. Guidance from specialists in cardiovascular preventive care is needed to maximize the effective use of resources.

Conclusions

Forty years of lipid clinic experience have created a new area of clinical specialization in lipid disorders. The subject has evolved from a recherché topic to a widely practiced one with a sound scientific and clinical base. The foregoing review attests the complexity of the problems facing physicians in this field. It is timely for practice in this area to be recognized as a registerable specialty within internal medicine.

Selected References

15. Lewis B, Tikkanen MJ. Low blood total cholesterol and mortality: causality, consequence and confounders. Amer J Cardiol 1994;73:80–5.

26. Watts GF, Lewis B, Sullivan DR. Familial hypercholesterolemia: a missed opportunity in preventive medicine. Nature Clin Practice 2007;4:2–3.

27. Marks D, Wonderling D, Thorogood M, Lambert H, Humphries SE, Neil HAW. Cost-effectiveness analysis of different approaches of screening for familial hypercholesterolaemia. Brit Med J 2002;324:1303–08.

28. Simon Broome Steering Committee on behalf of the Simon Broome Register Group. Mortality in treated heterozygous familial hypercholesterolaemia: implications for clinical management. Atherosclerosis 1999;142: 105–12.

38. Cholesterol Treatment Trialists (CTT) Collaborators. Efficacy and safety of cholesterol-lowering treatment: prospective meta-analysis of data from 90 056 participants in 14 randomised trials of statins. Lancet 2005; 366:1267–78.

SECTION IV

Nutrition, Hypertension, and Cardiovascular Disease

CHAPTER 33

From Abdominal Adiposity to Hypertension: Mechanisms and Clinical Implications

Albert P. Rocchini
University of Michigan, Ann Arbor, MI, USA

Introduction

Obesity, and visceral adiposity in particular, is often associated with systemic hypertension. This chapter describes the evidence that links obesity and visceral adiposity in particular, to hypertension, the potential mechanisms relating visceral obesity and the development of hypertension, and the clinical implications of the association of visceral obesity and hypertension.

Relationship between Obesity and High Blood Pressure

Epidemiologic Studies Linking Obesity to Hypertension

The association between obesity and hypertension has been recognized since the early 1900s. Many large epidemiologic studies document the association between increasing body weight and an increase in blood pressure [1–3]. For example, the Framingham study [1] documented that the prevalence of hypertension in obese individuals was twice that of average-weight individuals. This relationship was seen in all age-groups of both women and men. Based on this and many other population-based studies [1–3], we know that there is a very strong association between obesity and hypertension in both sexes, in all age-groups, and for virtually every geographical and ethnic group.

Nutritional and Metabolic Bases of Cardiovascular Disease, 1st edition.
Edited by Mario Mancini, José M. Ordovas, Gabriele Riccardi,
Paolo Rubba and Pasquale Strazzullo. © 2011 Blackwell Publishing Ltd.

Relationship of Weight Gain to Blood Pressure Level

There have been no studies in humans that have looked at the effect of weight gain on blood pressure. However, in the dog, it has been shown that weight gain is directly associated with an increase in blood pressure. In 1938, Cash and Wood demonstrated that weight gain caused dogs with renal vascular hypertension to further increase their blood pressure. More recently, Rocchini et al. [4] and Hall et al. [5] reported that normal mongrel dogs fed a high-fat diet gained weight and developed hypertension. In these dogs, the hypertension was associated with sodium retention, hyperinsulinemia, and activation of the sympathetic nervous system.

Effect of Weight Loss on Blood Pressure Level

Weight loss is associated with a lowering of blood pressure. Many clinical trials that have been published since the late 1970s have clearly documented the blood pressure-lowering effect of weight loss [6–8]. For example, the Hypertension Prevention Trial [7] documented that in individuals with borderline elevations in blood pressure a mean weight loss of 5 kg was associated with as much as a 5/3 mm Hg decrease in blood pressure. Thus, based on numerous weight loss studies, calorie restriction and weight loss are associated with a reduction in blood pressure. In addition, it is clear that even modest weight loss (i.e., 10% of body weight) improves blood pressure, and many individuals achieve normal blood pressure levels without attaining their calculated ideal weight.

A limitation with the use of studies documenting that weight loss is associated with a reduction in blood pressure is that most studies do not address the long-term effect of weight change on blood pressure in subjects who are again placed on unrestricted diets. Dornfield et al. [9] reported that over a follow-up of 1–4 years after weight loss, changes in blood pressure still correlate with changes in body weight. However, bariatric surgery data suggests that long-term weight loss may not reduce the incidence of hypertension. Sjostrom et al. [10] compared the incidence of hypertension and diabetes in 346 patients undergoing gastric surgery with 346 obese control subjects who were matched on 18 variables. After 8 years, the surgical group had maintained a 16% weight loss, whereas the control subjects had a 1% weight gain. These investigators demonstrated that the weight reduction in the surgical group had a dramatic effect on the 8-year incidence of diabetes but had no effect on the 8-year incidence of hypertension. They previously documented that surgical weight loss positively affected blood pressure at 2 and 4 years of follow-up, but that this effect on blood pressure was lost after 8 years of follow-up despite a maintained 16% weight reduction. These authors have speculated "that remaining obesity in the surgically treated patients could have induced a reappearance of hypertension during the course of the study independent of initial body weight and initial weight loss." Therefore, Sjostrom's study suggests that a relapse of hypertension after surgically induced weight loss does occur despite the maintenance of significant long-term weight loss and that the pathogenesis of recurrent hypertension is not well understood [10].

Effect of Body Fat Distribution on Blood Pressure

The definition of obesity also contributes to the controversy regarding the independence of obesity as an etiological determinant of hypertension. Obesity is defined not just as an increase in body weight but rather as an increase in adipose tissue mass. Adipose tissue mass can be estimated by multiple techniques such as skinfold thickness, body mass index (BMI, [weight in kg]/[height in meters]^2), hydrostatic weighing, bioelectrical impedance, water dilution methods, computed tomography (CT), and magnetic resonance imaging (MRI). In most clinical studies, BMI is usually used as the index of adiposity. Obesity is generally defined as a BMI of greater than $30 kg/m^2$. In 1956, Jean Vague reported that the cardiovascular and metabolic consequences of obesity were greatest in individuals whose fat distribution pattern favored the upper body segments. Since that observation, several population-based studies have demonstrated that abdominal obesity is a more important cardiovascular risk factor than BMI alone [3,11], thus, suggesting that increased visceral adipose tissue (VAT) as opposed to subcutaneous adipose tissue (SAT) relates better to the development of systemic hypertension. For example, Fox et al. [3] demonstrated in 3,001 participants from the Framingham Heart Study, that although both SAT and VAT are associated with the prevalence of hypertension, only VAT provides significant information above and beyond percent fat and waist circumference. Many investigators have demonstrated that the association of obesity to increased cardiovascular risk is also primarily related to abdominal adiposity [11]. Finally, in dogs that develop hypertension by being fed a high-fat diet, the increase in their abdominal circumference is significantly greater than that of their thoracic circumference [12]. MRI studies in these fat-fed dogs demonstrate a marked increase in omental and subcutaneous fat [13]. We also have preliminary data in dogs fed a high-fat diet that demonstrates a stronger relationship between the increase in blood pressure and the increase in abdominal circumference as compared to the increase in body weight.

Mechanism Whereby Obesity Might Cause Hypertension

Although there is a strong relation between hypertension, obesity, and abdominal obesity in particular, the mechanism whereby increased adiposity leads to the development of hypertension has not been completely elucidated. It is clear that obesity hypertension directly relates to abnormal renal sodium handling and that this alteration in sodium handling is predominately mediated through activation of the sympathetic nervous system and to a lesser extent through activation of the renin-angiotensin-aldosterone system. However, what is less clear is how obesity initiates the activation of the sympathetic nervous system.

Abnormal Renal Sodium Handling and Obesity Hypertension

There is ample human and animal data linking obesity hypertension to fluid retention. Many investigators have reported that obesity is associated with an increased cardiac output and blood volume. Rocchini et al. [8] demonstrated that prior to weight loss, the blood pressure of a group of obese adolescents was very sensitive to dietary sodium intake; however, after weight loss, the obese adolescent lost their blood pressure sensitivity to sodium. These investigators demonstrated that when compared to nonobese adolescents, the obese adolescents have a renal-function relation (plot of urinary sodium excretion as a function of arterial pressure) that has a shallower slope. The renal-function relationship is also normalized by weight loss (Figure 33.1).

In addition, abdominal adiposity is associated with altered renal tubular sodium handling. Strazzullo et al. [14,15] measured proximal and distal fractional sodium reabsorption in 702 participants of the Olivetti Heart Study. These investigators demonstrated in adult men that the metabolic syndrome was associated with an increased rate of proximal tubular sodium reabsorption. Similarly Barbato et al. [16] demonstrated that

increased proximal sodium reabsorption is associated with the metabolic syndrome in both white men and women; however, this relationship is not seen in people of African or South Asian origin, even though these two ethnic groups have a greater degree of insulin resistance and central adiposity. These investigators could not prove why alter proximal tubular sodium reabsorption was not observed in individuals of African or Asian origin; however they speculated that it could be due to differences in habitual sodium intake, differences in genetic background.

There is also animal data that suggests that sodium retention is associated with obesity hypertension. In a dog model of obesity-induced hypertension, Rocchini et al. [4] demonstrated that during the first week of the high-fat diet, the increase in sodium retention appeared to best relate to an increase in plasma norepinephrine (NE) activity, whereas during the latter weeks of the high-fat diet, an increase in plasma insulin appeared to be the best predictor of sodium retention. Rocchini also demonstrated that the hypertension associated with weight gain in the dog occurs only if adequate salt is present in the diet. Hall et al. [17] demonstrated that obesity-induced hypertension in the dog is associated with increased renal tubular sodium reabsorption since marked sodium retention occurred despite large increases in glomerular filtration and renal plasma flow. Ganger et al. [18] demonstrated

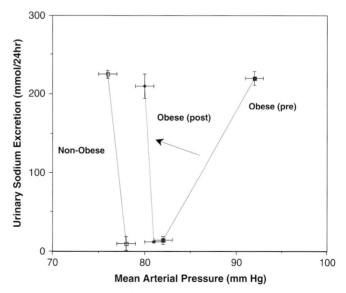

Figure 33.1 Renal-function relations for 18 nonobese and 60 obese adolescents before a weight loss program and the 36 obese adolescents who lost weight during a 20-week weight loss program. In comparison with the nonobese adolescents' renal function relation, the obese adolescents' renal function relation has a shallow slope (p < .001). In those who lost weight, the slope increased (arrow). This increase was due to a decrease in the mean arterial pressure during the 2 weeks of the high-salt diet. (Reproduced from Rocchini et al. N Engl J Med 1989;321:580–5, with permission.)

that dogs fed a high-fat diet develop an abnormal renal pressure-natriuresis relationship similar to that observed in obese adolescents.

The relationship between urinary sodium excretion and mean arterial pressure can be altered by intrinsic and extrinsic factors that are known to affect the ability of the kidney to excrete sodium. Factors that produce alterations in the renal-function curves are constriction of the renal arteries and arterioles, changes in glomerular filtration coefficients, changes in the rate of tubular reabsorption, reduced renal mass, and changing levels of renin-angiotensin activation, aldosterone, vasopressin, insulin, sympathetic nervous system activation, and atrial natriuretic hormone. Although both obese humans and animals can have compression of the kidney by the surrounding fat and that fat may penetrate the renal hilum into the sinuses surrounding the renal medulla [19], it is unlikely that fat-based structural changes in the kidney is the major pathophysiological cause of the renal sodium retention associated with obesity. Based on both human and animal data, activation of the renin-angiotensin-aldosterone system and that of the sympathetic nervous system are the most likely factors responsible for the altered renal function curves observed in obesity.

Renin-Angiotensin-Aldosterone System

The renin-angiotensin-aldosterone system is an important determinant of efferent glomerular arteriolar tone, and tubular sodium reabsorption. Its activity is modulated by dietary salt ingestion, blood pressure, and the sympathetic nervous system. Therefore, alterations in the renin-angiotensin-aldosterone system could be expected to alter pressure natriuresis. Enhanced activity of the renin-angiotensin-aldosterone system has been reported in obese humans and dogs [18,20,21]. Granger et al. [18] reported that plasma renin activity is 170% higher in obese dogs than in control dogs.

Aldosterone concentrations have been demonstrated to be abnormal in both human and animal obesity [4,21]. For example, Rocchini et al. [21] measured supine and 2-hour upright plasma renin activity and aldosterone in 10 nonobese and 30 obese adolescents before and after a 20-week weight loss program. The obese adolescents had significantly higher supine and 2-hour upright aldosterone concentrations. Although plasma renin activity was not significantly different between the two groups of adolescents, they observed that a given increment in plasma renin activity produced a greater increment in aldosterone in the obese adolescents. Compared with an obese control group, weight loss resulted in both a significant decrease in plasma aldosterone and a significant decrease in the slope of the posture-induced relation between plasma renin activity and aldosterone. Goodfriend and Calhoun [22] suggested that increased plasma free fatty acids (FFAs) produced in obese individuals may stimulate aldosterone production independent of renin.

Insulin also has been shown to influence the renin-angiotensin-aldosterone system in both normal subjects and in patients with diabetes. For example, Rocchini et al. [20] measured the increase in plasma aldosterone after graded increases in intravenous angiotensin II before and after euglycemic hyperinsulinemia in seven chronically instrumented dogs. Euglycemic hyperinsulinemia resulted in a significantly greater ($p < .01$) change in the angiotensin II–stimulated increments of plasma aldosterone than was observed when angiotensin II was administered alone. However, there was no dose-dependence of insulin's effect on angiotensin II–stimulated aldosterone. In addition, although weight gain significantly increased angiotensin II–stimulated aldosterone, with hyperinsulinemia the response was not significantly different than that observed in the dogs prior to weight gain.

Despite these results suggesting that obesity is associated with significant alterations in the renin-angiotensin-aldosterone system, Hall et al. [17] demonstrated that weight-related changes in blood pressure can occur in dogs independent of changes in angiotensin II, and de Paula et al. [23] demonstrated that the aldosterone antagonist, eplerenone, attenuated but did not prevent the sodium retention and hypertension associated with feeding dogs a high fat diet. Thus, although the renin-angiotensin-aldosterone system plays an important role in the pathogenesis of obesity hypertension, it is neither the major nor the sole mechanism responsible for the altered renal pressure–natriuresis relationship observed in obesity.

Sympathetic Nervous System

For over 20 years, it has been recognized that diet affects the sympathetic nervous system. Fasting suppresses sympathetic nervous system activity, whereas overfeeding with either a high-carbohydrate or a high-fat diet stimulates the sympathetic nervous system [24,25]. It is believed that the physiological consequence of the link between dietary intake and sympathetic nervous system activity is to regulate energy expenditure in a hope to maintain weight homeostasis. Landsberg [25] suggested that in obese individuals the sympathetic nervous system is chronically activated in an attempt to prevent further weight gain and that hypertension is a byproduct of the overactive sympathetic nervous system. Landsberg [25] proposed that obesity produces a compensatory sympathetic activation, which contributes to the cardiovascular morbidity associated with it. Microneurography, which directly measures sympathetic traffic to skeletal muscle, has consistently shown to be increased in obesity [26]. Previous studies in obese subjects have reported a positive association between sympathetic activity and increased blood pressure. We have preliminary data demonstrating that over six weeks of feeding dogs a high fat diet that although serial plasma NE concentrations only trended toward increasing ($p = .09$); however, using serial NE kinetic studies, we observed a significant ($p < .001$) increase in the rate of NE release from the sympathetic nerve terminals (NE_2). The most likely reason that we did not demonstrate a significant increase in plasma NE levels was because in addition to the increased rate of NE release from the sympathetic nerve terminals, we also observed a significant increase in NE clearance. In addition, after 6 weeks of the high-fat diet, there was a strong relationship between the increase in NE_2 and the increase in arterial pressure. In the fat-fed dog, Kassab et al. [27] demonstrated that renal denervation prevents both the sodium retention and the hypertension associated with weight gain but does not prevent insulin resistance. In addition, Eikelis et al. [28], using regional analysis of NE kinetics, demonstrated increased renal NE spillover in obese subjects. In both animal and human studies, pharmacologic blockade of the sympathetic nervous system prevents the increase in blood pressure and sodium retention associated with obesity [29,30].

Finally, Lohmeier et al. [31] demonstrated that fat feeding of dogs causes a marked increase in activity of the protein product of the immediate early gene *c*-fos in the baroreceptor sympathoexcitatory cells in the rostral ventrolateral medulla, a site known to be affected by both angiotensin II and leptin. Increased gene *c*-fos expression in the rostral ventrolateral medulla of obese dogs supports the observations that sympathetic activity to the kidney and other vascular beds is increased in obesity hypertension [27,28]. Thus, activation of the sympathetic nervous systems appears to be one of the major factors responsible for both the altered renal-function relationship and hypertension observed in obesity. However, what is still unknown is what is the factor or factors responsible for activation of the sympathetic nervous system in obesity.

Possible Mechanisms Responsible for Activation of the Sympathetic Nervous System in Obesity

Since increased VAT appears to be the best predictor of hypertension [3], it is likely that increased sympathetic activation is related to the metabolically active adipose tissue found in the visceral region. VAT is known to secrete FFAs, adipocytokines, and inflammatory cytokines into the portal circulation. Three possible mechanisms that may be responsible for the increase in sympathetic nervous system activity associated with obesity are increased FFA levels in the portal circulation, increased adipocytokines and inflammatory cytokines, and/or increased secretion of leptin.

Increased Portal FFA and Sympathetic Activation

Increased portal FFA may increase sympathetic activity through the development of insulin resistance and hyperinsulinemia. Arner et al. [32] first suggested that the release into the portal vein of FFAs originating from visceral fat might be responsible for the development of insulin resistance. There are a number of reports demonstrating that increasing FFAs by the infusion of a lipid emulsion leads, within hours, to substantial insulin resistance. Griffin et al. [33] demonstrated that FFAs interfere with insulin signaling at the level of a serine kinase cascade involving protein kinase C-θ, leading to defects in insulin signaling and glucose transport. Kabir et al. [34] demonstrated in dogs fed a moderate-fat diet for 12 weeks increased gene expression promoting lipid accumulation and lipolysis in visceral fat, as well as elevated rate-limiting gluconeogenic enzyme expression in the liver as evidence in favor of the portal FFA hypothesis. Their laboratory has previously shown that on this diet, the dogs develop an inability of insulin to completely suppress hepatic glucose production during euglycemic, physiologically hyperinsulinemic conditions.

Many investigators have documented that euglycemic hyperinsulinemia in both normal and obese humans and animals causes activation of the sympathetic nervous system as documented by increases in heart rate, blood pressure, and plasma NE [20,25,35]. It also has been shown that hyperinsulinemia in normal humans is associated not only with an increase in circulating catecholamines but also with an increase in sympathetic nerve activity [35]. However, it is unlikely in obesity that either hyperinsulinemia or insulin resistance is responsible for activation of the sympathetic nervous system or the subsequent development of hypertension since insulin resistance and hypertension are dissociated from each other [36]. When fat-fed dogs were treated with aspirin, an inhibitor of nuclear factor-κB (NF-κB) activation, insulin resistance did not develop as the dogs became obese, but the dogs still developed hypertension. Similarly, when fat-fed dogs were treated with α- and β-blockade using prazosin and atenolol, hypertension did not develop as the dogs became obese, but the dogs still developed insulin resistance. Finally, in humans, long-term weight loss induced by bariatric surgery corrects the insulin resistance and hyperinsulinemia but does not prevent the hypertension [10].

A second explanation for how increased portal FFA could lead to activation of the sympathetic nervous system is that there is a known feedback mechanism relating FFA production and the sympathetic nervous system, whereby delivery of FFAs into the circulation results in sympathetic activation and conversely, sympathetic activity stimulates lipolysis. Grekin et al. [37] demonstrated that chronic portal venous infusion of oleate solution and other long-chain fatty acids have a pressor effect that is mediated by the α-adrenergic component of the sympathetic nervous system. Thus, increased portal FFAs could be responsible for the initiation of both the hypertension and insulin resistance associated with obesity.

Increase Inflammatory Cytokines Levels in the Portal Circulation Leading to Sympathetic Activation

Visceral fat secretes substances such as tumor necrosis factor-α (TNF-α), interleukin-6 (IL-6), or decreased adiponectin that may induce both insulin resistance and activation of the sympathetic nervous system. TNF-α and other proinflammatory cytokines elicit a broad spectrum of biological responses via their peripheral and central nervous system effects. Because blood-borne cytokines are too large to readily cross the blood–brain barrier, one possible route by which circulating cytokines might stimulate sympathetic activation is through activation of visceral sensory afferent nerves, particularly the abdominal vagus [38]. In addition, systemically administered cytokines are known to increase splenic and lumbar sympathetic activity.

Adipocytokines secreted by visceral fat may also play a role in the sympathetic activation associated with obesity. Low levels of both ghrelin and adiponectin have been reported to be associated with hypertension. In addition Lin et al. [39] showed that ghrelin acts in the nucleus of the solitary tract to suppress renal sympathetic activity and to decrease arterial pressure.

In summary, the potential role of abdominally derived inflammatory cytokines and adipocytokines in obesity hypertension and activation of the sympathetic nervous system remains controversial because of the limited amount of available data on the interaction between these substances and arterial pressure.

Increased Secretion of Leptin as a Cause for Increased Sympathetic Activity in Obesity

Recent evidence from Eikelis and Esler [40] suggests that leptin may be the link between excess adiposity and increased cardiovascular sympathetic activity. Plasma leptin concentrations are known to correlate with the level of obesity. Since Eikelis et al.

[40] reported that the rate of leptin clearance from plasma and the plasma leptin half-life are unrelated to adiposity, the increase in plasma leptin observed in obesity is due to increased synthesis and not due to a decrease in leptin clearance.

Using simultaneous arteriovenous blood sampling, Eikelis et al. [28] demonstrated that the increase in plasma leptin concentration in obese individuals is not from either the heart (since there is no overflow of leptin into the coronary sinus) or the portal circulation (since there was no net release of leptin into the hepatic veins), but rather it is from peripheral adipose tissue and from the leptin produced in the brain and secreted into the systemic circulation.

Leptin and the sympathetic nervous system are intimately linked. There is a direct interaction between leptin and the sympathetic nervous system, leptin acting within the hypothalamus to cause activation of the central sympathetic outflow and stimulation of the adrenal medulla to release epinephrine. While leptin has been shown in animals to be associated with an increased sympathetic outflow to the kidney, adipose tissue, and skeletal muscle, Eikelis et al. [28] demonstrated in humans that of the measures of sympathoadrenal function tested, only total and renal NE spillover rates correlated with leptin secretion rate. In addition, Galletti et al. [41] demonstrated in a sample of originally normotensive men that circulating leptin level, independent of BMI and insulin resistance, was a significant predictor of the risk of developing hypertension over an 8-year period of follow-up. This data and the report of Kassab et al. [27] that renal sympathetic denervation prevents the fluid retention and hypertension in the fat-fed dog is consistent with but does not prove the hypothesis that leptin may be a major factor responsible for the increased sympathetic activation observed in obesity. However, since leptin has been shown to be equally if not more correlated to SAT compared to VAT, leptin does not complete fit the observation of Fox et al. [3] that hypertension is more associated with VAT than with SAT in obese individuals.

In summary, based on animal and human data the best hypothesis for the mechanism of obesity hypertension is that with increasing adiposity, the combination of FFA, adipocytokines, and inflammatory cytokines secreted from visceral adipocytes

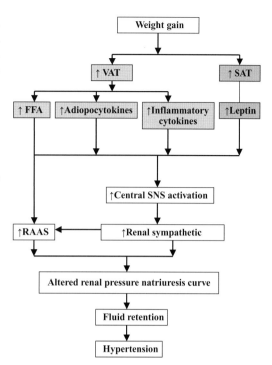

Figure 33.2 A schematic representation of the proposed mechanism of obesity hypertension. (VAT: visceral adipose tissue; SAT: subcutaneous adipose tissue; FFA: free fatty acid; RAAS: renin-angiotensin-aldosterone system; SNS: sympathetic nervous system.)

and leptin secreted from peripheral and brain adipocytes results in central activation of the sympathetic nervous system producing increased renal sympathetic activity that results in activation of the renin-angiotensin-aldosterone system, fluid retention, and ultimately in the development of systemic hypertension (Figure 33.2).

Therapeutic Implications

Weight loss is the cornerstone of hypertensive management in the obese individual. Weight loss in both adolescents and adults improves all of the cardiovascular abnormalities associated with obesity, including hypertension, dyslipidemia, and sodium retention, structural abnormalities in resistant vessels, and left ventricular hypertrophy and dysfunction. It is also important to realize that the method by which weight loss is accomplished is important. Although weight loss in general results in a drop in resting systolic/diastolic blood pressure and heart rate, when the weight loss is incorporated with physical conditioning, the greatest decrease in resting systolic blood pressure, peak exercise diastolic pressure, and heart rate can be achieved [42]. Similarly, a weight loss program that incorporates exercise along with caloric restriction produces the most favorable effects on insulin resistance, dyslipidemia and vascular reactivity [42]. Endurance training in obese and nonobese individuals improves insulin resistance, in part, by increasing muscle oxidative capacity and increasing capillary density.

Although weight loss and exercise are the cornerstones of blood pressure management in obese hypertensive individuals, most obese individuals are either unable or unwilling to lose weight or are unable to keep from regaining lost weight. Therefore, pharmacological therapy is frequently required in the hypertensive obese individual. When choosing an antihypertensive agent, it is important to remember that in addition to hypertension, most patients with obesity have other cardiovascular risk factors that ought to be taken into account. Based on the proposed mechanism of obesity hypertension outlined in Figure 33.2, the three major classes of antihypertensive medicines that might be expected to be efficacious in the treatment of obesity hypertension are: diuretics, blockers of the renin-angiotensin-aldosterone system, and sympatholytic agents.

Although thiazide diuretics are one of the most common antihypertensive agents, they are known to impair insulin sensitivity, glucose tolerance, and pancreatic insulin secretion and to increase total and LDL-C. Perhaps the best diuretic to be used in individuals with obesity hypertension is a mineralocorticoid receptor antagonist. de Paula et al. [23] demonstrated that eplerenone, a selective mineralocorticoid receptor antagonist, significantly attenuated the hypertension associated with feeding dogs a high-fat diet. However, Amador et al. [43] demonstrated that although spironolactone decreases arterial pressure in obese subjects it did not reduce heart sympathetic overactivity or left ventricular mass.

The angiotensin I–converting enzyme (ACE) inhibitors and angiotensin II receptor blockers are another class of antihypertensives that would be expected to be effective in treating obesity hypertension. Animal studies have demonstrated that block-

ade of the renin-angiotensin-aldosterone system can attenuate the hypertension associated with obesity [17,23]. In addition, ACE inhibitors also have been reported to improve glucose metabolism and insulin resistance in obese hypertensive individuals. Amador et al. [43] demonstrated that losartan, an angiotensin II receptor blocker, not only effectively lowers blood pressure in obese individuals but also causes regression of left ventricular hypertrophy and decreases cardiac sympathetic overactivity.

The third class of antihypertensives that would be expected to be effective in treating obesity hypertension is the sympatholytic agents. In both animal and human studies, blockade of the sympathetic nervous system with α- and β-adrenergic blockade prevents the increase in blood pressure associated with obesity [29,36]. However, β-blockers are known to impair insulin resistance, are associated with a twofold to threefold higher risk of diabetes mellitus and are associated with a significant lowering of HDL-C. On the other hand, α_1-blockers are reported to improve glucose metabolism and insulin resistance. However, the sympatholytic agents that appear to be most efficacious in obesity hypertension are the centrally acting α_2-agonists and the centrally acting selective imidazoline agonists. Rocchini et al. [29] have demonstrated that clonidine, a centrally acting α_2-agonist, not only prevented the hypertension associated with obesity in the dog but also prevented the development of insulin resistance. Giugliano et al. [44] demonstrated that transdermal clonidine was effective in reducing blood pressure and improving insulin resistance in hypertensive individuals with non-insulin-dependent diabetes mellitus. In addition, moxonidine, a centrally active imidazoline receptor agonist, improves hypertension, glycemic control, and endothelial dysfunction and also may reduce weight in obese hypertensive individuals [45].

Conclusions

Although weight loss is the cornerstone of hypertensive management in the obese individual, many individuals will also require pharmacologic therapy. When choosing an antihypertensive medication it is important to individualize the agent to the patient. Some agents such as thiazide diuretics and β-blockers can impair glucose tolerance and adversely alter plasma lipid levels, whereas ACE inhibitors, angiotensin II receptor blockers, and centrally acting sympathetic agents improve the hypertension, insulin resistance, and many of the other cardiovascular risk factors associated with obesity hypertension.

Acknowledgment

Supported in part by grants 1RO1 HL 52205, HL-18575, 2RO1-HL-35743, 2P60 AM 20572, and 2P01HL18575-24 from the National Institutes of Health.

Selected References

8. Rocchini AP, Key J, Bondie D, et al. The effect of weight loss on the sensitivity of blood pressure to sodium in obese adolescents. N Engl J Med 1989;321:580–5.

19. Hall JE. The kidney, hypertension and obesity. Hypertension 2003;41:625–33.

27. Kassab S, Kato T, Wilkins C, et al. Renal denervation attenuates the sodium retention and hypertension associated with obesity. Hypertension 1995;25[part2]:893–97.

29. Rocchini AP, Mao HZ, Babu K, et al. Clonidine prevents insulin resistance and hypertension in obese dogs. Hypertension 1999;33:548–53.

36. Rocchini AP, Yang Q, Gokee A. Hypertension and insulin resistance are not directly related in obese dogs. Hypertension 2004;43:1011–6.

CHAPTER 34

Role of the Adipose-Tissue Renin-Angiotensin-Aldosterone System in Obesity and Obesity-Associated Hypertension

Stefan Engeli

Hannover Medical School, Hannover, Germany

Introduction

The renin-angiotensin-aldosterone system (RAAS) is a complex system with many components. In brief, the precursor angiotensinogen (AGT) is cleaved subsequently by renin and the angiotensin-converting enzyme (ACE) yielding angiotensin II (Ang II). The principal receptors for Ang II are the membrane-bound angiotensin type I and type II receptors (AT_1 and AT_2). Although new components of the RAAS are still being discovered, their physiological and pathophysiological importance needs further clarification (e.g., ACE2, chymase, cathepsins, and other enzymes that process angiotensin peptides; several additional angiotensin peptides; new receptors such as AT_4, apelin, and renin receptors). Beside the well-known effects on sodium homeostasis and vascular tone, the RAAS is involved in physiological and pathophysiological processes such as tissue growth and hypertrophy, inflammation, and oxidative stress. Also, the RAAS interferes with glucose, lipid, and energy metabolism. Complexity to the field is added by interactions between the circulating systemic and local tissue RAAS, and tissue- and species-specific regulation of RAAS activity [1,2].

Adipose tissue is of great importance for metabolic regulation and metabolic disorders in obesity, partly because a complete local RAAS is present in adipose tissue. Evidence is accumulating on up-regulated RAAS activity in obesity, both on the systemic and the local adipose-tissue level [3,4]. Given the cellular composition of adipose tissue, possible target cells and effects for locally produced Ang II include pre-adipocytes (growth and differentiation), mature adipocytes (glucose and lipid metabolism, secretion of adipokines), mononuclear cells (chemotaxis, production of radical oxygen species, secretion of cytokines), smooth muscle cells and endothelial cells (blood flow regulation, proliferation), and sympathetic nerve endings (norepinephrine release). Clinical trials of ACE inhibitors and AT_1-receptor blockers have demonstrated significant reductions in cardiovascular and renal disease and suggest a beneficial effect on the development of new-onset diabetes [5]. Thus, one important question is whether these positive drug effects are attributable to an influence of RAAS blockade on the adipose-tissue RAAS. This chapter describes the adipose-tissue RAAS, the influence of obesity on the regulation of this system, and its potential role for obesity-associated metabolic disorders and hypertension.

Nutritional and Metabolic Bases of Cardiovascular Disease, 1st edition.
Edited by Mario Mancini, José M. Ordovas, Gabriele Riccardi,
Paolo Rubba and Pasquale Strazzullo. © 2011 Blackwell Publishing Ltd.

The Adipose-Tissue Renin-Angiotensin-Aldosterone System

All Components of the RAAS are Present in Adipose Tissue

The following components of the RAAS have been identified in adipose tissue:

- AGT
- Renin, several cathepsins
- ACE, chymase, neutral endopeptidase
- Ang II and some other Ang peptides
- Angiotensin receptors, renin receptor, aldosterone receptor

The expression of all these RAAS genes was also found in isolated human adipocytes (see [4] for a comprehensive review). In fact, expression and secretion of AGT by adipocytes had already been described when leptin was not even discovered [6]. Hormonal regulation especially of the AGT gene has been studied extensively, although mostly in mouse clonal pre-adipocytes [4]. A common feature of all murine and human cell culture models is the fact that AGT is not expressed in pre-adipocytes but is induced by early adipogenic events in a robust manner. Thus, AGT is a real adipokine that appears to be regulated by insulin, glucocorticoids, and tumor necrosis factor-α TNF-α [4,7]. Beside AGT, the regulation of AT$_1$-receptors was studied to some extent, and glucocorticoids were shown to induce AT$_1$-receptor gene expression in isolated human adipocytes [8].

The contribution of several enzymes to local formation of Ang II has been demonstrated *in vitro* with human adipocytes, but essentially nothing is known about the regulation of Ang II–forming enzymatic activity in animal or human adipose tissue [9]. Ang II secretion from subcutaneous adipose tissue into the circulation was demonstrated by measuring arteriovenous differences in lean and obese human volunteers [7]. However, it is unknown whether differences in RAAS activity exist between adipose-tissue depots. Although the RAAS is invariably present in adipose tissue, there are notable differences in the regulation and physiology of the adipose-tissue RAAS between humans and rodents. For example, the AT$_1$-receptor is the only receptor subtype present on human pre-adipocytes and adipocytes, but both AT$_1$- and AT$_2$- receptors have been identified in rodent adipose cells [4].

Obesity Influences the Adipose-Tissue RAAS

Several groups have examined the influence of obesity on the expression of RAAS genes in adipose tissue with differing findings that are thoroughly reviewed in [10]. These sometimes divergent findings are due to the large number of different models that were studied. In general, RAAS gene expression is higher in visceral adipose tissue compared to subcutaneous adipose tissue, but it is unknown whether this translates into higher rates of Ang II production. With the exception of AGT, RAAS gene expression in human adipose tissue is dependent on the presence of hypertension: Renin, ACE, and AT$_1$-receptor mRNA levels are only increased in adipose tissue of obese hypertensive subjects [8,11]. Although the AGT gene is typically down-regulated in adipose tissue of obese normotensive and hypertensive human subjects [12,13], AGT secretion from isolated human subcutaneous adipocytes was independent from body mass index (BMI) of the tissue donors [14]. The influence of obesity on AGT expression in rodent adipose tissue is dependent on the underlying genotype [15]. Diet-induced obesity in wild-type animals typically leads to up-regulation of AGT gene expression in adipose-tissue depots [16]. Especially in diet-induced obese rats, increased AGT gene expression in adipose tissue was associated with increased circulating AGT and Ang II levels [17]. This finding clearly raises the question of whether local secretion of AGT by adipocytes can contribute to circulating AGT levels.

Obesity and Hypertension

Adipocyte-Derived AGT Regulates Blood Pressure

Mice with a genetically deleted AGT gene suffer from salt wasting and hypotension due to the lack of circulating AGT/Ang II. Targeted AGT expression in adipocytes of these AGT-knockout mice leads to detectable circulating AGT levels and near-normal blood pressure. Furthermore, targeted AGT expression in adipocytes of wild-type animals raised circulating AGT and blood pressure above normal levels [18]. Unfortunately, no high-fat diet was given to these animals, so the data represent only a proof of principle but do not reflect the situation in obesity. Other groups, however, demonstrated the correlation between obesity, increased adipose-tissue AGT expression, increased plasma AGT, and hypertension in experimental animal models [17,19]. In both settings, high-fat feeding or raised corticosterone levels in adipose tissue, the hypertension of the animals could also be well treated by AT_1-receptor antagonists. Recent studies described for the first time that subcutaneous adipose tissue contributes significantly to circulating Ang II blood levels in humans, with 23% higher adipose-venous Ang II concentrations compared to arterial blood [7]. As in previous studies [13], however, no correlation was found by the authors between BMI and systemic or adipose-venous Ang II levels. Another group employed the same technique, arterio-adipose venous difference, and found that AGT is released from subcutaneous adipose tissue in obese subjects in response to β-adrenergic stimulation. This was associated with increased systemic renin activity and Ang II levels [20]. Thus, the secretion of AGT from adipose tissue and the ectopic cleavage into Ang II in nonadipose vascular beds appears to be more important for the relationship between obesity, adipose tissue, and hypertension than the local formation of Ang II in adipose tissue.

Weight Loss Decreases Blood Pressure and RAAS Activity

Reductions of plasma renin activity, aldosterone, and ACE activity upon weight loss have occasionally been reported. Furthermore, high renin levels predicted the decline in blood pressure induced by weight loss [21,22]. We have recently reported the influence of 5% body weight reduction on the circulating and adipose-tissue RAAS in 17 postmenopausal obese women [13]. Weight loss was achieved by a reduction in total calorie consumption, whereas food composition was not changed. Sodium and potassium intake and excretion were not significantly influenced by weight loss. A 5% body weight reduction in our study was associated by 4-cm reduction in waist circumference, a decrease in daily mean ambulatory blood pressure by 7/2 mm Hg, and a slight decrease of fasting insulin. This weight reduction was accompanied by reduced levels of circulating AGT, renin, aldosterone, and ACE and decreased expression of the AGT gene in adipose tissue. We found a highly significant correlation between the decline in AGT plasma levels with the reduction in waist circumference, with the decrease of AGT gene expression in adipose tissue, and with the reduction in systolic blood pressure. Reduction of waist circumference is an accepted surrogate for a reduction of visceral adipose tissue; thus, our data point to the link between adipose AGT and the circulating RAAS in obesity as already described.

If adipocytes contribute to circulating AGT levels in humans, then increased adipose-tissue mass itself would be sufficient to increase AGT plasma levels in the obese. Increased AGT expression on the adipocyte level is not a necessary requirement and has not been found in humans. We propose a negative feedback loop that controls adipocyte AGT expression in the situation of rising AGT plasma levels in the obese. Weight loss may add another regulatory mechanism that further reduces AGT expression in adipose tissue. The mechanisms that control AGT expression in the obese and reduce AGT expression during weight loss are not known. Salt intake, which is high in obese subjects because it typically accompanies high-fat diets, was studied in a highly controlled environment and we could exclude high sodium intake as a modulator of adipose AGT gene expression in healthy subjects [23].

Angiotensin II and Adipose-Tissue Cellularity and Metabolism

Angiotensin II has Differential Effects on Adipogenesis in Mice and Men

The process of differentiation that increases the number of mature adipocytes within a given adipose tissue depot is called adipogenesis. Adipogenesis is important to maintain adipose-tissue insulin sensitivity because newly differentiated small adipocytes are insulin sensitive, whereas old and enlarged adipocytes are not. Furthermore, an increase in adipocyte size is associated with increased secretion of pro-inflammatory molecules, whereas beneficial adipokines such as adiponectin or interleukin-10 (IL-10) are secreted less when adipocytes gain in volume [24]. Disturbances in adipogenic capacity have been demonstrated in human obesity and the insulin-sensitizing effects of thiazolidinediones are in part explained by the stimulation of adipogenesis in the subcutaneous adipose tissue. Ang II has a species-specific role in the regulation of adipogenesis: In murine clonal preadipocytes, Ang II stimulated prostacyclin release via AT_2-receptors and prostacyclin then acts as an adipogenic stimulator. *Ex vivo* incubation of rat WAT pads with Ang II or prostacyclin also increased the amount of stromavascular cells undergoing adipogenesis. These adipogenic effects of Ang II were abolished by aspirin, a potent inhibitor of the prostaglandin endoperoxide synthase [25]. In clear contrast to the findings in animal models, AGT or Ang II treatment of committed human pre-adipocytes inhibited adipogenesis, whereas blockade of the AT_1-receptor stimulated adipogenesis [26]. Furthermore, co-culture experiments demonstrated that mature human adipocytes inhibit preadipocyte differentiation by AT_1-receptor dependent mechanisms. Thus, we postulated a paracrine negative-feedback loop in which Ang II is secreted by mature adipocytes and inhibits further recruitment of pre-adipocytes. The anti-adipogenic mechanisms induced by Ang II are currently unknown, but interactions with insulin signaling, TNF-α and nuclear factor-κB activation, or peroxisome proliferator-activated receptor-γ (PPARγ) inhibition are the most likely candidates.

Angiotensin Receptors Influence Adipocyte Growth and Metabolism in Rodents

Whereas adipogenesis determines the number of mature adipocytes within a given depot, triglyceride storage determines the volume of an adipocyte. Impaired lipolysis, decreased energy expenditure, increased energy intake, or increased triglyceride synthesis (lipogenesis) may lead to enlarged adipocytes. In AT_1-receptor knockout mice, adipogenesis was not influenced, again suggesting that AT_2-receptors are more important in rodent models to promote adipocyte differentiation. Surprisingly though, the animals were protected against diet-induced obesity by high-fat feeding, most likely because brown adipose-tissue thermogenesis was increased [27]. In line with these observations, chronic treat-

ment of rats with the AT_1-receptor antagonist candesartan decreased body weight and adipocyte size, but not number, in several adipose-tissue depots [28]. Chronic treatment with telmisartan, another AT_1-receptor antagonist, also leads to protection against diet-induced weight gain and adipose-tissue growth. Again, increased brown adipose-tissue thermogenesis appears to be involved [29]. Together with several *in vitro* studies, activation of adipocyte lipogenesis by Ang II thus appears to be of importance [4].

When AT_2-receptors were knocked out in mice, decreased adipocyte size was observed, and again, these animals were protected against diet-induced obesity, this time because lipid oxidation rates in skeletal muscle were strongly increased. When subjected to fasting, a defect in lipid mobilization was observed in the animals that translated into reduced plasma free fatty acid levels. Studies with isolated adipocytes revealed an anti-lipolytic effect of Ang II that was mediated by AT_1-receptors [30,31]. These data are by far not conclusive, because Ang II infusion studies at least in rats consistently demonstrate weight loss, which speaks against anti-lipolytic and lipogenic effects of AT_1-receptors. Again, species differences have to be considered, because several metabolic and cardiovascular effects that are seen by Ang II infusion in rats cannot easily be translated to the findings obtained in mice [32]. Thus, a closer look to the findings in humans is necessary, which is facilitated by the fact that only AT_1-receptors are present in human adipose tissue.

AT₁-Receptor–Mediated Regulation of Blood Flow and Lipolysis in Humans

Interstitial Ang II, applied by microdialysis catheters, did not influence blood flow in subcutaneous abdominal adipose tissue but stimulated glycerol release [33]. Tonic AT_1-receptor blockade in obese human volunteers did not influence glucose supply to adipose tissue and also not lipolysis [34,35]. Thus, Ang II locally produced by adipocytes in humans appears to play no role for the regulation of blood flow and only a minor role for the stimulation of lipolysis in these studies. These findings were confirmed by others that demonstrated nitric oxide (NO)-independent vasoconstriction to circulating Ang II in the fasting state, with no role for locally produced Ang II. In contrast, postprandial vasodilation in subcutaneous adipose tissue was not influenced by Ang II [36]. Small effects on suppression of lipolysis by interstitially applied Ang II were reported by the same group with no difference between lean and obese subjects [37]. Taken together, these studies could not reveal an important effect of Ang II on adipose tissue metabolism in humans.

Influence of Angiotensin II on Adipokine Production

Adipocytes and other cells localized in adipose tissue (mostly monocytes/macrophages) secrete a host of substances into the circulation that are collectively called "adipokines." The secretory products of adipocytes range from metabolites to enzymes, hormones, cytokines, and chemokines. The dysbalance between beneficial and deleterious adipokines is currently thought to explain several metabolic and cardiovascular changes commonly seen in obesity (e.g., insulin resistance, inflammation, atherosclerosis, sympathetic activation). Ang II via AT_1-receptors is involved in the regulation of some of these adipokines. Leptin, the most prominent adipokine, is regulated by Ang II in a complicated manner: Isolated adipocytes *in vitro* secrete more leptin in response to Ang II, a finding true for rodent and human adipocytes [38]. In Ang II infusion studies in rats, however, leptin plasma levels decreased because Ang II stimulated norepinephrine release from peripheral sympathetic nerves and β-adrenergic receptors mediate a well-known inhibitory effect on leptin secretion from adipocytes [39]. In human isolated adipocytes, Ang II also increased the release of plasminogen activator inhibitor-1, IL-6, and IL-8 *in vitro*. These effects could always be blocked by the use of AT_1-receptor antagonists [40] and were also seen in mice adipocytes [27].

Adiponectin is an adipokine with protective effects on insulin sensitivity and atherosclerosis. The loss of adiponectin with the development of obesity and in type 2 diabetes is discussed as a major pathophysiological principle and several attempts were undertaken to raise adiponectin by pharmacological intervention. Ang II appears to play an indirect role for the decrease of adiponectin secretion in obesity. Treatment of isolated rat adipocytes with Ang II increased the production of radical oxygen species. Most likely, NADPH oxidase is involved in radical oxygen species production by adipocytes, and activation of NADPH oxidase by Ang II has extensively been described in vascular smooth muscle cells. Radical oxygen species down-regulated adiponectin secretion *in vitro*, and *in vivo* studies employing Ang II infusion also found decreased adiponectin levels in the blood and adipose tissue. The use of NADPH oxidase inhibitors and antioxidants was able to prevent the decrease of adiponectin in Ang II–infused rats[41]. A significant reduction of radical oxygen species production in adipose tissue, together with metabolic improvements and correction of the disturbed adipokine profile, was found in diet-induced obese mice treated with the AT_1-receptor antagonist olmesartan [42]. Thus, Ang II, via AT_1-receptors, plays an important role in the regulation of adipokine release from adipose tissue either by induction of radical oxygen species or directly by AT_1-dependent intracellular signaling. Whether adipokine-regulating Ang II comes from the circulation or must be produced locally within adipose tissue needs further experimental clarification.

Conclusion

The local RAAS in adipose tissue was the subject of intensive research over the last 20 years, but unfortunately, no clear picture has evolved what the true physiological and pathophysiological role it plays in obesity. This uncertainty predominantly comes from the fact that a large number of different animal models and cell culture systems has been studied and that several findings from one model could not be replicated in another. However, studies in obese humans and in diet-induced rodents, which resemble human obesity better than genetically modified animals, allow the following statements (Figures 34.1 and 34.2):

• More AGT is secreted from adipose tissue in obesity.

• AGT from adipose tissue contributes to blood pressure regulation, whereas local formation of Ang II in adipose tissue does not.

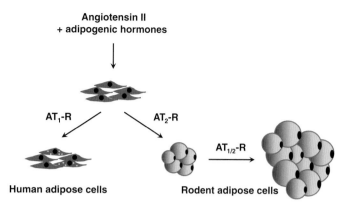

Figure 34.1 Differential role of angiotensin II on adipocyte differentiation and growth in humans and rodents.

- Increased circulating and adipose tissue AGT can be reduced by weight loss and the accompanying decrease in blood pressure correlates with this reduction.
- Human adipogenesis is inhibited by Ang II, which may contribute to local insulin resistance in adipose tissue.
- Ang II is a trophic factor for rodent adipocytes, but its metabolic effects in humans appear to be negligible.
- Ang II regulates leptin, adiponectin, and other adipokines in a deleterious manner.

Beside these findings, many questions remain open, among them the role for mineralocorticoid and renin receptors in adipocytes. Several studies have reported in the past beneficial effects of angiotensin receptor antagonists on insulin sensitivity, adiponectin plasma levels, and other obesity-related metabolic changes. It was recently discovered that some but not all angiotensin receptor antagonists are able to activate the nuclear receptor PPARγ in a manner different from thiazolidinediones [43,44]. These findings have further complicated the field of adipose-tissue RAAS research, because now AT_1-receptor dependent and independent effects of angiotensin receptor antagonists have to be differentiated. However, these findings also opened the door to new and exciting treatment options of patients with the metabolic syndrome.

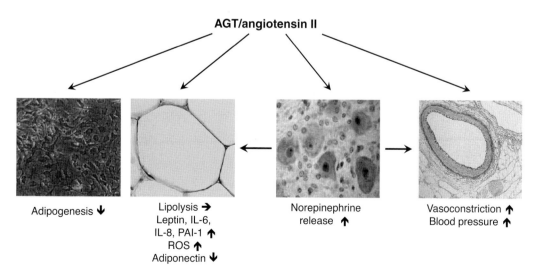

Figure 34.2 Certain actions of AGT/angiotensin II on adipose tissue physiology.

Selected References

2. Re RN. Mechanisms of disease: local renin-angiotensin-aldosterone systems and the pathogenesis and treatment of cardiovascular disease. Nat Clin Pract Cardiovasc Med 2004;1:42–7.

10. Engeli S. Role of the renin-angiotensin-aldosterone system in the metabolic syndrome. Contrib Nephrol 2006;151:122–34.

13. Engeli S, Böhnke J, Gorzelniak K, et al. Weight loss and the renin-angiotensin-aldosterone system. Hypertension 2005;45:356–62.

23. Engeli S, Boschmann M, Frings P, et al. Influence of salt intake on renin-angiotensin and natriuretic peptide system genes in human adipose tissue. Hypertension 2006.

35. Boschmann M, Engeli S, Adams F, et al. Influences of AT1 receptor blockade on tissue metabolism in obese men. Am J Physiol Regul Integr Comp Physiol 2006;290:R219–23.

CHAPTER 35

Relationship of Dietary Electrolyte Intake to Blood Pressure Regulation and Hypertension

Francesco P. Cappuccio
Warwick Medical School, University of Warwick, Coventry, UK

Introduction

Cardiovascular diseases (CVDs) are the leading cause of mortality, morbidity, and disability worldwide [1]. Although CVDs are proportionally more relevant in developed countries, currently 70% of the total number of cardiovascular deaths occurs in developing countries. Globally, high blood pressure causes 7 million premature deaths a year [1]. In particular, hypertension affects approximately 1 billion individuals [2]. The burden of hypertension-related diseases is likely to increase as the population ages [3]. Overall, high blood pressure is the most important and independent risk factor for myocardial infarction, heart failure, stroke, and kidney disease. Therefore, prevention and treatment of hypertension are a priority in both developed and developing countries.

Nonpharmacological interventions are essential to the primary prevention of high blood pressure and an important component of the treatment of hypertension. Lifestyle modifications are effective in reducing blood pressure, increasing the efficacy of pharmacological therapies, and reducing the global risk of CVD.

Nutritional and Metabolic Bases of Cardiovascular Disease, 1st edition.
Edited by Mario Mancini, José M. Ordovas, Gabriele Riccardi,
Paolo Rubba and Pasquale Strazzullo. © 2011 Blackwell Publishing Ltd.

Salt Intake

Effect of Lowering Dietary Salt Intake on Blood Pressure and Cardiovascular Disease

The amount of dietary salt is an important determinant of blood pressure levels and of hypertension risk in both individuals and populations. This relationship is direct and progressive without an apparent threshold. Thus, the reduction of dietary salt intake is one of the most important and effective lifestyle modifications to reduce blood pressure and control hypertension [4,5].

Randomized controlled clinical trials of moderate reductions in salt intake show a dose-dependent cause–effect relationship and lack of threshold effect within usual levels of salt intake [6]. The effect is independent of age, sex, ethnic origin, baseline blood pressure, and body mass. Prospective studies [7–10] with one exception [11] also indicate that higher salt intake predicts the incidence of cardiovascular events. Finally, participants in randomized clinical trials of long-term moderate reduction in salt intake (e.g., approximately 2.5 g of salt reduction) show a 30% reduction in cardiovascular events 10–15 years later [12].

Pooled estimates from meta-analyses of clinical trials on the effects of salt reduction on blood pressure levels indicate a fall in blood pressure of 7.1/3.9 mm Hg in hypertensive individuals and

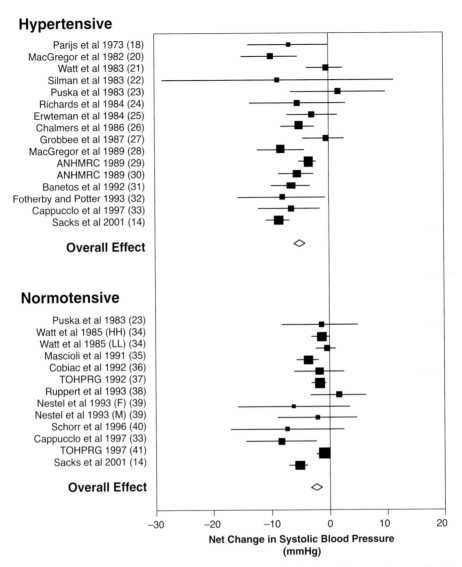

Figure 35.1 Effect of reduced sodium intake on systolic blood pressure in hypertensive and normotensive individuals (adapted from He and MacGregor [13], with permission). The size of the square is proportional to the total sample size. Bars indicate 95% confidence intervals.

3.6/1.7 mm Hg in normotensive individuals per 100 mmol reduction of 24-hour urinary sodium excretion (about 6 g of salt/day) [13,14] (Figure 35.1).

The response of blood pressure to dietary changes in salt intake, as to other environmental stimuli, may vary between individuals. This phenomenon has been termed *salt sensitivity*, and it is likely to be due to the degree of response of the renin-angiotensin system [15,16]. The weaker the response of this system to a change in sodium intake, the larger the response of the blood pressure will be. This phenomenon explains why the blood pressure–lowering effect of salt reduction is larger in hypertensive individuals, elderly, and "low-renin" black populations. Indeed, although a significant reduction of blood pressure induced by reduced salt intake has been observed in children and adolescents as well, this response increases with age and is largest in the elderly [17]. Furthermore, the blood pressure fall observed in the elderly as a result of a dietary salt reduction may reduce the need for anti-hypertensive medication. These observations are relevant to the prevention of hypertension-related diseases in developed countries, where the majority of strokes occur in the elderly and individuals with blood pressure levels below the treatment threshold for hypertension [18]. Nevertheless, several anti-hypertensive drugs blocking the renin-angiotensin system (e.g., angiotensin-converting enzyme inhibitors [ACE], β-blockers, angiotensin II receptors antagonists [ARBs], and renin inhibitors) have an additive effect on blood pressure reduction in those patients already on a reduced salt diet [19]. People of black African origin also show a greater blood pressure response when dietary salt is reduced [16]. In two separate studies in Nigeria and Ghana, a moderate reduction in salt intake was associated with a significant reduction in blood pressure [20,21]. In areas such as sub-Saharan Africa, the prevalence of hypertension is increasing, the health care resources are scarce, and thus the identification of people with hypertension is still haphazard. The effectiveness of a reduction in salt intake at a population level might prove extremely important for policy makers.

The major benefit of salt reduction is the lowering of blood pressure. It has been argued that the blood pressure reduction realistically achievable at a population level (i.e., 1–3 mm Hg in systolic blood pressure) is small, not clinically significant, and with long-term benefits remaining unclear [22]. However, a meta-analysis of 61 prospective studies estimated that even a reduction of 2 mm Hg in systolic blood pressure would determine a 10% reduction in stroke mortality and a 7% reduction in mortality from coronary heart disease (CHD) or other cardiovascular causes, meaning a large number of premature deaths and disabilities avoided [23]. Finally, recent evidence from randomized clinical trials suggests a 30% reduction in CVD mortality following a moderate reduction in salt intake [12] (Figure 35.2). Other benefits of a moderate reduction in salt intake include regression of left ventricular hypertrophy, reduction in proteinuria, and glomerular hyperfiltration, reduction in bone mineral loss with

age and osteoporosis, protection against stomach cancer and stroke, and protection against asthma attacks and possibly against cataracts [24].

In light of the present evidence, reduction of dietary salt intake appears a plausible population-wide recommendation for the prevention and treatment of hypertension [4,5]. A decrease of dietary salt to no more than 5 g/day (~2.0 g or ~80 mmol of sodium) represents a reasonable goal at a population level. However, this reduction will be only feasible in Western societies if efforts are made by the food industry, manufacturers, and restaurants to decrease the amount of salt added to processed food [25]. In fact, in these societies, a large proportion of salt intake (75%–80%) comes from processed food and bread [26]. On the contrary, in developing countries where the prevalence of hypertension continues to increase, more traditional health promotion strategies would be applicable and nutritional education might have an important effect in these settings [18,21,27].

Public Health Strategies to Reduce Salt Intake in Developed Countries

In developed countries, the estimated prevalence of hypertension is, on average, 28% in North America (Canada and United States) and 44% in western Europe [28]. Community-based intervention trials to reduce blood pressure by means of salt reduction are scanty. For example, a community-based intervention trial in Portugal over 2 years involved a whole town receiving a health education program to reduce salt intake while another town was not given any advice and used as a control [29]. Average blood pressure fell by 3.6/5.0 mm Hg at 1 year and 5.0/5.1 mm Hg at 2 years. In developed countries the majority of an individual's salt intake is not added by the person but is already present in foods. Indeed, given that 75%–80% of salt intake comes from salt added to bread and processed foods [28], a population-wide strategy involving the food industry would be more effective in the long term. The North Karelia Project is a meaningful example to support this concept. The program was launched in 1972 in Finland to prevent noncommunicable diseases and, primarily, to reduce mortality and morbidity from CVDs [30]. The interventions implemented during this trial were extensive: Collaborations with the community, the health

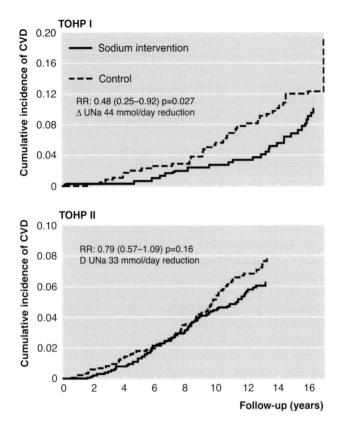

Figure 35.2 Long-term effect of dietary sodium reduction on the incidence of cardiovascular outcomes (adapted from Cook et al. [12], with permission). TOHP I and II combined relative risk (RR): 0.70 (0.53–0.94) $p = .018$. (CVD: cardiovascular disease; TOHP: Trials of Hypertension Prevention.)

services, and the food industry were added to a mass media campaign. Over 25 years, the age-adjusted mortality rate from CVD among men aged 25–64 years fell by 73%. These results show that a comprehensive and collaborative program involving the food industry and the health and community services is essential to successfully implement strategies of primary prevention of CVDs in developed countries.

A complementary approach to lower salt intake, in developed countries, may reside in the use of salt substitutes.

In summary, in developed countries comprehensive population strategies to reduce the average levels of salt intake are required. The expected benefits of a modest reduction in blood pressure across the whole population would be significant, especially on stroke, CHD, and all other cardiovascular conditions for which high blood pressure is a causative risk factor. The benefits would be greater in the elderly, because they have a much higher stroke incidence (greater absolute risk); additionally, in this age-group, the majority of strokes occur at levels of blood pressure not always requiring drug therapy (more stroke events attributable to the effect of blood pressure).

Public Health Strategies to Reduce Salt Intake in Developing Countries

In developing countries, noncommunicable diseases are increasingly becoming an important threat to the health of populations [1]. Worldwide, stroke is second only to ischemic heart disease as a cause of death, and most of these deaths occur in developing countries [31]. Likewise, in areas such as sub-Saharan Africa the prevalence of hypertension is elevated and comparable to figures from developed regions [2,27]. Thus, preventing the impending epidemic of CVD in these countries is critical, as they are facing a rapid demographic change and already experiencing a "double" burden of disease, that is, communicable and noncommunicable. In the 30-year period from 2000 to 2030, the population of elderly persons is projected to double in many sub-Saharan African countries.

Salt consumption in developing countries is becoming more common as urbanization increases. However, interventions to reduce salt intake at a population level have not been extensively studied in these countries. The population approach to reduce salt consumption is particularly relevant in developing countries due to the cost-effectiveness of these measures [32]. Furthermore, in countries of sub-Saharan Africa where effective healthcare provision for chronic diseases is haphazard, a population strategy to limit salt consumption might prove extremely effective. It can be predicted that the same reduction in salt intake obtained with a behavioral intervention will be more effective in black African origin populations than in white populations due to the higher salt sensitivity of people of black African origin and because most of the salt ingested is added to food by the consumer, whereas processed food is used relatively scarcely compared to developed countries [18]. Two short-term trials in sub-Saharan Africa have confirmed that simple, cost-effective and culturally adapted behavioral and educational interventions to reduce blood pressure can be successfully implemented [20,21]. Concerns about population-wide strategies to limit salt consumption in developing countries pertain to the perceived risk of counteracting worldwide policies directed to the prevention of iodine deficiency disorders (IDD) through universal salt iodization. Therefore, there is an urgent need to consider alternative vehicles for the deliveries of iodine to populations [33].

In summary, in developing countries, which are experiencing an increasing burden of CVD, multiple risk factor interventions and community-based programs of primary prevention should be encouraged. In particular, public health measures to promote dietary changes such a reduction in salt intake should be strongly recommended given that the prevalence of hypertension is likely to increase in these countries.

Dietary Approach to Stop Hypertension (DASH) Diet

Expert reports [4,5] emphasize the importance of adopting a dietary regimen resembling the so-called "DASH" diet as one major lifestyle modification to prevent and treat hypertension. The DASH dietary plan provides large intakes of fruit, vegetables, and low-fat dairy products; comprises whole grains, poultry, fish and nuts; and has limited amounts of red meat, sweets, and sugar-containing beverages. Thus, in comparison with habitual diets of Western societies, the DASH dietary pattern provides higher intakes in potassium, magnesium, calcium, fiber, and proteins and lower intakes in total fat, saturated fat, and cholesterol. The blood pressure–lowering effect of this diet is the result of the combined effects of these nutrients when consumed together in food, rather than of the specific effect of a single nutrient [34,35]. A full report of the results of this 11-week program can be found in Chapter 42.

In a sister trial, 412 participants were randomly allocated to two dietary regimens, a control diet and the DASH combination diet [36]. Within these two dietary regimens, participants were randomly assigned to three decreasing levels of salt consumption, defined as high (~9 g of salt or 150 mmol or 3.5 g of sodium per day), intermediate (<6 g of salt or 100 mmol or 2.3 g of sodium per day), and low (<3 g of salt or 50 mmol or 1.6 g of sodium per day). Each feeding period lasted 30 consecutive days. Overall, findings indicate that (i) the DASH diet lowers blood pressure independent from the level of salt intake; (ii) the blood pressure lowering effect of a reduction in salt intake occurs by reducing the salt intake even to levels below the currently recommended limit (i.e., <6 g/day); (iii) the effects of salt reductions are observed in all major subgroups [37]; (iv) greater lowering effects on blood pressure may derive from the combination of the two interventions than from adopting either the DASH diet or low salt diet individually. In fact, the difference of systolic blood pressure between the DASH-low salt group and the control-high salt group was a substantial reduction of 7.1 mm Hg in participants without hypertension and 11.5 mm Hg in participants with hypertension. The last finding resembles the effect of a single-drug therapy in hypertensive individuals. Thus, the combination of the DASH diet and reduced salt intake represents an alternative to drug therapy for individuals with mild hypertension and willing to comply with long-term dietary changes.

Table 35.1 Meta-analysis of the effects of potassium supplementation on blood pressure.

	Systolic blood pressure		Diastolic blood pressure	
	Net change	95% CI	Net change	95% CI
All trials				
1991 – Cappuccio et al. [39]	−5.9	−5.2 to −6.6	−3.4	−2.8 to −4.0
1997 – Whelton et al. [40]	−3.1	−1.9 to −4.3	−2.0	−0.5 to −3.4
2003 – Geleijnse et al. [14]	−2.4	−1.1 to −3.7	−1.6	−0.5 to −2.6

Potassium Intake

The INTERSALT cooperative study was one of the earlier epidemiologic investigations to estimate the effect of potassium intake on blood pressure levels. This study tested both the within- and cross-population association between 24-hour urinary sodium, potassium, and sodium/potassium ratio, reflecting the amount of dietary intake of these micronutrients, and blood pressure levels. Within the centers, a reduction in systolic and diastolic blood pressure of 3.4/1.9 mm Hg was related to a higher potassium intake of 50 mmol/day. Furthermore, the sodium/potassium ratio was positively and significantly related to the blood pressure levels of individuals in both men and women. These relationships were more marked with increasing age [38].

Numerous clinical trials have reported on the effect of potassium supplementation on blood pressure levels in both normotensive and hypertensive individuals. Although results have not always been consistent, pool estimates from meta-analyses support a significant inverse association between potassium intake and blood pressure levels [14,39,40] in both normotensive and hypertensive individuals (Table 35.1).

The effect of potassium supplementation on blood pressure is independent of the baseline potassium status; it appears similar in women and men, whereas it is stronger among hypertensive individuals and individuals of black African origin. Furthermore, the effect is dependent on the concurrent intake of dietary sodium and vice versa. This means that this effect is larger in individuals on a high-sodium diet and smaller in individuals on a low-sodium diet; conversely, the lowering effect of a reduction in dietary sodium intake on blood pressure is larger in individuals on a low-potassium diet and smaller in individuals on a high-potassium diet. Accordingly, the ratio of urinary sodium-potassium excretion is more closely related to changes in blood pressure levels than either urinary sodium or potassium excretion individually.

Fruit, vegetables, pulses and nuts are the main sources of dietary potassium in the form of inorganic or organic salts. These foods, especially fruit and vegetables, are rich in potassium as well as in other essential micronutrients; therefore, diet is a suitable strategy to increase the levels of potassium intake and prevents the need for supplements. Several randomized controlled trials have reported on the lowering effects on blood pressure of dietary interventions providing large intakes of potassium [34]. The increase in potassium intake from natural dietary sources may represent a feasible and effective measure to reduce the need for anti-hypertensive medication. Siani et al. randomized hypertensive individuals to either a dietary intervention, which specifically aimed at increasing potassium intake, or to the control group. As a result of the dietary intervention, potassium intake increased and blood pressure could be controlled using less than 50% of the initial pharmacological therapy in 81% of the patients in the intervention group compared with 29% of the patients in the control group [41].

The mechanisms responsible for the lowering effect of increased potassium intake on blood pressure are not fully understood. High potassium intake might exert a vascular protective effect and reduce the development of atherosclerosis. It may also reduce arteriolar thickening in the kidney. Moreover, potassium infusion increases acetylcholine-induced vasodilatation, and this effect is inhibited by the consequent infusion of the nitric oxide synthase inhibitor L-NMMA (L-nitromonomethylarginine). This suggests that potassium could lower blood pressure by a NO-dependent vasodilatation. Conversely, potassium depletion in humans is accompanied by sodium retention and calcium depletion and also by an altered response to vasoactive hormones. These metabolic effects together with the direct vasoconstrictive effects of hypokalemia might be the cause of the augmentation in blood pressure during a decrease of potassium intake.

Calcium Intake

Association between Calcium Intake and Blood Pressure in Observational Studies

A large number of epidemiologic studies have looked at the possible association between dietary calcium intake and blood pressure levels (see [42–44] for review). Most of the studies have been cross-sectional, examining the association between dietary calcium and blood pressure as an outcome at one point in time. Similarly, some studies have also used a case-control design with hypertension as the disease. A limited number of studies have been prospective. Although there might be an indication for an inverse association between dietary calcium and blood pressure, controlled clinical trials were carried out to test causality.

Effect of Calcium Supplementation on Blood Pressure in Clinical Trials

At least five increasingly larger meta-analyses have been performed [45–49] and one large trial also has been carried out (Trials of Hypertension Prevention [TOHP]) [50]. Since the original meta-analysis by Cappuccio et al. [45] based on a small overall sample size ($n = 391$), the trials have increased over time leading to the latest meta-analysis by Griffith et al. [49], with a much larger sample size ($n > 4,000$). The five meta-analyses differ for important aspects regarding the inclusion criteria. Whilst the first three studies [45–47] limited the pooled analysis to randomized and placebo-controlled trials, the latest [49] was inclusive of all trials of calcium sup-

plementation of 2 weeks duration or longer. This choice allowed the inclusion of trials not controlled versus placebo, with the likelihood of a bias towards an overestimate of effect. They estimate a fall in blood pressure of −1.4 mm Hg (95% confidence interval [CI], −2.2 to −0.7) for systolic and −0.8 mm Hg (−1.4 to −0.2) for diastolic for approximately an oral calcium supplement of 1,000 mg/day. A more conservative estimate is reported by Allender et al. [47] in placebo-controlled trials only (−0.89 mm Hg [−1.74 to −0.05] for systolic and −0.18 mm Hg [−0.75 to +0.40] for diastolic). In spite of these important differences in inclusion criteria, the results of the different meta-analyses are compatible with each other, although the confidence intervals have narrowed with the increase in the sample sizes (Figure 35.3). The TOHP study was the sole large intervention trial that could stand alone in the comparison of effect sizes, given its large sample size. The trial did not show an effect on blood pressure of oral calcium supplementation (−0.5 mm Hg [−1.8 to +0.9] systolic and +0.2 mm Hg [−0.7 to +1.1] diastolic).

Calcium Supplementation in Pregnancy and Preeclampsia

In the early 1980s, Belizan et al. [51,52] were the first to describe an inverse relationship between calcium intake and gestational hypertension and preeclampsia. Early randomized clinical trials of calcium supplementation in pregnant women also suggested that the epidemiological inverse relationship between calcium intake and maternal blood pressure could be causal [53]. However, small sample sizes limited the assessment of effects on important maternal and neonatal outcomes and the highly selected populations of high-risk South American young women of low socioeconomic background and low calcium intake (known to have a disproportionately high incidence of preeclampsia), limited the generalizability of the early findings to the wider population of pregnant women in Europe and in the United States.

In response to the need for a more definitive evaluation of calcium supplementation to prevent preeclampsia, the Calcium for Preeclampsia Prevention (CPEP) trial was undertaken in the United States in 4,589 healthy nulliparous

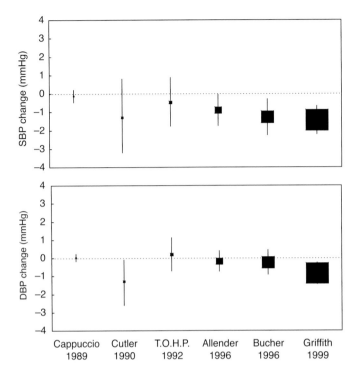

Figure 35.3 Effect of calcium supplementation on blood pressure in clinical trials: summary of the pooled results of meta-analyses of clinical trials of oral calcium supplementation and changes in blood pressure [45–49] and the results of a large trial [50]. The size of the square is proportional to the total sample size. Bars indicate 95% confidence intervals. (SBP: systolic blood pressue; DBP: diastolic blood pressure.)

women who were 13–21 weeks pregnant [54]. They were randomized to receive either 2,000 mg/day of elemental calcium or placebo for the remainder of their pregnancy. Outcomes of interest were pregnancy-associated hypertension, pregnancy-associated proteinuria, preeclampsia, eclampsia, obstetrical complications, and perinatal outcomes, such as growth retardation, neonatal distress, and perinatal deaths. Calcium supplementation did not reduce the incidence or severity of preeclampsia or delay its onset. There were no differences between treatment groups in the prevalence of pregnancy-associated hypertension without preeclampsia or of all hypertensive disorders. The mean systolic and diastolic pressures during pregnancy were similar in both groups. Calcium supplementation did not reduce the numbers of preterm deliveries, small-for-gestational age births, or fetal and neonatal deaths. The conclusions of the CPEP trial were that calcium supplementation during pregnancy does not prevent preeclampsia, pregnancy-associated hypertension or adverse perinatal outcomes in healthy nulliparous women in the United States, therefore, not supporting the earlier

claims of a policy of calcium supplementation in pregnancy.

Magnesium Intake

Association between Magnesium Intake and Blood Pressure in Observational Studies

The possible association between dietary magnesium intake and blood pressure has also been intensively studied [55]. A recent overview of observational epidemiological studies identified at least 29 studies relating dietary magnesium intake to blood pressure. The majority were cross-sectional, employing a wide variety of tools for assessing dietary magnesium (24-hour dietary recalls, food-frequency questionnaires, food records). They had been carried out in different parts of the world and included young, middle-aged, and elderly populations as well as children. Individual estimates are either negative or null, pointing to a possible negative association between dietary magnesium intake and blood pressure. However, as mentioned earlier, great caution should be used in interpreting and generalizing pooled results from observational studies.

Effect of Magnesium Supplementation on Blood Pressure in Clinical Trials

A few clinical trials on the effects of magnesium supplementation on blood pressure have been reported [42]. Some were carried out in hypertensive patients either on treatment with diuretics, which lead to magnesium wasting, or in conjunction with potassium supplementation or sodium restriction. Two small controlled trials did not detect any effect of magnesium supplementation on blood pressure.

Magnesium in Drinking Water and Cardiovascular Risk

Recently there has been renewed interest in the potential protective effect of hard drinking water on CVD. Furthermore, it has been suggested that low magnesium content of drinking waters might be associated to increased cardiovascular health risks [56,57]. A recent long-term prospective analysis from the British Regional Heart Study, however, has clearly indicated no cardiovascular benefits from high water hardness and specifically individual magnesium intake through diet or drinking water [58]. The results indicate that neither high water hardness, nor high calcium or magnesium intake appreciably protect against CHD or CVD.

Selected References

17. Cappuccio FP, Markandu ND, Carney C et al. Double-blind randomised trial of modest salt restriction in older people. Lancet 1997;350:850–4.

19. Cappuccio FP, Siani A. Nonpharmacologic treatment of hypertension. In: Crawford MH, Di Marco JP, Paulus WJ, eds. Cardiology. Mosby;2004, p. 523–32.

25. Cappuccio FP. Salt and cardiovascular disease. Br Med J 2007;334:859–60.

40. Whelton PK, He J, Cutler JA, et al. Effects of oral potassium on blood pressure. Meta-analysis of randomized controlled clinical trials. JAMA 1997;277:1624–32.

43. Cappuccio FP, Elliott P, Allender PS, et al. Epidemiologic association between dietary calcium intake and blood pressure: a meta-analysis of published data. Am J Epidemiol 1995;142:935–45.

CHAPTER 36

Genetic Susceptibility and Metabolic Bases of BP Salt Sensitivity

Ferruccio Galletti & Pasquale Strazzullo
Federico II University, Naples, Italy

Introduction

Salt-sensitivity of blood pressure (BPSS) may be defined as the interindividual difference in the blood pressure (BP) response to changes in habitual dietary sodium chloride (NaCl) intake.This phenomenon implies the existence of interindividual differences in the slope of the pressure-natriuresis relationship in such a way that the subjects with the highest BPSS have the steepest regression line [1]. While ideally SSBP should be estimated using a single carefully standardized protocol, the majority of the studies available have used different methods, such as the BP response to short-term dietary NaCl restriction or the BP response to saline infusion or to diuretic administration (Figure 36.1). The heterogeneity of the methods adopted in different studies conceivably impairs the possibility to make reliable comparisons between their results. Based on these considerations, we refer here to allelic variants of genes that are likely to have an impact on the pressure-natriuresis relationship even when a precise demonstration of an association with an abnormal BP response to sodium intake was not provided.

A most valuable tool for the understanding of the concept of BPSS is given by the monogenic forms of hypertension so far recognized. These hypertensive syndromes are caused by well-characterized genetic mutations occurring at a single locus and share the common feature of being associated with major alterations in renal tubular sodium handling [2]. Although monogenic hypertension accounts for less than 1% of the overall prevalence of hypertension in humans, its existence is strongly supportive of the hypothesis that much more common subtle genetic alterations in the numerous structures involved in the control of renal sodium and water handling make a contribution to the individual susceptibility to hypertension. More recently, several allelic variants of candidate genes for BPSS have been described. Most of these genes encode for proteins involved with sodium transport through the renal tubular epithelia or with the endocrine/paracrine regulation of renal tubular sodium handling.

Monogenic Hypertension

Mendelian forms of hypertension are caused by single gene mutations that are little influenced by environmental factors. The monogenic forms of hypertension affect either electrolyte transport in the distal nephron, or the synthesis or activity of mineralocorticoid hormones, leading to the common pathogenic mechanisms of increased distal tubular reabsorption of sodium and chloride, volume expansion and hypertension.

The classical monogenic forms include:

1) The Liddle's syndrome, characterized by development of hypertension at an early age, together with hypokalemia and suppression of both PRA

Nutritional and Metabolic Bases of Cardiovascular Disease, 1st edition.
Edited by Mario Mancini, José M. Ordovas, Gabriele Riccardi,
Paolo Rubba and Pasquale Strazzullo. © 2011 Blackwell Publishing Ltd.

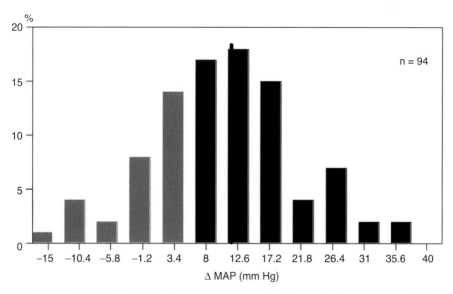

Figure 36.1 Frequency distribution of the blood pressure response to the Grim test for the assessment of salt-sensitivity. (Reproduced from Galletti F, J Hypertension 1997;15:1485–9, with permission.)

and aldosterone, and caused by mutations in the carboxyl-terminus of the β- or γ-subunits of the renal epithelial sodium channel.

2) The glucocorticoid remediable aldosteronism, also known as familial hyperaldosteronism, an autosomal dominant form of low renin hypertension involving a rare mutation in the aldosterone synthase/11β-hydroxylase gene (HSDβ2).

3) The apparent mineralocorticoid excess syndrome (AME), caused by a deficiency of 11β-hydroxysteroid dehydrogenase, featuring an alteration in the relative excretion of cortisol and cortisone metabolites.

On the other hand, Gitelman's syndrome is a form of monogenic hypotension associated with a renal tubular disorder resulting from defective absorption of sodium chloride in the distal convoluted tubule caused by loss-of-function mutations in the gene encoding for a sodium-chloride-cotransporter at the distal convoluted tubule.

Role of Genetic Variation in BP Homeostasis

Candidate Gene Approach

By the classical candidate gene approach, a large number of relatively common genetic variants were found to be associated with higher BP and increased susceptibility to hypertension. For some of these polymorphic variants, direct or circumstantial evidence of an impact on BPSS was obtained.

Variants of Genes Encoding for Renin-Angiotensin System Components or Mineralocorticoid Hormones

Both the insertion/deletion polymorphism of the angiotensin-converting enzyme gene (ACE I/D) and the 11-G534A polymorphism of HSDβ2 were significantly associated with the BP response to high salt intake in patients with hypertension [3]. Another recent case-control study detected a significant relationship of both polymorphisms to high BP, although it was not able to show an association with the response to a test of salt sensitivity [4]. The possible association of several relatively common polymorphisms of the renin-angiotensin-aldosterone system with renal sodium handling and BP was investigated in an unselected sample of adult male population ($n = 918$) participating in the Olivetti Heart Study in southern Italy. The authors evaluated the effects of the angiotensinogen (AGT) M235T, the angiotensin II type 1 receptor (AT1R) A1166C, the CYP11B2 C-344T substitutions, and the ACE I/D insertion. While none of the polymorphisms analyzed was significantly associated with BP or with altered renal sodium handling, it was observed that a group of 28 individuals featuring triple homozygosity for the M allele of AGT M235T, the A allele of AT1R A1166C, and the C allele of CYP11B2 C-344T plus an ACE D/D genotype showed markedly and highly significantly reduced lower fractional excretion of lithium, sodium, and uric acid as compared to all other allelic combinations, suggesting an enhanced rate of proximal tubular sodium reabsorption. This same group also carried a substantially greater risk of hypertension [5]. These results highlight the importance of paying careful attention to the possibility of gene–gene interaction in the study of complex disorders such as high BP.

Given that rare mutations in the gene encoding for aldosterone synthase lead to Mendelian forms of hypertension as discussed above, the aldosterone synthase gene (CYP11B2) has been the focus of interest in hypertension research for many years, although with conflicting results. On the assumption that populations accustomed to high salt intake are a good model for the investigation of the genetic impact on salt-sensitivity, a recent study investigated the association of the -344T/C, K173R and intron-2 conversion polymorphisms of CYP11B2 with circulating aldosterone levels and hypertension in normotensive and hypertensive highlanders living in the Himalayan valley whose daily salt consumption averaged 17 g/day [6]. Of the three variants examined, the intron-2 conversion allele showed significant association with both BP and plasma aldosterone to renin ratio. Very recently, Makhanova et al. investigated BP salt sensitivity in a mouse model (AS(hi/hi)) featuring a moderately increased expression of aldosterone synthase. In this model, BPSS appeared to be increased, raising speculation that even relatively minor alterations in aldosterone synthase gene expression might contribute to hypertension and cardiovascular complications also in man during high-salt intake [7].

As mentioned above, mutations in the HSD11B2 gene, encoding for the kidney isoenzyme of 11β-hydroxysteroid dehydrogenase, cause the AME syndrome. Presently, the AME syndrome is felt to be a continuum disorder in which defects of 11-HSDβ2 gene encoding mutant cDNA result in varying degrees of enzymatic impairment. Thus, the HSD11B2 is an obvious candidate gene for so called "essential" hypertension. Consistently with this interpretation, deficient cortisol inactivation and increased excretion of urinary cortisol metabolites was reported in patients with essential hypertension [8]. The detection of heterozygous [9] and homozygous [10] mutations associated with mineralocorticoid hypertension, the presence of short alleles of CA-repeat microsatellites associated with salt-sensitive hypertension [11] and the demonstration of microsatellite A7/A7 in salt-sensitive normotensive subjects [12] suggest that the 11-HSDβ2 isoform may have an important role in essential hypertension and in BP salt sensitivity.

Variants of the Genes Encoding for α, β, and γ-adducin

Adducin is a heterodimeric cytoskeleton protein consisting of an α-subunit and either a β- or a γ-subunit. The α-adducin subunit is involved in the activity of the sodium-potassium pump in renal tubular cells, thus playing a key role in renal sodium reabsorption and possibly in BPSS. Hypertensive patients carrying the Gly460Trp variant of the α-adducin gene were shown to exhibit a reduction in endogenous lithium and uric acid clearance suggesting an increased rate of sodium reabsorption in the proximal tubule [13,14]. The biochemical alteration underlying the greater avidity of the tubular epithelium for sodium might be an enhanced Na,K-ATPase activity caused by a gain-of-function interaction between the mutated α-adducin molecule and the Na,K pump [15]. Efendiev et al. [16] have recently shown that the insertion of the MHS rat allelic variant or of the rare human variant of α-adducin into renal epithelial cells of MNS rats reproduces the hypertensive phenotype with failure to suppress Na,K-ATPase activity in isolated proximal convoluted tubular cells by natriuretic signals, such as dopamine stimulation. The α-adducin mutation seems to interfere with the process of Na,K-ATPase endocytosis in response to dopamine, thus determining the exposure of a greater number of pump units at any given time. These results support previous findings in humans indicating that α-adducin polymorphism affects the pressure-natriuresis relationship and the rate of sodium transport in the proximal tubule [14]. A study of renal hemodynamics in relation to α-adducin polymorphism was carried out by Beeks et al. in hypertensive patients undergoing two different dietary sodium regimens. It was observed that effective renal blood flow and glomerular filtration rate were lower in patients homozygous for the α-adducin rare 460Trp allele compared with patients with the Gly460Gly genotype on low sodium diet, while no differences were found at the higher sodium intake. Moreover, plasma atrial natriuretic peptide levels were significantly greater in patients with the Trp460Trp genotype, possibly as a compensatory response to the trend to renal sodium and water retention [17].

A systematic overview of the studies on gene polymorphisms impacting on renal sodium handling, renin-angiotensin-aldosterone system activity and BPSS has been carried out recently [18]. In these studies, the BP response to sodium chloride was measured either as the BP change occurring upon change in dietary sodium intake or as the response to the Grim and Weimberger 3-day protocol involving volume expansion and contraction maneuvers. The review suggested a rather consistent association of the α-adducin polymorphism G460T with salt-sensitive hypertension and with a low-renin status [13].

Many recent works reported the finding of significant interactions between genetic variability in the α-adducin molecule and other genetic polymorphisms. In a study of 125 Han nuclear families in northern China, Wang et al. [19] found that systolic BP was significantly higher in ACE D/D compared with ACE I/I individuals, but only among participants carrying the α-adducin TrpTrp and the aldosterone synthase CC genotype. Pedrinelli et al. reported that microalbuminuria was more frequent in patients with the ACE D/D variant, but only in those with an α-adducin Gly460Gly background, while α-adducin polymorphism was not associated with the rate of albumin excretion [20]. A study by Tamaki et al. [21] showed that the combination of AGT M235T Thr/Thr and α-adducin G460T genotype was associated with higher susceptibility to hypertension. In another population-based cross-sectional study of a large rural community in Japan, Yamagishi et al. investigated the association of the α-adducin G460T polymorphism with BP according to habitual dietary salt intake, as estimated by 24-hour urine collection and dietary questionnaire.

Although the authors found no between-genotype difference in BP levels in the whole population, upon stratification for sodium intake, systolic BP was significantly higher in subjects homozygous for the Trp allele than in the GlyGly group among men with higher urinary sodium excretion, supporting a role of this allelic variant in salt-sensitive hypertension. In a multilocus case-control study of genotypes and haplotypes predisposing to myocardial infarction, a lower frequency of the α-adducin G460T Trp allele was reported in myocardial infarction survivors aged less than 75 years compared with controls of the same age [22]. According to the authors, this finding might be attributed to premature death of the Trp allele carriers supporting previous findings demonstrating an association between coronary events and this allelic variant in hypertensive patients [23,24]. Finally, an epistatic interaction has been suggested between the α- and the γ-adducin gene in never-treated hypertensive patients [25] as well as in European populations in relation to pulse pressure [26].

Variants in Other Candidate Genes Involved in Sodium Transport

The epithelial sodium channel (ENaC) expressed in aldosterone-responsive epithelial cells of the kidney and colon plays a critical role in the control of sodium balance, blood volume, and BP. Mutations in ENaC may cause both severe salt-wasting syndromes and severe forms of salt-sensitive hypertension [27]. The interaction between ENaC single-nucleotide polymorphisms and salt intake might significantly affect BP salt-sensitivity. A few years ago a missense mutation (T594M) in the beta-subunit of the human ENaC gene, detected only in people of African descent, was implicated in causing impaired renal sodium excretion and salt-sensitive hypertension [28]. Nevertheless, a subsequent study did not confirm these associations nor was it possible to confirm that the extent of BP fall induced by the ENaC-blocker amiloride in black individuals is predicted by T594M allelic variation [29].

The serum glucocorticoid-inducible kinase 1 (SGK1) is an aldosterone- and insulin-dependent positive regulator of ENaC density at the plasma membrane and exerts a significant role in the regulation of ion transport and sodium excretion [30]. Therefore, the SGK1 gene was considered a candidate for salt-sensitive hypertension. SGK1-knockout mice exhibit an impaired ability to decrease urinary sodium upon dietary NaCl restriction and display a tendency to lower BP [31]. Busjahn et al. [32] reported an association between the SGK1 gene locus and diastolic BP in twins. Two single-nucleotide polymorphisms in exon 8 and intron 6 were related to BP. Unfortunately, these findings were not confirmed by a more recent study conducted in a relatively large population of several hundred patients with end-stage renal disease [33].

Variants of Genes Involved in the Dopaminergic System

The dopaminergic system plays an important role in the regulation of renal sodium and water handling and in the maintenance of fluid and electrolyte balance as stimulation of dopamine-like receptors (D_1 and D_5) inhibits Na,K-ATPase–mediated sodium transport in the kidney and the gut. Thus, genetic-based variation in the function of this control system is likely to affect BPSS and susceptibility to hypertension.

In Dahl salt-sensitive (DSS) and spontaneously hypertensive rats (SHRs) and in humans with essential hypertension, the D_1-like receptor–mediated inhibition of epithelial sodium transport was found to be impaired because of an uncoupling of the D_1-like receptor from its G-protein/effector complex [34]. The defective transduction of the renal dopaminergic signal would be caused by gain-of-function variants of G protein-coupled receptor kinase type 4 (GRK4: R65L, A142V, A486V). The GRK4 locus is linked to and GRK4 gene variants are associated with essential hypertension, especially in salt-sensitive subjects. The presence of three or more GRK4 variants was recently reported to impair the natriuretic response to dopaminergic stimulation [35]. Single nucleotide polymorphisms of a G-protein–coupled receptor kinase, GRK4-gamma, were associated with increased activity of this enzyme: The resulting increase in receptor phosphorylation resulted in the uncoupling of the dopamine-1 receptor from its G-protein/effector enzyme complex in renal proximal tubular cells

[36]. This same study showed that transgenic mice expressing the polymorphic variant became hypertensive.

Polymorphisms of Nitric Oxide Synthase Gene

Many studies have reported associations between genetic variability in the nitric oxide synthase (eNOS) gene and susceptibility to cardiovascular diseases. Recently, Miyaki et al. investigated the T786C polymorphism in a sample of healthy Japanese men in relation to BP and to 24-hour urinary sodium excretion. They observed a marginally higher BP in the carriers of the rare C allele, but their more impressive finding was a significant interaction between the mutation and the subject's urinary sodium excretion, in as much as the individuals who carried the mutation and who were in the upper quartile of urinary salt excretion had a definitely higher systolic and diastolic BP than the rest of the study population [37]. It remains to be determined whether dietary salt reduction prevents the rise in BP in the subjects carrying this unfavorable genotype. Two other variants of eNOS—the Glu298Asp in exon 7 and the 27 bp variable number of tandem repeats (VNTR) within intron 4—were investigated in a small group of healthy Hispanic individuals from Venezuela [38]. The authors reported that the 4a/b genotype was significantly associated with reduced NO production and a greater BP response to salt restriction. Neither this polymorphism nor the Glu298Asp variant was associated with BP. Very recently it has been reported that in a DOCA-salt model of volume-expanded low-renin hypertension, endothelium-specific GTP cyclohydrolase I overexpression, inducing greater eNOS activity, significantly lowers BP [39].

Variation in Other Candidate Genes

A higher prevalence of hypertension was reported in individuals carrying the rare Arg40Ser variant of the glucagon receptor (GCGR) gene [40,41]. In a large sample of an Italian male adult population, the carriers of this genetic variant (3.8%) had a high prevalence of hypertension and a significantly reduced fractional excretion of lithium and uric acid, again suggesting an enhanced rate of proximal tubular sodium reabsorption [21]. The mechanistic explanation for this finding is based on the notion that, normally, the large glucagon-induced hepatic production of cyclic adenosine monophosphate (cAMP) is followed by a substantial spillover of cAMP into the systemic circulation. Circulating cAMP significantly affects proximal tubular function promoting sodium, phosphate, and water diuresis. In subjects carrying the Gly40Ser substitution, an impaired hepatic cAMP production occurs: In turn, the cAMP concentration in the blood is expected to be reduced and so its influence on renal proximal sodium transport, with resultant defective natriuresis and a modification of the pressure-natriuresis relationship [41].

The C825T polymorphism of the beta-3 subunit of G-protein (GNB3) was related to an increased activity of the Na+/H+ exchanger isoform 1 (NHE-1) through the synthesis of an anomalous hyperactive protein [42]. In another study, the TT genotype was associated with lower plasma renin activity and higher BP [43]. Studies exploring its possible association with salt-sensitivity and susceptibility to hypertension gave contrasting results [42,44,45]. In a recent study, Nieto Martin et al. found no association between this polymorphism and SSBP or prevalence of hypertension; nevertheless, they observed that plasma sodium concentration was higher and plasma potassium was lower in TT than in CC patients, a finding suggesting that increased NHE-1 activity is indeed associated with the less common allelic variant of the gene [46]. The study of possible association of polymorphic variants of the gene coding for another isoform (the NHE3) of the sodium/hydrogen exchanger with hypertension and sodium balance gave negative results [47].

Rodent models made knockout for the gene encoding for adrenomedullin (ADM) were found to develop hypertension, which was attenuated by ADM infusion or ADM gene transfer [48]. The A/G polymorphism in the ADM promoter at -1984 position was reported to cause the appearance of a binding site for the glucocorticoid receptor, which stimulates the transcription of several genes[49]. In a recent study of a family-based population of over 400 Chinese individuals [50], the carriers of the G-allele in comparison with AA individuals had lower systolic and pulse pressure as well as lower urinary sodium excretion, probably indicating a lower habitual sodium intake. In a subsample study, the authors detected significantly higher ADM plasma levels in association with the GG genotype.

Earlier studies implicated members of the P450 CYP2C and CYP4A gene subfamilies in the control of renal function and BP [51–53]. A recent work [54] has shown that disruption of cytochrome P450, family 4, subfamily a, polypeptide 10 (Cyp4a10) gene causes a salt-dependent type of hypertension in mice. Cyp4a10–/– mice fed low-salt diets were normotensive but became hypertensive when fed normal or high-salt diets. They had a dysfunctional kidney epithelial sodium channel and became normotensive when administered amiloride, a selective inhibitor of this sodium channel. These studies establish a physiological role for the arachidonate monooxygenases in renal sodium reabsorption and BP regulation, and demonstrate that a dysfunctional Cyp4a10 gene causes alterations in the kidney epithelial sodium channel activity [54].

Members of the cytochrome P450 3A (CYP3A) subfamily catalyze the metabolism of endogenous substrates, environmental carcinogens, and various drugs and therapeutic agents. In particular, the CYP3A4 and CYP3A5 genes play an especially important role in pharmacogenetics. Moreover, CYP3A enzymes convert circulating cortisol to 6-b-hydroxycortisol, which plays a role in sodium transport in the kidney and is hypothesized to result in defective renal sodium excretion [55]. By a comparative genomics approach using three ethnically diverse populations, Thompson et al. reported that remarkable interpopulation differences exist with regard to frequency spectrum and haplotype structure. The CYP3A5*1/*3 polymorphism was genotyped in 11,000 individuals from 52 world-wide population samples. The results reveal an unusual geographic pattern whereby the CYP3A5*3 frequency shows extreme variation across human populations and is significantly correlated with distance from the equator. The authors also showed that an unlinked variant, AGT M235T, also implicated in hypertension as described above, exhibits a similar geographic distribution and is significantly correlated in frequency with CYP3A5*1/*3. According to these scientists, these results suggest that variants that influence salt homeostasis were the targets of a shared selective pressure that resulted from an environmental variable correlated with latitude [56].

Genome-wide Scan and Quantitative Trait Loci Approach

Genome-wide scans to identify chromosomal loci presumably linked to hypertensive phenotypes have been carried out with variable results. The large genetic and phenotypic heterogeneity of high BP has made the search for genetic loci consistently linked to BP and to susceptibility to hypertension a particularly difficult task. An original approach to circumvent these difficulties has been that of stratifying hypertensive patients by their response to different classes of antihypertensive drug, so trying to disentangle possibly different mechanisms of hypertension. By applying this methodology to the British Genetics of Hypertension Study population, composed of more than 2,000 hypertensive white affected sibling pairs, Padmanabhan et al. showed a significant linkage in sibling pairs who were concordant for non-response to drugs that inhibit the renin-angiotensin axis on chromosome 2p and suggestive linkage for sibling pairs concordant for nonresponse to diuretics or Ca-channel blockers on chromosome 10q. The authors speculated that the chromosome 2p locus might contain a gene for salt-sensitive hypertension and/or a pharmacogenetic locus affecting drug response [57].

Interesting results have come from the search for quantitative trait loci (QTLs) associated with the transmission of salt-sensitivity/hypertension phenotypes. As mentioned above, Efendiev et al. [16] showed that the insertion of the MHS rat allelic variant or of the rare human variant of α-adducin into renal epithelial cells from MNS rats reproduces the hypertensive phenotype. The identification of QTLs for BP and the revelation of their functional role and of their interactions is fundamental for the understanding of the pathogenesis of essential hypertension. A number of BP QTLs were identified in the DSS strain of rat [58]. Recently, Charron et al. detected several BP QTLs within a segment of Dahl rat chromosome 10, which is homologous to a section of human chromosome 17. They also found that the three BP QTLs are epistatic to one another in their effects on BP, a finding that may contribute to elucidate the relationships among homologous human QTLs in population studies [59,60]. Similarly, epistatic interactions were demonstrated between three QTLs for BP located on chromosome 2 of the Dahl SS rat in other works by the same group [61,62]. Another recent study examined BP variation before and after a salt-loading experiment in the intercross (F2) progeny from a cross between the Brown-Norway normotensive rat strain and the SHR [63]. After baseline measurements, the rats were given a diet that included water with 1.0% NaCl for 13 days, after which SBP, DBP, MAP, and HR were remeasured under anesthesia. By using univariate and multivariate mapping models for detection of genes putatively relevant to BP variation under salt loading, a new relevant QTL involved in the responsiveness to salt was identified on a region close to marker R589 in chromosome 5.

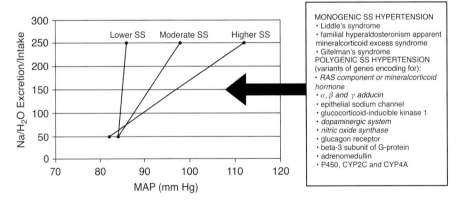

Figure 36.2 Interindividual differences in salt sensitivity expressed as the slope of the pressure-natriuresis relationship. SS: salt sensitivity; MAP: mean arterial pressure. (Adapted from Cowley AL. Am J Clin Nutr 1997;65(Suppl):587S–93S, with permission.)

Future work is expected to focus on fine mapping and identification of the causative variant responsible for the QTL signal.

Conclusions

The search on the genetic bases of BPSS and salt-sensitive hypertension has achieved significant results not only with regard to the description of rare monogenic forms of hypertension but also to the unraveling of the impact of several relatively common genetic variants on BPSS and susceptibility to hypertension (Figure 36.2). However, in order to achieve significant improvements in this area, fundamental requirements are the careful characterization of well defined phenotypes and the adoption of large homogenous study populations. In the case of BPSS, it would be important also to reach a consensus on the evaluation of the BP response to sodium intake and to improve the technical evaluation of renal tubular sodium handling through better standardization of the available methodology and the introduction of more advanced methodologies. The implementation of collaborative studies involving multiple forms of expertise should be pursued for more rapid and substantial achievements.

Selected References

2. Luft FC. Hypertension as a complex genetic trait. Semin Nephrol 2002;22(2):115–26.

5. Siani A, Russo P, Cappuccio FP, et al. Combination of renin-angiotensin system polymorphisms is associated with altered renal sodium handling and hypertension. Hypertension 2004;43:598–602.

13. Bianchi G, Ferrari P, Staessen JA. Adducin polymorphism detection and impact on hypertension and related disorders. Hypertension 2005;45:331–40.

21. Strazzullo P, Iacone R, Siani A, et al. Altered renal sodium handling and hypertension in men carrying the glucagon receptor gene (Gly40Ser) variant. J Mol Med 2001;79:574–80.

27. Strazzullo P, Galletti F. Genetics of salt-sensitive hypertension. Curr Hypertens Rep 2007 Mar;9(1):25–32.

CHAPTER 37

Are Sodium and Potassium Intake Independent Predictors of Cardiovascular and Cerebrovascular Events?

Pasquale Strazzullo[1], Gianvincenzo Barba[2], & Renato Ippolito[1]

[1] Federico II University of Naples, Naples, Italy
[2] Institute of Food Science, National Research Council, Avellino, Italy

Dietary Sodium and Cardiovascular Risk

Interaction of Dietary Sodium Intake with Blood Pressure and Other Recognized Cardiovascular Fisk Factors

The role of dietary sodium chloride (NaCl) has been extensively studied in relation to its effects on the cardiovascular and the renal apparatus and to its interaction with the individual genetic susceptibility to the effects of salt on BP [1–2]. The amount of NaCl in "naturally" available foods is modest [3] and it has been the growing use of NaCl for food preservation that has led to a progressive increase in its consumption in the most recent part of the mankind evolution [4].

Ecological studies have highlighted the association between average habitual NaCl and prevalence of hypertension in different populations [5]. According to INTERSALT data, a 100-mmol difference in habitual daily salt intake was associated with a 10/6 mm Hg higher blood pressure (BP) over 30 years [6].

The causality of the association between salt intake and BP was strongly supported by the results of

Nutritional and Metabolic Bases of Cardiovascular Disease, 1st edition. Edited by Mario Mancini, José M. Ordovas, Gabriele Riccardi, Paolo Rubba and Pasquale Strazzullo. © 2011 Blackwell Publishing Ltd.

a carefully conducted experimental study in chimpanzees. In that study, switching from the habitual low-salt diet of these animals to a high-salt diet for 5 months led to a substantial increment of their BP, which was shown to be reversible upon return to a "normal" level of salt consumption [7].

Controlled clinical trials of the effect of dietary NaCl reduction on BP in man are numerous and have been the object of several meta-analyses. The most recent one has reviewed 20 trials of at least 4-week duration involving a total of 802 hypertensive patients and 11 trials on 2,220 normotensive individuals. The meta-analysis showed that in hypertensive patients a mean NaCl reduction of 78 mmol per day (4.6 g of salt) was associated with an average BP decrease of 5.1/2.7 mm Hg, while in normotensive individuals a similar salt intake reduction brought to a 2.0/1.0 mm Hg fall in BP [8]. Another very recent meta-analysis has investigated the effect of NaCl reduction for at least 2 weeks on BP in children and adolescents [9]. In 10 such studies involving 966 children and adolescent participants, salt consumption was reduced on average by 42% and a statistically significant BP fall of 1.2/1.3 mm Hg was detected.

In addition to its effects on BP, several experimental studies have suggested that elevated habitual salt intake might promote target organ damage by different mechanisms, such as an increase in the production of free oxygen radicals and oxidative stress [10], an increase in arterial wall stiffness [11], and a rise in platelet aggregability [12].

The fact that the susceptibility to the effect of NaCl on BP is different between individuals (salt sensitivity of BP) has been the object of intensive, albeit on practical grounds unproductive, debate. In fact, the large majority of individuals experience a larger or smaller decrease in BP upon moderate reduction in NaCl intake [13,14]. While genetic susceptibility certainly plays a role in this response, there is clear evidence that metabolic and neurohormonal factors are also very important in this regard, in particular the elevated sympathetic tone, the activation of the renin-angiotensin-aldosterone system and the hyperinsulinemia associated with abdominal adiposity [15–20]. In addition, overweight and obese individuals tend to have a particularly high dietary salt intake (20bis, Strazzullo et al.). Together, this may provide a plausible reason for the tighter association observed in some studies between salt intake and morbidity or mortality for cardiovascular disease (CVD) in obese individuals (see later).

Dietary Sodium and Cardiovascular Disease

Tunstall-Pedoe et al. investigated the prospective association between a number of metabolic and dietary factors and the rate of coronary heart disease (CHD) and death in 11,629 men and women participating in the Scottish Heart Health Study and followed for an average of 7.6 years [21]. In this population featuring a high average sodium intake, a significant association was detected between sodium intake determined at entry by food frequency questionnaire (FFQ) and risk of all CHD events in women (age-adjusted hazard ratio [HR] for highest vs. lowest quintile: 1.16). A positive but not significant trend was observed also in men. There was no relation with CHD deaths and a trend to an inverse relation with all cause deaths in men. Similar results were provided by the analysis of 24-hour urinary sodium excretion [22].

Alderman et al. examined mortality rates in sex-specific quartiles of sodium intake and sodium/calorie ratio in a representative sample of 11,348 U.S. adults (aged 25–75 years) participating in the first National Health and Nutrition Examination Survey (NHANES I) for whom an evaluation of dietary habits had been obtained by a single 24-hour recall at baseline in 1971–1975 [23]. Vital status was determined up to June 1992 through interview, tracing, and searches of the national death index. There were 3,923 deaths, of which 1,970 were attributed to CVD. The authors reported a significant inverse association between age- and gender-adjusted all-cause mortality and sex-specific quartiles of sodium intake (lowest to highest quartile: 23.2 vs. 19.0 per 1,000 person-years). This relationship, however, was neutralized when dietary sodium was indexed to dietary calorie intake. A similar pattern was obtained for CVD mortality. In a multivariate regression analysis that included a number of potential confounders, among which age, gender, body mass index (BMI), BP, and history of hypertension and CVD, sodium intake were again inversely associated with all-cause mortality but not with CVD deaths. By contrast, the sodium/calorie ratio was directly associated with both all-cause and CVD mortality. Drawbacks of this study were the inclusion of subjects with previous CVD and the evaluation of sodium intake only at baseline, using a single 24-hour dietary recall, with an average reported salt intake surprisingly low for a Western population (about 5 and 3 g/day, in men and women, respectively).

The NHANES I population was also the basis for the follow-up investigation carried out by He et al. [24], although the sample included in the analysis (*n* = 9,485) differed from that used by Alderman et al. because of the exclusion of individuals with clinical evidence or past history of cardiovascular and cerebrovascular disease. The evaluation of sodium intake was again based on a single 24-hour dietary recall performed at baseline. Whereas sodium intake was not significantly associated with CVD risk among non-overweight persons, among overweight participants a 100-mmol higher sodium intake, even when indexed to calorie intake and upon adjustment for most conventional cardiovascular risk factors, was associated with a 44% (95% C.I.=14%–81%) increase in CHD mortality, 61% increase in CVD mortality, and 39% increase in mortality from all causes.

The study by Tuomilehto et al. was based on random population samples of North Karelia and Kuopio (eastern Finland) and Turku-Liomaa (southwest) recruited in 1982 and 1987 and followed up to the end of 1995. The final sample consisted of 1,221 men and 1,312 women who had completed a 24-hour urine collection and had cardiovascular risk factor data at entry [25]. The analysis of this population indicated that a 100-mmol higher urinary sodium excretion at baseline was associated with significantly higher CHD incidence (HR = 1.34), higher CHD death rate (1.56), higher CVD death rate (1.36), and higher death rate from all causes (1.22) upon adjustment for age, smoking, serum total cholesterol and high-density lipoprotein (HDL)-cholesterol (HDL-C), systolic BP, and BMI. The trends were similar in both sexes, but statistical significance about the effects of sodium intake was achieved only in men. Also in this study, as in the one by He et al. [24], a significant interaction was detected between urinary sodium excretion and BMI with respect to CVD and total mortality: Sodium predicted mortality in men who were overweight.

Cohen et al. conducted a statistical analysis of findings from 7,154 individuals participating in the NHANES II, who provided a 24-hour dietary recall at baseline and were followed on average for 13.7 years. Estimated sodium intake was on average relatively low (about 6 g/day) as observed in the previous NHANES I reports, and apparently unrelated to BMI. Upon adjustment for most conventional risk factors for CVD, the individuals reporting a sodium intake below 2,300 mg/day, compared with those with a greater intake, had HRs for CVD mortality of 1.37 and HR for all-cause mortality of 1.28. No such associations, however, were observed for persons younger than 55 years, for non-whites, or for the obese. Likewise, no association was detected between sodium intake and incidence of CHD or cerebrovascular disease [26].

The Rotterdam study was a population-based prospective investigation of a sample of men and women 55 years and older in the Netherlands with a median follow-up time of 5.5 years. An analysis of the relationship of sodium and potassium intake to cardiovascular morbidity and mortality was performed on all the subjects who died or experienced a nonfatal myocardial infarction or stroke

during follow-up (n = 1,182) and in 1,448 randomly selected controls [27]. Since the participants only provided overnight timed urine collections at baseline, only an estimate of the sodium/potassium ratio could be obtained. This ratio was unrelated to CVD events or mortality in the whole population; however, when restricting the analysis to participants free of CVD at baseline and with BMI over 25, it was significantly associated with all-cause mortality (relative risk [RR] = 1.19) after adjustment for multiple confounders. There was no relationship, however, between the urinary sodium/potassium ratio and CVD mortality.

In the first and second Trials of Hypertension Prevention (TOHP I and TOHP II, respectively), the effect of nonpharmacological intervention on BP was tested in 30- to 54-year-old adult individuals with prehypertension at baseline. A total of 744 participants in TOHP I and 2,382 participants in TOHP II were randomized to a sodium reduction intervention or control group for 18 months (TOHP I) and 36–48 months (TOHP II). In TOHP I (which ended early in 1990), the net decrease in 24-hour sodium excretion from baseline to end of the study was 44 mmol and net, statistically significant, changes in BP were −1.7/−0.8 mm Hg [28]. In TOHP II (ending March 1992), the sodium reduction group achieved a net decrease in sodium excretion of 40 mmol/24 hr with a borderline significant decrease in the incidence of hypertension [29]. Follow-up information on CVD outcomes and death was obtained after 10–15 years for 2,415 participants in the original intervention studies (77%). After adjustment for age, clinic site of original examination, demographic features, and baseline BMI and urinary sodium excretion, a significantly lower RR of CVD was observed in the participants randomized to the sodium reduction group compared to controls. The results were similar when the two trials were analyzed separately. The final follow-up questionnaire administered in 2004 to 2005 to event-free participants in the two studies indicated that those who had been randomized to the active intervention group still maintained a reduced sodium diet compared to those in the control group. Strengths of this study were the repeated measurements of urinary sodium excretion during the intervention phase and the reasonably long follow-up time. Its weaknesses were the less than complete rate of follow-up and the lack of direct measurement of BP, weight, and sodium after termination of the intervention study [30].

Dietary Sodium Intake and Stroke

A cohort of 7,895 men of Japanese ancestry aged 45–68 years was followed for 10 years in the island of Oahu (Hawaii). There were 238 cases of stroke (154 thromboembolic, 65 hemorrhagic,19 of unknown type). Whereas elevated BP was the main risk factor for all types of stroke, no significant relationship was detected with dietary salt intake evaluated at baseline by a single 24-hour dietary recall [31].

In Taiwan, a cohort of 8,562 individuals of both genders (age range 36–79 years) were followed for up to 4 years during which time 104 first-ever strokes were identified. The annual incidence was as high as 3.3 per 1,000 subjects. In multivariate analysis, hypertension and daily consumption of foods with a very high salt content were significant risk factors for stroke (total) with risk ratios of 1.9 and 1.3, respectively. Habitual food intake was evaluated by a questionnaire administered at baseline [32].

The evaluation of sodium intake was likewise based on a 24-hour dietary recall obtained in the study by He et al. in which a separate analysis of normal weight ($n = 6,797$) and overweight participants ($n = 2,688$) was carried out. Sodium intake was not associated with the risk of stroke among non-overweight persons whereas among overweight participants a 100-mmol higher sodium intake predicted a significantly greater incidence (32%) and higher mortality (89%) from stroke upon multivariate adjustment [24].

In the study by Tuomilehto et al., conducted on a random sample of population of a few Finnish provinces ($n = 2,533$), no significant relationship was observed between sodium intake (estimated by 24-hour urine collection) and risk of stroke in either men or women recruited in 1982 and 1987 and followed until the end of 1995 [25].

In the Takayama study, a population-based prospective investigation conducted in Japan, 13,355 men and 15,724 women were enrolled (after exclusion of subjects with history of CVD) and followed for an average of 7 years. The participants' usual diet at entry was evaluated by the use of a val-

idated food frequency questionnaire. The habitual dietary salt intake in this population was on average over 12 g/day. Upon stratification of the participants by tertiles of sodium intake and adjustment for age, BMI, smoking, alcohol, physical activity, history of hypertension and diabetes, and intakes of potassium protein and vitamin E, statistical associations were detected between sodium intake and mortality from total and ischemic stroke. The association was stronger and highly significant in men and borderline significant in women. It was strengthened in persons with a BMI over 23 [33].

In the above-mentioned Rotterdam study, the analysis of the relationship between the sodium/potassium ratio determined on overnight urine collections provided at baseline and subsequent incidence of stroke found no statistically significant association [27].

Conclusions

An overall assessment of the results of the cohort studies that evaluated the relationship of habitual dietary sodium intake to morbidity and mortality from CVD shows a prevalence of studies indicating a direct association between salt intake and cardiovascular risk. In particular, with regard to the incidence of CHD and stroke, an equal number of studies proved a statistically significant direct association or were not able to show any association, with no study suggesting an inverse relationship. As far as total CVD and all-cause mortality the evidence was inconclusive. Based on the results of three large studies, the hypothesis has been made of a particularly unfavorable interaction between high sodium intake and overweight with respect to cardiovascular outcomes [24,25,33].

It must be noted that all the studies available are affected by substantial methodological limitations of which the most important is the very inaccurate evaluation of the habitual sodium intake of participants, this having been estimated by either a food questionnaire or a 24-hour urine collection provided at entry into the study in a single occasion. This limitation substantially reduces the potential to detect a true biological association between the exposure factor (salt intake) and the study outcomes.

Recently, on the basis of a comparison between the outcomes of studies conducted in populations with relatively low NaCl intake versus those with higher intakes, a J-shaped relationship was proposed between sodium intake and risk of CVD [34]. This model would suggest substantial benefit from sodium intake reductions at least in population with average intakes higher than 5 g/day. It should be noted that an average consumption well above this figure is common to the large majority of both developed and developing countries.

In conclusion, there is a prevalence of prospective studies indicating an unfavorable effect of high sodium intake on risk of stroke and CHD, but further evidence needs to be accumulated in order to come to definitive results.

Dietary Potassium and Cardiovascular Risk

Several studies suggested that a potassium-rich diet may protects against CVD. First-generation studies mainly focused on the relationships between dietary potassium and BP, whereas later studies investigated the possible effects of potassium on vascular function and structure in order to seek biological plausibility for an influence of dietary potassium intake on cardiovascular morbidity and mortality even independently of changes in BP. In addition, the results of longitudinal epidemiological studies, in which the association between dietary potassium and cardiovascular morbidity and mortality was evaluated, will be briefly reviewed.

Dietary Potassium and Blood Pressure

Several epidemiologic studies have detected an inverse relationship between dietary potassium intake and BP both within and across populations [35]. In the INTERSALT study, dietary potassium intake was associated with lower BP values after adjustment for age, gender, BMI, alcohol intake, and sodium excretion [36]. A few studies provided a 'quantitative' estimate of the protective effect of a potassium-rich diet against the development of hypertension. In the Nurses' Health Study, controlling for age, BMI, and alcohol intake, a potassium intake at baseline greater than 3.2 g/day was associated with an RR of 0.77 of developing hypertension in

4 years compared with an intake lower than 2 g/day [37]. In the Health Professionals Study, participants with a potassium intake greater than 3.6 g/day had a reduced risk of hypertension in 4 years (RR = 0.65) in comparison with those on a lower intake (2.4 g/day or less) [38]. A meta-analysis of randomized controlled trials of potassium supplements indicated that an increase in potassium intake of at least 20 mmol/day (0.5 g/day) was associated with significant falls in BP [39]. This antihypertensive effect was more pronounced in the presence of an elevated sodium intake and in blacks in comparison to whites. Another recently published meta-analysis of five trials ($n = 425$; 8–16 weeks of follow-up) indicated that potassium supplementation resulted in a large, but statistically nonsignificant, reduction in systolic (-11.2 mm Hg) and diastolic (-5.0 mm Hg) BP in comparison to control [40].

In the evaluation of available data, however, it must considered that the response to potassium supplementation is slow to appear, and therefore, the duration of intervention plays a crucial role for effects to be detected [41]. Indeed, in a randomized controlled trial from our group, potassium supplementation was effective in reducing BP in hypertensive patients after 24 weeks of intervention [42].

In addition, there may be a difference in response whether potassium supplementation is provided as a pharmacological preparation or as part of the habitual diet. We carried out a long-term randomized controlled trial to evaluate the effects of increased potassium intake attained by a rise in fruit, vegetable and legume consumption. The results showed that, at the end of 1-year follow-up, in the patients assigned to the potassium-rich diet, BP control was achieved with less than half the amount of drugs needed in the control group [43].

The nutritional strategies aiming at enhancing dietary potassium intake have been recently reviewed [44,45]. Overall, the results of the studies of oral potassium supplementation suggest that a causal relationship exists between the higher potassium intake and the BP fall observed in most clinical trials and that the antihypertensive effect of potassium is clinically meaningful. Moreover, the significant BP decrease observed also in trials in normotensive individuals is consistent with a potential of this type of intervention in hypertension prevention. Oral potassium supplementation is generally very well tolerated and has not been associated to any detectable adverse effect. The ratio of sodium to potassium intake may be even more important than the individual intakes of the two electrolytes.

Potassium and Vascular Function

The protective role of dietary potassium against CVD has been mostly investigated in terms of its effects on BP regulation. However, a number of experimental studies confer biological plausibility to the hypothesis that an elevated potassium intake has a direct protective role against vascular damage. A high potassium diet was able to dramatically reduce the elevated death rate associated with feeding stroke-prone spontaneously hypertensive rats (SHR-SP) a high-sodium diet [46]. In Dahl salt-sensitive rats, increased potassium intake counteracted the sodium-induced renal damage [47] as well as the release of endothelium- and macrophage-derived growth factors [48], suggesting an antiproliferative effect of potassium. The effect of potassium on oxidative endothelial stress was examined by measuring lipid peroxides in the aortic wall and in the plasma of SHR-SP exposed to a high potassium intake: a significant reduction in lipid peroxide accumulation [49] was detected together with lower endothelial permeability [50] and decreased macrophage adherence to the vascular wall [51]. In *in vitro* experiments, increasing potassium concentration in the medium (to values within the physiological range) reduced reactive oxygen species (ROS) generation by endothelial cultures and human white blood cells [52,53] and caused a significant inhibition of vascular smooth muscle cell proliferation [54]. Furthermore, a recent study suggested that potassium supplementation provides neuroprotection (reduction of ischemic cerebral infarct size by reversing cerebral artery hypertrophy) in SHR-SP [55], whereas in DOCA/salt rats, a potassium-rich diet was associated with a reduction of cardiac and renal hypertrophy, independently of changes in BP [56].

Taken together, these results are consistent with the epidemiologic findings and suggest that the favorable influence of dietary potassium on vascular function might occur independently of its effect on BP control.

Dietary Potassium and Coronary Heart Disease

A few studies investigated whether dietary potassium exerts a protective role against the occurrence of CHD events. Some of them, in particular, investigated the relationship of habitual fruit and vegetable consumption, the most important sources of potassium in the diet, to morbidity and mortality from CHD [57,58].

In the Women's Health Study [57], the incidence of CVD (including myocardial infarction, stroke, CHD, and cardiovascular-related deaths) was prospectively investigated in 39,876 women whose intake of fruit and vegetables was evaluated at baseline. During 5-year follow-up, 418 incident cases of CVD were documented, including 126 myocardial infarctions. A 32% reduction of the risk of cardiovascular events was detected after adjustment for age, smoking, and drug treatment, increasing the daily consumption of fruit and vegetables from 2 to 10 servings per day. Similarly, higher intakes of fruit and vegetables were associated with a lower, though not statistically significant, incidence of myocardial infarction.

The Kuopio Ischemic Heart Disease Risk Factor Study prospectively investigated all-cause and cardiovascular-related mortality (follow-up 13 years) in 1,950 male adults without previous history of CVD, in relation to the estimated consumption of fruits and vegetables. All-cause mortality was significantly lower among men in the highest quintile of consumption of fruits and vegetables (fully adjusted model: RR = 0.66), but risk reduction did not reach statistical significance when only cardiovascular-related deaths were considered [58].

In the aforementioned analyses, the possible role of potassium was indirectly estimated by the consumption of fruit and vegetables. However, other epidemiological prospective studies evaluated more specifically the association between dietary potassium intake and CVD risk. This was the case for the analysis of the NHANES I by Bazzano et al., carried out in a sample of 9,805 individuals, in whom the incidence of cardiovascular events ($n = 1,847$) was documented over a very long (19 years) follow-up period [59]. The potassium-rich diet did not show a statistically significant protective effect (RR = 1.01) against the risk of developing CHD in this study.

Table 37.1 Cohort studies on dietary sodium and potassium intake and risk of stroke.

Author (year)	N	Gender	Follow-up (yr)	No. of events	Hazard Ratio* (95% CI)
Dietary sodium intake and risk of stroke (highest vs. lowest intake)					
Tuomilehto (2001)	2,436	M+F	6	84	1.13 (0.84–1.51)
Nagata (2004)	29,079	M/F	7	M 137	2.33 (1.23–4.45)
				F 132	1.70 (0.96–3.02)
					Relative risk* (95% CI)
Kagan (1985)	7,895	M	10	238	not reported
Hu (1992)	8,562	M+F	4	104	1.8 (1.2–2.7)[b]
He (1999)	9,479	M+F	19	NW[c] 430	0.99 (0.81–1.21)
				OW[d] 250	1.39 (1.09–1.77)
Geleijnse (2007)	795	M+F	5	181	1.08 (0.80–1.46)
Dietary potassium intake and risk of stroke (high vs. low intake)					
Khaw (1987)[a]	859	M+F	12	24	0.60 (0.44–0.82)
Ascherio (1998)	43,738	M	8	328	0.62 (0.43–0.88)
Iso (1999)	85,764	F	14	690	0.69 (0.50–0.95)
Bazzano (2001)	9,805	M+F	19	927	0.76 (0.58–1.01)
Geleijinse (2007)	795	M+F	5	181	1.02 (0.71–1.46)

*Adjusted for the main cardiovascular risk factors.
[a]End-point = mortality.
[b]Adjusted for age.
[c]Normal-weight participants.
[d]Overweight participants.

In the Rotterdam Study, sodium and potassium intake were examined in relation to CVD and mortality in an unselected sample of subjects 55 years and older, who were followed for 5 years. Dietary sodium and potassium intakes were estimated by daily urinary excretion of the two cations and, in a larger sample, by dietary questionnaires. There was no consistent association between the daily urinary excretion of potassium and CVD mortality. However, dietary potassium intake estimated by food frequency questionnaire was associated with a lower risk (RR = 0.71) of death from all causes in normotensive subjects without previous history of CVD [27].

Dietary Potassium and Stroke

Table 37.1 briefly summarizes the results of the main epidemiological studies that investigated the association between dietary potassium intake and the risk of stroke [60].

The first such study was published in 1987. Among the 859 men and women composing the Rancho Bernardo study cohort, at the end of the 12-year follow-up observation, stroke-associated mortality was significantly lower among participants in the upper tertile of dietary potassium intake [61]. In particular, a 10-mmol increase in daily consumption of potassium was associated with a 40% reduction in the risk of stroke-associated mortality. This issue was also investigated in the analysis of the data of the NHANES I. In this study, an inverse, statistically significant association between dietary potassium and stroke-related mortality was detected among black men and hypertensive men [62]. The previously mentioned Rotterdam Study [27] evaluated the association between the incidence of cardiovascular events and the dietary intake of potassium, estimated either by 24-hour urinary excretion of the cation or by dietary questionnaire (in a larger sample). As shown in Table 37.1, dietary potassium intake did not significantly affect the incidence of stroke.

In the Health Professionals' Study, carried out in a large male population, the RR of stroke was significantly lower in men in the upper quintile of potassium intake (median daily intake = 4.3 g) as compared to those in the bottom one (median daily intake = 2.4 g): No significant difference was noted in the reduction of risk for ischemic stroke as compared with total stroke among participants consuming a potassium-rich diet [63].

The relationship between dietary potassium intake and stroke in women was evaluated in the large Nurses' Health Study population in which a 30%, borderline statistically significant, reduction of the risk of stroke in women in the highest quintile of potassium consumption was observed [64]. The previously quoted study by Bazzano et al. showed that the risk of stroke was significantly higher among participants on potassium-poor diet, that is, consuming less than 34.6 mmol of potassium per day [59]. Finally, in a recently published study carried out in individuals older than 65 years [65], both low serum potassium level in diuretic users and low dietary potassium intake in those not taking diuretics were associated with increased risk of stroke (RR = 2.37).

Conclusions

Experimental, epidemiologic, and clinical evidence supports the hypothesis that the adoption of a high-potassium diet represents an effective non-pharmacological measure for the treatment of mild hypertension and an useful tool to reduce antihypertensive drug consumption in people with BP values exceeding the threshold for pharmacological treatment. This is particularly true in selected hypertensive subgroups, such as African American individuals and patients unable or unwilling to reduce their habitual sodium intake.

As far as the possible preventive role of a high potassium intake against the occurrence of CVD, while together the available data do not clearly support a protective role of dietary potassium against the occurrence of CHD, in most studies greater dietary potassium intake was shown to confer significant benefit against all-cause mortality and against morbidity and mortality from stroke.

The existing body of evidence from animal studies does suggest a biological plausibility for this effect and makes the case for seeking additional information from human studies in order to confirm the role of dietary potassium in the prevention of cardiovascular morbidity and mortality.

Selected References

17. Strazzullo P, Galletti F, Barba G. Altered renal handling of sodium in human hypertension: short review of the evidence. Hypertension 2003;41:1000–5.
24. He J, Ogden LG, Vupputuri S, et al. Dietary sodium intake and subsequent risk of cardiovascular disease in overweight adults. JAMA 1999;282(21):2027–34.
25. Tuomilehto J, Jousilahti P, Rastenyte D, et al. Urinary sodium excretion and cardiovascular mortality in Finland: a prospective study. Lancet 2001;357:848–51.
30. Cook NR, Cutler JA, Obarzanek E, et al. Long term effects of dietary sodium reduction on cardiovascular disease outcomes: observational follow-up of the trials of hypertension prevention (TOHP). BMJ 2007;334(7599): 885.
45. Siani A, Strazzullo P. Dietary potassium and cardiovascular disease: clinical applications. J Cardiovasc Risk 2000; 7:15–21.

CHAPTER 38

Metabolic and Dietary Influences on Sympathetic Nervous System Activity

Elaine Ku, Jeanie Park, Tanzina Nasreen, & Vito M. Campese
University of Southern California, Keck School of Medicine, Los Angeles, CA, USA

Introduction

Sympathetic nervous system (SNS) activity and regulation have been studied in multiple metabolic conditions, including diabetes, insulin resistance, metabolic syndrome, and human obesity. These conditions are characterized by an increased risk of cardiovascular disease (CVD) and hypertension, all of which are likely influenced by SNS overactivity. The mechanisms underlying SNS overactivity in these conditions are not fully understood, but experimental and human studies implicate factors such as hyperinsulinemia, hyperleptinemia, elevated levels of angiotensin II, reactive oxygen species (ROS), inflammation, and dietary factors. Furthermore, these factors may also contribute to the perpetuation of the metabolic disorder itself, illustrating the importance of understanding the mechanisms and considering the SNS as a potential therapeutic target in these conditions. This chapter will review SNS function and potential mechanisms underlying SNS overactivity in diabetes, insulin resistance, obesity, and metabolic syndrome.

Diabetes, Insulin Resistance, and the Role of Hyperinsulinemia

Patients with diabetes are known to be at increased risk for CVD. Heightened SNS activity might con-

Nutritional and Metabolic Bases of Cardiovascular Disease, 1st edition.
Edited by Mario Mancini, José M. Ordovas, Gabriele Riccardi,
Paolo Rubba and Pasquale Strazzullo. © 2011 Blackwell Publishing Ltd.

tribute to the development and pathogenesis of cardiovascular risk, given the correlation between sympathetic hyperactivity, hypertension, and the occurrence of CVD in diabetics. A majority of studies in the literature have shown the presence of sympathetic hyperactivity in diabetic populations without autonomic neuropathy, although some controversy still surrounds this issue. The use of microneurographic recordings of muscle sympathetic nerve activity (MSNA) in real time has been validated in study populations as a reliable measurement of central sympathetic outflow [1]. Huggett et al. observed that diabetic patients without autonomic neuropathy had higher baseline MSNA levels than nondiabetics, and the presence of diabetes further augmented sympathetic hyperactivity in hypertensive patients [2]. Even the nondiabetic offspring of patients with non-insulin-dependent diabetes mellitus (NIDDM) exhibited an elevated baseline level of sympathetic outflow that correlates closely with their degree of insulin resistance [3], suggesting that hyperinsulinemia may be a putative trigger of this excessive SNS activity.

Studies in healthy individuals maintained at euglycemia while receiving insulin infusions simulating both physiologic and supraphysiologic levels of insulinemia have elicited a rise in muscle, but not skin, SNS activity similar to that seen in diabetics [4]. These results suggest that hyperinsulinemia, as opposed to hyperglycemia, may be the actual trigger of sympathetic outflow. The exact mechanisms by which insulin influences SNS activity is not yet known but may be mediated through direct effects on the central nervous system, or through a baroreceptor-mediated elevation in SNS outflow in response to insulin-stimulated hypotension [5,6].

On the contrary, a few studies have demonstrated a diminished SNS response to hyperinsulinemia in diabetics, particularly in those with long-standing disease [7]. A small study of insulin dependent diabetics showed lower levels of MSNA in response to insulin infusions than in control subjects [8]. The relative sympathetic non-responsiveness in select populations of diabetics has not been solidified, but this phenomenon could be explained as either a maximally stimulated SNS from chronic hyperinsulinemia that obviates any further increase in response, or an early form of autonomic neuropathy [8].

Several studies on the circadian rhythm of sympathetic tone in diabetic populations have also shown an overall increase in sympathetic tone throughout the day, with a diminished parasympathetic tone during the night [7,9,10]. In heart rate variability studies using spectral analysis and 24-hour electrocardiogram (EKG) monitoring, sympathetic hyperactivity was found to be highest in non-diabetic populations with insulin resistance, as opposed to known diabetics [7]. Analysis of the offspring of diabetics with and without impaired fasting glucose also showed an association between sympathetic hyperactivity and a family history of diabetes, with the degree of sympathetic hyperactivity correlated closely to the degree of insulin resistance [11]. Previous studies have shown that patients with evidence of autonomic dysfunction are more likely to develop diabetes, even when confounders such as age, sex, body mass index (BMI), and health risk factors are accounted for [12]. Altered sympathovagal balance with a loss of normal autonomic circadian rhythm may explain the higher incidence of cardiovascular events in diabetics, since these populations lack the normal protective effects of the para-SNS during nocturnal hours [7]. Thus, earlier diagnosis of insulin resistance and treatment targeted at decreasing sympathetic hyperactivity and restoring normal autonomic circadian function may decrease the mortality of such at-risk populations.

The question, then, is whether sympathetic hyperactivity precedes hyperinsulinemia, or whether hyperinsulinemia triggers sympathetic hyperactivity. Landsberg et al. proposed that sympathetic hyperactivity in the obese precedes hyperinsulinemia, and hyperinsulinemia leads to increased thermogenesis as a evolutionary defense mechanism against obesity [13]. One of the criticisms of their proposal, however, is that sympathetic hyperactivity has been demonstrated in nonobese individuals [14]. Alternatively, chronic SNS overactivity, particularly directed to the muscle, may precede and lead to the development of insulin resistance and diabetes by decreasing blood flow to skeletal muscle beds, and thereby reducing glucose delivery and uptake by muscle cells [15] showed in a longitudinal study that sympathetic hyperactivity precedes the development of hyperinsulinemia, but one of the limitations of their study was the use of plasma norepinephrine levels as a measure of sympathetic activity: Plasma norepinephrine levels is an indirect marker of sympathetic nervous activity that can be influenced by other factors such as the clearance rate of norepinephrine in the plasma [16]. In a study conducted on dogs fed a high-fat diet with and without clonidine, clonidine administration prevented the development of insulin resistance despite weight changes, again suggesting that central sympathetic nervous activity may play a role in the pathogenesis of insulin resistance [17]. Thus far, the "chicken or the egg" question remains unanswered, and further research will need to be conducted to fully answer this question.

Obesity and the Sympathetic Nervous System

Obesity is a growing worldwide epidemic, and in itself, is a significant risk factor for cardiovascular mortality. Obesity is associated with SNS overactivity, independent of arterial blood pressure, and SNS hyperactivity is one pathogenic mechanism underlying obesity-related hypertension [18,19]. In a case-control matched study of lean versus obese normotensive individuals, MSNA was found to be uniformly higher in obese subjects when compared to lean controls [20]. Individuals with hypertension and obesity were found to have cumulatively higher levels of MSNA than either individuals with obesity or hypertension alone [21]. Similarly, in healthy individuals, MSNA levels correlated closely with percent body fat and body mass index; individuals who had a BMI > 27 were found to have MSNA levels as high as double that of nonobese individuals [22]. However, this relationship between percentage body fat and MSNA level was not replicated in a study of Pima Indians, and Abate et al. previously showed that BMI correlated positively with MSNA in white men, white women, and black women, but not in black men [23], suggesting that genetic and racial factors also contribute to sympathetic regulation in the obese [24]. In addition, a differential effect of the SNS on various organs in the body has been noted, with increased renal and muscular, but subnormal levels of cardiac, sympathetic activity being noted in the obese [25].

Weight gain in healthy, lean individuals has also been shown to correlate with an increase in SNS activity. Several studies have shown that the consumption of standardized, hypercaloric diets designed to induce modest weight gain results in short-term elevations in sympathetic nervous activity, as demonstrated by elevated norepinephrine turnover rates and MSNA, independent of changes in dietary sodium [26–28]. Furthermore, the effect of weight gain on MSNA was reversible with weight loss induced by use of hypocaloric diets [27]. The relationship between the type of body fat and the sympathetic activity has also been examined. Alvarez et al. showed that the degree of visceral, but not subcutaneous fat, correlated closely to the degree of MSNA activity, even though plasma levels of leptin were found to be more closely correlated to subcutaneous fat [29]. However, other studies have shown no relationship between visceral fat and MSNA [28]. The exact relationship between body fat type and sympathetic activity is still controversial.

Multiple theories have been proposed for the mechanistic relationship between sympathetic hyperactivity and obesity. Since many obese individuals have insulin resistance, hyperinsulinemia has been proposed by some as the putative trigger for sympathetic hyperactivity in obesity, especially since overeating leads to increased plasma insulin levels [25]. In addition, obese individuals have high leptin levels that act on the central nervous system to increase SNS outflow. Leptin, a protein secreted primarily by white adipose tissue, acts centrally to decrease appetite and food intake [30], increase energy expenditure and thermogenesis [31,32], and increase sympathetic outflow [25,33]. Animal studies have shown that mice injected with leptin demonstrate increased sympathetic innervation in brown adipose tissue, the adrenal glands, and the hindlimbs, an effect that is independent of any changes in plasma insulin [34]. Furthermore, Zucker rats with mutated leptin receptors fail to demonstrate any change in sympathetic activity, even with injection of high levels of leptin into the plasma [34]. These studies point at a possible role for leptin in the regulation of sympathetic nervous activity and the pathogenesis of obesity-related hypertension.

Hyperleptinemia and insulin resistance are features of human obesity [25,35,36], and both leptin and insulin levels correlate with MSNA levels in humans [36], suggesting a causal link. Furthermore, renal norepinephrine spillover has been shown to correlate with plasma leptin levels in men with different levels of obesity [37].

Metabolic Syndrome and the Sympathetic Nervous System

Metabolic syndrome is defined by the World Health Organization as the coexistence of insulin resistance with two of the following: hypertension, hypertriglyceridemia, low high-density lipoprotein (HDL)-cholesterol, BMI greater than 30, or abdominal obesity. Metabolic syndrome and obesity are associated with an increased risk of diabetes and CVD [38], and recent studies have shown that sympathetic neural discharge is increased in metabolic syndrome [18,35]. MSNA has been shown to be elevated in nondiabetic humans with metabolic syndrome, and is further augmented by the presence of hypertension [18]. Mechanisms underlying sympathetic activation in metabolic syndrome have not been fully elucidated. Since many of the features of metabolic syndrome overlap those associated with diabetes and obesity, the mechanisms eliciting SNS overactivity may be similar in these disorders. Some potential mediators of sympathetic activation in metabolic syndrome includes hyperinsulinemia, fatty acids, hyperleptinemia, angiotensin II, and renal afferent nerves [19].

Dietary Influences on the Sympathetic Nervous System

Salt Intake

The influence of dietary salt intake on cardiovascular morbidity has remained an issue of great debate in the literature. A high-salt diet is thought to increase the risk of developing hypertension and CVD in prone individuals, although no studies have shown definitively that reducing salt intake alters cardiovascular morbidity [39,40]. Most of the studies on the influence of salt intake on the SNS have been based on animal studies and demonstrate that high salt intake is associated with increased SNS activity. Dietary salt is thought to sensitize the rostral ventrolateral medulla (RVLM), the control center for sympathetic activity, and heighten sympathetic response. In one study, rats given saline solutions exhibited exaggerated blood pressure responses thought to be secondary to sympathetic hyperactivity, an effect postulated by the authors to be affected through the predisposition of neurons in the RVLM to excitation through salt exposure, although the exact cause is unknown [41]. In a similar study, rats drinking sodium chloride had higher sympathetic nervous activity levels in the renal and splanchnic systems in response to glutamate injections into the RVLM, but this effect was only observed if rats were given sodium chloride in their diet for more than one week [42].

Brooks et al. proposed that dietary salt intake exerts its effects on the SNS by disturbing the balance between sympathoexcitatory and sympathoinhibitory influences on the rostral ventrolateral medulla [43]. The increase in dietary salt intake is postulated to decrease angiotensin II levels, a sympathoexcitatory factor in the brain [44,45]. Brooks et al. also hypothesizes that in normal, nonhypertensive individuals, the sympathoinhibitory effects of dietary salt intake predominate and angiotensin II levels fall in response to sodium, leading to decreased sympathetic activity. In contrast, in salt-sensitive hypertensive individuals, angiotensin II levels do not fall as expected, resulting in increased sympathetic activity that may contribute to worsening hypertension [43]. This hypothesis has been validated in a rat study, where injection of angiotensin II resulted in sympathoexcitation, but pretreatment of rats with candesartan (an an-

giotensin receptor blocker) blunted the expected sympathoexcitatory response [46]. Furthermore, in spontaneously hypertensive rats (SHRs), social stress triggered increased sympathetic nervous activity and enhanced dietary salt appetite compared to control rats, but this enhancement of salt appetite in SHRs was inhibited by the administration of both reserpine and clonidine [47]. Inhibition of sympathetic hyperactivity in response to dietary salt intake may explain improvements in blood pressure in some populations of hypertensives who appear to have salt-sensitive disease [39]. Thus, the SNS may play a role in both the pathogenesis and continual propagation of hypertension both through increase of salt-sensitivity and/or through and enhancement of dietary salt intake in certain salt-sensitive populations [48].

Few direct studies on the effect of dietary salt on the sympathetic nervous activity have been conducted in humans. Since plasma osmolality is mainly dependent on sodium levels in the body, plasma osmolality may represent a reasonable surrogate marker of dietary salt influence on the autonomic nervous system. In humans, assessment of MSNA following infusions of hypertonic versus isotonic saline have shown that increases in plasma osmolality also increase sympathetic nervous activity, a change that is independent of changes in circulatory volume [49]. Studies on rats have demonstrated that the response of sympathetic outflow to changes in plasma osmolality is also independent of vasopressin activity [44]. The paraventricular nucleus of the hypothalamus (PVH) is thought to control plasma osmolality, and the PVH may initiate an enhancement of sympathetic outflow through its interactions with the RVLM as demonstrated in animal studies, but more studies need to be conducted to confirm that this is also true in humans [45].

Potassium Intake

Multiple studies have shown the benefits of a high-potassium diet in the treatment of hypertension [50,51]. The mechanisms underlying the beneficial effects of dietary potassium intake on blood pressure are not entirely clear, and the possible mechanistic role of potassium intake on modulation of the SNS remains controversial. A high-potassium diet ameliorates the pressor effect of high sodium intake in salt-sensitive hypertension, and animal studies suggest that the hypotensive effect is mediated by inhibition of central sympathetic outflow, particularly that directed to kidneys [52,53]. Furthermore, a high-salt diet combined with a low-potassium diet was associated with inappropriate sympathetic activation [54]. In humans, potassium supplementation lowered blood pressure in salt-loaded hypertensive patients and was associated with a reduction in plasma norepinephrine, suggesting that potassium intake decreased blood pressure by decreasing sympathetic activity [53]. However, in another study of salt-loaded hypertensive patients, the reduction in blood pressure with potassium supplementation was associated with concomitant increases in plasma norepinephrine levels, suggesting that the hypotensive effect of dietary potassium was volume mediated, and the increase in sympathetic activity was in turn a compensatory mechanism [55]. Similarly, MSNA was found to be lower in normotensive and borderline hypertensive humans on a *low*-potassium diet, despite its association with higher blood pressures. Whether sympathetic activity is lowered with dietary potassium intake in salt-sensitive hypertension and is the mediator of blood pressure reduction, or instead is higher with dietary potassium as a reflex to increased sodium excretion, is currently unknown, and warrants further investigation in the future.

Dietary Fat and Carbohydrates

The fat versus carbohydrate composition of diets also appears to affect sympathetic nervous activity. One rat study has shown that diets high in fat composition appear to increase sympathetic innervation of the heart, but not brown adipose tissue, which may explain the subsequent development of obesity and risk of hypertension [24]. High fat feeding has also been correlated with elevated levels of insulin and leptin in rats [56], which in turn may stimulate central SNS outflow. High carbohydrate dietary intake has also been found to stimulate sympathetic activity in human studies as measured by MSNA, a mechanism that may be secondary to the effects of insulin on the SNS with carbohydrate intake [57].

Selected References

19. Hall JE, DA Hildebrandt, J Kuo. Obesity hypertension: role of leptin and sympathetic nervous system. Am J Hypertens 2001;14(6 Pt 2):103S–15S.

21. Grassi G, Seravalle G, Dell'Oro R, et al. Adrenergic and reflex abnormalities in obesity-related hypertension. Hypertension 2000;36(4):538–42.

25. Esler M, Rumantir M, Wiesner G, et al. Sympathetic nervous system and insulin resistance: from obesity to diabetes. Am J Hypertens 2001;14(11 Pt 2):304S–9S.

37. Eikelis N, Schlaich M, Aggarwal A, et al. Interactions between leptin and the human sympathetic nervous system. Hypertension 2003;41(5):1072–9.

48. Campese VM, Romoff MS, Levitan D, et al. Abnormal relationship between sodium intake and sympathetic nervous system activity in salt-sensitive patients with essential hypertension. Kidney Int 1982;21(2):371–8.

CHAPTER 39

Improved Nutrition: Key to Solving the Populationwide Blood Pressure Problem

Jeremiah Stamler
Northwestern University, Chicago, IL, USA

This chapter is an overview of 25 years of research, primarily by its authors, on relations of multiple dietary factors to blood pressure (BP).

The Population-wide Blood Pressure Problem

Adverse BP is one of the established major factors causing the epidemic occurrence of cardiovascular diseases (CVDs) worldwide. The relation of BP to CVD (coronary heart disease [CHD], stroke, heart failure, etc) is continuous, graded (curvilinear), strong over the whole range of BP, systolic and diastolic, and independent of other major risk factors (Figure 39.1 and Table 39.1) [1,2]. This is the case for women and men at all adult ages, worldwide, in industrialized and developing countries;

In collaboration with Ian J. Brown[2], Paul Elliott[2], Martha L. Daviglus[1], Alan R. Dyer[1], Dan Garside[1], Linda Van Horn[1], Lawrence J. Appel[3], Queenie Chan[2], Ioanna Tzoulaki[2], Hugo Kesteloot[4], Katsuyuki Miura[5], Nagako Okuda[6], Hirotsugu Ueshima[5], & Liancheng Zhao[7]

[1] Northwestern university, Chicago, 1L, USA
[2] Imperial College, London, UK, [3] Johns Hopkins Medical Institutions, Baltimore, MD, USA, [4] Katholieke Universiteit, Leuven, Belgium, [5] Shiga University of Medical Science, Shiga, Japan, [6] The First Institute for Health Promotion and Health Care, Tokyo, Japan [7] Fuwai Hospital and Cardiovascular Institute, Chinese Academy of Medical Sciences Beijing, Peoples Republic of China

Nutritional and Metabolic Bases of Cardiovascular Disease, 1st edition. Edited by Mario Mancini, José M. Ordovas, Gabriele Riccardi, Paolo Rubba and Pasquale Strazzullo. © 2011 Blackwell Publishing Ltd.

for all ethnic and socioeconomic strata. Considered separately, systolic BP (SBP) relates more strongly to CVD risk than diastolic (DBP), as unequivocally demonstrated by the extraordinarily precise MRFIT data on approximately 350,000 men ages 35–57 years surveyed in 18 U.S. cities from 1973 to 1975 and followed for 25 years (Figure 39.1) [1]. Therefore, the focus here is on SBP, in considering impact of multiple dietary factors on BP.

In youth and young adulthood (e.g., at ages 18–29 years), as shown repeatedly by epidemiologic studies in many countries, population average SBP/DBP is at or below the generally accepted cutpoint for normal BP, that is, $\leq120/\leq80$ mm Hg (Table 39.2) [3]. However, in middle and older age—due to the rise in BP with age (SBP more steeply than DBP) that occurs in the great majority of people—population average SBP is well above normal, in the prehypertensive (121–139 mm Hg) or hypertensive (≥140 mm Hg) range (Table 39.2) [3]; prevalence rates of prehypertension and hypertension are high, at epidemic levels; prevalence rates of normal BP are low; most of the population is at inordinate risk of CVD morbidity, disability, and death, with resultant impaired life expectancy. In many populations of varied ethnicity, people in lower socioeconomic strata (SES) have this set of problems to an aggravated degree [2].

Throughout the world, the emphasis in medical care and public health efforts to deal with the BP problem has been overwhelmingly or exclusively on

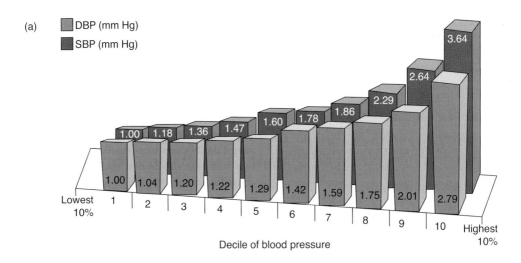

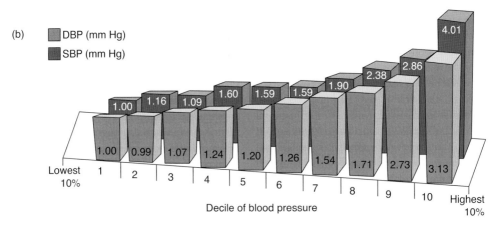

Figure 39.1 Relation of SBP and DBP decile, considered separately to relative risk of 25-year mortality from (a) CHD, (b) stroke; 347,978 men screened for MRFIT, ages 35–57 years at baseline and without a history of hospitalization for heart attack. SBP deciles are defined by the following cut points: <112, 112–117, 118–120, 121–124, 125–128, 129–131, 132–136, 137–141, 142–150, ≥151 mm Hg; DBP deciles: <71, 71–75, 76–78, 79–80, 81–83, 84–85, 86–88, 89–91, 92–97, ≥98 mm Hg [1].

identification, evaluation, and treatment of people with high BP (SBP ≥ 140 and/or DBP ≥ 90 mm Hg, or SBP ≥ 160 and/or DBP ≥ 95 mm Hg), that is, on the proverbial "tip of the iceberg" of the population-wide BP problem. As four decades of experience with this high-risk strategy have demonstrated, it is by itself, however important and necessary, inadequate to solve the problem. It is a late, reactive (not proactive) strategy. It entails waiting for people to develop high BP as BP rises with age over the adult decades, then finding and treating them—a never-ending process. It means relying on costly, com-plex long-term drug treatment of tens of millions of people for the foreseeable future. Since it en-compasses no strategic component for prevention of high BP, it offers no approach to the resolution (i.e., elimination or ending) of the epidemic of ad-verse BP levels. For hypertensive people so man-aged, its capabilities are limited. The BP reduc-tions achieved are almost always incomplete, and BP is only rarely reduced to normal levels (SBP/DBP ≤120/≤80 mm Hg). It is further limited in that its focus is only on hypertensive people; it offers no approach to reducing CVD risks for the tens of

Table 39.1   Serum total cholesterol (TC), SBP, smoking, and hazard ratio for CHD death, MRFIT men.

Men ages 35–44 at baseline (N = 149, 339)

TC (mg/dl)	SBP (mm Hg)				
	≤120	121–129	130–139	140–159	160+
Nonsmokers at baseline					
<180	1.00	1.38	2.45***	4.09***	10.25***
180–99	1.78*	2.50**	2.95***	4.79***	12.64***
200–19	1.96**	2.26***	3.14***	5.63***	8.57***
220–39	2.68***	2.84***	5.47***	7.61***	21.72***
240+	3.66***	6.64***	8.65***	13.18***	26.77***
Cigarette smokers at baseline					
<180	3.35***	3.10***	7.55***	10.32***	37.61***
180–99	5.78***	6.86***	7.82***	12.82***	24.74***
200–19	5.69***	7.28***	10.22***	18.99***	22.25***
220–39	7.94***	10.74***	14.74***	23.16***	41.23***
240+	14.53***	19.09***	20.36***	34.46***	52.26***

Men ages 45–57 at baseline (N = 198, 639)

TC (mg/dl)	SBP (mm Hg)				
	≤120	121–129	130–139	140–159	160+
Nonsmokers at baseline					
<180	1.00	1.32	2.09***	2.64***	5.31***
180–99	1.38*	1.79***	2.30***	3.95***	6.87***
200–19	1.43**	2.02***	2.89***	3.88***	7.69***
220–39	1.97***	2.33***	3.32***	5.42***	8.36***
240+	2.75***	3.57***	4.81***	7.07***	12.05***
Cigarette smokers at baseline					
<180	2.50***	3.32***	3.79***	6.74***	10.30***
180–99	2.77***	3.95***	5.45***	7.98***	11.80***
200–19	3.64***	4.05***	6.47***	9.24***	17.55***
220–39	4.72***	6.05***	7.28***	11.83***	18.09***
240+	5.65***	7.30***	9.59***	13.09***	19.28***

All analyses exclude persons with history of myocardial infaration at baseline; follow-up 25 years, men ages 35–44 at baseline, 3,345 CHD deaths; men ages 45–57, 12,354 CHD deaths.
*$p < .05$; **$p < .01$; ***$p < .001$.
Hazard ratio, adjusted for age, race, and diabetes, substratum of nonsmokers with TC < 180 mg/dl and SBP ≤ 120 mm Hg set at 1.00.
SBP: systolic blood pressure; CHD: coronary heart disease.

millions at higher risk due to prehypertensive BP levels.

Recognition of these critical problems inherent in an exclusive high-risk strategy has led recently to modifications of public policy: expansion of strategy to embrace also primary prevention of ad-verse BP levels, i.e., a two-pronged strategy: (1) population-wide primary prevention of adverse BP levels, and (2) focused public health and medical care efforts for people who already are hypertensive [4]. The population-wide primary prevention effort involves people of all ages, beginning with

Table 39.2 Mean SBP and DBP, U.S. population, NHANES III, Phase 1 (1988–91), by age, ethnic group, and gender.

	Mean SBP (mm Hg)				Mean DBP (mm Hg)			
Age (yrs)	Black men	Black women	White men	White women	Black men	Black women	White men	White women
18–29	119	108	117	106	72	65	70	65
30–39	122	115	119	110	78	73	77	70
40–49	128	123	122	114	82	76	79	72
50–59	136	132	127	123	84	76	79	74
60–74	140	142	134	132	79	73	75	70

NHANES: National Health and Nutrition Examination Survey.
Source; Burt et al. [3].

young women (preconception), involving the pregnant woman to protect both her and her fetus, and proceeding then from infancy forward (i.e., it includes as a key component primordial prevention [5]). Its goal is to achieve a significant downward shift in population average SBP/DBP to favorable levels at all ages, i.e., to end the rise in BP with age and solve the problem of epidemic adverse BP levels. This is a population-wide goal that cannot be addressed by pharmacologic means. It requires reduction/elimination of the exposures to adverse lifestyles producing this epidemic.

In fact, data are indeed available from population studies, cross-sectional and prospective, indicating that the increases in SBP and DBP experienced by most people during adult decades are *not* programmed in the genome, as inevitable human developments. Many isolated populations have been identified who have no such rise (Figure 39.2) [6], at least not until with migration they undergo lifestyle changes. Undoubtedly, the currently common BP increases with age are consequences of adverse environmental exposures in populations generally susceptible genetically. Within these populations so exposed over the life span to multiple environmental factors tending to increase BP, interindividual differences in BP response occur, due both to differences in degree of exposure and in susceptibility, the latter likely due in the main to interindividual differences in multiple genetic pathways influencing BP. But the central qualitative phenomenon is that in the face of multiple persistent adverse mass exposures, most people are more or less susceptible genetically to adverse environmental influences

on BP. The basic reason for this probably is that the adverse lifestyle exposures, dietary et al. are recent and unprecedented experiences for the human species; hence, there has been no opportunity for evolutionary genetic adaptation to them.

Is it realistic to project/undertake such population-wide efforts to improve lifestyles and thereby BP levels/distributions? On this, one good example is worth a thousand words. Since 1960, multifaceted efforts were undertaken in the United

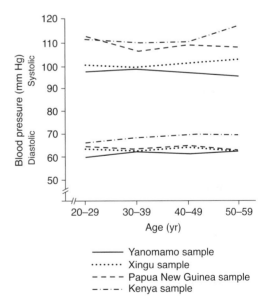

Figure 39.2 Line graphs of systolic and diastolic blood pressures by 10-year age-groups, women and men combined, four remote population samples, INTERSALT Study. (Reproduced from Mancilha-Carvalho et al. [6], with permission.)

States to reduce intake of dietary lipids, in order to decrease average serum cholesterol and rates of CHD/CVD. Over the ensuing decades, population total fat intake declined from over 40% of total calories to about 33%; saturated fat, from about 17% to 11%; dietary cholesterol, from over 700 mg/day to about 300 mg/day (130 mg/1,000 kcal) [2,7,8]. By the year 2000, adult population average serum cholesterol was down from 1960 levels of about 240 mg/dl to 200 mg/dl, and a national health goal for the year 2000 was achieved. Successive National Health and Nutrition Examination Surveys (NHANES) also indicated a modest downward trend for BP independent of drug treatment for high BP. Those favorable trends were accomplished despite countervailing influences on serum cholesterol and BP of the waxing obesity epidemic during the last decades of the twentieth century. Concurrently, U.S. CHD/CVD death rates declined more than 50% and life expectancy increased for adult men and women. Thus, it can be done.

Historical/Anthropological Notes

In clinical medicine, for actuarial purposes, in population surveys, BP measurement is a modern procedure, of the last 100 or so years. Its prerequisite was the noninvasive indirect method, invented by Riva-Rocci in the last decade of the nineteenth century [9]. Nonetheless, recognition of dietary-CVD/BP relations dates back 4,500 years, to the Chinese Yellow Emperor's classic of internal medicine *Nei Ching*: "Hence if too much salt is used for food, the pulse hardens. . ." [10]. A hard pulse is, of course, a cardinal sign of high BP.

This observation was only a few millennia after the human species made the transition from food gathering to food production, generally abandoned its traditional nomadic lifestyle, settled on the land as cultivators/herders and, hence, for the first time came to grips with the challenge of creating and storing surplus food. As nomadic food gatherers, humans had little need/use for food surpluses, actually a nuisance for nomads to transport in any quantity. Food (tubers, berries, other fruits, nuts, etc.) was collected daily by the women as families/tribes went along, as was game by the male hunters (successfully on some days at least!), and it was generally consumed as they went along. How-

ever, settled food producers had to have a safely stored surplus or one bad harvest or an epidemic disease in the flock threatened starvation and destruction. Two methods emerged to store food: drying and salting. These became foundations of the new-type food supply sustaining much greater population growth and development of towns and cities—in short, civilization, with its further transition from preliteracy to literacy, prehistory to history. Hominid/hominoid/human biological evolutionary adaptation proceeded over the course of two to four million years of nomadic food gathering; the landmark socioeconomic transition to food production occurred just a few *thousand* years ago, too recently to enable substantial genetic adaptation. Thus, the species evolved in salt-poor Africa on a habitual low-salt nomadic fare and was splendidly adapted to this circumstance, i.e., to maintaining its electrolyte-based extracellular fluid internal environment (0.9% NaCl, via the ancient oceans where multicellular complex organisms first evolved), while habitually consuming little salt in a warm climate. The human kidney remains remarkably capable of reabsorbing every millimole of filtered Na and Cl (cf. data on the Yanamamo Indians of Brazil, with virtually no NaCl in their 24-hour urine collections) [6]. However, there was too little time for evolutionary adaptation to high salt intake, belatedly introduced as a food additive to preserve food. The human kidney was and is generally slow and incomplete in clearing large amounts of consumed salt, a homeostatic adjustment accomplished by most people with associated expansion of plasma/extracellular fluid volume, and BP increase. Hence, epidemic occurrence of adverse BP levels, one of the adverse consequences of lifelong exposure to high salt as a food additive/preservative [11].

There is, of course, a short P.S. to this important particular of the adverse lifestyle–adverse BP relationship: With the invention in the twentieth century of the electric refrigerator/freezer to preserve food, need ceases for salt as a food preservative. Only the destructive aspects of the high salt additive habit remain—for society an anachronism that needs to be retired to the museum of food history.

In light of the Yellow Emperor's prescient insight of 4,500 years ago, it is relevant intellectually to note that not until the first half of the twentieth century did a few pioneer Western clinicians note that high BP could be controlled by a low-salt diet: Ambard and Beaujard in France in 1904 [12], Allen and Sherrill in the United States in 1922 [13], and Kempner in the United States in 1948 [14]. Subsequently, further trials demonstrated that reduced salt intake lowered SBP/DBP of prehypertensive as well as hypertensive adults, younger and older [15,16]. Also, the Rotterdam randomized controlled trial in infants yielded results of special relevance in terms of possible lifetime beneficial effects on BP of early exposure to lower salt intake [17,18]: a group of almost 250 newborns fed a diet lower in salt by about 30% for six months developed SBP lower by 2.1 mm Hg compared to a control group (17). Fifteen years later, those fed less salt in early infancy (follow-up 35%) had significantly lower SBP by 3.6 mm Hg (adjusted for confounders), although there was no further intervention post 6 months of age [18]. These data underscore the relevance of a strategic emphasis on primordial prevention of adverse BP by favorable lifestyle from preconception/conception/pregnancy/birth/weaning on.

Other dietary-BP relations were noted in the initial decades after indirect BP measurement became available, that is, higher BP levels in obese compared to lean people, and in habitual heavy drinkers. Also, insurance company actuaries noted early on that adults with high BP were at greater risk of CVD, premature death, and impaired life expectancy [19]. In the 1960s and 1970s, extensive prospective data became available from the first generation of population-based epidemiologic studies demonstrating the continuous, graded, strong, independent, predictive relation of BP to CHD/CVD risk, as well as the similar relation of serum total cholesterol (TC) to CHD/CVD risk [20–24]. The latter finding was noted to be concordant with clinical, pathologic, and animal experimental data implicating cholesterol—dietary and serum—as a pivotal etiologically significant risk factors in the etiopathogenesis of severe atherosclerosis, the pathologic lesion that (with its complications, e.g., thrombosis) was responsible for most cases of the then waxing CHD epidemic. It was also recognized that the BP–CHD and the TC–CHD relationships were remarkably similar (virtually superimposable) in quantitative contour—curvilinear, continuous, graded, strong (Table 39.1) [2]. As with BP, extensive data became extant showing for U.S. adult population samples substantial rises with age in average TC levels to values of about 240 mg/dl, in contrast to findings in developing country population samples and in Japan, where average TC levels were lower in youth/young adulthood and little rise occurred with age (average levels in middle age, $\leq$180 mg/dl) [20–24].

In those years, as these data accumulated, an as yet unexplained dichotomy in research activity emerged: The developing discipline of CVD epidemiology focused on the high average TC levels in middle age of U.S./northern Europe/western Europe populations, and the contrasting lower average TC levels of East Asian (e.g., Japanese) and Mediterranean (e.g., Italian) populations, and the corresponding high and low CHD death rates. However, little was said about high average BP levels in middle age in countries such as Japan and Italy, high hypertension rates, and high stroke rates, much higher than for the United States, for example. The obvious question was posed and addressed in cited Western populations of the possible role of dietary factors in accounting for high mean TC levels, the steep TC rise with age, and the epidemic of hypercholesterolemia. However, the seemingly equally obvious equivalent question went neglected on the possible role of dietary factors in accounting for rise in BP with age and the epidemic of hypertension. By 1970 [23], CVD epidemiologic research, in concert with metabolic ward [25] type and animal controlled dietary experiments, had clearly shown that dietary saturated fat, dietary cholesterol, and positive caloric balance with weight gain all drove serum TC levels upward, whereas intake of polyunsaturated fat and water-soluble fiber had the opposite effect (evidence on the adverse effects on serum TC of dietary trans-fats came later, in the 1990s). These research advances became the foundation for expert public policy statements advising the general population to improve eating patterns for the primary prevention/control of hypercholesterolemia and CHD, for example, in the United States, from the Inter-Society Commission for Heart Disease Resources (ICHD) [23]. However, no such research assault developed in those years to elucidate influences of multiple dietary factors on BP. Thus, in 1970, the ICHD expert group (set up to make state-of-the-art recommendations on the primary prevention of hypertension) concluded (in contrast to the atherosclerotic disease group) that it could make no evidence-based recommendations, not even on the possible roles of prevention/control of overweight/obesity, high salt intake, and excess alcohol consumption [26].

Perhaps ongoing work on the history of CVD epidemiology will dig up reasons for this one-sided development in knowledge on relations of dietary factors to the two major endogenous risk factors, TC and BP.

Only in the 1980s was this research gap vigorously addressed, largely as a result of the First Ten Day Advanced International Seminar on CVD Epidemiology and Prevention, in Finland in 1982; the result was the INTERSALT Study [11,27–31].

INTERSALT, Phase 1

INTERSALT is a standardized cooperative basic epidemiologic study of 10,079 men and women ages 20–59 years in 52 diverse population samples in 32 countries on five continents [11,27–31]. In its first phase, focus was on relations to SBP and DBP of timed 24-hour urinary excretion of Na and K. Relations to BP of BMI, alcohol intake, and 24-hour urinary Ca and Mg also were assessed. Each local center was asked to recruit 200 people ages 20–59 years, 25 each of 8 age-sex strata, as random or chunk samples of defined populations. Center staffs were trained and certified for all standardized procedures at regional training sessions. The surveys proceeded based on centrally prepared materials, including common protocol, manual of operations, forms, and equipment. The study was designed, organized, and led by Coordinating Centers in Chicago and London; data storage, editing, and analyses were done mainly in London; analyses of 24-hour urine specimens for Na, K, Ca, Mg, and creatinine were done at a Central Laboratory in Leuven, Belgium. All work, local and central, was carried out with specified comprehensive ongoing quality control measures. Data analyses were both within population and across population (ecologic).

The cross-population (ecologic) analyses ($N = 52$ samples) yielded significant findings for the five prior hypotheses tested on Na and BP: Sample median timed 24-hour urinary Na excretion (i.e., sample median Na/NaCl intake) is related directly to 1) sample slope of SBP with age, 2) sample slope of DBP with age, 3) sample median SBP, 4) sample median DBP, and 5) sample prevalence rate of high BP (Table 39.3) [11].

Table 39.3 INTERSALT Study—ecologic (cross-population) data ($N = 52$ population samples). Multiple linear regression coefficients for sample 24-hour median sodium excretion and blood pressure: Tests of the INTERSALT prior ecologic hypotheses.

Dependent variable	Adjusted for age and sex	Adjusted for age, sex, BMI, and alcohol
SBP slope with age (mm Hg over 30 yr with 100 mmol/day greater Na intake)	9.0***	10.2***
DBP slope with age (mm Hg over 30 yr with 100 mmol/day greater Na intake)	6.3***	6.3***
Median SBP (mm Hg with 100 mmol/day greater Na intake)	7.1***	4.5***
Median DBP (mm Hg with 100 mmol/day greater Na intake)	3.8**	2.3†
Hypertension prevalence (% with 100 mmol/day greater Na intake)	6.2**	4.8*

*$p < .05$; **$p < .01$; ***$p < .001$.
†$p = .08$.
BMI: body mass index; SBP: Systolic blood pressure; DBP: diastolic blood pressure.

The within-population analyses for all 10,079 INTERSALT participants yielded significant direct relations to SBP of 24-urinary Na, Na/K, BMI, and heavy alcohol use (≥300 ml of absolute alcohol per week), and significant inverse associations with K and Mg (Table 39.4) [11]. The Na-BP relation prevailed for both non-overweight and overweight strata, without significant interaction. Findings were qualitatively similar for men and women. Regression coefficients were larger with age (40–59 vs. 20–39) for SBP and DBP on Na, Na/K, and K [11,30,31].

With removal of hypertensive persons from analyses, size of Na-SBP regression coefficient changed little, indicating that the Na-SBP relation ("salt sensitivity") prevailed qualitatively for most people, not only for the minority with high BP, in these diverse population samples [11]. These significant INTERSALT findings lend support to the conclusion, based on many other research data sets (epidemiologic, clinical interventional, animal experimental), that relations of dietary salt, potassium, caloric balance (body mass), and alcohol intake to BP are etiologically significant. It was, therefore, concluded that further work on other dietary factors and BP can proceed from this foundation, with recognition that these four variables must be measured and controlled for in analyses.

Other INTERSALT analyses showed that the inverse relation between educational attainment and BP, repeatedly shown for U.S. population samples, prevails for many populations worldwide [32]. For the first time, these analyses demonstrated that education-correlated differences in BMI, alcohol use, and dietary Na and K explain higher average BP levels of less educated people. These findings underscored the importance of further work on other nutrients, foods, and their metabolites that may also relate to higher BP in less educated individuals.

Based on INTERSALT multiple regression coefficients, combined impact on BP of the four key variables studied was quantitated and estimates made of potential of improved levels of these variables to shift SBP and DBP distributions downward (Table 39.4) [11]. Implications were also set down as to estimated resultant lower population rates of CVD incidence and mortality and annual savings of lives [11,33,34]. Potential benefits were shown to be sizable and hence of considerable significance for medical care and public health.

Table 39.4 INTERSALT Study—within population data on individuals $N = 10,074$ men and women from 52 population samples. Estimated differences in SBP and DBP for specified differences in 24-hour Na and K excretion, BMI, and alcohol intake.

Variable	SBP (mm Hg)		DBP (mm Hg)	
Na (100 mmol lower)	−3.1		−0.1	
Without BMI		6.0		−2.5
K (50 mmol higher)	−3.4		−1.8	
BMI (2 units lower)	−1.6		−1.2	
Alcohol (nil vs. ≥300 ml/wk)	−0.5		−0.3	
Sum	−8.6	−11.5	−3.4	−5.9

Individual-level regression models adjusted for sample, age, sex, and the other variables, except Na adjusted with/without BMI. Na, K, corrected for reliability estimated from repeated measures on 8%.

Regression estimates for alcohol intake are multiplied by 0.15 since 15% of the participants reported alcohol intake of ≥ 300 ml/wk.

SBP: systolic blood pressure; DBP: diastolic blood pressure; BMI: body mass index.

INTERSALT, Phase 2

Based on these main phase 1 findings, the INTERSALT investigators inferred that relations of dietary factors to BP were *not* entirely subsumed by calorie balance, alcohol, and electrolytes. The further hypothesis was formulated and tested that dietary protein intake of individuals was independently related to their BP; timed 24-hour urinary total nitrogen and urea N were used as indices of total protein intake [35]. Total nitrogen (N) excretion in 24-hour urine is a known measure of total protein intake. For 10,020 participants ages 20–59 years, urea N made up most of total N (about 82%); the rank-order correlation coefficient between these two variables was 0.97, with similar results for men and women and for each of the 52 samples [35].

For all participants and those ages 40–59 years, regression of SBP and DBP on the urinary markers of dietary protein, with control for multiple other factors, demonstrated a consistent significant inverse relationship for *total N* and *urea N* ($p < .01$) [35]. As with Na and BP, coefficients for SBP and DBP regressed on *total N* and *urea N* were much larger for persons ages 40–59 years than 20–39 years. These findings on total dietary protein intake and BP did not answer important questions on relations of dietary vegetable protein, dietary animal protein, and specific dietary amino acids to BP; INTERSALT lacked data to address these questions.

Multiple Risk Factor Intervention Trial (MRFIT) Epidemiologic Analyses

For MRFIT epidemiologic analyses on dietary factors and BP, use was made of data collected during the 6 years of the trial on its two groups, usual care (UC) and special intervention (SI), rather than baseline data only, since only one 24-hour dietary recall per participant was done at baseline, whereas 4–5/man were done during the trial, so that attenuation of true relations by regression dilution bias was much less [36]. In multivariate analyses, averages of yearly SBP and DBP for six trial years for 11,342 men were regressed on average dietary intake (as amount/day and caloric density) from 4–5 recalls, separately for UC and SI men, then with pooling of coefficients of the two groups, weighted by inverse of variances. First, each dietary factor was considered separately, with control for multiple nondietary BP-related variables. In addition to BMI and alcohol, other dietary variables significantly related to SBP ($p < .01$) included Na, Na/K, starch (directly), caffeine (inversely); significantly related to DBP, Na, Na/K, dietary cholesterol, Keys dietary lipid score all directly, and inversely Mg, K, caffeine, and protein [37]. With inclusion in regression models of sets of several dietary variables for which there was not a high-order intercorrelation problem, SBP and DBP were significantly related to BMI, alcohol, Na/K, dietary cholesterol, and starch and inversely to caffeine; DBP was inversely related to protein and PFA/SFA [38]. Estimated combined effects of several dietary variables on both SBP and DBP were of a magnitude as to have potential importance for prevention and control of the population-wide BP problem.

Chicago Western Electric Study

For 1,804 men ages 40–55 years at baseline in 1957 in the Western Electric Study, dietary data were collected at baseline and again 1 year later, and BP was measured at baseline and annually for the next 9 years. The Bertha Burke in-depth interview with cross-checks was used to assess usual eating pattern during the preceding 28 days [7]. The Generalized Estimating Equation (GEE) method for longitudinal analyses was used to assess relations between baseline nutrients, foods/food groups, other variables, and change in BP over time [39]. For baseline age, BMI, and alcohol intake, there were consistent significant positive relations to SBP change; for educational attainment, a significant inverse relation. With specific macronutrients considered one at a time, for vegetable protein, but not for animal or total protein, there was a significant inverse relation to SBP change ($p < .05$) as there was also for carbohydrate and PFA/SFA; for Keys dietary lipid score and dietary cholesterol, there was a significant positive relation to SBP change [39]. In models with two macronutrient variables considered together (as well as age, BMI, alcohol, Ca, education, cigarettes), for dietary cholesterol or Keys score, there was a significant positive relation to SBP change; for vegetable protein, significant or borderline significant inverse relations; and for Ca, nonsignificant inverse relation. In other analyses, vegetables, fruits, and fish had inverse relations to BP change [40]. These all too sparse prospective findings are limited by absence from the Western Electric file of dietary and urinary data on intake of Na and K.

INTERMAP

INTERMAP Aims, Premises, Design, Methods

INTERMAP is an international cooperative basic epidemiologic investigation on the role of multiple dietary factors and their urinary metabolites in the etiology of unfavorable BP levels prevailing for most middle-aged and older individuals [41]. Its basic premises are: multiple nutrients (macro/micro), multiple foods, their metabolites have small independent influences on BP of individuals that in combination summate as sizable clinically and epidemiologically relevant effects. To detect impact of single nutrients, foods, food groups, and metabolites on BP of individuals, standardized high-quality data are needed on large, diverse population samples. Accordingly, INTERMAP surveyed in-depth—with four multipass 24-hour dietary recalls, two timed 24-hour urine collections, eight BP measurements, extensive questionnaire data, etc.—4,680 men and women ages 40–59 years from 17 random population samples consuming diverse diets in Japan, Peoples Republic of China (PRC), United Kingdom, and United States (eight diverse U.S. samples totaling 2,195 people). Throughout, it used state-of-the-art, high-quality, standardized assessment methods and standardized country-specific data on the nutrient composition of foods (83 nutrients), biochemical measurements, and statistical methods [42–44]. Its general aim is to achieve a major advance in knowledge on relations of multiple dietary factors/urinary metabolites to BP of individuals (men and women) of varied ethnic and sociodemographic backgrounds.

To date, several INTERMAP papers have been published on independent relations to BP of specific nutrients (macronutrients and micronutrients) [45–51]. Each report generally deals with the relation to BP of one or more nutrients considered singly (with control for multiple possible confounders, nondietary and dietary). Extensive descriptive statistics on the INTERMAP cohort and its substrata have been components of these and other papers, including on nutrients consumed and the main food sources supplying them [42–51].

Dietary protein and BP: In analyses on INTERMAP, prior hypothesis no. 1, on dietary protein and BP, vegetable protein intake (%kcal) by individuals was inversely related to their SBP and DBP; animal protein intake tended to be directly related to BP ($N = 4,680$, i.e., all INTERMAP participants) [45]. In the subgroup of 491 persons in the highest quartile of vegetable protein intake/lowest quartile of animal protein intake (country-specific), 5 (of 18) dietary amino acids were significantly higher as percent of total protein than for the subgroup of 471 participants in the lowest quartile of vegetable protein intake/highest quartile of animal protein intake, for example, first and foremost, glutamic acid (the most common dietary amino acid): for the foregoing two subgroups, 22.8% and 18.3% of total protein (t for difference = 30.0).

Dietary glutamic acid and BP: These data served as the basis for further research on possible inverse relations to BP of individuals of their dietary intake of glutamic acid and of the four

other amino acids (cystine, proline, phenylalanine, serine) predominating in vegetable protein [51]. Consistently, dietary glutamic acid (% total protein) related inversely to BP in serial multiple linear regression analyses involving all 4,680 participants and preselected substrata. This finding prevailed with each of the four other cited dietary amino acids included one-by-one with glutamic acid in multivariate controlled analyses. Intake of each of the four other amino acids—cystine, proline, phenylalanine, serine—was not consistently related independently to BP in these models [51].

Dietary PFA (total, omega-3, omega-6) and BP: In analyses related to other INTERMAP prior hypotheses, inverse relations to BP of individuals were shown for dietary total polyunsaturated fatty acids (PFAs), omega-6 PFA and its main component linoleic acid, omega-3 PFA and its vegetable and marine components (linolenic acid and the sum of three long-chain omega-3 PFAs) [46,47]. PFA/saturated fatty acid (SFA) ratio related only low order to BP.

Dietary starch and BP: With control for multiple possible dietary confounders, attenuation occurred in a dietary starch (% kcal)-BP inverse (not direct) relation observed with control only for nondietary possible confounders [50]. The MRFIT observation of an independent direct relation of dietary starch to BP [38] was not reproduced in analyses for all 4,680 INTERMAP participants and in analyses for substrata, such as all U.S. individuals, U.S. men, or U.S. high-risk men (comparable to the MRFIT cohort).

Dietary iron, red meat, and BP: In other similar analyses, total iron (Fe) and non-heme iron intakes (mg/24 hours) related inversely to BP [49]. In most of the several multivariate models routinely used in these analyses, a low-order direct relation was found of heme Fe to BP. Red meat intake (grams/24 hours) was directly related to BP in successive multivariate regression models; beef intake (grams/24 hours) similarly, lower order. These latter data, on relation of a food group (red meat) and a food (beef) to BP, are the first of their kind to date from INTERMAP, as distinct from nutrient-BP data.

Dietary minerals (Ca, Mg, P) and BP: INTERMAP has also published findings on the relations of calcium (Ca), magnesium (Mg), and phosphorus (P) intakes (mg/1,000 kcal) to BP [48]. For Ca and Mg, inverse relations to BP were shown consistent with other results from both observational studies and randomized trials. In contrast, prior data are sparse on dietary P and BP. For INTERMAP participants, dietary P related inversely to BP in serial regression analyses controlled for multiple possible confounders, nondietary and dietary. Since intakes of these three minerals (mg/1,000 kcal) are highly correlated, interpretation of data must be guarded on their relation to BP with any two or all three together in regression models. To further assess this matter of the independence of their relation to BP, each person was classified as above/below median intake of his/her country/gender group; SBP and DBP levels were then compared for persons above and below the median in intake of these three minerals; sizes of the BP differences supported the inference that their influences on BP are combinative, that is, partially independent [48].

Dietary factors and the higher BP of less educated individuals: Other analyses related to an INTERMAP prior hypothesis on the role of multiple dietary factors in accounting for higher BP in less educated persons [52] (see above, INTERSALT report on this) [32]. Since the 2,195 U.S. INTERMAP participants manifested this inverse relation much more strongly (independent of ethnicity) than Japanese, PRC, U.K. participants, the analyses focused on the American subcohort. Several dietary factors, with differing intakes across U.S. educational strata, accounted for the inverse education-BP relation, that is, 24 hour Na and K intake, alcohol intake, vegetable protein intake, Keys dietary lipid score, and mineral intake (Ca, Mg, P, Fe) [52].

Dietary factors and lower BP of southern than northern Chinese: Similar analyses were used to assess the role of dietary factors in accounting for the repeatedly observed lower average SBP/DBP levels of southern compared to northern Chinese [53] (a finding in conspicuous contrast to the U.S. north–south pattern, witness the U.S. southern "strokebelt.") INTERMAP analyses demonstrated multiple south–north differences in nutrient intake that accounted for lower southern average SBP/DBP, specifically from multivariate

models, much lower salt intake and higher dietary K, Mg south than north, and lower BMI. With control for these variables, SBP/DBP differences were reduced from $-7.6/-6.9$ ($p < .001$) to $-1.7/-1.6$ (p 0.20 and 0.21) [49].

INTERMAP metabolomics research: As noted briefly above, INTERMAP aims encompass not only relations of nutrients, foods, food groups, and food patterns to BP, but also metabolite-BP relations. For this latter purpose, nuclear magnetic resonance (NMR) scanning was done on all INTERMAP urine specimens (10,000 + NMR scans, 7,100 peaks/scan). Review of this metabolomics aspect of the INTERMAP work is beyond the scope of this chapter; for an overview on this work (methodologic and substantive), including reported data to date on urinary metabolite-BP relations, see the 2008 paper in *Nature* [54].

The foregoing INTERMAP reports do not deal systematically with the matter—of key importance for medical care and public health—of the estimated combined quantitative effects on BP of the multiple dietary variables assessed. Such INTERMAP data are presented here for the first time.

Estimated population-wide combined effects on BP of improved intakes of dietary electrolytes (Na, K), elimination of heavy drinking, and lower BMI—the INTERSALT model: For all 4,680 INTERMAP participants, 24-hour urinary sodium excretion, reflecting intake, was high; averaging 181 mmol; for men, 198; for women, 164. Based on these findings, data from INTERSALT (Table 39.4), and data from trials on reduced salt intake, estimates were made of the effect on SBP of a 110 mmol/day reduction in Na intake, i.e., to an average level of 71 mmol/day for all participants, 88 for men, 54 for women. With 24-hour average urinary potassium excretion 53 mmol overall, 57 for men, 49 for women, estimates were made of the influence on SBP of a 60 mmol/day increase, to a level of 113 overall, 117 for men, 109 for women. These values for Na and K, yielding a Na/K ratio well under 1.0, are in accord with data (biomedical and anthropologic) on the Na and K composition of the fare of preliterate hunter gatherers experiencing little or no rise in BP during adulthood (see Figure 39.2). As to alcohol

Table 39.5 INTERMAP findings on individuals, INTERSALT multivariate model: Estimated populationwide lower average SBP with more favorable intakes of sodium and potassium, no heavy alcohol intake, and more favorable body mass index, all INTERMAP participants ($N = 4,680$).

		Estimated lower average SBP (mm Hg)					
		All (N = 4,680)		Men (N = 2,359)		Women (N = 2,321)	
Variable	Improvement in Level	A	B	A	B	A	B
Sodium—mmol/24 hr	−110	−3.0***	−0.8†	−1.8***	−0.1	−5.2***	2.2**
Potassium—mmol/24 hr	+60	−3.8***	−3.9***	−3.4***	−4.2***	−4.2***	−3.6**
Heavy alcohol intake	Prevalence—None	−3.3***	−3.7***	3.9***	−4.1***	−2.5*	−3.2**
		(−0.6†)	(−0.6)	(−1.0)	(−1.0)	(−0.2)	(−0.3)
BMI-kg/m²	−4 units	—	−3.5***	—	−3.6***	—	−3.4***
Sum	—	−7.4	−8.8	−6.2	−8.9	−9.6	−9.5

Uncorrected for regression dilution bias; controlled for age, gender, sample, dietary supplement use, special diet, CVD/DM diagnosis, family history of high BP, physical activity.
Heavy alcohol intake: men >26 g/day (>2 drinks/day), women >13 g/day (>1 drink/day); prevalence of heavy alcohol intake: all — 17.0%; men — 25.4%; women — 8.4%.
†Estimate of populationwide effect, i.e., 3.3×0.17 (prevalence of heavy drinking).
A: Without BMI in the model.   B: With BMI in the model.
*$p < .05$ **$p < .01$ ***$p < .001$ †$p < .10$.
SBP: systolic blood pressure; CVD: cardiovascular disease; DM: diabetes mellitus; BP: blood pressure; BMI: body mass index.

intake, with 17% prevalence rate overall of heaving drinking (men, 25.4%; women, 8.4%) (>26 g alcohol/day for men, >13 g/day for women, i.e., >2 and >1 drink/day, respectively), the estimate was made of the population-wide SBP effect of elimination of all heavy drinking. With BMI averaging 26.4 kg/m² (26.4 for men, 26.3 for women), the estimate was made of the influence on BP of a 4 kg/m² BMI reduction, to a population-wide average of 22.4 kg/m², i.e., within the normal range by both western criteria (<25.0 kg/m²) and Asian (WHO) criteria (<23.0 kg/m²).

With these more favorable patterns, in the three-factor model (without BMI) SBP was estimated to be on average lower by 7.4 mm Hg for all 4,680 INTERMAP participants (6.2 mm Hg for men, 9.6 mm Hg for women), a gender difference due to the greater impact on SBP of Na for women than men (test for gender × Na interaction; $p < .001$) (Table 39.5). In the four-factor model including BMI, this estimate was 8.8 mm Hg (8.9 for men, 9.5 for women). With inclusion of BMI in this multivariate model, relation of Na to BP—sizable and significant in the three-factor model ($p < .001$)—was atten-

uated, a finding also recorded by INTERSALT [11]. Likely reasons for this are, first, Na and BMI are positively correlated ($p = .28$), hence possible overadjustment with BMI in the four-factor model; second, with addition to the model of BMI, a variable measured with high reliability, attenuation of the relation to BP of Na, a variable measured with less reliability (even based on two 24-hour urine collections) [55] (see also below for further comments on biases tending to produce underestimates of nutrient-BP relations). INTERMAP by design made no corrections for reliability in any of its analyses, given the complexities of the factors—random and non-random (systematic)—possibly contributing to limitations in reliability of the nutrient data [55–58]. Thus, the INTERSALT (Table 39.4) and INTERMAP (Table 39.5) data, which are similar qualitatively, are quantitatively not comparable.

Estimated population-wide combined effects on BP of improved intakes of electrolytes (Na, K), minerals (Ca, Mg, P), non-heme iron, vegetable protein, PFA elimination of heavy drinking, and lower BMI: Based on its data on 83 nutrients/person derived from four in-depth multi-pass 24-hour dietary recalls and two timed 24-hour urine specimens on each participant, INTERMAP is able to go beyond the INTERSALT model in estimating combined effects of multiple nutrients on BP. For this purpose, eight multiple linear regression models were assessed, without and with BMI, involving various combinations of dietary vegetable protein, Ca, Mg, P, and non-heme Fe, plus Na, K, heavy drinking, and PFA (exclusive of arachidonic acid, related low-order directly to BP). (In all these models for all 4,680 INTERMAP participants, relations of omega-3 and omega-6 PFA were low order with p values more than .10; hence, these two variables

were not included in the combined estimate of lower SBP with improved pattern for all variables.) Multiple models were assessed particularly since colinearity is a problem with the dietary variables under consideration, for example, partial correlation coefficients: vegetable protein and Mg 0.56, Ca and Mg 0.46, Ca and P 0.71, Ca and non-heme Fe 0.42, Mg and P 0.69.

For all 4,680 INTERMAP participants, in the models without BMI, improved Na and K intakes and elimination of heavy drinking (the INTERSALT components of the models), all contributed sizably to estimated lower SBP, combined estimated effect

Table 39.6 Estimated populationwide lower average systolic BP$^\triangle$ with more favorable electrolyte (Na, K), mineral (Ca, Mg, P), non-heme iron (Fe), PFA, vegetable protein intake, no heavy alcohol intake, normal BMI, eight multivariate analyses, INTERMAP Study—all 4,680 INTERMAP participants.

| | | Estimated populationwide lower average SBP$^\triangle$ (mm Hg) | | | | | | | |
| | | Multivariate models without BMI | | | | Multivariate models with BMI | | | |
Variable	Improvement in level	Model 1A	Model 2A	Model 3A	Model 4A	Model 1B	Model 2B	Model 3B	Model 4B
Sodium (mmol/24 hr)	−110	−2.8***	−2.8***	−2.7***	−2.8***	−0.7‡	−0.7‡	−0.7	−0.7‡
Potassium (mmol/24 hr)	+60	−2.1*	−2.0*	−1.7*	−1.8*	−2.8***	−2.7***	−2.8***	−2.8***
Calcium (mg/1,000 kcal)	+240	−1.9*	−1.4**	−1.8**	−1.1*	−1.4*	−1.2**	−1.2‡	−1.1
Phosphorus (mg/1,000 kcal)	+232	−0.2	—	+0.8	—	−0.5	—	−0.2	—
Magnesium (mg/1,000 kcal)	+76	—	—	−2.6***	−1.5*	—	—	−0.8	−0.2
Non-Heme Fe (mg/1,000 kcal)	+4.1	—	−1.2*	—	−1.5***	—	−0.9‡	—	−1.3**
PFA (% kcal)	+4.1	−0.4	−0.5	−0.4	−0.5	−0.6	−0.6	−0.6	−0.7
Vegetable protein (% kcal)	+2.8	−2.3***	−1.7***	—	—	−1.2**	−0.8‡	—	—
Heavy alcohol intake^X	Prevalence:	−2.8	−2.9	−3.2	−3.1	−3.3	−3.3	−3.5	−3.4
	None	(−0.5)***	(−0.5)***	(−0.5)***	(−0.5)***	(−0.6)***	(−0.6)***	(0.6)***	(0.6)***
BMI (kg/m^2)	−4	—	—	—	—	−3.4***	−3.4***	−3.5***	−3.5***
Sum† (all variables)		−10.2	−10.1	−8.9	−9.7	−11.2	−10.9	−10.4	−11.0
Sum† (Na, K, alcohol, BMI)		−5.4	−5.3	−4.9	−5.1	−7.5	−7.4	−7.6	−7.7

$^\triangle$Uncorrected for regression dilution bias; controlled for age, gender, sample, family history of high BP, physical activity, diagnosis of CVD/diabetes, use of special diet, dietary supplement use.

^{X}Heavy alcohol intake: men >26 g/day (>2 drinks/day); women >13 g/day (>1 drink/day); prevalence: 17.0%

†Estimate for no heavy drinking adjusted for its prevalence rate at INTERMAP field survey (17.0%), see value in parentheses in table above.

Non-heme Fe: non-heme iron; BMI: body mass index; BP: blood pressure; CVD: cardiovascular disease.

Mean (sd) for variables: Na 181.1 (72.4) mmol/24 hr; K 53.2 (20.0) mmol/24 hr; Ca 319.4 (149.1) mg/1,000 kcal; P 564.4 (132.7) mg/1,000 kcal; Mg 146.5 (38.5) mg/1,000 kcal; non-heme Fe 6.6 (2.3) mg/1,000 kcal; total PFA minus arachidonic acid 6.5 (2.1)% kcal; vegetable protein 6.6 (2.2) % kcal; energy 2,148.4 (624.5) kcal/day based on mean of data from four 24-hour dietary recalls or two 24-hour urine collections (Na,K); mean (sd) SBP and DBP 118.9 (14.7) mm Hg and 73.8 (10.0) mm Hg based on eight measurements (two at each of four visits).

*p < .05; **p < .01; ***p < .001; ‡p < .10.

about 5 mm Hg (Table 39.6, columns 1–4). With inclusion in these models of triad combinations of the other five nutrients, improved vegetable protein, Ca, Mg, non-heme Fe (but not P) contributed to lower SBP; estimated total effect was SBP lower by 8–9 mm Hg, i.e., lower by 3–4 mm Hg additional compared to the INTERSALT model. With inclusion of BMI in the model, (Table 39.6, columns 5–8), the combined contribution of the four

INTERSALT variables was 7–8 mm Hg; as before, estimated Na effect was attenuated as was Mg effect. Estimated SBP reduction overall was about 10 mm Hg, i.e., 2–3 mm Hg additional effect of the non-INTERSALT variables (particularly vegetable protein, Ca, non-heme Fe).

In corresponding analyses for INTERMAP subcohorts, results were similar to the foregoing (Table 39.7), with the exception that for non-intervened

Table 39.7 Summary: Estimated populationwide lower average systolic BP$^\triangle$ with more favorable electrolyte, mineral, non-heme Fe, PFA, vegetable protein intakes, no heavy alcohol intake, normal BMI, eight multivariate models, INTERMAP data for specified cohorts.

	Estimated cohort-wide lower average SBP$^\triangle$ (mm Hg)							
	Multivariate models without BMI				Multivariate models with BMI			
Cohort and number of participants	Model 1A	Model 2A	Model 3A	Model 4A	Model 1B	Model 2B	Model 3B	Model 4B
All (N = 4,680)	−10.2^{X}	−10.1	−8.9	−9.7	−11.2	−10.9	−10.4	−11.0
	−5.4†	−5.3	−4.9	−5.1	−7.5	−7.4	−7.6	−7.7
Nonintervened (N = 2,238)	−11.6	−10.9	−10.4	−10.9	−13.3	−12.3	−12.4	−13.1
	−6.1	−5.9	−5.7	−5.7	−8.2	−8.1	−8.5	−8.5
Nonhypertensive (N = 3,671)	−7.2	−6.9	−6.4	−7.0	−8.3	−8.1	−7.9	−8.3
	−3.4	−3.2	−3.2	−3.4	−5.1	−5.0	−5.5	−5.7
Western (U.K. and U.S.A). (N = 2,696)	−10.5	−10.7	−9.1	−9.9	−10.6	−10.6	−9.9	−10.5
	−5.1	−4.9	−4.5	−4.7	−6.5	−6.4	−6.7	−6.9
East Asian (Japan + PRC) (N = 1,984)	−9.5	−8.5	−8.6	−8.2	−13.5	−12.6	−12.8	−12.8
	−6.6	−6.8	−6.3	−6.3	−11.0	−11.1	−10.9	−11.0
Men (N = 2,359)	−9.9	−9.4	−8.3	−9.0	−12.5	−11.8	−11.3	−11.9
	−4.7	−4.9	−4.0	−4.3	−7.9	−8.0	−7.8	−7.9
Women (N = 2,321)	−11.7	−12.2	−10.4	−11.6	−10.5	−11.3	−9.9	−11.1
	−7.6	−7.3	−7.1	−7.5	−8.3	−8.3	−8.6	−8.8

$^\triangle$All models uncorrected for regression dilution bias; controlled for age, sample, gender (except for separate analyses for men and women), use of special diet, use of dietary supplement, diagnosis of CVD/diabetes, physical activity, family history of high BP; all models include 24-hour excretion of sodium and potassium (mmol), heavy alcohol intake (yes, no) defined as >26 g/day (>2 drinks/day) for men and >13 g/day (>1 drink/day) for women; Models 1B–4B include BMI (kg/m^2); Models 1A and 1B also include dietary calcium and phosphorus (mg/1,000 kcal) and vegetable protein (% kcal); Models 2A and 2B, dietary calcium, non-heme iron (mg/1000 kcal), vegetable protein; Models 3A and 3B, calcium, phosphorus, magnesium (mg/1,000 kcal); Models 4A and 4B, calcium, magnesium, non-heme iron; for values used as more favorable dietary intake levels, and for mean (sd) levels at INTERMAP field survey, see Table 39.6. Estimate for cessation of all heavy drinking adjusted for its prevalence rate at INTERMAP field survey: All 4,680, 17.0%; Nonintervened participants, 19.2%; nonhypertensive, 16.7%; Western (U.K. and U.S.A.), 13.4%; East Asian (Japan and PRO), 21.9%; men, 25.4%; women, 8.4%. Nonintervened participants: No reported use of a special diet or dietary supplement; no diagnosis of CVD/diabetes; no drug treatment for high BP, CVD, diabetes. Nonhypertensive: SBP <140 mm Hg and DBP <90 mm Hg and no reported drug use for high BP.
^{X}Sum of estimated lower average SBP based on more favorable levels of all variables in the model.
†Sum of estimated lower average SBP based on more favorable levels of four INTERSALT variables: dietary sodium, potassium, alcohol, and BMI.

participants, SBP difference with more dietary PFA was greater (about 1.5 mm Hg) (data not tabulated). For these 2,238 non-intervened participants (not consuming a special diet, not using dietary supplements, not diagnosed as having CVD or diabetes, not taking medication for high BP, CVD, diabetes), estimated lower SBP was only slightly, not markedly, greater than for all 4,680. These data support the judgment that possible bias due to intervention was modest.

For 3,671 nonhypertensive participants, effect sizes were all substantial. For example, in the models with BMI (Table 39.7, columns 5–8), SBP was lower by 7–8 mm Hg overall and 5–6 mm Hg with the four INTERSALT variables only. These data indicate that these dietary factors *influence BP population-wide*, that is, they are not confined to people with high BP.

Correspondingly, findings were similar for IN-TERMAP western (United Kingdom and United States) and East Asian (Japan and PRC) participants (Table 39.7). These data indicate that these findings on multiple dietary factors and BP are *widely generalizable*. Concordantly, findings were similar for men and women; the above cited greater effect of Na reduction for women than men tended to produce more of an overall SBP effect for women than men especially in the analyses without BMI.

All these estimations of effect on SBP of improvement in these dietary variables are underestimates, for several reasons [11,55–58]: 1) regression-dilution bias–even with four high-quality 24-hour dietary recalls and two timed 24-hour urine collections, limitations remain in the reliability of nutrient data, resulting in imperfect ordering (classification) of individuals and thus biasing true associations toward zero; 2) in multiple linear regression analyses of BP on Na and other nutrients measured with limited precision in INTERMAP, possible decrease in the estimates of their effects on BP due to inclusion of BMI, measured with very high precision; 3) in multiple regression analyses of BP on Na with inclusion of BMI, the possibility of overadjustment because part of the BMI association may be due to the positive correlation of BMI with Na (higher Na intake by obese people); 4) in regard to electrolyte (Na, K) intakes assessed based on 24-hour collection, bias due to non-reported incompleteness in urine collection by some partici-

pants, varying in degree; 5) in regard to nutrients assessed by 24-hour dietary recalls, biases due to deliberate (nonrandom) underreporting or over-reporting by some participants, e.g., due to their judgments of what is "bad" or "good" for them to eat—as well as random misreporting, quantitative and qualitative; 6) modification, random and nonrandom, by some participants of their usual eating pattern on the days prior to the 24-hour recalls, possibly biased as to occurrence in people with higher BP; 7) effects of antihypertensive medication on BP; 8) the cross-sectional nature of the INTERMAP Study (such as INTERSALT), i.e., lack of prospective data on long-term influences of the dietary variables on BP, possibly resulting in sizable underestimation of at least some nutrient-BP relations, as suggested by INTERSALT ecologic data on estimated impact of 100 mmol/day higher Na intake on 30-year slope of SBP with age—10 mm Hg (Table 39.3, row 1).

Randomized Trials on Prevention and Control of High BP by Nutritional Means

The Chicago-based Primary Prevention of Hypertension Trial, the first of its kind, demonstrated ability to reduce 5-year incidence of hypertension by 50% with reduction of NaCl intake, weight, and alcohol intake [59]. The Hypertension Control Program, with use of the same intervention, tested the ability to maintain nonhypertensive BP without drug treatment in hypertensive persons with BP that was previously well controlled pharmacologically. After 4 years, 40% of those treated by nutritional means alone were able to remain off medication with nonhypertensive BP, compared with only 5% in the control group [60]. These trials, together with other national cooperative trials—the Treatment of Mild Hypertension Study (TOMHS) [61,62], the Trials of Hypertension Prevention (TOHP) [63–66], the two DASH feeding trials [67,68], and the OMNIHEART feeding trial [69]—have all demonstrated the ability to improve BP level with multiple dietary interventions.

The DASH and OMNIHEART trials have been particularly important because of their key design features, *feeding* of participants, rather than just counseling them [67–69]. With this approach, high-level adherence to the study diet was achieved, akin to the situation in metabolic ward studies. These feeding trials were of crucial importance not only because they involved both prehypertensive and hypertensive adult men and women, most of them either African Americans or non-Hispanic whites, but also because the DASH combination diet involved multiple modifications in food intake, such as increased fruits, fruit juices/vegetables/nuts, seeds, legumes/low-fat and fat-free dairy products/fish, and decreased intake of beef, pork, ham /fats, oils, salad dressings/snacks and sweets, with resultant multiple putatively favorable modifications in intakes of both macronutrients and micronutrients (Table 39.8) [67,68]. In addition, in the DASH-Sodium Feeding Trial [68], a two-step reduction in salt intake was a design component, from control level of 144 mmol Na/day to 107 and then 67. For the first time in Americans with prehypertension and stage 1 hypertension, this enabled assessment of the combinative effects of the DASH diet plus sodium reductions, assessed to be 8.9 mm Hg overall (Table 39.9) (compare INTERMAP estimates in Table 39.7). The design of this second DASH feeding trial also enabled estimation of the contribution of the step-1 and step-2 sodium (salt) reduction to SBP decline—2.1 and 6.7 mm Hg, respectively, for persons on the control diet; the step 2 decline of 6.7 mm Hg with Na intake 67 mmol Na/day, significantly greater and steeper than the step-1 fall of 2.1 mm Hg [68]. The OMNIHEART feeding trial added valuable further knowledge in showing modest incremental BP reductions with modification of the DASH diet to include higher protein intake (particularly from vegetable sources) or higher monounsaturated fat intake [69].

The DASH-Na/OMNIHEART and Mediterranean eating patterns: As noted by researchers, science writers, and policy makers, the DASH-Sodium/OMNIHEART feeding trials demonstrated the merits in regard to both BP and serum cholesterol/lipids of an eating pattern resembling several aspects of "classical" Mediterranean fare (circa the 1950s) [70–74]. The feeding trials also addressed aspects of this eating pattern that, based on current scientific knowledge, can be assessed as suboptimal, e.g., in the DASH-sodium feeding trial, but not in "classical" Mediterranean fare, low not high salt intake; moderate not high

Table 39.8 Foods and nutrients, DASH combination diet compared to control diet.

Variable	Control diet	Combination diet
Food groups: menu analysis (servings/day)		
Fruits and juices	1.6	5.2
Vegetables	2.0	4.4
Grains	8.2	7.5
Nuts, seeds, legumes	0.0	0.7
Low-fat and fat-free dairy	0.1	2.0
Regular-fat dairy	0.4	0.7
Poultry	0.8	0.6
Fish	0.2	0.5
Beef, pork, ham	1.5	0.5
Fats, oils, salad dressings	5.8	2.5
Snacks and sweets	4.1	0.7
Nutrients: menu analysis		
Protein (% kcal)	13.8	17.9
Carbohydrate (% kcal)	50.5	56.5
Total fat (% kcal)	35.7	25.6
SFA (% kcal)	14.1	7.0
MFA (% kcal)	12.4	9.9
PFA (% kcal)	6.2	6.8
Cholesterol (mg/day)	233	151
Fiber (mg/day)	9[b]	31[b]
Magnesium (mg/day)	176	480
Calcium (mg/day)	443	1,265
Potassium (mg/day)	1,752	4,415
Nutrients: 24-hour urinary excretion		
Potassium (mmol)	39	75
Magnesium (mg)	70	98
Calcium (mg)	137	146
Phosphorus (mg)	739	851
Urea nitrogen (mg)	9,026	11,583
Sodium: DASH-1 (mmol)	138	136
Sodium: DASH-Na (mmol)		
Higher	141	144
Intermediate	106	107
Lower	64	67

From DASH-Na, total daily calorie intake averages 2,576 (sd 493) and 2,576 (sd 511) [68].

In both DASH trials, during the 8-week [66] and 90-day [67] intervention periods, weight was stable in both groups, in accordance with the design provision for isocaloricity; average BMI values were about 28–29 kg/m^2 (sd 4–5 kg/m^2). Also by design, participants were either nonusers of alcoholic beverages or light drinkers, e.g., in the DASH-Na trial 43%–44% were drinkers, who reported an average of 0.4–0.5 drinks/day (sd 0.4).

[a]Data are from the first DASH feeding trial [63] unless otherwise specified.

[b]Not available from DASH-1 menu analyses; data are nutrient targets; DASH-Na reported values were 17.3 and 35.0 g/day [68].

Table 39.9   Effect on SBP of reduced sodium (salt) intake and DASH diet, DASH-sodium feeding trial.

Feeding period	SBP (mm Hg)	Change in SBP (mm Hg)
Control with 144 mmol Na/day	133	—
Control with 107 mmol Na/day	131	−2.1
Control with 67 mmol Na/day	126	−6.7
DASH with 67 mmol Na/day	124	−8.9

SBP levels are approximations, read off the published graph on these data; changes in SBP are as published in the graph legend [68].

Participants: U.S. adult men and women average age 48 years, most African American and non Hispanic white, with SBP 121–159 and DBP 81–99 mm Hg, i.e., prehypertensive and stage 1 hypertensive.

intake of seed oils, including olive oil; modest not high intake of alcohol; and high protein, especially vegetable protein, intake. With an additional focus on *whole grain* breads, pasta, and rice, the DASH/OMNIHEART eating pattern can reasonably be designated as Mediterranean fare updated for the twenty-first century and for all people (Table 39.10). It is a fare not only with a Mediterranean but also with an East Asian, South Asian, and Latino flare (its roots: poor people's foods) [70–74], that

Table 39.10   Mediterranean eating style for the twenty-first century: food emphases and deemphases.

Emphases
1 Vegetables, salt free or low in salt
2 Beans (legumes) nuts/seeds salt free
3 Fruits
4 Whole-grain breads/cereals low in salt
5 Whole-grain pasta/rice low in salt
6 Fish, shellfish, lean poultry low in salt
7 Lean unprocessed red meats (beef, pork, lamb, veal) low in salt, once or twice weekly
8 Fat-free or low-fat dairy products and egg whites
9 Olive oil/seed oils in modest amounts
10 Wine (if desired) in moderation

All foods/dishes salt-free or low-salt; recipes low-oil or oil-free; all portion sizes modest.

Deemphases
As in the DASH eating pattern: high-fat/high-salt/processed animal, dairy, and marine products, egg yolks, solid (hard) fats (e.g., butter/lard/hard margarines), sugars/sweets/soft drinks/baked goods high in fats/sugars/calories.

is, it involves a range of foods/condiments readily applicable for the preparation of recipes in the best traditions of the delights of the table.

Conclusions

The first and foremost conclusion from the extensive data amassed over the last quarter century is that across the population (i.e., for most people) multiple dietary factors do indeed influence BP, independent or partially independent of each other. Like serum cholesterol, BP responds significantly and sizably to multiple favorable modifications in food intake. This substantial favorable response has been demonstrated by population-based epidemiologic studies and randomized trials for women and men, East Asians and Westerners, African Americans and non-Hispanic white Americans, persons of lower and higher socioeconomic status, and non-hypertensive and hypertensive strata. Clearly, the findings are widely generalizable. While in cross-sectional observational studies of any one nutrient, effect size is apparently small (possibly deceptively so in terms of decades-long effects), combined effects are substantial and clinically and epidemiologically relevant. The data show the way for the solution of the mass BP problem, that is, population-wide improved nutrition based on a set of evidence-based specific recommendations in regard to foods and food groups (Tables 39.8 and 39.10) and nutrients/alcohol/weight:

1   Low salt intake (50 mmol Na/day = 1,150 mg Na or 2,900 mg NaCl, still about five times physiologic need [71]; the research data clearly show that the still prevailing advisory, up to 100 mmol/day, is unsound and needs to be updated to 50 mmol.

2   High potassium intake (>100 mmol/day).

3   Normal weight (BMI 18.5–24.9 kg/m^2).

4   For people who use alcohol, daily intake of no more than 13 g/day (women) or 26 g/day (men).

Beyond the by-now classical four INTERSALT variables:

5   High vegetable protein/total protein intake.

6   High mineral—calcium, magnesium, phosphorus—intakes.

7   High non-heme iron intake.

8   High fiber intake, at least 25 g/day.

9   Moderate total fat intake, no more than 25% of total calories.

10   Low saturated fat intake, less than 7% kcal.

11 Moderate intake of monounsaturated fatty acids (MFAs) and the desirable PFAs (linoleic acid, omega-6 PFA, vegetable/marine omega-3 PFAs), about 8% MFA and 8% PFA.

12 Low dietary cholesterol –<200 mg/day, <100 mg/1,000 kcal.

13 Low intake of processed sugars (<20 g/day).

The research effort to clarify the relations of multiple nutrients/foods/food groups/food patterns to BP is ongoing. Although much has been learned, information gaps remain to be filled in. Further knowledge will probably lead to additions/refinements in the above recommendations. However, the evidence for the foregoing is extensive, varied, and substantial. *High BP is not essential.*

People buy and eat foods and beverages, not nutrients, so foods/food patterns are the bottom line (see Table 39.8), the DASH-low sodium pattern, and Table 39.10, the Mediterranean food pattern (emphases/de-emphases) for the twenty-first century.

These nutrient/food recommendations have multiple merits: They favorably influence both BP and serum cholesterol/lipids, and by virtue of their high ratio of nutrients to calories and low caloric density, they are eminently suitable along with increased exercise for maintaining/achieving normal weight (controlling the obesity epidemic) while eating a delightful fare, that is, without "going on a diet" (a disastrous approach).

Low risk: Established major risk factors for the CHD/stroke/CVD epidemic are adverse eating/drinking patterns, diet-dependent high BP/high TC, adverse lipid fractions/diabetes/overweight/obesity, aided and abetted by sedentary lifestyle–and, of course, cigarette smoking [2]. The recommendations above when implemented can end the mass occurrences of most of these five. That is, they can take us toward achieving *low risk; favorable levels of all major CVD risk factors, from conception on* with resultant conversion of CVD *from epidemic to endemic (rare) disease* [2,75–78].

To achieve this, enlightened national public policy is essential, with adequate sustained resources for implementation. Above we said and illustrated that it can be done, and we close on that theme.

Acknowledgments

Most of the research reported here (including both observational epidemiologic research and randomized trials) was supported by the U.S. National Heart, Lung, and Blood Institute, National Institutes of Health, with complementary support in many individual countries involved in international cooperative studies (INTERSALT/INTERMAP). All these studies were accomplished by virtue of the dedicated service of many colleagues, as well as the fine cooperation of their participants. Please see the cited papers for details on both research grant support and coworkers.

Selected References

1. Elliott P, Stamler J. Primary Prevention of High Blood Pressure. In: Marmot M, Elliott P, eds. Coronary Heart Disease Epidemiology: From Aetiology to Public Health. 2nd ed. London: Oxford University Press; 2005; p. 751–68.

11. Stamler J. The INTERSALT Study: background, methods, findings, and implications. Am J Clin Nutr 1997; 65(2 Suppl);626S–42S.

40. Miura K, Greenland P, Stamler J, Liu K, Daviglus ML, Nakagawa H. Relation of vegetable, fruit, and meat intake to 7-year blood pressure change in middle-aged men. The Chicago Western Electric Study. Am J Epidemiol 2004; 159:572–80.

41. Stamler J. Guest Ed. Special Issue: INTERMAP – International study of macro- and micronutrients and blood pressure. J Hum Hypertens 2003;17:585–775.

45. Elliott P, Stamler J, Dyer AR, Appel L, Dennnis B, Kesteloot H, Ueshima H, Okayama A, Chan Q, Garside DB, Zhou B, for the INTERMAP Cooperative Research Group. Association Between Protein Intake and Blood Pressure. Arch Intern Med 2006;166:1–9.

CHAPTER 40

Alcohol and Coffee Intake, BP, and Cerebrovascular Disorders

Tanika N. Kelly[1] *& Jiang He*[1,2]

[1]Tulane University, School of Public Health and Tropical Medicine, New Orleans, LA, USA
[2]Tulane University, School of Medicine, New Orleans, LA, USA

Introduction

Hypertension and stroke are important public health challenges worldwide [1,2]. Hypertension is the most important risk factor for stroke, which is the second leading cause of death and leading cause of long-term disability worldwide [3]. In addition, hypertension is the leading cause of the global burden of disease and premature deaths [4]. Understanding the effects of lifestyle risk factors on hypertension and stroke will assist in developing strategies for their prevention.

Alcohol and caffeine are widely used in the general population worldwide due to their psychoactive properties and widespread availability [5,6]. Caffeine is an important component of coffee, tea, soda, and energy drinks, and alcohol can be found in a variety of beverages, including beer, wine, and hard liquors [6,7]. Given the widespread use of alcohol and caffeine, even small effects of these substances on common health problems could have very serious public health consequences. Both observational studies and clinical trials have assessed the relationships of alcohol and caffeine with blood pressure and stroke risk. While the results of individual reports have sometimes been conflicting, in total, there is strong evidence that alcohol and caffeine intake plays an important role in the etiology of hypertension and stroke.

Nutritional and Metabolic Bases of Cardiovascular Disease, 1st edition.
Edited by Mario Mancini, José M. Ordovas, Gabriele Riccardi,
Paolo Rubba and Pasquale Strazzullo. © 2011 Blackwell Publishing Ltd.

Alcohol and Blood Pressure

Hypertension is a common disorder that affects roughly 26% of the world's adult population [2]. It is also the leading risk factor for cardiovascular disease (CVD) and premature deaths worldwide [8,9]. Interestingly, the potential hemodynamic effects of alcohol consumption were recognized as early as 1861 [10]. Since then, many observational studies and clinical trials have been conducted to better understand the acute and long-term influence of alcohol consumption on blood pressure and hypertension risk.

Observational Studies

Effect of Heavy Alcohol Consumption

In 1915, Lian described a positive relationship between alcohol consumption and the prevalence of hypertension in French soldiers [11]. Many observational studies have replicated these findings, providing persuasive evidence that heavy alcohol consumption increases both systolic and diastolic blood pressure [12–14]. Data from the INTERSALT study showed that men who drank 300–499 ml (approximately 24–40 drinks) of alcohol per week had systolic and diastolic blood pressures 2.7 and 1.6 mm Hg, respectively, higher than nondrinkers. Similarly, compared to female nondrinkers, women who drank 300 ml (approximately 24 or more drinks) of alcohol per week or more had systolic and diastolic blood pressures that were increased by 3.9 and 3.1 mm Hg, respectively [15]. In 1999, a meta-analysis of three cohort studies by Corrao et al.

identified a 40% increased risk of hypertension for each 25-g (equivalent to 2 alcoholic beverages) increase in alcohol consumed per day [16]. These data indicate that heavy alcohol consumption increases blood pressure level and risk of hypertension.

Effects of Light to Moderate Alcohol Consumption

The association between light to moderate alcohol consumption and risk of hypertension is more inconclusive. Some prospective studies have noted beneficial effects of light to moderate alcohol drinking on blood pressure [17–20], while others have demonstrated null or even deleterious effects [17,19–21]. In addition, the association between light to moderate alcohol consumption and blood pressure may differ by gender or racial groups. Many epidemiological studies have observed U- or J-shaped relationships between alcohol and blood pressure levels among women, with the lowest average blood pressures among light female drinkers [13,17,20,22,23]. A meta-analysis of 11 observational studies conducted in 1996 showed a significant 15% decreased risk of hypertension in female drinkers who consumed less than 2.9 drinks/day compared to those who abstained from drinking [20]. In contrast, some observational studies have identified a significant, positive dose–response relationship between alcohol consumption and blood pressure in men [17,24].

The association between light to moderate alcohol consumption and risk of hypertension also varies by race. An analysis from the Atherosclerosis Risk in Community Study indicated that low to moderate amounts of alcohol does not increase risk of hypertension in whites, whereas it was associated with increased risk in African Americans [21]. Similarly, a study by Strogatz et al. identified a dose–response relationship between alcohol consumption and blood pressure in African American men and women [25]. However, a study by Klatsky et al. showed a more consistent positive dose–response relationship between alcohol and blood pressure in whites compared to African Americans [23,26]. Clearly, more research is needed to delineate the relationship between blood pressure and light to moderate alcohol consumption in different race and gender groups.

Effect of Alcoholic Beverage Types

The association between alcoholic beverage types and blood pressure has been examined by several investigators with conflicting results. It has been hypothesized that the vasodilator antioxidant phenols found in red wine may have a beneficial effect on endothelial function [27]. A study by Brenn et al. found an inverse association between wine and blood pressure but a positive association between beer consumption and blood pressure. In contrast, Sesso et al. identified similar positive associations of both beverage types [17,28]. Other studies have identified significant positive associations between both beer and wine and blood pressure, but with wine having lesser increasing blood pressure effects [23,29].

Clinical Trials

Short-Term Effects of Alcohol Consumption

Clinical trials have been used to examine whether a causal relationship between the short-term effect of alcohol consumption and blood pressure may exist. Many of these studies have investigated the effect of alcohol reduction on systolic and diastolic blood pressure levels [30–32]. A meta-analysis by Xin et al. examined 15 randomized trials lasting a median of 8 weeks with a median alcohol reduction of 76%. They identified a significant decrease of 3.3 mm Hg systolic and 2.0 mm Hg diastolic blood pressures associated with alcohol reduction (Figure 40.1) [32]. Similarly, a systematic review by Dickinson et al. observed significant decreases of 3.8 and 3.2 mm Hg systolic and diastolic blood pressures, respectively, in response to alcohol restriction [33]. Other trials have examined the effects of alcohol administration on changes in blood pressure [34–36]. A systematic review conducted in 2005 found significant increases in systolic and diastolic blood pressure of 2.7 and 1.4 mm Hg, respectively, associated with alcohol intake [36]. These data suggest a causal role for alcohol consumption on increased blood pressure.

Effects of Alcoholic Beverage Types

The only controlled-trial conducted to examine the effects of beverage types on blood pressure was conducted among 24 men and found similar increases in systolic blood pressure associated with red wine

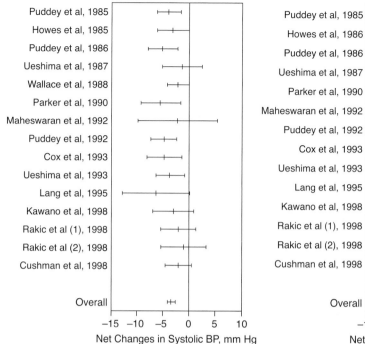

Figure 40.1 Average net change in systolic (left) and diastolic (right) blood pressure and corresponding 95% confidence intervals related to alcohol reduction intervention in 15 randomized controlled trials. (Reproduced from Xin et al. [32], with permission.)

and beer [27]. The authors suggested that factors such as patterns of alcohol intake and diet may confound the relationship between beverage type and blood pressure in observational studies.

In summary, the accumulated evidence points to a significant causal relationship between heavy alcohol consumption and increased blood pressure. However, many questions remain unanswered. Long-term randomized controlled-clinical trials will be necessary to delineate the effects of light-to-moderate alcohol consumption on blood pressure and hypertension risk. In addition, the interactions between gender, race, and alcohol on blood pressure should be further explored. Finally, more research is needed to compare the effect of alcoholic beverage types on blood pressure levels and risk of hypertension.

Alcohol and Stroke

Alcohol consumption has been associated with the risk of stroke in observational studies [37] . Un-

fortunately, randomized controlled trials examining the relationship between alcohol consumption and stroke incidence and mortality have not been conducted due to ethical, logistic, and behavioral challenges [38]. Therefore, inferences regarding this association must be based on well-designed prospective cohort studies, with consideration of their inherent limitations.

Alcohol Consumption and Total Stroke

Observational studies have linked heavy alcohol consumption to an increased risk of total stroke [37,39,40]. However, the relationship between light to moderate alcohol consumption and stroke has been demonstrated to vary between study populations. In the United States and other Western populations, researchers have generally found significant J-shaped relationships between alcohol consumption and total stroke, with an apparent reduced risk of stroke among those who are light to moderate alcohol drinkers [41,42]. In contrast, some studies conducted in Asian populations have

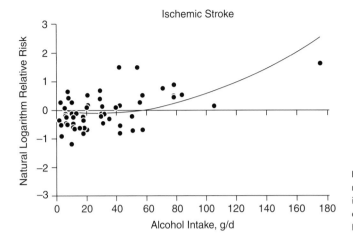

Figure 40.2 Scatterplot of log relative risk and meta-regression curve of ischemic stroke associated with alcohol consumption. (Reproduced from Reynolds et al. [37], with permission.)

found statistically significant linear relationships between alcohol consumption and stroke incidence and mortality [43,44]. Investigators have postulated that these differences may exist because stroke is not just one disease, but rather a combination of its two major subtypes, hemorrhagic and ischemic stroke [45]. Alcohol may have unique relationships with these two stroke subtypes, and discrepancies in the association between alcohol and total stroke between populations may result from differences in the frequency of stroke subtypes. For example, hemorrhagic strokes account for less than 20% of all strokes in Western populations [46], while they make up 30%–40% of incident strokes and 50% of stroke deaths in Asian populations [47]. Thus, the relationship between alcohol intake and total stroke may be more reflective of alcohol's association with ischemic stroke in Western populations as compared to Asian populations [40]. To further examine this issue, many researchers have considered alcohol's influence on ischemic and hemorrhagic stroke separately.

Alcohol Consumption and Ischemic Stroke

Studies in various populations have identified reduced overall risks of ischemic stroke associated with light to moderate alcohol consumption and increased risk associated with heavy alcohol consumption [41,42,48–50]. A meta-analysis of 35 observational studies confirmed these findings, noting a significant J-shaped association between alcohol consumption and the relative risk of ischemic stroke (Figure 40.2) [37]. In this study, alcohol intakes of less than 12 g/day and 12–24 g/day (roughly equal to one or less or one to two drinks per day, respectively) were associated with 20% and 28% reduced risks of ischemic stroke, respectively, while intake of greater than 60 g/day (equivalent to 5 drinks/day) was associated with a 69% increased risk of ischemic stroke.

Biological mechanisms have been postulated to explain the apparent J-shaped relationship between alcohol and ischemic stroke. The deleterious effects of alcohol consumptions at higher dosages have been attributed to alcohol-induced increases in blood pressure, hypercoaguable states, and cardiac arrhythmias [51,52]. In contrast, the protective effect of light-to-moderate alcohol consumption on stroke risk may be mediated by increased high-density lipoprotein (HDL)-cholesterol levels and prostacyclin-thromboxane ratios and decreased platelet aggregability and fibrinolytic activity [48,51,53].

Alcohol Consumption and Hemorrhagic Stroke

Ironically, the antithrombotic effects of alcohol, which may be protective against ischemic stroke, along with alcohol's ability to elevate systolic and diastolic blood pressure may result in a positive, dose-dependent association between alcohol intake and hemorrhagic stroke [54]. In fact, several studies have identified significant linear relationships

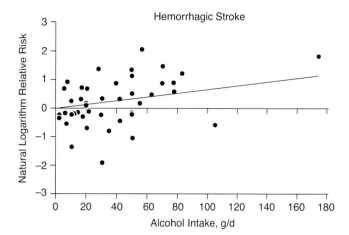

Figure 40.3 Scatterplot of log relative risk and meta-regression curve of hemorrhagic stroke associated with alcohol consumption. (Reproduced from Reynolds et al. [37], with permission.)

between alcohol consumption and hemorrhagic stroke (Figure 40.3) [37,55,56]. The 2003 meta-analysis by Reynolds et al. observed a significant positive association, with a 2.2-fold increased risk of hemorrhagic stroke associated with alcohol intake greater than 60 g/day (equivalent to five drinks) [37]. Despite the significant linear trend, light-to-moderate drinkers were not at a significantly increased risk of hemorrhagic stroke [37]. Similarly, in a cohort of 22,071 male physicians, Berger et al. examined the effects of light-to-moderate drinking on hemorrhagic stroke and found comparable risks of hemorrhagic stroke in light-to-moderate drinkers and nondrinkers [41]. Sankai et al. observed a nonsignificant increased relative risk of 1.4 among light-to-moderate drinkers and a significant sevenfold increased risk of hemorrhagic stroke among heavy drinkers [57]. However, data from the Honolulu Heart Program showed a statistically significant increased risk of hemorrhagic stroke that more than doubled among light drinkers and nearly tripled in heavy drinkers compared to non-drinkers [56]. Thus, while there is some consensus that the relationship between alcohol consumption and hemorrhagic stroke is linear, with significantly increased risk of stroke among heavy drinkers, there is still some question as to whether or not light-to-moderate drinking significantly elevates hemorrhagic stroke risk.

Effect of Alcoholic Beverage Types

There has been some evidence to suggest that red wine, beer, and hard liquors may each have different effects on stroke risk. In particular, researchers have advocated the idea of a "French paradox," proposing that red wine in moderate amounts may be especially protective against stroke. Its polyphenolic compounds have been hypothesized to decrease stroke incidence and mortality through their antioxidant, antithrombotic, and antiatherogenic effects [58]. Data from several studies have supported this hypothesis, showing a more protective effect of red wine on stroke as compared to beer or hard liquors [59–62]. Mukamel et al. showed a significant, inverse association between red wine consumption and ischemic stroke, with 23% and 46% decreased risks among those who drink 0.1–9.9 g/day (less than one drink) and greater than or equal to 10 g/day (roughly one or more drinks) of alcohol, respectively, compared to those who drank none. However, they did not find an association between either white wine, beer, or hard liquor, and ischemic stroke [62]. Similarly, reports by Malarcher et al. and Djousse et al. did not find associations between either beer or hard liquor and stroke risk [59,61]. In contrast, Sacco et al. describe a similar and significantly protective effect of moderate wine, beer, and liquor consumption on stroke risk [48]. However, it should be pointed out that red wine and white wine were not distinguished in this study [48]. Thus, while several observational studies point to a more protective effect of red wine on stroke risk compared to other types of alcoholic beverages, contradictory findings have been reported, and the evidence is inconclusive. It has been speculated that factors associated with red wine, including drinking pattern and consumption with food, may confound its association with stroke [60]. Further studies that carefully control for important confounding variables will be necessary to clearly delineate this association.

In summary, data from observational studies suggests that heavy alcohol consumption increases the risk of total, ischemic and hemorrhagic stroke. In addition, light-to-moderate alcohol consumption was generally associated with a reduced risk of ischemic stroke and had a null effect on hemorrhagic stroke. Data also suggests that red wine may have an additional protective effect on stroke but further research is warranted.

Caffeine and Blood Pressure

As one of the world's most popularly consumed substances, caffeine is also the most widely used psychoactive substance [6,63]. Caffeine's influence on blood pressure has been examined in prospective cohort studies to assess its long-term impact, as well as in clinical trials to determine its short-term effects. Interestingly, the results of observational and experimental studies have not always been congruent. Understanding these discrepancies will be important to derive reasonable conclusions regarding the association between caffeine intake and blood pressure.

Observational Studies

Because approximately 75% of caffeine is consumed as coffee in the United States [64], most observational studies have focused on the long-term effects of coffee use on blood pressure and hypertension risk [65–68]. Some observational studies have suggested that coffee intake slightly increases blood pressure levels [66,68], while other studies have indicated that coffee intake may actually decrease hypertension risk [65,67]. In a cohort of 1,017 men with a median follow-up of 33 years, Klag et al. showed that one cup of coffee per day was correlated with small but significant increases of 0.19 mm Hg systolic and 0.27 mm Hg diastolic blood pressure, which were comparable to results by Jenner et al. [66,68]. Despite observed increases in blood pressures, Klag et al. did not find a significant association between coffee consumption and incident hy-

pertension in multivariable adjusted analyses [68]. More recently, Winkelmayer et al. examined this association among women in the Nurses' Health Study (NHS) and concluded that there was considerable evidence to refute the claim that coffee drinking was associated with an increased risk of developing hypertension [65]. This study found a significant inverse trend in the relationship between coffee and hypertension risk. In addition, Uiterwaal et al. found a significant 33% reduction in hypertension among women that consumed greater than six cups of coffee per day compared to those who drank greater than zero to three cups per day [67].

While coffee is by far the most commonly studied caffeine containing product and the focus of nearly all observational studies, Winkelmayer et al. were able to assess the effects of total caffeine, tea, and soda intake on hypertension risk in the NHS [65]. They observed an inverse U-shaped association between total caffeine intake and hypertension risk. While coffee exhibited an inverse association with hypertension, findings for tea were inconclusive, and a significant positive relationship between cola and hypertension were observed. Although these findings are of great interest, these data need to be replicated in other longitudinal cohorts.

Clinical Trials

Coffee, tea and caffeine tablet intake increases blood pressure in short-term clinical trials [69,70]. A meta-analysis of clinical trials conducted by Jee et al. showed significant increases of 2.4 mm Hg systolic and 1.2 mm Hg diastolic blood pressure associated with a median coffee consumption of 5 cups/day and trial duration of 56 days (Figure 40.4) [69]. A meta-analysis conducted in 2005 by Noordzij et al. showed a significant increase of 1.22 mm Hg systolic and a nonsignificant increase of 0.49 mm Hg diastolic blood pressure associated with a median coffee intake of 750 ml/day (4.8 cups) and a median of 42 days study duration [70].

Clinical trials also show that caffeine alone may have greater pressor effects than coffee. Compared to systolic and diastolic blood pressure increases of 1.22 and 0.49 mm Hg, respectively, for coffee, Noordzij et al. observed increases of 4.16 and 2.24 mm Hg, respectively, for caffeine in their 2005 meta-analysis [70]. They postulate that caffeine tablets

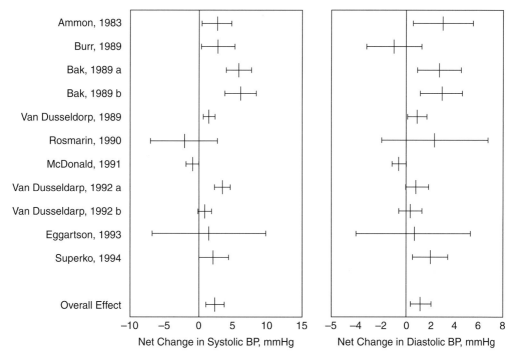

Figure 40.4 Net change in systolic and diastolic blood pressure associated with coffee drinking in 11 clinical trials. (Reproduced from Jee et al. [69], with permission.)

may exert a stronger effect than coffee for reasons of bioavailability or due to coffee's, but not caffeine's, antagonizing effect on alcohol-induced hypertension. It has also suggested that there are other compounds in coffee that may attenuate the pressor effects of caffeine [71]. For example, coffee contains flavanoids, potassium, and magnesium, which may help explain its beneficial effects [72].

Clinical trials that have investigated the effects of tea on blood pressure have had mixed results [73,74]. While a study by Bingham et al. identified a significant decrease in blood pressure in the first week of tea intervention compared to the first week of placebo [74], Hodgson et al. showed a significant acute increase in blood pressure associated with tea intervention compared to placebo [73]. However, neither study observed significant alterations in blood pressure associated with tea intervention over a longer period [73,74]. These data suggest that the acute effects of tea consumption on blood pressure may not translate into long-term blood pressure changes. However, the Bingham and Hodgson studies were conducted for a period of 1 month or less, and trials of longer duration will

be needed to fully assess the long-term effects of tea consumption.

Observational Studies versus Clinical Trials

While clinical trials have documented short-term pressor effects of coffee consumption, observational studies have found no increased risk of hypertension associated with its long-term use. Several reasons for these discrepancies have been suggested. In a 2006 review, Hamer indicated that coffee may acutely increase blood pressure levels, which is evident in short clinical trials, but this effect may decrease with habitual use [72]. The hypothesis of caffeine tolerance is supported in a trial by Lovall et al., who found that caffeine intake for 5 days reduced blood pressure response to repeated acute doses [75]. In addition, there appears to be a large variability in caffeine tolerance, ranging from no tolerance in some individuals to complete tolerance among others [76]. Therefore, at the population level, one may not expect to see the same increases in blood pressure associated with habitual coffee intake that they would when examining coffee's acute effects.

To the contrary, it has been argued that the lack of association between coffee consumption and hypertension in longitudinal studies may be due to methodological issues that are common in observational designs [63]. James argued that poor measurement of coffee intake could lead to a dilution of the association between coffee and hypertension [63]. In addition, it has been suggested that those with heightened blood pressure may be advised to decrease coffee consumption, which may dilute the actual association [72]. Nurminen et al. pointed out that blood pressure has often been taken during fasting in prospective studies [77]. Since caffeine deprivation has been associated with decreased blood pressure in habitual coffee drinkers, this may have lead to an underestimate of their regular blood pressure levels, which again could result in a reduced or inverse association between blood pressure and coffee [77].

In summary, experimental evidence clearly indicates that caffeine has acute pressor effects, ingested in coffee or alone in tablet form. However, the long-term effects of caffeine intake are still unclear. There is some evidence that habitual coffee use may not significantly increase hypertension risk, but because of the methodological limitations of observational designs, this conclusion is by no means unequivocal. Moreover, further research examining the effects of other caffeine-containing products such as tea and soda is essential due to their widespread usage and potential adverse effects on blood pressure.

Caffeine and Stroke

While the effect of caffeine on coronary heart disease has been studied extensively [78,79], there is scant data on the relationship between caffeine and stroke risk from observational studies [80–85]. In addition, no randomized clinical trials have examined the effect of caffeine on the risk of stroke.

Most observational studies have examined the effects of caffeinated coffee and tea on the risk of stroke and showed conflicting results [80–85]. Two of these studies were able to examine this relationship by stroke subtype, and the results were also inconsistent [80,83]. Hakim et al. identified a positive and significant linear trend in the association between coffee intake and ischemic thromboembolic stroke in a Japanese American cohort of nonsmoking hypertensive men. They found a twofold increased risk of incident stroke among participants that drank 24 oz/day of coffee compared to nondrinkers [83]. In contrast, a study of 29,133 Finnish male smokers by Larsson et al. found a significant inverse association between coffee consumption and ischemic stroke, with a 23% decreased risk of stroke among those consuming at least 8 cups/day of coffee compared to those who drank less than two. This study did not identify an association between coffee consumption and risk of hemorrhagic stroke [80].

Findings from prospective studies examining the association between tea consumption and stroke incidence have also been conflicting. Larsson et al. found a significant inverse trend in the association between tea and ischemic stroke incidence, with a 21% reduced risk of stroke among participants who drank 2 or more cups of tea per day compared to those who drank none, which were similar to results by Keli et al. [80,93]. However, several other cohort studies reported no association between tea and stroke risk [82,94,95].

Since coffee and tea have been shown to contain cardioprotective compounds, it has been hypothesized that both may decrease stroke incidence and mortality. For example, coffee has been demonstrated to improve insulin sensitivity [86,87]. Furthermore, coffee and tea contain antioxidants which may prevent the oxidation of low-density lipoprotein (LDL)-cholesterol and, hence, the formation of atherosclerotic lesions [80,88]. On the other hand, coffee and tea have been shown to acutely increase blood pressure levels, and a meta-analysis of clinical trials showed a positive, dose-dependent relationship between unfiltered coffee and LDL-cholesterol levels [69,73,89]. In addition, coffee consumption has also been shown to increase plasma homocysteine levels, which has long been linked to increased stroke risk [90–92].

In summary, there is a paucity of data describing the effects of caffeine on stroke risk, and existing reports are incongruent. Whether these discrepancies are due to methodological issues, population heterogeneity, or other study differences is still unclear. Further observational studies that carefully measure caffeine intake, control for confounding factors, and examine the risks of hemorrhagic and ischemic stroke subtypes separately will be necessary to help delineate this association.

Conclusion

Due to their widespread consumption and potential public health impact, understanding the effects of alcohol and caffeine on common conditions such as hypertension and stroke is critical. To date, much about the health influences of alcohol and caffeine is known, but questions still remain. Current data suggests that heavy alcohol consumption increases blood pressure levels, as well as the risk of hypertension and stroke. Light-to-moderate drinking appears to moderately reduce the risk of ischemic stroke but its effect on the risk of hypertension and hemorrhagic stroke is inconclusive. Furthermore, the lack of data about the effect of alcoholic beverage types on blood pressure and stroke represents a gap in our current knowledge. Clinical trials have clearly demonstrated an acute pressor effect of caffeine, but its longitudinal association with blood pressure is not clear. In addition, little is known about the long-term effects of caffeine consumption on the risk of stroke. In general, heavy alcohol and caffeine consumption should be avoided for cardiovascular health. On the other hand, light to moderate alcohol consumption might reduce the risk of ischemic stroke.

Selected References

7. Beilin LJ, Puddey IB. Alcohol and hypertension: an update. Hypertension 2006;47:1035–8.

33. Dickinson HO, Mason JM, Nicolson DJ, et al. Lifestyle interventions to reduce raised blood pressure: a systematic review of randomized controlled trials. Journal of Hypertension 2006;24:215–33.

64. Cornelis MC, El-Sohemy A. Coffee, caffeine, and coronary heart disease. Current Opin Clin Nutr Metabolic Care 2007;10:745–51.

71. Higdon JV, Frei B. Coffee and health: a review of recent human research. Crit Rev Food Sci Nutr 2006;46:101–23.

78. Sofi F, Conti AA, Gori AM, et al. Coffee consumption and risk of coronary heart disease: a meta-analysis. Nutr Metabolism Cardiovasc Dis 2007;17:209–23.

CHAPTER 41

Fruit and Vegetable Consumption, Hypertension, and Risk of Stroke

Lydia A. Bazzano[1] *& Domnica Fotino*[2]

[1]Tulane University, School of Public Health and Tropical Medicine, New Orleans, LA, USA
[2]Tulane University, School of Medicine, New Orleans, LA, USA

Introduction

Stroke is a major cause of death, disability, and financial burden, remaining the third leading cause of death and disease burden, with 15 million people suffering a stroke each year worldwide. Of these 15 million people, one-third die and one-third are permanently disabled [1]. This is the most common cause of disability in the majority of developed countries. For those who remain disabled, the cost was estimated to be 38 million disability-adjusted life-years (DALY) in 1990 and is projected to increase to 61 million DALYs by the year 2020 [1]. While some risk factors are genetic, many others are modifiable, with the leading risk factor for stroke of any type being hypertension. In fact, out of every 10 people who die from stroke, 4 could have been prevented by better control of blood pressure [1]. Other modifiable risk factors that strongly influence the incidence of strokes are cigarette smoking, poor diet, diabetes mellitus and elevated cholesterol levels. Although the incidence of stroke has decreased in developed countries, the worldwide numbers are increasing due to the aging population.

Hypertension, independently *and* as a risk factor for stroke, continues to be a major cause of morbidity and mortality worldwide. From data collected in 2000, roughly one-quarter of the world's population is afflicted by this misleadingly silent disease, and by 2025 closer to 29% of the world, a total of 1.56 billion people, are predicted to be affected by hypertension [2]. Hypertension is thought to be accountable for one-third of strokes in the United States and is a major risk factor for coronary heart disease, the world's leading cause of morbidity and mortality. Certain global regions are noted to be more affected by hypertension than others. Among men worldwide, Latin American and Caribbean men having the highest prevalence of hypertension at 44.5%. Among women, those from former socialist economies having the highest prevalence of hypertension at 45.9% [2]. The lowest prevalence of hypertension for men and women is found in Asia and the Pacific islands (excluding China and India).

Several factors contribute to the ongoing epidemic of hypertension. While increasing longevity is part of the cause, many environmental factors play a role in the development and persistence of hypertension. Obesity, poor diets, sedentary lifestyles, and other lifestyle risk factors are separately and together responsible for much of the prevalence of hypertension. In this chapter, we focus specifically on the potential preventive role of fruit and vegetable intake in the development of hypertension and stroke.

Classification of Hypertension and Stroke

The Sixth Report of the U.S. Joint National Committee for Detection, Evaluation, and Treatment of

Nutritional and Metabolic Bases of Cardiovascular Disease, 1st edition.
Edited by Mario Mancini, José M. Ordovas, Gabriele Riccardi,
Paolo Rubba and Pasquale Strazzullo. © 2011 Blackwell Publishing Ltd.

High Blood Pressure (JNC VI) was published in 1997 and recommended a classification of blood pressure that was adopted by the World Health Organization—International Society of Hypertension [3,4]. This classification scheme was updated in the Seventh Report, published in 2003 [5]. These criteria are for individuals who are not on anti-hypertensive medication and who are not acutely ill. The classification is based on the average of two or more blood pressure readings after an initial screening visit. When systolic blood pressure and diastolic blood pressure fall into different categories, the higher category should be selected to classify the individual's blood pressure. According to JNC VII criteria, normal blood pressure is defined as a systolic blood pressure less than 120 mm Hg and a diastolic blood pressure less than 80 mm Hg. Those with a systolic blood pressure between 120 mm and 139 mm Hg or diastolic blood pressure between 80 and 89 mm Hg are designated as having prehypertension. Hypertension is characterized by a confirmed elevation of systolic (≥ 140 mm Hg) or diastolic (≥ 90 mm Hg) blood pressure. Hypertension is further characterized into two stages according to the patient's level of systolic and diastolic blood pressure. Stage 1 is the milder (systolic 140 to 159 mm Hg and/or diastolic 90 to 99 mm Hg) and most common form of hypertension. It accounts for approximately 80% of hypertension. Stage 2 hypertension includes those with systolic blood pressure ≥ 160 mm Hg and/or diastolic blood pressure ≥ 100 mm Hg. Isolated systolic hypertension is defined as systolic blood pressure of 140 mm Hg or greater and diastolic blood pressure below 90 mm Hg and staged appropriately.

Strokes are generally separated into two categories, ischemic and hemorrhagic. The vast majority of strokes in Western countries, roughly 80%, are ischemic which implies that insufficient blood reaches the brain to provide oxygen or nutrients. This kind typically results from thrombosis, embolism or low blood pressure. The most common cause for ischemic strokes is atherosclerosis. The remaining 20% in Western countries are hemorrhagic which implies bleeding or hemorrhage in a certain area of the brain. This kind of stroke typically results from hypertension and vascular malformations in the blood vessels of the brain. The proportion of strokes that are ischemic as opposed to hemor-rhagic strokes differs widely across the globe. In some Asian countries, such as China and Japan, the proportions of ischemic and hemorrhagic strokes can be nearly equal.

Issues Related to the Assessment of Fruit and Vegetable Consumption

Day-to-day variation in an individual's dietary intake about his or her true mean intake is termed intra-individual variation, while variation between the true mean intakes of individuals within a population is termed inter-individual variation [6]. Intra-individual variation in diet has important consequences for the statistical analysis of nutritional data. Reductions in the magnitude of correlation coefficients often occur because of large intra-individual variations nutrient intake. This phenomenon results in a reduction in the power of a study to test relationships between diet and disease [6].

Because of the difficulty of measuring dietary intake in free-living populations, the magnitude of associations between diet and disease is often small compared to associations in other epidemiologic fields, perhaps because everyone is exposed to diet from birth and accurate measurement of the exposure is extremely difficult. It is far more common to find risk estimates of 0.8 to 1.2 than to find a twofold or greater estimate of risk. Very strong risk estimates are so uncommon that they may be considered suspicious, but weak associations are often viewed with caution because they may be explained by bias. In nutritional studies, weak associations may have important public health implications because exposures to dietary factors are so common.

Persons who consume large amounts of fruits, vegetables, legumes, and nutrients such as folate and potassium (much of which is provided by these food items), may have other lifestyle factors which could reduce their risk of cardiovascular disease (CVD). Despite adjustments for these shared characteristics, imperfect measurement and unmeasured characteristics may still affect study findings. Thus, randomized controlled trials, which are not affected by such shared characteristics, provide the best evidence of a causal relationship between diet and disease.

Influence of Fruit and Vegetable Consumption on Risk Factors for Stroke

Serum Cholesterol

Consumption of fruits and vegetables has been inversely associated with serum cholesterol levels in some epidemiologic studies. For example, using the National Heart Lung and Blood Institute's Family Heart Study, Djoussé et al. noted that average low-density lipoprotein (LDL)-cholesterol level was significantly and inversely linked to consumption of fruit and vegetables [7]. In the Dietary Approaches to Stop Hypertension (DASH) trial, a diet high in fruits and vegetables was associated with a reduction in LDL compared to a control diet; however, the association did not reach standard levels of statistical significance [8]. In the Indian Diet Heart Study, fruit and vegetable consumption decreased LDL concentrations by approximately 7% [9]. In a randomized trial among persons who had suffered acute myocardial infarction, fruit and vegetable intake was associated with a reduction in LDL after 12 weeks of intervention [10].

Beans, peas, and other legumes, also commonly called pulses, and sometimes included as vegetables, have also been shown to lower cholesterol levels. For example, soybean protein in particular has been shown to reduce serum total and LDL-cholesterol levels in a meta-analysis of 29 clinical trials [11]. Legume intake other than soybean has also been associated with a reduction in serum cholesterol in clinical studies [12–17] For example, Anderson et al. conducted a controlled study of oat and bean supplemented diets in the treatment of hypercholesterolemia. After a period of time on a control diet, 20 hypercholesterolemic men were randomly allocated to oat-bran or bean supplemented diets for three weeks on a metabolic ward. Both control and test diets were formulated to provide the same amounts of energy, fat, and cholesterol, but test diets had double the amount of total and three times more soluble fiber than the control diet. Over the course of three weeks, oat-bran diets decreased serum cholesterol concentrations by 19% ($p < .001$) and calculated LDL-cholesterol by 23% ($p < .01$). Bean diets decreased serum cholesterol concentrations by 19% ($p < .001$) and LDL-cholesterol by 24% ($p < .001$). In another study, the substitution of chick peas for wheat flour decreased serum cholesterol levels by 22% after 55 weeks [17]. In Chinese participants, consumption of 30 g of dried legumes daily over a 3-month period resulted in a 16% decrease in serum cholesterol in hyperlipidemic patients, whereas in normal volunteers an 8.7% decrease was observed [14]. Similarly, substitution of 140 g of dried beans (kidney, pinto, chick pea, green and red lentils) daily for other sources of starch over a 4-month period in hyperlipidemic patients resulted in a 7% decrease in total cholesterol and a 25% reduction in serum triglycerides [13]. A meta-analysis of 11 clinical trials examining the effects on legumes other than soybeans demonstrated a 7.2% reduction in total cholesterol, 6.2% reduction in LDL-cholesterol, and a 16.6% reduction in triglycerides with no effect on HDL-cholesterol [18]. Legumes are a significant source of soluble fiber which may be partially responsible for their hypercholesterolemic effects. A substantial body of evidence relates soluble fiber to reduced cholesterol levels and a lower risk of coronary heart disease [12,19,20]. A recent meta-analysis of 67 controlled trials in which participants consumed between 2 and 10 g of soluble fiber per day suggests that high intakes of soluble fiber result in small but significant decreases in total and LDL-cholesterol, while triglycerides and HDL-cholesterol are not significantly affected [20]. Other constituents of legumes including oligosaccharides, isoflavones, phospholipids, saponins, and known and unknown phytochemicals may also be part of the cholesterol-lowering effects of these foods [18].

Obesity

Obesity is one of the most prevalent risk factors for hypertension and stroke. In recent decades the prevalence of obesity has increased to epidemic proportions worldwide with more than 1 billion adults classified as overweight, and at least 300 million of them obese as defined by a body mass index (BMI) of 30 or greater [21]. To date, however, relatively few studies have examined the relationship between fruit and vegetable intake and body weight or risk of obesity. A 2004 review of this topic identified 15 cross-sectional studies and one prospective cohort study in adults; however, only one of these studies had as a primary objective to examine the relationship between fruit and vegetable intake and body weight [22]. Overall, 8 of the 16 observational studies identified an inverse association between intake of fruits and vegetables and body weight in adults [22].

Even fewer studies have examined the effects of a diet high in fruits and vegetables on body weight using randomized controlled trials. Shintani et al. examined the effects of providing a traditional Native Hawaiian diet, rich in fruits and vegetables, on food intake and body weight in overweight Hawaiians [23]. During the 3-week intervention period, participants decreased their daily caloric intake and lost an average of 7.8 kg, while rating the diet as moderately to highly satiating. These findings suggest that participants on the traditional Hawaiian diet were able to consume enough food, in particular fruits and vegetables, to avoid feeling deprived. In a similar study conducted by Shintani et al., obese participants were provided with the same diet but energy contribution from fat was increased to 12% [24]. Participants lost an average of 4.9 kg during the 3-week intervention.

Fruit and Vegetable Intake and Hypertension

Dietary modification has long been known to aid in the control of hypertension, and fruit and vegetable intake, in particular, has been shown to reduce blood pressure in a variety of settings, including randomized controlled trials [25–27]. Several decades ago, it was noted that persons with vegetarian diets consistently had lower blood pressure levels than those with omnivorous diets [28]. In trials of vegetarian diets, replacing animal products with vegetable products reduced blood pressure in normotensive and hypertensive adults [26,27]. However, fewer investigations have specifically examined whole fruit and vegetable intake and hypertension. An examination of 1,710 men, 41–57 years of age, followed for 40 years demonstrated that intake of fruits and vegetables was inversely associated with age-related rise in blood pressure over the course of the study [29]. Similarly, in a cohort of 2,341 persons, after adjustment for potential confounders, higher fruit and vegetable consumption was associated with lower systolic and diastolic blood pressure at baseline examination ($p < .02$ for both) and a lower 5-year increase in systolic (-2.1 mm Hg

in the fourth compared with the first quartile; $p < .004$) and diastolic blood pressure (-0.7 mm Hg in the fourth compared with the first quartile; $p < .03$) [30].

DASH was one of the most influential randomized controlled trials to examine fruit and vegetable intake and the development of hypertension. The DASH trial showed that a diet supplemented with fruits and vegetables lowered blood pressure in a multiethnic population [25]. In the DASH study, 459 adults with systolic blood pressure of less than 160 mm Hg and diastolic blood pressure between 80 and 95 mm Hg were randomly assigned to receive the control diet, a diet rich in fruits and vegetables, or a combination diet rich in fruits, vegetables, and low-fat dairy products with reduced saturated and total fat, for 8 weeks [25]. Sodium intake and body weight were maintained at constant levels. The fruits and vegetables diet reduced systolic blood pressure by 2.8 mm Hg ($p < .001$) and diastolic blood pressure by 1.1 mm Hg ($p = .07$) compared to the control diet. The combination diet showed even greater reductions in systolic and diastolic blood pressures.

In another intervention study, Singh and colleagues randomized 72 participants to a diet supplemented with guava fruit or to continue their usual diet [31]. They found a significant decrease in mean systolic and diastolic pressures (7.5/8.5 mm Hg net decrease, respectively) among participants on the guava supplemented diet. Several more intervention studies have combined increases in fruits and vegetables with other dietary interventions, weight loss, and increases in physical activity, thus obscuring the specific effects of fruit and vegetable intake on blood pressure.

Fruit and Vegetable Intake and Risk of Stroke

Prospective cohort studies provide the best estimate of long term stroke risk reduction that could be associated with a dietary pattern high in fruits and vegetables. Several prospective cohort studies have looked at the effect of fruit and vegetable intake on risk of stroke, taking hypertension into consideration. The evidence regarding fruit and vegetable intake and stroke has been reviewed previously by Ness and Powles in 1999, and most recently by

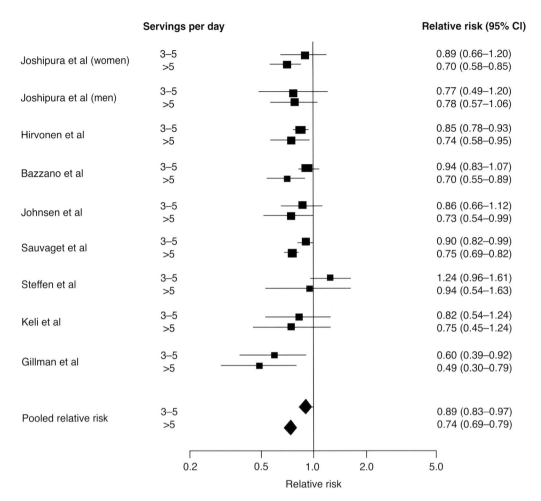

Figure 41.1 Forrest plot showing risk of stroke for three to five and more than five servings of fruit and vegetables per day compared with less than three servings. (Adapted from He FJ , Nowson CA, MacGregor GA. Lancet 2006;367:320–5, with permission.)

He et al. [32,33]. Eight prospective cohort studies evaluating intake of fruits and vegetables and risk of stroke have been conducted since the review by Ness and Powles, and of those, five have found significant inverse relationships between fruit and vegetable consumption and risk of stroke [34–38], and another three had inverse findings that trended toward significance [39–41].

He et al. conducted a meta-analysis synthesizing the results of nine cohort studies examining fruit and vegetable intake in relation to stroke risk [33]. These nine studies included 257,551 participants from the United States, Europe, and Japan [34–42]. The authors identified a 26% risk reduction (pooled relative risk 0.74; 95% confidence interval 0.69 to 0.79) for those who consumed more than three to five servings per day of fruits and vegetables compared to less than three servings per day (Figure 41.1). For those who consumed three to five servings per day only some subgroups were noted to benefit, and 11% of strokes were prevented [33].

Nutrients and Bioactive Aspects of Fruit and Vegetables

Potassium

Potassium may have an important role in the effect of fruit and vegetable consumption on incidence and mortality from CVDs. Epidemiologic studies have identified an inverse association between dietary intake of potassium and blood pressure level within and across populations [43]. In one of the largest studies, the INTERSALT study, 10,079 participants in communities from 32 countries were examined. The investigators identified a strong, inverse relationship between dietary intake of potassium and blood pressure: for every 50 mmol/day decrease in urinary excretion of potassium there is on average an increase by 3.4 mm Hg and 1.9 mm Hg for systolic and diastolic blood pressure, respectively [44].

In addition, randomized controlled trials have documented that potassium supplementation lowers blood pressure in both hypertensive and normotensive persons [45]. A meta-analysis of 33 randomized controlled trials of potassium supplementation showed a significant reduction in mean (95% confidence interval) systolic and diastolic blood pressure of -3.11 mm Hg (-1.91 to -4.31 mm Hg) and -1.97 mm Hg (-0.52 to -3.42 mm Hg), respectively [45]. In hypertensive subjects, the systolic blood pressure was decreased by 4 mm Hg and diastolic blood pressure by 2.5 mm Hg, while the normotensive population had a decrease in systolic blood pressure of 1.8 mm Hg and in diastolic blood pressure of 1.0 mm Hg. Conversely, a low dietary potassium intake has been associated with elevated blood pressure levels. In a randomized, crossover trial of potassium depletion in ten normotensive men, participants fed a low potassium diet (10 mmol/day) significantly increased mean arterial blood pressure (4 mm Hg increase, $p <$ .05) [46]. In a second randomized, crossover trial examining dietary potassium depletion (from consumption of 96 mmol/day to 16 mmol/day of potassium) in 12 hypertensive subjects, the same research group reported significant increases in blood pressure, both systolic (7 mm Hg increase, $p = .01$) and diastolic (6 mm Hg increase, $p = .04$), after feeding a low potassium diet [47]. Such evidence suggests that a diet rich in fruits and vegetables and hence high in potassium may protect against increased risk of stroke via lowering blood pressure. Yet another study suggested the possibility of reducing antihypertensive medication requirement by as much as 50% at the end of one year by increasing potassium intake by at least 30 mmol/day [48].

Several studies have reported an inverse relationship between dietary potassium intake and risk of stroke or stroke mortality. Xie et al. conducted an ecologic analysis which indicated an inverse relationship between 24-hour urinary excretion of potassium and stroke mortality among 27 populations [49]. In a population of 859 male and female retirees in Southern California, Khaw and Barrett-Conner identified a strong inverse association between potassium intake and stroke mortality [50] Ascherio et al. also documented an inverse relationship between the risk of stroke and dietary potassium intake in a cohort of 43,738 male health professionals [51]. In the NHANES I, dietary potassium was inversely associated with risk of stroke after adjustment for established CVD risk factors [52].

Fiber

The relationship between dietary fiber intake and risk of stroke has not been well studied. At least one large prospective study identified an inverse association between cereal fiber and risk of stroke [53]. Dietary fiber has been shown to delay the absorption of carbohydrates after a meal and thereby decrease the insulinemic response to dietary carbohydrates [54]. Experimental studies have also shown that higher levels of insulin may promote dyslipidemia, hypertension, abnormalities in blood clotting factors, and atherosclerosis [55]. In addition, water-soluble dietary fiber has been shown to decrease both total cholesterol and LDL-cholesterol while not affecting levels of high-density lipoprotein [56]. While the cholesterol-lowering effects of dietary fiber are usually though too be modest, they may play a role in the inverse association between dietary intake of fiber and stroke risk. Moreover, epidemiologic studies and randomized controlled trials have suggested inverse associations between dietary fiber and other CVD risk factors such as blood pressure, waist-to-hip ratio, fasting insulin, 2-hour post glucose insulin, levels of triglycerides, and levels of fibrinogen [57,58]. Several studies also indicate that increased dietary fiber may act to increase satiety and therefore assist with weight regulation and the prevention of obesity, a common risk factor for both hypertension and stroke [59].

Antioxidants and Phytochemicals

Antioxidants are substances that inactivate reactive oxygen species and therefore significantly delay or prevent oxidative damage, and atherosclerosis is thought to proceed in part due to the oxidation of lipids in atherosclerotic plaques. Fruits and vegetables are rich sources of antioxidants including vitamin E, vitamin C, polyphenols, flavonoids, and carotenoids that may help prevent atherosclerosis and subsequent cerebrovascular diseases. Dietary supplements of specific antioxidants including vitamins C, E, and β-carotene were tested in randomized controlled trials that on the whole did not show significant benefit in secondary prevention of CVDs [60]. Recently, other antioxidant compounds such as lycopene and flavonoids have received attention [61,62]. Dietary lycopene, which is derived in large part from tomato products, was significantly and inversely associated with relative risk of CVDs in a cohort of 39,876 middle-aged women [61]. Polyphenolic compounds from pomegranate juice have been shown to inhibit LDL-cholesterol peroxidation, and dietary supplementation of pomegranate juice to atherosclerotic mice has significantly inhibited the development of plaques and streaks in these animals [62,63]. Antioxidants received from whole foods such as fruits and vegetables and in juices may act in combination with each other and/or other phytochemicals within the foods to provide their protective effects.

While each of the components described above may play a protective role with respect to CVD, it is their combined effects that we see in a diet rich in whole fruits and vegetables. The biochemical complexity of fruits and vegetables as a delivery system for protective nutrients and functional components should not be underestimated. Hence, it is important to emphasize the consumption of whole fruits and vegetables rather than specific nutrients or supplements in any dietary recommendation to prevent hypertension and stroke.

Conclusions

In conclusion, fruit and vegetable consumption plays an important role in the reduction of hypertension as well as stroke. According to one estimate, increasing individual fruit and vegetable consumption to 600 g/day could reduce the global burden of disease by 1.8%, and reduce the burden of ischemic stroke by 19% [64]. Because hypertension and ischemic stroke are such common and potentially deadly diseases worldwide, primary prevention of even a small part of the growing number of cases using dietary means would result in millions of lives saved and significant reductions in health care expenditures in most nations. Dietary modification should be an important element of any public health intervention aimed at the prevention of hypertension and stroke in adults.

Selected References

30. Dauchet L, Kesse-Guyot E, Czernichow S, et al. Dietary patterns and blood pressure change over 5-y follow-up in the SU.VI.MAX cohort. Am J Clin Nutr 2007;85: 1650–6.

33. He FJ, Nowson CA, MacGregor GA. Fruit and vegetable consumption and stroke: meta-analysis of cohort studies. Lancet 2006;367:320–5.

34. Bazzano LA, He J, Ogden LG, et al. Fruit and vegetable intake and risk of cardiovascular disease in US adults: the first National Health and Nutrition Examination Survey Epidemiologic Follow-up Study. Am J Clin Nutr 2002; 76:93–9.

58. Whelton SP, Hyre AD, Pedersen B, Yi Y, Whelton PK, He J. Effect of dietary fiber intake on blood pressure: a meta-analysis of randomized, controlled clinical trials. J Hypertens 2005;23:475–81.

64. Lock K, Pomerleau J, Causer L, Altmann DR, McKee M. The global burden of disease attributable to low consumption of fruit and vegetables: implications for the global strategy on diet. Bull World Health Organ 2005; 83:100–8.

CHAPTER 42

Complex Dietary Patterns and Blood Pressure

Alfonso Siani[1] *& L. Aldo Ferrara*[2]

[1] Institute of Food Sciences, National Research Council, Avellino, Italy
[2] Federico II University, Naples, Italy

Introduction

Industrialized countries pay since long time a heavy tribute to cardiovascular diseases (CVDs) in terms of morbidity and mortality. In the past two decades there has been an increasing burden of CVD in many developing countries so that CVD represent now the leading cause of mortality, morbidity, and disability worldwide [1]. Unfortunately, both prevalence and incidence of CVD are expected to rise further mainly because of population aging. Never perhaps as in the case of CVD, primary prevention may be more effective than treatment. While waiting for more conclusive identification of genetic traits predisposing to CVD and related conditions, a growing body of evidence has accumulated concerning the risk factors involved in the pathogenesis of CVD. Seventy-five percent of the global burden of CVD results from smoking, high blood cholesterol, and high blood pressure (BP) or their combination. In particular, high BP is a powerful predisposing factor for CVD, stroke, heart failure, renal failure, and deaths [1–4]. Specifically, hypertension affects approximately 1 billion individuals worldwide, thus representing the most common cardiovascular condition in the world. In addition, it is implicated in 13% of all deaths worldwide [1,2,5]. The prevalence of hypertension is likely to increase as the population ages, as suggested by recent data from the Framingham Hearth Study,

whereby normotensive individuals at 55 years of age have a 90% lifetime risk to develop hypertension [6]. Furthermore, high BP is less frequently an isolated risk factor but is more often accompanied by a cluster of other risk factors grouped under the definition of metabolic syndrome [7].

Therefore, the development of effective strategies for the prevention and treatment of high BP is of utmost importance for healthcare providers and public health bodies. Elevated BP results from environmental factors, genetic factors, and mutual interactions among these factors. Of the environmental factors that affect BP (diet, sedentary lifestyle, and psychosocial factors), dietary factors have a prominent role in BP regulation [8]. It follows that nutrition has a great potential role in the prevention of hypertension and its sequelae. Although the extent of BP reduction from dietary manipulation is somewhat greater in hypertensive than in non-hypertensive individuals, even an apparently small reduction in BP could have a great beneficial impact on the whole population [8].

Well-established lifestyle modifications that effectively lower BP are reduced salt intake, weight loss, and moderation of alcohol consumption (among those who drink) [8]. Over the past decade, increased potassium intake and adoption of dietary patterns based on the Dietary Approaches to Stop Hypertension (DASH) diet have emerged as effective strategies that also lower BP, while more limited evidence indicates the beneficial effect of other complex dietary patterns such as vegetarian diets and the Mediterranean diet [8].

Nutritional and Metabolic Bases of Cardiovascular Disease, 1st edition.
Edited by Mario Mancini, José M. Ordovas, Gabriele Riccardi,
Paolo Rubba and Pasquale Strazzullo. © 2011 Blackwell Publishing Ltd.

Importance of Dietary Patterns

Whereas hundreds of studies explored the possibility to reduce BP through dietary modifications based on a single intervention or nutrient, there are less, though conclusive data, demonstrating that not only single dietary components but also the overall dietary pattern may have great influence on BP. Achieving unequivocal evidence of a protective or adverse role of a complex dietary pattern is indeed difficult for a number of reasons. The most important one is the large variation in dietary patterns both within and between populations that is likely to contribute to the biological variability, deriving from the interaction between genetic background, food components, and multiple pathogenic mechanisms, which make the same nutrient or food eliciting dissimilar responses in different individuals. Furthermore, the accurate estimate of the usual intake of foods and nutrients is hampered by methodological inadequacies that reduce the likelihood to detect true biological associations. Finally, long-term randomized controlled trials in the nutritional area are difficult to implement, in particular when complex dietary variations are investigated. The classical investigations over dietary factors and CVD risk have included the assessment of food and/or nutrient intake by food histories and food composition tables or by the measurement of nutrient concentrations in the blood or other tissues. Very often, inaccuracies in the estimate of intake and confounding by different factors have made it difficult to attribute associations with risk to specific nutrients or foods [9]. In other cases, the results of these studies have led to hypotheses regarding specific nutrients/foods thought to induce protective or negative effects. Actually, it may well be that it is the synergism between the various components of certain foods or food combinations that produces the health benefits observed. Notwithstanding these pitfalls, there are few doubts that, for instance, populations or individuals consuming mostly plant-based diets have lower BP than those following typical Western diets with elevated intakes of saturated fats [10]. Ecological observations have been supported by findings of several epidemiologic studies and randomized controlled trials, which have confirmed the important role of dietary patterns in the regulation of BP levels [11].

To this regard, it has been recently observed in a hypertension outpatient setting that not only total energy intake but also food components are able to beneficially affect BP levels in addition to drug treatment. In 307 hypertensive patients who had been on a low energy regimen with a body weight reduction of 5 ± 3 kg, with a significant BP reduction by $31/15 \pm 7/4$ mm Hg, only those who did not regained the lost weight were able to maintain an optimal BP control over time without increasing the dosage of antihypertensive drugs. When the weekly consumption of the single foods was analyzed, an inverse significant correlation was observed between systolic BP (SBP) or diastolic BP (DBP) and the number of weekly servings of fish ($r = -0.122$ for SBP and -0.104 for DBP, $p < .05$) or of vegetables ($r = -0.162$ for SBP and -0.103 for DBP, $p < .05$). On the other hand, a positive correlation between SBP or DBP was observed with the number of weekly servings of cheese ($r = 0.209$ for SBP and 0.191 for DBP, $p < .001$) or salami ($r = 0.157$ for SBP and 0.167 for DBP, $p < .005$) [12].

The aim of this chapter is to review present knowledge relating complex dietary patterns to the prevention and treatment of high BP. We focus specifically on two dietary patterns habitually consumed by different populations/individuals in different parts of the world—the vegetarian diets and the Mediterranean diets and an experimental diet that largely went into use, that is, the DASH diet.

Vegetarian Diet

Anthropological and historical considerations of the diet of primitive men [13] as well as observational data on population groups where diets are plant-based [14–15] clearly support the benefits on BP levels derived from the adherence to a vegetarian dietary regimen with no or very little amount of animal-based products [10]. Notably, when these individuals migrate to industrialized countries therefore changing their diet and lifestyles, their BP, and risk of hypertension increase [16]. However, even within industrialized societies, lifestyles and diet influence BP. To date, the most definitive and well-controlled observational data on the effects of vegetarian diets on BP come from studies of Seventh-Day Adventists. The Seventh-Day Adventists are expected, by religious belief, to abstain from alcohol, nicotine, and caffeine and to follow a vegetarian diet supplemented with eggs and dairy products. In a cross-sectional analysis on a large cohort of 34 192 California Seventh-Day Adventists, the prevalence of hypertension was nearly double among Adventists who followed a diet similar to a typical American diet than in vegetarian Adventists [17]. After adjustment for body weight, the effect was somewhat reduced, suggesting that the adherence to a vegetarian diet may be associated to lower body mass. Moreover, the Adventists showed a trend toward lower mortality from cancer, heart disease, and diabetes than non-Adventists living in the same communities. Cross-cultural studies have shown that the age-related increases in BP typically observed in developed societies is less evident in individuals adopting a vegetarian dietary style [18].

In summary, data from observational studies indicate that the SBP of vegetarians is 3–14 mm Hg lower and the DBP is 5–6 mm Hg lower than that of nonvegetarians. Vegetarians also show lower prevalence of hypertension than nonvegetarians (2%–40% vs. 8%–60%, respectively) [10].

The number of randomized controlled trials of the effect of vegetarian diets on BP is quite small [10]. Overall they are supportive of the BP-lowering effects of vegetarian diets in both normotensive and hypertensive individuals. However, in most clinical studies, the adjustment for body weight reduced the effect of the intervention on BP, indicating that weight loss may be one of the mechanisms leading to the reduction of BP, while apparently a reduction of sodium intake was not responsible for the observed effect.

Vegetarian diets are characterized by high intake of fruits, vegetables, legumes, and nuts, thus resulting in a relatively high polyunsaturated to saturated fat ratio, relatively low fat content and high potassium, magnesium, and fiber content, all factors possibly cooperating to the BP-lowering effect [19]. Additionally, the vegetarian lifestyle is often associated in Western societies to increased physical activity, abstention from alcohol and smoke, and adoption of relaxation techniques, possibly favorably acting on BP regulation.

In conclusion, although the evidence suggests a BP-lowering effect of a vegetarian diet, the high degree of intercorrelation among different dietary and nondietary components hampers the identification of the factor or factors responsible for this effect. However, although specific recommendations for a vegetarian diet in the prevention/treatment of high BP cannot be made, this diet is largely consistent with most guidelines for the prevention and treatment of hypertension and CVD.

Mediterranean Diet

The Mediterranean diet, first explored in the 1960s in the Seven Countries Study, is considered the golden standard of healthy nutrition and it is associated with decreased morbidity and mortality, especially from cardiovascular causes [20–22]. The protective effects of the traditional Mediterranean diet on coronary heart disease morbidity and mortality rates are well known and this diet has consistently been associated with better health and longevity [23–26]. The traditional Mediterranean diet is low in animal and dairy products as well as saturated fatty acids and cholesterol; it is rich in plant food, legumes, fiber, and antioxidant vitamins, whereas olive oil is the main fat source.

Several studies supported the hypothesis that the Mediterranean diet may favorably influence health status, but only few epidemiologic observations dealt with its effects (if any) on BP, suggesting in general a positive effect of this dietary pattern on BP levels or prevalence of hypertension [27–29].

Although this suggestion is attractive, epidemiologic observations may not give insight into cause–effect relationship, also considering the complexity of the interplaying factors. However, experimental evidence of a relationship between the Mediterranean diet and BP has been provided by a set of intervention trials conducted about 25 years ago in the framework of an international collaborative project involving Finland and Italy. The aim of the project was to investigate the effects of mid-term dietary manipulation (namely type and amount of dietary fats) on serum lipids and BP in populations with largely different dietary patterns (northern Karelia, Finland and Cilento, southern Italy).

The first study was carried out in northern Karelia, a region characterized by a particularly high rate of CVD and by a high intake of saturated fat intake with a low polyunsaturated to saturated fatty acid (P/S) ratio [30]. Fifty-four middle-aged normotensive volunteers participated in the trial, which consisted of a two week baseline period, a 6-week dietary intervention, and a 6-week switch-back period. During the intervention period, the composition of the habitual diet was modified with regard to fat quality and amount. Saturated fatty acids from animal food were reduced and replaced mainly by polyunsaturated fatty acid, resulting in a very high P/S ratio. As a result of the intervention, the proportion of energy derived from fat decreased from 39% during baseline to 24% during the intervention period, with a compensatory 10% increase in energy from carbohydrates. Dietary P/S increased from 0.15 to 1.18 during the intervention. During the switch-back period, participants resumed their habitual diet. At the end of the intervention, a significant decrease was observed in both SBP and DBP ($-7.5/-2.8$ mm Hg) compared to the baseline period. When participants resumed their habitual diet, their BP increased progressively, reaching the initial values at the end of the switch-back period. In the course of this study, the intake of both sodium and potassium was kept constant. The change in BP was associated with a significant decrease in total cholesterol, LDL-cholesterol, HDL-cholesterol, and apolipoprotein B.

A second trial was conducted again in northern Karelia, aiming at reproducing the results of the first study under better-controlled conditions and at comparing the effects on BP of changes in dietary fats and salt intake [31]. In brief, fifty-seven couples (normotensive or untreated mildly hypertensive subjects) were randomly allocated to one of the three groups: (1) low-fat diet, (2) low-sodium diet, and (3) control diet. While the control diet derived 38% of total energy from fat, the low-fat diet derived only 25% of energy from fat, with a P/S of 1.0. The low-salt diet was similar to the control diet but contained approximately 80 mmol of sodium per day instead of 190 mmol/day. This study also consisted of three periods: baseline, 2 weeks; intervention, 6 weeks; and switch-back, 4 weeks. The results of this controlled trial confirmed those of the former study. In group I (low-fat diet), a significant BP decrease was observed (8.9/7.6 mm Hg) during the intervention period, with a subsequent rise to baseline values after switchback. The BP changes in group II (low-salt) and III (control diet) were small and not significantly different from each other.

As part of the same international collaborative project, an intervention trial was implemented in a rural area of southern Italy [32,33]. The study was designed to investigate in a free-living situation the changes induced in the BP and serum lipid levels of a group of middle-aged men and women by manipulation of their customary Mediterranean-style diet. During the last decades of the last century, current trends in Italy were indeed marked by a gradual evolution from the traditional Mediterranean diet toward Westernized dietary patterns. The Cilento region was selected for this study because at the time of the study the inhabitants still maintained to a great extent traditional lifestyles and diet, in particular the use of olive oil as the only visible fat employed in cooking.

The design of the study was similar to that of the two Finnish trials, with a 2-week baseline period and two consecutive 6-week intervention and switch-back periods; the participants, 29 men and 28 women, were normotensive volunteers. The goal of dietary intervention was, in this case, to raise to 40% the fat contribution to total energy intake and to lower the P/S ratio about 0.2. This dietary modification was obtained by substituting foods rich in saturated fatty acids such as butter, dairy cream, cheese, and meat for specific items of the habitual diet: olive oil, cereals, and vegetables.

During the intervention the consumption of saturated fatty acids was increased by 70% and, by consequence, P/S decreased significantly (baseline was 0.44, intervention 0.22 and switchback 0.40). SBP increased gradually during the intervention period, with final values significantly higher as compared to the baseline. DBP increased to a lesser extent but was significantly higher compared with that observed at the end of the switch-back period (Figure 42.1) [33]. A rapid decrease in BP levels to pre-intervention values was observed after return to the customary diet. The increase in the saturated fat content of the diet was associated with a remarkable increase in total cholesterol of 15% and LDL-cholesterol of 19% (Figure 42.2) [32].

The joint results of the studies conducted in Finland and Italy support the concept that modifications of complex dietary patterns diet may influence BP. In particular, the current trend toward replacing the traditional diet with patterns typical of Western industrialized societies may have a deleterious impact on cardiovascular risk in Mediterranean populations.

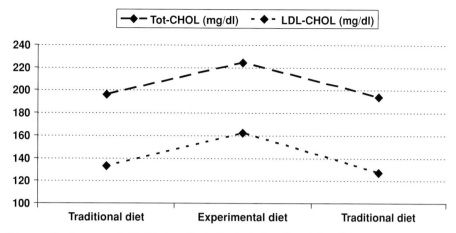

Figure 42.1 From Mediterranean diet to Western: The Pollica Study. Systolic and diastolic blood pressure during dietary intervention. (Modified from Strazzullo et al. [33].)

More recently, the possible beneficial effect of the monounsaturated olive oil, typical visible fat of the Mediterranean diet, was investigated in a group of 23 hypertensive patients regularly followed in an outpatient setting [34]. All patients were on stable antihypertensive treatment and had not changed their body weight in the last 6 months. The goal of the study was to evaluate whether a dietary approach based on the use of olive oil (40 g daily for men and 30 g for women) as the main source of lipid was able to interfere with BP control over long time in comparison to a dietary regimen whose lipid source was mainly represented by a similar amount of polyunsaturated sunflower oil. The study was a randomized single-blind clinical trial and consisted of three phases: a 1-month run-in, a 6-month intervention period with monounsaturated or polyunsaturated dietary treatment and a 6-month intervention period with the alternative dietary approach. Body weight did not change over both treatments. At the end of the olive oil dietary intervention, a significant reduction in the baseline dosage of antihypertensive drugs was detected (−48%, 95% confidence interval [CI], −25 to −71), while no change was observed at the end of the polyunsaturated treatment (−4%, 95% CI, −24 to 17), the difference between the effects of the two dietary periods being statistically significant ($p < .005$). Despite the reduction of drug dosage, also BP levels were significantly reduced at the end of the olive oil period in comparison to the sun-

flower oil (127/84 ± 14/8 mm Hg vs. 135/90 ± 13/8 mm Hg, $p < .05$ for SBP and $p < .01$ for DBP). Among the nonlipid component of the virgin olive oil, it is possible that the poly-phenols with antioxidant properties may improve the endothelial function and contribute to the effect on BP. These results, also confirmed by other studies [35], further suggest the usefulness of the Mediterranean diet for BP control, not only in comparison to the saturated fats, as shown by the Finnish Italian collaborative studies but also in comparison to the polyunsaturated fatty acids, which are widely used in the world as substitute of saturated fats.

Dash Diet

The most significant contribution to the nutritional management of hypertension through modification of dietary patterns derived from the DASH [36] and DASH-Sodium trials [37]. The effectiveness of a dietary regimen similar to that adopted in the DASH trials has been emphasized in recent authoritative reports [8,38]. DASH is an experimentally designed diet that emphasizes fruits, vegetables, and low-fat dairy foods. Compared to the typical American diet, it also includes more whole grains, poultry, fish, and nuts, and lower amounts of fats, red meat, sweets, and sugar-containing beverages. Looking at nutrient intakes, the DASH diet is poorer in total and saturated fat and cholesterol

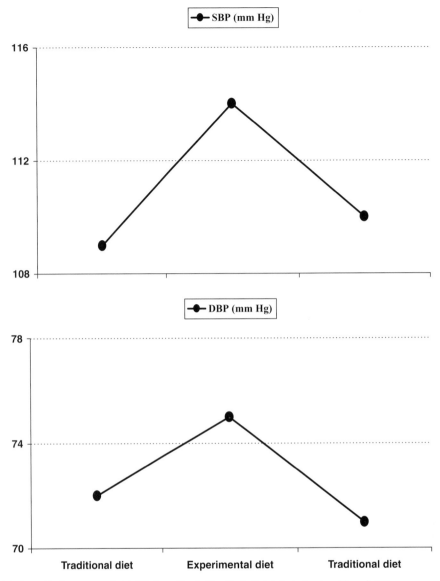

Figure 42.2 From Mediterranean diet to Western: The Pollica Study. Total cholesterol and low-density lipoprotein-cholesterol levels during dietary intervention. (A. Siani, personal archive.)

and richer in potassium, magnesium, calcium, and fiber in comparison to the habitual Western diet.

Actually, it may well be that the BP lowering effect observed with modification of complex dietary patterns is the result of the synergism between the various components of certain foods or food combinations rather than of the specific effect of a single nutrient. The purpose of the DASH trial was indeed to test the effects on BP of a change in di-

etary patterns, rather than the effects of a change in a single nutrient, as generally tested in previous trials [36]. This trial was an 11-week intervention program including 459 adults with ($n = 133$) and without hypertension ($n = 326$). For 3 weeks, participants followed a control diet that was low in fruit, vegetable, and dairy products. The fat content was tailored on the average consumption in the United States. Then, for the next 3 weeks, participants were randomly allocated in three groups and each group was fed three different diets. One group was fed the same control diet, the second group a diet richer in fruit and vegetables but similar to the control diet for other nutrients, and the third group was fed the DASH diet, which is a diet rich in fruit and vegetables, low-fat or fat-free dairy products, and reduced saturated and total fat content. The sodium intake was held constant in the three groups. Alcohol intake and body weight did not change during the trial or among the groups. Overall, the findings indicated a gradient in the reduction in BP among the diets. The complete DASH diet significantly reduced SBP and DBP by 5.5/3.0 mm Hg, respectively, compared to the control diet, whereas the fruit and vegetables diet significantly reduced SBP and DBP but to a lesser extent (2.8/1.1 mm Hg, respectively) compared to the control diet. A larger BP reduction was observed in hypertensive individuals, that is, 11.4/5.5 mm Hg for SBP and DBP, respectively, compared to the control diet. Interestingly, the BP-lowering effects of the DASH diet occurred within the first 2 weeks of the trial. Further subgroup analyses showed significant effects of the DASH diet in all major subgroups (sex, race, age, body mass index, etc.), although the effects were more evident among African Americans (6.9/3.7 mm Hg) than in whites (3.3/2.4 mm Hg) [39].

An appendix of the DASH trial evaluated the additive effect of a reduction in sodium intake to the DASH combination diet [37]: an account of its results is given in Chapter 35 of this book.

The information obtained by the DASH trials was further implemented in the setting of the Optimal Macronutrient Intake Trial to Prevent Heart Disease (OmniHeart) [40]. This randomized dietary intervention aimed to to compare the effects on BP and serum lipids of three dietary regimens, each reduced in saturated fat: a carbohydrate-rich diet (58% of total calories), similar to the DASH diet; a diet rich in protein, approximately half from plant sources; and a diet rich in unsaturated fat, predominantly monounsaturated fat. The intervention periods lasted 6 weeks and body weight was held constant. SBPs were lowered in each of the three intervention groups compared with baseline. However, BPs were further lowered in the two dietary regimens providing a partial substitution of carbohydrates (10% of total kcal) with either pro-

teins or unsaturated fats (1.4 and 1.3 mm Hg, respectively). Thus, these findings indicate that, along with known determinants of BP (i.e., micronutrients [sodium and potassium], body weight, alcohol consumption, and the DASH diet), macronutrients and the qualitative composition of diet are also important factors to consider for the prevention and management of hypertension.

As a follow-up to these controlled trials of nutritional intervention, the PREMIER trial tested the individuals ability to lower BP by implementing established guidelines for treating hypertension, including the DASH diet in addition to the established recommendations [41]. Traditionally, the lifestyle modifications for the control of BP include weight loss, if overweight, reduction of intake of salt, increase of aerobic physical activity, limitation of intake of alcohol, abolition of smoking, and control of stress. PREMIER used a lifestyle counseling approach and randomized more than 800 participants with above-optimal BP, including stage 1 hypertension (120–159 mm Hg SBP and 80–95 mm Hg DBP), and who were not on antihypertensive medications. They were randomly allocated to one of three intervention groups: (1) "established," a behavioral intervention that implemented established recommendations; (2) "established plus DASH," which also implemented the DASH diet; and (3) an "advice only" control group. At the end of the trial (after 6 months), in the group assigned to lifestyle modification only, the established group, the mean net reduction in BP was 3.7/1.7 mm Hg, compared to the control group, although for the group that followed the established recommendations together with the DASH diet, the mean net reduction in BP was 4.3/2.6 mm Hg, compared to the control group. Thus, these findings point to the everyday feasibility and effectiveness of comprehensive lifestyle modifications as preventive and therapeutic measures for both non-hypertensive individuals with above-optimal BP and hypertensive individuals who are not receiving antihypertensive drug treatment.

Conclusion

High BP is a largely diffused chronic condition impacting both developed and developing countries, with increasing risk associated with the ageing of the population. Substantial and undisputed evidence supports the concept that multiple dietary factors affect BP homeostasis and may have favorable effects on high BP prevention and treatment. Besides the "classical" nutritional approaches (weight loss, reduced salt intake, increased potassium intake, moderation of alcohol consumption among drinkers), there is a clear-cut evidence of the effectiveness of the DASH dietary pattern in lowering BP, particularly in hypertensive individuals and in African Americans. There is also consistent evidence in favor of the beneficial effect of other complex dietary patterns, like the vegetarian diets and the traditional Mediterranean diet. More research is indeed needed to substantiate the findings obtained by observational studies or short-term intervention trials with larger randomized intervention studies.

In conclusion, the role of nutrition in the prevention of high BP and its sequelae with high impact on public health and socioeconomic costs must not be disregarded and may indeed be even stronger than that supported by present scientific evidence

Selected References

10. Berkow SE, Barnard ND. BP regulation and vegetarian diets. Nutr Rev 2005;63:1–8.

33. Strazzullo P, Ferro-Luzzi A, Siani A, et al. Changing the Mediterranean diet: effects on blood pressure. J Hypertens 1986;4:407–12.

37. Sacks FM, Svetkey LP, Vollmer WM, et al, For the DASH-Sodium Collaborative Research Group. Effects on blood pressure of reduced dietary sodium and the Dietary Approaches to Stop Hypertension (DASH) diet. New Engl J Med 2001;344:3–10.

38. Svetkey LP, Simons-Morton D, Vollmer WM, et al. Effects of dietary patterns on BP: subgroup analysis of the Dietary Approaches to Stop Hypertension (DASH) randomized clinical trial. Arch Intern Med 1999;159: 285–93.

40. Appel LJ, Sacks FM, Carey VJ, et al, for the OmniHeart Collaborative Research Group. Effects of protein, monounsaturated fat, and carbohydrate intake on BP and serum lipids: results of the OmniHeart randomized trial. JAMA 2005;294:2455–64.

CHAPTER 43

Role of Obesity and Metabolic Alterations in Hypertensive Renal Disease and in Chronic Kidney Disease

Carmine Zoccali, Daniela Leonardis, & Francesca Mallamaci

Nephrology, Hypertension and Renal Transplantation Unit, and National Research Council—IBIM
Clinical Epidemiology of Renal Diseases and Hypertension, Reggio Calabria, Italy

Introduction

In economically developed countries, body weight excess and frank obesity are considered the most concerning epidemic of the third millennium [1]. In the United States, the prevalence of such diseases increased from 23% to 30.5% [2] just in 12 years, and recent observations show that the epidemic is still in an expanding phase, particularly among the youngest generations and in males [1]. The metabolic syndrome, a cluster of risk factors (i.e., the simultaneous presence of three risk factors in a list including central obesity, hypertriglyceridemia, low high-density lipoprotein [HDL]-cholesterol [HDL-C], fasting hyperglycemia, and hypertension) largely driven by overweight and obesity, affects a very large proportion of the general population. In the United States, about one-quarter of people who are 20 years or older and about four-tenths of the population older than 60 years is affected by this syndrome [2]. Central obesity predisposes to insulin resistance, which triggers sympathetic overactivity and sodium retention ultimately leading to hypertension. Systemic inflammation is another major consequence of visceral fat accumulation [3]. Hypertension, hyperglycemia, dys-

lipidemia, and inflammation are notoriously conducive to coronary heart disease (CHD) and to the full range of major atherosclerotic complications [4]. In recent years, substantial evidence has been accrued showing that well beyond cardiovascular disease (CVD), overweight and obesity are also directly or indirectly implicated in the mounting epidemic of chronic kidney disease (CKD) and end-stage renal disease (ESRD) [5]. CKD is a recently introduced definition of renal disease that has been internationally accepted. It is based on simple biochemical tests including a creatinine-based estimate of the glomerular filtration rate (GFR). CKD is diagnosed when structural or functional abnormalities of the kidneys persist for more than 3 months and it is categorized into five stages of increasing severity [6]. Data derived from the National Health and Nutrition Examination Survey III (NHANES III) show that about 1 out of 10 adult Americans exhibit CKD. Estimates in Asia and Australia indicate that the problem is of the same magnitude in those continents. In Europe, several surveys have now been completed and these studies indicate that CKD is of concern also in the European Union countries [7]. CKD is a dangerous clinical condition for two reasons: because renal impairment may be a prelude to the development of ESRD (i.e., the disease stage where dialysis and transplantation are needed), and because it amplifies the risk for

Nutritional and Metabolic Bases of Cardiovascular Disease, 1st edition.
Edited by Mario Mancini, José M. Ordovas, Gabriele Riccardi,
Paolo Rubba and Pasquale Strazzullo. © 2011 Blackwell Publishing Ltd.

cardiovascular complications. Patients with stage 4/5 CKD have a death risk for cardiovascular complications that is two to four times higher than that of the coeval general population, and those with ESRD, a 100 times higher risk [8] which is largely independent of classical factors [9]. There is coherent, undisputable evidence that treatment can prevent or delay kidney disease progression and resulting cardiovascular complications, but this knowledge has rarely been translated into public health policies.

The vast majority of patients with CKD present a renal histology picture characterized by various degrees of intimal fibroplasia of medium and small size arterial vessels, arterial jalinosis, glomerular ischemia and obsolescence, focal glomerulosclerosis, interstitial fibrosis, and tubular atrophy. Although some features are more common in some conditions (i.e., intimal fibroplasia in hypertension, focal glomerulosclerosis in obesity, and mesangial expansion or Kimmelstiel-Wilson nodules in diabetic nephropathy), nephrosclerosis appears to be a common background in diseases that are presently responsible for the CKD epidemics, namely arterial hypertension, diabetes, and obesity. This review discusses the link between classical hypertensive renal disease (nephrosclerosis) in a broader context encompassing risk factors for hypertension and obesity-driven metabolic risk factors for CKD that frequently coexist with hypertension and that produce renal damage also independently of high blood pressure (BP). The main focus is on the multiple links existing between risk factors that compound the metabolic syndrome (here held as a pure prognostic risk factors cluster rather than as an etiological entity [10]) and CKD considering these risk factors in both an isolated and a combined manner. Diabetic nephropathy is exhaustively covered in the current literature [11,12] and thus is only occasionally touch upon in this review.

Obesity and CKD: BP and beyond

Observational studies now provide a solid knowledge base for the association of excess body weight and CKD. Well-conceived analyses based on the Kaiser Permanente clinical database adjusting for BP, diabetes, and other risk factors [13] demonstrated that overweight persons have a 72% escess

risk for ESRD. The risk for ESRD is progressively higher at increasing body mass index (BMI) levels, and in extremely obese individuals, such risk is five times higher than in persons with normal body mass. Similar associations were reported in a study in Japan [14] and in a Swedish nationwide, population-based, case-control study [15]. Thus, there is a strong link between obesity and CKD and ESRD, and this link is incompletely accounted for by hypertension and type 2 diabetes. Visceral fat, insulin resistance, and inflammation are nicely inter correlated in cross-sectional studies in CKD patients [16]. However, until now there is no cohort or intervention study testing whether the association between waist circumference or waist/hip ratio and CKD or ESRD underlies a causal connection.

Clinical Epidemiology of Metabolic Syndrome Components and CKD

The separate and combined relationship between the metabolic syndrome components and CKD has been only sparsely investigated. In a survey in non-diabetic native Americans (The Inter-Tribal Heart Project), the metabolic syndrome was associated with a twofold increased prevalence of microalbuminuria [17]. In NHANES III analyses adjusting for age, race, ethnicity, sex, anti-inflammatory drug use, education, physical inactivity, smoking and BMI, the independent excess risk for CKD of hypertension, low HDL Cholesterol, hypertriglyceridemia, fasting hyperglicemia and large waist circumference ranged from 16% (serum glucose > 110 mg/dl) to 239% (BP >130/85 mmHg) [18]. However the combined effect of these risk factors was less than additive (Figure 43.1) suggesting that the pathways whereby these risk factors are conducive to CKD overlap to an important extent. Although the cross-sectional design of NHANES III study by Chen [18] does not allow making inferences about causality, this is the first study suggesting that at population level even mildly elevated BP (>130/85 mm Hg) or mild hyperglycemia may portend an increased risk for CKD and microalbuminuria. Furthermore, NHANES III confirms previous observations in the Modification Diet Renal Disease (MDRD) cohort indicating that low HDL-C levels predict faster CKD progression [19]. On the other hand, both high serum triglyceride and low

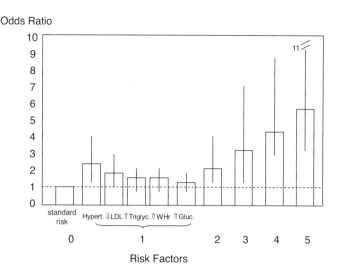

Odds Ratio

Risk Factors

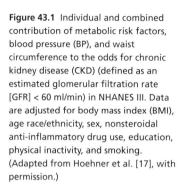

Figure 43.1 Individual and combined contribution of metabolic risk factors, blood pressure (BP), and waist circumference to the odds for chronic kidney disease (CKD) (defined as an estimated glomerular filtration rate [GFR] < 60 ml/min) in NHANES III. Data are adjusted for body mass index (BMI), age race/ethnicity, sex, nonsteroidal anti-inflammatory drug use, education, physical inactivity, and smoking. (Adapted from Hoehner et al. [17], with permission.)

HDL-C levels predicted an increased risk for renal dysfunction in a community study (the Atherosclerosis Risk in Communities study [ARIC]) in people 54–64 years of age [20]. Observational findings in these studies implicating dyslipidemia in CKD are corroborated by a large combined analysis of three major pravastatin trials [21] and by a secondary analysis of an atorvastatin-based trial [22], indicating that lipid lowering may help to preserve glomerular filtration rate in patients with coronary heart disease. Importantly, in line with experimental data in animal models, the NHANES III study by Chen et al. [18] also suggested that visceral fat, as defined on the basis of a larger than normal waist circumference, is implicated in chronic kidney disease.

Very limited information based on follow-up or longitudinal studies is available at this time. In the above-mentioned ARIC study, the multivariable adjusted odds ratio (OR) of developing CKD over a 9-year follow-up period in patients with the metabolic syndrome was 1.43 [23]. After adjusting for the subsequent development of diabetes and hypertension, metabolic syndrome entailed a 24% excess risk for incident CKD. Insulin resistance and hyperinsulinemia in the absence of diabetes were associated with CKD in another NHANES III cross-sectional analysis [23]. Collectively, these data suggest that renal dysfunction may start independently of hypertension or diabetes in patients harboring risk factors that are also components of the metabolic syndrome and supports the contention that, hypertension and diabetes apart, also other metabolic risk factors may underlie the current CKD epidemics.

Redefining the Problem of Hypertensive Nephropathy as a Cause of CKD and ESRD

As previously alluded to, nephrosclerosis is a common histologic picture in hypertension, diabetes, hypercholesterolemia, and obesity. Renal registries data point to hypertensive nephrosclerosis as to the main factor explaining the expansion of the dialysis population of the last few decades. However, knowledge supporting a cause-and-effect relationship between hypertension and the ascendancy of ESRD is flimsy, particularly in whites [24]. The definition of hypertensive nephrosclerosis does not take into proper account the fact that risk factors for hypertension and CKD (such as obesity and diabetes) may cause nephrosclerosis by BP dependent and independent mechanisms. Over 50% of hypertensive patients are obese and vice versa, and the risk for diabetes in morbidly obese individuals is seven times higher than in normal weight subjects [25]. Studies published so far do not allow discriminating the independent effect of hypertension on kidney structure and function from those of obesity and diabetes. As previously mentioned, features commonly observed in classical nephrosclerosis are also frequently seen in these two diseases. On the other hand, glomerulomegaly and focal glomerulosclerosis are currently considered features peculiar to nephropathy associated with obesity [26]. However, information on renal histopathology in the obese has been mainly derived from studies in case series with an over-representation of proteinuric patients [27]. Intriguingly, at comparable levels of proteinuria, obese patients display less severe podocyte damage and progress at a slower pace than patients with the idiopathic form of focal glomerulosclerosis (FGS) [28]. Most likely, glomerulomegaly and FGS in the obese with proteinuria underlie altered renal microcirculatory control eventuating in high glomerular flow and hyperfiltration (see below). These alterations occur at an early stage in obesity [29] and the contention that glomerulomegaly is a precocious renal alteration in the obese is also supported by the finding that obese kidney donors (i.e., subjects with minimal or no clinical evidence of renal dysfunction) display a glomerular surface area higher than that in well-matched non-obese donors [30].

Although knowledge on the quantitative relationship between risk factors implicated in kidney damage and ESRD is still limited, evidence derived from clinical series in patients with immunoglobulin A (IgA) nephropathy [31], renal agenesis [32], or nephrectomy [33], or in recipients of kidneys harvested from overweight or obese donors [34] supports the hypothesis that obesity is an important factor in the progression and perhaps even in the initiation of CKD. Indeed in all of the above-mentioned studies, a higher BMI (including a higher BMI in kidney donors) portended a relatively faster renal function loss.

Why and How Metabolic Factors and Obesity Damage the Kidney?

Inflammation in Overweight, Obesity, and Hypertension

Metabolic and immune pathways evolved in an interdependent manner and in part share the same cellular mechanism(s) [35]. Stimulation of the immune system activates metabolic pathways that mobilize stored body fuels and in parallel suppresses pathways conducive to energy storage, such

as the insulin signaling pathway [36]. This adaptive response serves to provide the energy input required to mount and sustain the inflammatory response. Starvation suppresses the immune system, while overfeeding and fat excess have an opposite influence on this system. Tumor necrosis factor-α (TNF-α) was the first biochemical link discovered between the adipose tissue and immune mechanisms/inflammation. Fat cells express a large series of inflammatory genes involved in adaptive and innate immunity. These include leptin, a hormone central to immunosuppression associated with starvation, and a large repertoire of "adipokines" (adiponectin, resistin, visfatin, and other cytokines), which contribute to the regulation of insulin sensitivity and the innate immune response [37,38]. The macrophage, a prototypical innate-immunity cell, has similarities with the adipocyte because it expresses gene products typical of the adipocyte, such as the cytoplasmic fatty acid—binding protein adipocyte lipid—binding protein 2 (aP2) and peroxisome proliferator-activated receptor-γ (PPARγ) [39]. Macrophages have large lipid-storage capabilities. On the other hand, preadipocytes may differentiate into fully functional macrophages [40]. It is important to note that in obese patients these two cell types, the macrophage and the adipocyte, co-localize in the adipose tissue [41] forming an integrated system integrating the innate immune response and metabolic regulation. The causal importance of fat mass, particularly visceral fat mass, in driving systemic inflammation is demonstrated by a variety of intervention studies of weight loss in obese patients. In a meta-analysis including medical and surgical interventions currently applied to induce weight loss [42], reduction in body weight was consistently associated with a decline in C-reactive protein (CRP) level across a wide range of weight loss. Importantly, also hypertension per se is associated with inflammation. Plasma interleukin-6 (IL-6) is directly related with BP in apparently healthy men [43]. Essential hypertensives show a propensity at mounting amplified inflammatory responses to hypertensive stimuli like angiotensin II [44]. Angiotensin II, through nuclear factor-κB (NF-κB), activates the major cytokine cascade, including TNF-α, IL-6, and monocyte chemoattractant protein (MCP-1) [45,46]. Increased vascular superoxide anion production and altered vascular relaxation are hallmarks of angiotensin II induced hypertension [47]. The association between inflammation and cardiovascular damage in experimental models and in humans seems to be causal in nature, because a variety of studies with ACE inhibitors or angiotensin II type-1 (AT1) receptor blockers demonstrated that these drugs improve target organ damage and reduce the plasma levels of a variety of inflammation markers as well [48].

Inflammation and CKD

Inflammation appears associated with metabolic risk factors and obesity not only in patients with atherosclerosis but also in patients with CKD [49,50], and it is well known that patients with atherosclerotic complications are at a higher risk of CKD and vice versa. That inflammation driven by metabolic factors be implicated in renal damage is nicely suggested by a recent study showing that low-density lipoprotein (LDL) receptor gene and other genes regulating lipid metabolism (fatty acid binding protein-3 and sterol regulatory element binding protein) as well as inflammatory genes (TNF-α and its receptors, IL-6 signal transducer, and interferon-γ) and genes implicated in insulin resistance (glucose transporter-1 and vascular endothelial growth factor) are overexpressed in glomeruli of patients with obesity-related nephropathy [51]. Although investigations on the link between adipokines and kidney damage have been started only in recent years, there is mounting evidence that lipid accumulation and alterations in fat cells cytokines can translate into inflammatory changes in the kidney.

Lipids and Kidney Damage

A parallelism between atherosclerosis and glomerulosclerosis was suggested about 20 years ago by Diamond who envisaged the foam cell, the lipid overloaded macrophage, as the pivotal factor both in atherosclerosis and in glomerulosclerosis [52]. The proinflammatory and toxic effects of lipids on the kidney are summarized in Figure 43.2. Free fatty acids (FFAs) accumulation increases the synthesis of triglycerides and very LDLs (VLDLs), which gives rise to atherogenic LDL and oxidized LDL in the liver. Hyperinsulinemia and hyperglycemia [53] induce organ damage by a variety of mechanisms including protein kinase C activation, oxidative stress, NF-κB activation, and other mechanisms eventuating in inflammation, apoptosis, and cell necrosis [54,55]. The transcription of many lipogenic genes is controlled by sterol-regulator element-binding proteins (SREBPs). SREBP-1 regulates fatty acid

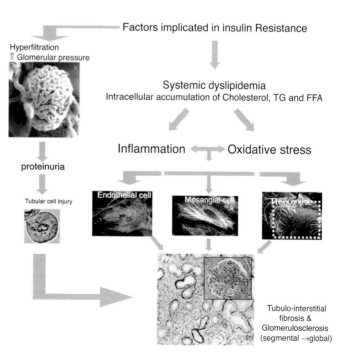

Figure 43.2 Hypothetic mechanisms whereby metabolic factors cause renal damage. Isolated dyslipidemia may directly start the pathogenetic chain leading to tubulointerstitial damage and glomerulosclerosis. Insulin resistance is a multifactorial phenotype which may be generated by altered major cytokines and adipokines profile (i.e., high IL-6, TNF-α, and MCP-1, low adiponectin, and high resistin). Intracellular accumulation of triglycerides may impair insulin sensitivity. High angiotensin and leptin resistance can contribute to reduce insulin sensitivity. High leptin may per se engender kidney damage. Mechanisms summarized in the figure are described in more detail in the main text.

synthesis, whereas SREBP-2 is mainly involved in the control of cholesterol synthesis [56]. PPARs are present in virtually all organ systems, including the kidney [57]. When stimulated, these receptors promote adipogenesis and insulin sensitivity. Thiazolidinediones, a class of drugs with PPARγ agonist property, are currently used to treat insulin resistance in type 2 diabetics. As discussed below, both alterations in SERBP and in PPAR appear relevant to organ damage in experimental models. High-fat feeding in the obesity-prone mice triggers obesity, hyperglycemia, and hyperinsulinemia [58]. These mice show renal triglyceride and cholesterol accumulation in glomerular and tubule-interstitial cells as well as overexpression of SREBP-1 and SREBP-2 proteins, PAI-1, type IV collagen, and fibronectin and develop glomerulosclerosis and proteinuria [53,58]. FFA accumulation is responsible endothelial dysfunction in a well-established model of visceral obesity as the Zucker rat [59].

VLDL, intermediate-density lipoprotein (IDL), and LDL all enhance IL-6, TNF-α, and transforming growth factor-β synthesis and induce mesangial cell proliferation [60]. Oxidized LDL stimulates extracellular matrix and MCP-1 and PAI-1 synthesis in these same cells [61]. IGF-I determines triglyceride accumulation in mesangial cells, which transform into foam cells and such a transformation impairs their ability to phagocyte and migrate [62]. Importantly, up-regulation of mesangial cell VLDL receptors (and hence enhanced triglyceride entry) and down-regulation of triglyceride efflux from mesangial cells may be triggered by a reduction in PPARδ [63]. In proteinuric nephropathies, and in full-blown nephrotic syndrome, albumin-saturated FFAs appear causally implicated in tubulointerstitial inflammation [64]. Overall, these studies support a role of lipotoxicity in renal damage in dyslipidemia and in obesity.

Classical Cytokines

Besides T cells and macrophages, IL-6 is ubiquitously represented in fat cells, being well expressed in both adipocytes and macrophages in visceral and peripheral adipose tissue. This cytokine is an autacoid—it acts locally, in proximity of the site where it is synthesized—and a hormone because it acts at distance where it exerts a variety of effects including amplification of the inflammatory pro-

cess, stimulation of energy mobilization, hyperthermia, and other effects including insulin resistance [65,66]. Circulating IL-6 is much increased in obese subjects and it predicts incident type 2 diabetes independently of other risk factors [67]. Interestingly, IL-6 increases TGF-β1 (TGF-β1) receptor activity, and by this action, it may favor fibrosis. IL-6 is a marker of progressive renal function loss in patients with IgA nephropathy [68] and may be involved in renal damage in obesity, a condition characterized by high circulating levels of this cytokine.

Like IL-6, TNF-α is abundantly synthesized by macrophages in adipose tissue where it modulates insulin sensitivity by multiple mechanisms such as inactivation of insulin receptor and insulin receptor substrate-1, lipolysis, and lipogenesis [36]. Furthermore TNF-α blunts secretion of an important insulin sensitizer-like adiponectin [69]. TNF-α has been shown to mediate inflammation and scarring in experimental crescentic glomerulonephritis [70], in acute renal failure in endotoxemia [71], and in renal fibrosis [72]. Similarly to IL-6, TNF-α may exert toxic effects on virtually all renal cells species including endothelial, mesangial, and epithelial cells. However, it should be emphasized that until now there is no study specifically testing the involvement of this cytokine or of IL-6 in the nephropathy associated with metabolic syndrome or with obesity in man.

Adipokines

Besides IL-6 and TNF-α, the adipose tissue makes up a variety of substances that may be implicated in kidney damage including plasminogen activator inhibitor-1 (PAI-1) and MCP-1. These factors may produce tissue damage by a direct proinflammatory mechanism or may act because implicated in insulin resistance [73].

Leptin is a fundamental adipose tissue hormone that modulates appetite and energy expenditure via pathways that modulate neuropeptide Y in the hypothalamus. Circulating levels of leptin are strictly proportional to fat mass, but obese subjects are resistant to the anorexigen effect of leptin [74]. Receptors for leptin are well expressed in the kidney [75]. In mesangial cell cultures of obese mice lacking the functional full-length leptin receptor (Ob-Rb), this adipokine enhances glucose uptake and augments TGF-β2 expressions, which eventually increases collagen production [76]. In the rat, leptin stimulates TGF-β1 mRNA expression in glomerular endothelial cells and is able to produce glomerulosclerosis and proteinuria by BP independent mechanisms [77]. This adipokine is implicated in hypertension and sodium retention secondary to obesity because it potently activates the sympathetic system, including sympathetic activity in the kidney [78]. Leptin is currently considered as a pro-inflammatory factor and a pro-oxidant implicated in endothelial dysfunction and atherosclerosis. Accordingly, the obese leptin-deficient mouse is protected from atherosclerosis despite the presence of other risk factors [79]. Hence, endothelial dysfunction represents an additional mechanism whereby this adipokine may induce renal damage. Collectively these observations suggest that, also independently of hypertension, leptin may be involved in glomerulosclerosis in obese patients.

Adiponectin is an adipose tissue cytokine with well characterized insulin-sensitizing, anti-inflammatory, and anti-atherogenic properties. Adiponectin is inversely associated with body weight, with serum triglyceride, and LDL-C levels and with various inflammation biomarkers. Plasma adiponectin concentration increases after weight loss [80,81]. Atherogenic changes characterize the adiponectin-deficient transgenic mice [83]. Hypoadiponectinemia is associated with endothelial dysfunction and with coronary events in patients with cardiac disease [82] or with ESRD [83]. Despite the evidence that adiponectin is a vasculoprotective factor is overwhelming, it remains much debated whether this adipokine is cardiovasculoprotective or not in patients with CKD and ESRD [84]. Disparate results in the current literature mainly reflect differences in the study populations, background risk factors, and degree of statistical adjustment [84]. Very recent experimental studies strongly implicate low adiponectin in the pathogenesis of renal disease in obesity. Albuminuria correlates inversely with plasma adiponectin in obese patients [85] and the adiponectin-knockout mouse exhibits increased albuminuria and fusion of podocyte foot processes [85]. In cultured podocytes, adiponectin increases the activity of adenosine monophosphate (AMP)-activated protein kinase (AMPK), and both adiponectin and AMPK activation reduce podocyte permeability to albumin and podocyte

dysfunction by decreasing oxidative stress. Furthermore, the adiponectin-deficient mouse treated with adiponectin shows normalization of albuminuria, improvement of podocyte foot process effacement, increased glomerular AMPK activation, and reduced urinary and glomerular markers of oxidant stress [85]. These intriguing results in a transgenic model and parallel observations in obese subjects suggest that adiponectin may prevent albuminuria, possibly by reducing oxidant stress in podocytes.

Renal Hemodynamic Factors, Glomerular Hypertension and the Renin-Angiotensin System

Substantial evidence has been accrued that the renin-angiotensin system and aldosterone are up-regulated in obesity [86]. This phenomenon is attributable to sympathetic over activity (see above) and/or to hyperinsulinemia and/or to enhanced synthesis of angiotensinogen in visceral fat. Both angiotensinogen and AT1 receptor mRNA are over-expressed in visceral adipose tissue as compared subcutaneous adipose tissue [87]. Weight loss in obese women is accompanied by a decrease in plasma angiotensinogen which is highly correlated with waist circumference reduction [88].The renin-angiotensin system is of paramount importance in renal disease generation and progression in obesity because of its interference with glomerular hemodynamics (see below) and with inflammatory mechanisms. In a transgenic model of obesity, angiotensin II blockade significantly reduces TNF-α, MCP-1, and oxidative stress and prompts increases in adiponectin levels [89]. Thus, inflammation and derangement in adipokines levels may be additional mechanisms whereby the renin angiotensin system is conducive to renal damage in obese persons.

As previously alluded to, hyperfiltration is commonly found in obese persons. Due to high sympathetic activity, high levels of angiotensin II, and hyperinsulinemia, obese persons display enhanced sodium reabsorption in the proximal tubule and are unable to rapidly increase sodium excretion [29]. Enhanced proximal salt reabsorption determines a reduced delivery of sodium to the macula densa and, therefore, promotes afferent vasodilatation and enhanced renin synthesis. As a result of high local angiotensin II levels, the efferent arteriole is constricted in the obese. Glomerulomegaly and focal glomerulosclerosis represent the anatomical counterparts of glomerular hyperfiltration-hypertension. Brenner theory linking low nephron number at birth with reduced intrauterine growth [90] provides an explanation for why some individuals (those with a reduced nephron number) appear particular prone at developing progressive renal damage later in life when overweight and obesity and other risk factors supervene. Severe obesity may alter renal hemodynamics also by mechanical compression of renal vein [91]. Furthermore, morbidly obese patients frequently display sleep apnea, a sleep disorder engendering systemic and pulmonary hypertension [92]. Right ventricular overload in the obese with sleep apnea [93] may per se trigger and/or amplify venous hypertension in the kidney. Both left ventricular dysfunction (via reduced cardiac output) and right ventricular dysfunction (via increased venous pressure) may eventually impair renal perfusion thereby further aggravating CKD in the obese.

Prevention and Treatment of CKD Secondary to Metabolic Factors and Hypertension

Metabolic risk factors and body weight excess—obesity—independently contribute to nephrosclerosis, the most common histology pattern seen in patients with CKD. Lipotoxicity, inflammation, and disturbances in the control of renal microcirculation all concur in engendering kidney damage in this condition, but the precise causal involvement of these factors is still unknown. Interventions aimed at preventing overweight and obesity are fundamental for decreasing the burden of hormonal, inflammatory and hemodynamic factors implicated in the epidemics of cardiac and renal diseases. A meta-analysis has shown that regardless of how it is achieved (by bariatric surgery, behavioral interventions, or drug treatment), weight loss ameliorates the metabolic profile and reduces the inflammatory burden in obese patients [42]. However, the long-term effects of bariatric surgery are still unknown. Angiotensin antagonists have an almost ideal pharmacological profile for prevention and treatment of CKD progression in obesity but this contention is not supported by specific trials in this population. Thiazolidinediones, a class of PPARγ agonists, improve insulin sensitivity and hyperglycemia, but a higher risk of progression toward heart failure has been reported in patients treated with rosiglitazone [94]. Pravastatin and atorvastatin showed cardiovascular and nephroprotective actions [21,22] in CKD patients in secondary analyses performed in databases of large cardiovascular trials (see Chapter 23) and should be considered a useful therapeutic option in patients with metabolic syndrome, obesity, and CKD.

Selected References

9. Zoccali C. Traditional and emerging cardiovascular and renal risk factors: an epidemiologic perspective. Kidney Int 2006;70:26–33.

13. Hsu CY, McCulloch CE, Iribarren C, et al. Body mass index and risk for end-stage renal disease. Ann Intern Med 2006;144:21–8.

15. Ejerblad E, Fored CM, Lindblad P, et al. Obesity and risk for chronic renal failure. J Am Soc Nephrol 2006;17:1695–1702.

38. Zoccali C, Mallamaci F, Tripepi G. Adipose tissue as a source of inflammatory cytokines in health and disease: focus on end-stage renal disease. Kidney Int Suppl 2003;S65–8.

84. Zoccali C, Mallamaci F. Adiponectin and renal disease progression: another epidemiologic conundrum? Kidney Int 2007;71:1195–7.

CHAPTER 44

Current Experience and Future Perspectives for Worldwide Reduction of Dietary Salt Intake

Naomi M. Marrero[1], Feng J. He[2], & Graham A. MacGregor[2]
[1]St. George's, University of London, London, UK
[2]Barts and The London School of Medicine & Dentistry, Queen Mary University of London, London, UK

Introduction

Cardiovascular disease (CVD) (strokes, heart attacks, and heart failure) is the largest cause of death and disability in the world. There are three major causes of CVD: raised blood pressure, raised cholesterol, and cigarette smoking. However, raised blood pressure is the single most important cause, accounting for 62% of stroke and 49% of coronary heart disease worldwide [1]. Importantly, the risk of CVD is not confined to those with raised blood pressure, but throughout the range, starting at a systolic pressure of 115 mm Hg [2]. This means that the majority of the global adult population is at risk from their blood pressure.

There is much evidence from epidemiologic [3], migration [4], intervention [5], treatment [6], genetic [7], and animal studies [8,9] that dietary salt (sodium chloride) plays an important role in regulating blood pressure, and our current high salt intake is largely responsible for the rise in blood pressure with age. Many randomized trials have demonstrated that a modest reduction in salt intake lowers blood pressure significantly in both hypertensive and normotensive individuals [6,10–13]. Population-based intervention studies have shown that a reduction in population salt intake lowers blood pressure in the population [5,14]. A de-

crease in population blood pressure even by a small amount would have a significant impact in reducing CVD. Indeed, a recent meta-analysis of 12 prospective cohort studies with over 15,000 participants who were followed up for between 3.5–19 years, showed that a 5 g/day increase in salt intake was associated with a 17% increase in CVD risk [15]. Similarly, outcome trials have demonstrated that a reduction in salt lowers CVD risk. A follow-up study of individuals with prehypertension who took part in two large randomized trials, the Trial of Hypertension Prevention (TOHP) I and II, demonstrated that a 25%–30% reduction in salt intake from approximately 10 g/day caused a 25% decrease in cardiovascular events [16].

Currently, salt intake is unnecessarily high in many countries around the world. Several countries, such as the United Kingdom and Finland, have successfully carried out salt-reduction programs and salt intake has fallen in these countries. In this chapter, we provide an update on the current experience of worldwide salt reduction programs and future perspectives for worldwide reduction of dietary salt intake.

Salt Intake around the World

Adults

In most regions of the world, salt intake far exceeds the World Health Organization (WHO) recommendation of 5 g/day. Several methods have been

Nutritional and Metabolic Bases of Cardiovascular Disease, 1st edition.
Edited by Mario Mancini, José M. Ordovas, Gabriele Riccardi, Paolo Rubba and Pasquale Strazzullo. © 2011 Blackwell Publishing Ltd.

used to estimate dietary salt intake, such as food diaries [14], food frequency questionnaire [17], dietary recall [18], spot urinary sodium/creatinine ratio [19], overnight urinary sodium [20], and 24-hour urinary sodium excretion [3]. However, it has been shown that most of these methods are unreliable and the most accurate method is to measure urinary sodium from complete 24-hour urine collection. The INTERSALT (International Study on Salt and Blood Pressure) study [3] collected 24-hour urine samples from 10,079 individuals in 52 adult population groups across 32 countries, providing the largest dataset on dietary salt intake patterns around the world. Of the 52 centers, 48 (92%) had an average salt intake that was above the WHO recommendation, and only 4 centers from isolated populations had salt intake below the recommended level. The mean salt intake for the 48 centers ranged from 6.0 g/day in the Black Goodman population in the United States to 14 g/day in Tianjin, China. The INTERSALT study was done more than 20 years ago. Since then, salt intake is likely to have increased, particularly in many developed countries, due to the increasing consumption of processed foods that are generally very high in salt.

The INTERMAP study (International Study of Macronutrients and Micronutrients and blood pressure) [21] studied diverse populations in four countries (China, Japan, United Kingdom, and United States) in the late 1990s. Although salt intake was higher in Asian than Western countries, salt intake in all countries was well above the WHO-recommended level, as illustrated in Table 44.1.

In a few countries, because of the successful public health campaign, salt intake has decreased over recent years. For example, in Finland, salt intake fell from an average of approximately 12 g/day in 1979 to less than 9 g/day in 2002 as measured by 24-hour urinary sodium [22]. In the United Kingdom, the average salt intake was 9.5 g/day in 2001 [23] and reduced to 8.6 g/day in 2008 [24].

Children

Most of the studies examining salt intake in population groups have been done in adults and there is a considerable lack of data on salt intake in children. In the 1980s, a number of small studies in Europe [25–27], the United States [28,29], and China [30] collected 24-hour urine (from one single 24-hour urine collection in most studies to seven collections) from children and adolescents and measured urinary sodium. These studies showed that salt intake varied with age and was generally high in children, for example, 3.8 g/day for 4- to 6-year-old British boys and girls [25], 8.4 g/day for 8- to 9-year-old Hungarian boys [26], 10.0 g/day for 12- to 16-year-old rural Chinese boys and girls [30]. These studies were done at a time when the consumption of processed foods by young people was not high. Since then, salt intake in children in developed countries is likely to have increased due to the dramatic changes in dietary habits, such as an increasing consumption of processed, takeaway, restaurant, and fast foods. Recently, Schreuder et al. reported 24-hour urinary sodium data from a group of children aged 7 to 8 years in Amsterdam and showed that 24-hour urinary sodium increased by more than 50% over a 10-year period, from 65 mmol/24-hour (3.7 g of salt) in 1993–1995 to 101 mmol/24-hour (5.8 g of salt) in 2003–2005 [31]. If these results were expressed as for an adult with a 70-kg body weight, salt intake would be 12 g/day in 1993–1995

Table 44.1 Salt intake (mean ±SD) as measured by 24-hour urinary sodium in four countries.

Country	Salt intake in men		Salt intake in women	
	gram/day	% of WHO recommendation	gram/day	% of WHO recommendation
China	14.1 ± 6.1	280	12.1 ± 5.2	240
Japan	12.1 ± 3.3	240	10.7 ± 3.1	215
United Kingdom	9.3 ± 3.0	185	7.3 ± 2.3	145
United States	10.5 ± 3.6	210	8.2 ± 2.8	165

Adapted from Zhou et al. [21].

and increased to 16 g/day by 2003–2005. Although this group of children is not a random sample of the general pediatric population, it is likely that children's salt intake in most developed countries has followed a similar trend.

Major Sources of Salt Intake

In many countries, particularly developed countries, dietary habits have changed considerably over the past 50 years, and in both adults and children, there have been major shifts in eating behavior. For example, in the United States, the amount of food that children consumed from restaurants and fast-food outlets increased by approximately 300% between 1977 and 1996 [32]. Similar trends have been shown in adults [33]. Additionally, with individuals becoming more time pressured, less time is spent on cooking and more processed, snack and convenience foods are being consumed. Therefore, it will come as no surprise that surveys have shown that in developed countries, such as the United States, an increasing proportion of household food income is spent on food prepared away from the home [34]. Processed, restaurant and fast foods are very high in salt and contribute to 75%–85% of salt intake [35]. For example, in the United Kingdom, cereals and cereal products including bread, breakfast cereals, biscuits and cakes, meat and meat products, soups, pickles, sauces, and baked beans are the main contributors to salt intake [23].

In some developing countries, there has also been an increase in the consumption of processed foods, an increase in the number of fast-food outlets, and an increase in the amount of money spent on food eaten away from the home over recent years. However, for the majority of the world's developing population, most of the salt consumed comes from salt used to pickle foods, salt added during cooking and from sauces or seasonings. For example, in rural China about 75% of salt intake comes from salt added during cooking, with soy sauce providing a further 8% [36].

Current Salt Intake Recommendations

Salt intake recommendations vary considerably between countries. In many African countries, for example, there are no dietary salt recommendations.

In other countries such as Greece and Hungary, recommendations are very vague and general, i.e. avoid foods that contain a lot of salt [36]. In most developed countries, however, there are very specific recommendations. In the UK [37], USA, Australia, Canada, Ireland, New Zealand [36] and the Netherlands [38], it is recommended that the general adult population consume no more than 6 g/day of salt. In Portugal the recommendation is to consume no more than 5 g/day of salt [36]. The WHO has also reviewed all of the evidence and recommended that salt intake around the world should be reduced to 5 g/day or less [39].

Most of the recommendations that have been set are well below the average salt consumption of the population but are far higher than the physiological requirement of approximately 0.25 g/day for an adult. The recommendations reflect what is achievable and not what is optimal. Both epidemiologic studies and randomized trials have demonstrated a dose response relationship between salt intake and blood pressure. Well-controlled randomized trials have clearly shown that a reduction in salt intake from the current levels of 9–12 g/day to the recommended levels of 5–6 g/day lowers blood pressure significantly in both hypertensive and normotensive individuals; however, a further reduction to 3–4 g/day has an additional effect [12,13,40].Moreover, the association between blood pressure and CVD risk is continuous, meaning the lower the blood pressure, the lower the risk of CVD [41]. In view of these, it is clear that the current public health recommendations to reduce salt intake to 5–6 g/day will have a major effect on blood pressure and CVD but are not ideal. A further reduction to 3 g/day will have a much greater effect and should, therefore, become the long-term target for population salt intake worldwide.

For children, only a few countries have set a target level of salt intake. For example, in the United Kingdom, the Scientific Advisory Committee on Nutrition (SACN) recognized that health benefits would be gained from a reduction in average salt consumption in children. In 2003, SACN recommended target salt levels for infants and children on a sliding scale by age (Table 44.2). Like those in adults, these targets do not represent an optimal or ideal level of salt consumption but they represent achievable population goals [37].

Table 44.2 SACN recommendations on salt intake for children.

Age	Target average salt intake (g/day)
0–6 months	<1
7–12 months	1
1–3 years	2
4–6 years	3
7–10 years	5
11–14 years	6

Worldwide Actions Occurring on Salt

Currently there is considerable variation in the amount of action being taken to reduce salt intake in populations around the world. Many, but not all, countries have produced recommendations about how far salt intake should be reduced. However, the recommendations alone without any supporting salt reduction activities will have no impact at all on the amount of salt consumed. For example, since the 1980s, it has been advised that salt intake should be reduced to 6 g/day in the United States; however, despite these recommendations the use of salt actually increased by approximately 55% per person from the mid-1980s to the late 1990s [42].

Through its regional directorates, the WHO is starting salt-reduction strategies [36]. The European Union is also following and eleven countries have signed up to make a 16% reduction in salt intake over 4 years [43]. Several countries, such as Finland and the United Kingdom, have already successfully carried out salt reduction programs. However, many other countries, particularly developing countries where approximately 80% of global blood pressure–related disease burden occurs [44], have not even developed a salt reduction strategy. It is important that each country in the world determines what its salt intake is and what the major sources of salt are in the diet, and then implements a strategic approach to lowering salt intake in the population to the target level.

United Kingdom

The United Kingdom is one of the countries leading the way and setting the example for other countries

in salt reduction strategies. In 1994, an independent advisory panel, COMA (the Committee on Medical Aspects of Food and Nutrition Policy), appointed by the government reviewed all of the evidence and recommended that salt intake in adults should be reduced to 6 g/day or less [45]. However, the recommendations on salt were rejected as some food companies had threatened to withdraw funding from the political party in power. As a result of the rejection of the salt reduction recommendations by the Chief Medical Officer with no reasons given [46], 22 scientific experts on salt and BP in the UK set up an action group, Consensus Action on Salt and Health, known as CASH [47,48]. The aims of CASH are:

1 To ensure the body of evidence from the scientific community about the dangers of excessive salt consumption becomes translated into policy by the Government and relevant professional organizations.

2 To reach a consensus with the food manufacturers and suppliers that there is strong evidence that salt is a major cause of high blood pressure and has other adverse health effects, thereby persuading food processors and suppliers to universally and gradually reduce the salt content of processed foods.

3 To educate the public in becoming more salt aware in terms of understanding the impact of salt on their health, checking labels when shopping and avoiding products with high levels of salt [47].

Since CASH was set up in 1996, it has been very successful in raising the awareness of the importance of salt and, within a few years, persuaded the U.K. Department of Health to change its stance on salt, finally resulting in the new Chief Medical Officer endorsing the original recommendations of the COMA report to reduce salt intake to less than 6 gram/day in adults. Before this endorsement, CASH had already persuaded a major supermarket and several food companies to reduce the amount of salt they added to their foods by 10%–15%, an amount that can not be detected by the human salt taste receptors [49]. Two years later, CASH ensured that the newly setup U.K. Food Standards Agency took on the task of reducing salt intake in the United Kingdom, and their independent SACN again confirmed that there was a very strong scientific case to reduce salt intake in the whole population [37].

The UK Strategy: a Model for Other Countries

The first step for all countries who want to carry out a salt reduction policy is to measure or estimate salt intake. For example, in the United Kingdom, a random sample of the adult population collected 24-hour urine samples and this showed that the average 24-hour urinary sodium excretion was 9.5 g/day of salt in 2001 [23]. From knowledge of dietary intake in the United Kingdom, it was then possible to roughly calculate what proportion of this salt intake is added by the consumer, that is, in the form of added salt, stock cubes, sauces, pickles, etc., and how much is contributed by the food industry as a whole, that is, where the consumer has no control over the amount of salt, for example, in supermarkets, fast food, restaurants, takeaways.

In the United Kingdom, it was roughly estimated that 15% of the total 9.5 g of salt consumed (i.e., 1.4 g) was added either at the table or during cooking. Approximately 5% was naturally present in the food (i.e., 0.5 g), and the rest, 80% (i.e., 7.6 g), was not in the hands of the consumer and was added by the food industry either in processed, canteen, restaurant food, etc. From these figures it can then be worked out (Table 44.3) that if the target in a particular country is 6 g, which is the recommendation in the United Kingdom, the reduction in salt intake that is needed is from 9.5 to 6.0 g (i.e., 3.5 g), which is an approximate 40% reduction. This means that the public would have to reduce the amount of salt they add to foods themselves by 40% and the food industry would need to reduce the amount of salt added to all foods by 40%. It was also estimated in the United Kingdom that only 15% of food was eaten outside the home, such as restaurant, canteen, etc., and therefore the main target in the initial phase of salt reduction should be on foods that were bought in supermarkets. These foods, where salt was added, were split into more than 80 different categories. The Food Standards Agency set target levels for each food category that the food industry needed to achieve within a certain time period. The aim was to reduce the salt added to food by small amounts, that is, 10%–20%, which cannot be detected by human salt taste receptors and, furthermore, cause no technical or safety issues to the food in question. After a 1- to 2-year gap, a further 10%–20% reduction could be made and this could be followed by a further reduction after a further one to two years.

In addition to the efforts in reducing the salt content of processed foods, there has been a huge consumer awareness campaign including adverts on the television, in the tabloids, on buses, on posters and in magazines. The campaign has been run in three stages [50]. The first stage was to raise awareness that too much salt is bad for health. Stage 2 alerted adults to the fact that they should be consuming no more than 6 g of salt per day. The main messages of the final stage focused on the fact that 75% of salt consumed comes from processed foods and therefore consumers should check the labels and choose lower salt options. Several million pounds has been spent on this advertising campaign. Since the start of the campaign the Food Standards Agency has carried out research to track the progress of the campaign. It found that the number of people aware that they should be eating no more than 6 g salt per day rose from 3% to 34% in just 1 year [51]. Similarly, there had been a rise in the number of people making an effort to reduce their salt intake with 20 million people saying they were cutting down on the amount of salt they ate [51].

Table 44.3 United Kingdom strategy for reducing salt.

Source	Salt intake (g/day)	Reduction needed	Target intake (g/day)
Table/cooking (15%)	1.4	40% reduction	0.9
Natural (5%)	0.5	No reduction	0.5
Food industry (80%)	7.6	40% reduction	4.6
	Total: 9.5		Target: 6.0

Clear labeling of the salt content of food is essential so that consumers can see at a glance how much salt is in any food they purchase. A front of pack signpost labeling system [52] has been developed, which is being implemented by many supermarkets where there is a color-coding of green, amber, and red for low, medium, and high amounts of salt, fat, sugar, and calories, as well as the amount of salt per portion and per 100 g, and the recommended intake for an adult for the whole day. This type of label is much preferred by consumers to others as they can see at a glance whether a product has a little or a lot of salt. It has already been shown to have a dramatic effect on the purchase of foods, particularly when they are in the red category.

Success of the U.K. Salt-Reduction Strategy

The U.K. salt-reduction strategy started in 2003/2004 and has worked successfully on a voluntary basis with many processed foods bought in supermarkets containing 20%–30% less salt by 2008. For example, one of the major supermarkets in the United Kingdom announced in 2006 that over the past 5 years it had removed over 1,000 tons of salt from its own-label food products, stating that "the average weekly shop could now have 24% less salt than exactly the same basket of groceries did a year earlier" [53]. Since then, this announcement of salt reduction has been extended to many other products.

Additionally, many of the major brand manufacturers, such as Kellogg's, Heinz, and Unilever, have reduced the salt concentration of their foods. A number of caterers are also working towards the salt targets. For example, McDonalds has reduced the amount of salt in its products by between 14% and 75% and is continuing to make further reductions [54].

Looking at individual food categories the results are also very positive. There have been significant reductions across a broad range of product categories that included everything from bread and breakfast cereals to soups and meal sauces. For example, a survey revealed that the average salt level of ready meals on sale in U.K. supermarkets reduced by 45% between 2003 and 2007. In fact, in 2007 84% had already reached the Food Standards Agency's 2010 targets for salt content [55].

As a result of the successful salt reduction strategy, the adult daily salt intake in the United Kingdom has already fallen. A random sample of the population where 24-hour urines were collected showed that salt intake fell from an average of 9.5 g/day in 2001 to 8.6 g/day by May 2008 [24]. This may seem a small change, but it was on the back of a previously increasing salt intake and it marks the beginning of a reversal of an increasing trend that is occurring in most other countries with the greater consumption of processed food.

Salt intake will fall further as increasing reductions in salt added to food are being made by the food industry, particularly as new targets are have been set for over 80 categories of food. It is anticipated, with these new targets, that salt intake will reach the current recommendation of an average of 6 g/day by 2012 [56]. An important aspect of this policy is that it particularly focuses on the most disadvantaged in the community as the biggest reductions in salt added to food have been made in the cheapest foods as part of the policy. The amount of salt added to children's food is also being reduced. This means that the salt added to food is being reduced across the board, and therefore, people do not essentially need to change the foods they eat, their salt intake will fall without them necessarily being aware of it. At the same time, consumers who want to can avoid the most highly salted products and reduce their salt intake even further.

Having successfully shown that the amount of salt can be reduced in foods bought in supermarkets, this message is now being spread out to restaurants, takeaways, caterers, canteens, prisons, hospitals, and fast-food outlets.

Finland

In the late 1970s, Finland was one of the first countries to initiate a systematic approach to decrease salt intake in the population through mass media campaigns, co-operation with the food industry and implementing salt labeling legislation [42,57]. Since the 1980s, many food companies have reduced the sodium content of their food products by replacing conventional table salt with a sodium-reduced, potassium- and magnesium-enriched mineral salt known as Pansalt. Furthermore, in the early 1990s, the Ministry of Trade and Industry and the Ministry of Social Affairs and Health, set new salt labeling legislation for all the food categories which made a substantial contribution to the salt intake of the Finnish population. Foods that are high in salt are required to carry a "high salt content" warning and if a food product contains a low level of salt the product is allowed to display a low salt label. These different measures have resulted in a significant reduction in salt intake of the Finnish population, from an average of approximately 12 g/day in 1979 to less than 9 g/day in 2002 as measured by 24-hour urinary sodium [22]. Accompanying this reduction in salt intake there has been a reduction of over 10mmHg in both systolic and diastolic blood pressure and a corresponding decrease of 75%–80% in both stroke and coronary heart disease mortality [42]. Since both BMI and alcohol consumption have increased during this period, this can largely be explained by the reduction in salt intake. A reduction in fat intake and an increase in potassium intake via the use of reduced-sodium, potassium and magnesium-enriched salt, an increased consumption of fruit and vegetables, and a reduction in smoking rate in men have also contributed to the fall in CVD.

Other Countries

Following the success of the U.K. campaign group CASH, the World Action on Salt and Health (WASH) group was established in 2005 to encourage action on salt reduction worldwide [58]. The aim of the group is to improve the health of populations throughout the world by achieving a gradual reduction in salt intake. Like CASH, WASH works to reduce salt in the diet worldwide by exerting pressure on multinational food companies to reduce the salt content of their products. WASH is supported by more than 300 international members, who are mainly experts in hypertension. WASH members in each country are being encouraged to set up their own country division of WASH, to work together on a localized level to lower salt intake specifically in their own population. For example, in 2007 an Australian Division of World Action on Salt and Health (AWASH) was established. It has launched a national campaign to lower the salt intake of the Australian population to 6 g/day by 2012. The main objectives of the campaign known as Drop the Salt! are to lower salt in food by 25%, increase consumer awareness

about the benefits of a low-salt diet, and promote clear labeling of foods that makes the salt content immediately apparent to the consumers [59].

In Ireland, a nutrition committee of the Food Safety Authority of Ireland (FSAI) concluded, in 2005, that the scientific evidence supports a link between salt intake and raised blood pressure [60]. Subsequently the FSAI set the goal to reduce salt intake in the population from 10 g/day to 6 g/day. The strategic approach includes consumer awareness efforts, as well as action by the food industry to lower the salt content of their food products, where to-date substantial reductions have been made in the salt content of food.

In Canada the first Chair in Hypertension Prevention and Control was appointed in 2006. The Chair is supported by a number of health-related organizations as well as scientists. Together, they lobby the government and public food sector for policies to reduce the addition of salt to food [61]. The food industry is already lowering salt in foods. For example a number of whole grain bread products have had their salt levels reduced by 25%.

Many other countries are stepping up their activity. In the Netherlands the dietary guidelines were revised in 2006 stating that salt intake should be reduced to 6 g/day [38]. The Dutch Consumer Organization (Consumentenbond) has also initiated a number of activities to raise awareness about the harmful effect of too much salt on health. In addition, both the French Food Standards Agency (AFFSA) and the Swedish Food Standards Agency have now considered the evidence and have a program in place for reducing the salt content of food in both France and Sweden in a similar way as in the United Kingdom.

In the United States, there has been consistent advice to reduce salt intake to 6 g/day since the 1980s. For example, in January 2000, a large meeting was organized by the National Heart, Lung and Blood Institute in Washington where all of the evidence on salt was reconsidered. There was representation both from the food industry and Salt Institute. The conclusion of this meeting was that "Americans consume more sodium than they need and a population wide strategy of reducing salt in the food supply is an important public health strategy that can lower BP among populations" [62]. In 2007, The American Medical Association (AMA) published a report calling for a major reduction in the salt content of processed and restaurant foods [63]. The AMA also pressed the FDA (U.S. Food and Drug Administration) to cease the rule that allows salt and its component sodium to be treated as "generally recognized as safe." In a petition to the FDA in 2005, the Center for Science in the Public Interest (CSPI) called for tougher regulations on salt [64]. However, despite this, little action had been taken until recently. In January 2010, the National Salt Reduction Initiative (NSRI), a partnership of more than 40 cities, states and national health organizations, set out a strategy to reduce salt intake in the American population by 20% over 5 years and 40% over 10 years. To guide this reduction the NSRI has developed voluntary 2- and 4- year interim targets for cutting salt levels in different categories of packaged and restaurant foods [65]. Most recently the Institute of Medicine (IOM) released a report 'Strategies to Reduce Sodium Intake in the United States' [66]. The Report recommends that the FDA should set standards for the salt levels that food manufacturers, restaurants and food service companies can add to their products in the United States. Following IOM's report 16 food companies in the United States, including Kraft foods and HJ Heinz Co, have pledged to cut the amount of salt in some of their products.

Future Perspectives

Raised blood pressure is a global burden, and many individuals with high blood pressure do not actually know they have it. For example, a survey in England revealed that one-third of adults with high blood pressure were not aware they had the condition [67]. Additionally, because the risk of blood pressure on CVD starts at systolic pressure of 115 mm Hg, which is considered normal, a large proportion of the population are at high risk of CVD. This confirms that population-wide salt reduction initiatives to reduce blood pressure on a global basis are warranted. This will cause a downward shift in population blood pressure, preventing many cardiovascular events. It has also been demonstrated from cost-effectiveness analyses that reducing salt intake in developing and developed countries will have very large beneficial health effects at a low cost [68]. Therefore, it is expedient for all countries to

adopt a very clear strategy to lower salt intake in the population. Depending on where the major sources of salt come from this strategy needs to be tailored specifically to each country's population.

Establish Salt Intake Recommendations

Many countries need to start at the beginning, that is, estimate salt intake by measuring 24-hour urinary sodium excretion in a random sample of the population, and establish official salt intake recommendations. However, as mentioned previously, the recommendations alone will have very little impact unless there are some corresponding salt reduction activities. To achieve the recommended levels of salt intake for adults and children, a substantial reduction in the current average salt intake of the population is required.

Goals need to be set, with a time-frame in which to achieve these goals. For example in the United Kingdom, the aim is to lower salt intake in the population to 6 g/day by 2012. Depending on the current salt intake of the population, these goals may differ between countries, that is, the higher the salt intake, the longer time may be needed to achieve the target.

The first step in accomplishing this goal will be to identify those foods that are the major sources of dietary salt in the population. This will support the development of more effective policies and interventions.

Food Industry Action

For those countries where most of the salt comes from processed foods, the policy could be the same as that in the United Kingdom. The U.K. effort is a prime example of how product reformulation to lower the salt content of foods can be very effective in countries where processed foods contribute significantly to the salt intake of the population. The United Kingdom has also demonstrated how the government and industry can work effectively together to reduce salt intake. It illustrates to the rest of the world how a public health campaign can be successful alongside the co-operation of the food industry. In addition to lowering salt content in processed foods, there should also be an objective to lower salt in all other foods where the addition is not under the control of the consumer, such as in canteen, restaurant, and fast foods. For example, in the United Kingdom, one of the major school meal providers has reduced the salt content of meals in primary schools by 38% since 2002.

A short-term solution could be to replace salt with a mineral salt in all manufactured foods, as has been done in Finland. However, due to the metallic, bitter taste of salt substitutes, only 25%–40% of the sodium can be replaced with other mineral salts to avoid overtly noticeable impacts on the flavor of food. The best long-term strategy is to gradually lower the salt content of all manufactured foods where it has been added.

International companies should be required to apply a global salt policy to reduce the salt content of all of their products to the lowest possible level in all countries where they are marketed. At the moment, there is a very large variation in the amount of salt added to the same branded products in different countries or regions of the world [58]. This variation is entirely random. This illustrates once again how easy it would be for the food industry to reduce the amount of salt they add to food, particularly as they could do this straightaway to their branded products to the lowest level in the world.

Many international companies argue that the reason for differences in the salt content of the same product between countries is due to consumer taste preferences; for example, individuals in some countries prefer saltier products. However, in countries such as the United Kingdom and Finland where consumers were previously habituated to products with a higher salt content, there have been no reduction in sales and no complaints about taste when salt has been reduced. The salt should be removed in small quantities, for example, 10%–20% reductions at a time, which cannot be detected by human salt taste receptors, so that consumers do not notice. As salt intake falls, the specific salt taste receptors in the mouth become much more sensitive to lower concentrations of salt and this adjustment takes approximately 1 or 2 months. This means that lower concentrations of salt then taste as salty as the previous higher concentrations. It is therefore very unlikely that the lowering of salt concentrations in foods will lead to rejection of the foods. Indeed, all of the evidence suggests that once salt intake is reduced, individuals much prefer food with less salt and reject the highly salted foods they ate previously.

Despite all of the evidence supporting the health benefits of a reduction in the salt content of processed foods, some food manufacturers are resistant to cooperate. Cost is a major obstacle for food manufacturers (Figure 44.1). Historically, salt was added

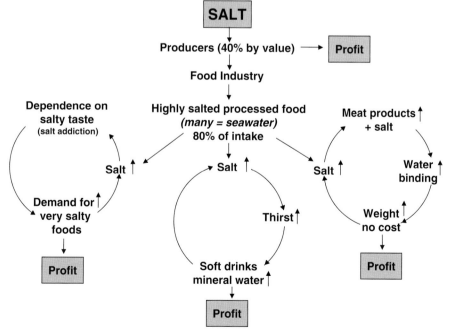

Figure 44.1 The commercial importance of salt in processed food.

to preserve foods. However, due to the development of the refrigerator and the freezer, salt is no longer required to preserve foods. The main reason now for adding salt to a wide range of processed foods is that it makes cheap, unpalatable food edible at no cost. Additionally, for processed meat, salt acts with polyphosphanates to bind water so the product's weight can be increased at no cost. It is also a major determinant of thirst and any reduction in salt intake would cause large reductions in soft drink, mineral water, and beer consumption. Some of the largest food companies in the world also manufacture soft drinks. Therefore, it is obviously apparent why so many food and drink companies are reluctant to lower the salt content of their products.

To ensure that the salt content of processed food products is reduced, maximum salt-content targets need to be set for the food industry. In the first instance, these targets should be voluntary. However, if these targets are not achieved within a certain timeframe, then the government should consider statutory regulation. Assessment and monitoring of policy implementation uptake is, therefore, fundamental.

Consumer Awareness Campaign

In addition to food industry action, there needs to be a public health campaign to highlight the dangers of too much salt, encouraging consumers to cut back on salt by reducing the amount of salt they add to food and most particularly to check product labels choosing lower salt options.

However, in countries where the majority of salt comes from processed foods, a consumer awareness campaign alone will have limited impact as it has been shown that dietary advice alone results in very little change in salt intake, and even if a small reduction is achieved it is usually not maintained over time. This highlights the difficulty for the individuals to self-willingly lower salt intake, as most dietary salt comes from processed foods and the consumer has absolutely no control over and quite often is unaware of the large amount of salt hidden in these foods.

Labeling

Changes in the environment should make it easy for the consumer to choose foods with the lowest salt content. In addition to making available foods with the lowest possible salt content, this should include the use of a clear labeling system.

In many countries there is no mandatory requirement to label the sodium/salt content of a product, and if sodium or salt is labeled, it is often difficult and confusing for the general consumer to interpret labels to know whether a product is high or low in salt. For example, some food products have sodium labeled per 100 g, and for the consumer to find out the amount of salt per portion, he would have to divide sodium by 100, multiply by product weight, and then multiply by 2.5.

Clear labeling is vital for the consumer to easily identify whether a food is high in salt so that an informed decision can be made about the purchase of the item. It should be a mandatory minimum requirement for the salt content to be expressed per 100 g and per serving, for example, "one serving of X grams of this product contains Y grams of salt." It should also state the recommended intake for adults, or if the product is specifically marketed at children, the amount of salt that that particular age group should consume.

The United Kingdom's traffic light labeling system has been accepted by major supermarkets and is the most preferred labeling by consumers compared with other types of labels. Consumer research has shown that it has a significant effect on the purchase of foods [52]. The traffic light labeling should be adopted by all other countries.

Developing Countries

It was estimated that between 2006 and 2015, if salt intake was reduced in developing countries by as little as 15%, 8.5 million cardiovascular deaths could be prevented, at an estimated cost of $0.04 to $0.32 per person [69].

In most developing countries where the majority of salt is added by the consumer, where it is used predominantly to preserve meat and fish, and in seasoning or sauces used during cooking and at the table, a different strategy needs to be implemented. Community-based interventions such as a public health campaign to highlight the dangers of consuming too much salt have been shown to be effective in countries such as China, Jamaica, and Nigeria at reducing salt intake [14,70]. Salt intake was reduced by about 30% by implementing simple changes in the diet, such as avoiding salty food and not adding salt at the table. Intervention measures included leaflet distribution, an advertising campaign in supermarkets and health professionals gave practical advice to patients.

Although the majority of salt comes from salt added during cooking or at the table, in many regions sauces such as soy sauce, fish sauce, and miso can contribute a significant amount of salt to a person's diet. Therefore, the salt content of these foods should be lowered.

The use of salt substitutes is another feasible intervention that could be introduced in areas, where most dietary salt comes from home-cooked rather than processed food. In a region of rural north China where the majority of salt comes from home pickled foods and salt added during cooking, normal salt was substituted with a reduced sodium, high-potassium salt substitute. This significantly lowered blood pressure by 3.7 mm Hg [71]. Another study in a group of elderly veterans in Taiwan showed that switching from regular salt to potassium-enriched salt had a long-term beneficial effect on CVD mortality and medical expenditure [72]. For a period of 31 months, kitchens in veteran retirement homes used either potassium-enriched salt (intervention group) or regular salt (control group). Those in the intervention group had a 40% reduction in CVD mortality, lived 0.3–0.9 years longer and spent significantly less on inpatient care for CVD than the control group. These beneficial effects have been attributed to the major increase in potassium and the moderate decrease in salt intake.

Children

Although raised blood pressure and CVD mainly occur in adults, blood pressure in children has been shown to follow a tracking pattern; that is, those individuals with a higher level of blood pressure during childhood are more likely to present with high blood pressure later in life. It is, therefore, important to start interventions during childhood on modifiable risk factors to lower blood pressure. A meta-analysis of salt-reduction trials in children showed that a modest reduction in salt intake causes immediate falls in blood pressure [73]. There is very limited data on salt consumption in children and there are only a few countries, such as the

United Kingdom, that have salt intake recommendations for children. It is important to find out salt consumption levels in children, where the major sources of salt are in children's diet and then set an achievable target level for children.

It is also important to lower salt intake in children as eating habits and preferences are established during childhood. Therefore, exposing children to salty foods when they are young will habituate their taste preferences to salty foods as they grow up.

A reduction in salt intake in children can be achieved by a gradual and sustained reduction in the amount of salt added to children's foods by the food industry. A comprehensive school meals program, for example, the one recently announced by the U.K. government [74], combined with advice to parents and children, will also help reduce salt.

Conclusion

The scientific body of evidence to support a reduction in salt intake in the whole population is strong. It is vital that all countries adopt a coherent and workable strategy to reduce salt intake. In most developed countries, approximately 80% of salt comes from processed food [35], and the amount of salt added to food by the food industry must be reduced. In these countries, reducing salt intake is one of the easiest changes in the diet to implement, as it does not require consumers to change their dietary practices, but it requires the food industry to make gradual and sustained reductions in the amount of salt they add to food. In other countries where most of the salt consumed comes from salt either added during cooking or from sauces, a public health campaign is needed to encourage consumers to use less salt, perhaps a combination of both, as in developing countries more and more processed food is being consumed. In several countries salt-reduction programs have already been carried out successfully and salt intake has fallen [24,40]. Other countries should follow these examples and start taking action now. A modest reduction in population salt intake worldwide would result in a major improvement in public health, similar to the provision of clean water and drains in the late nineteenth century in Europe.

Selected References

36. Reducing salt intake in populations. WHO Forum and Technical Meeting on Reducing Salt Intake in Populations. http://www.who.int/dietphysicalactivity/reducingsalt/en/index.html (Access verified August 7 2008).

57. Pietinen P, Valsta LM, Hirvonen T, et al. Labelling the salt content in foods: a useful tool in reducing sodium intake in Finland. Public Health Nutr 2008;11: 335–40.

63. Dickinson BD, Havas S. Reducing the population burden of cardiovascular disease by reducing sodium intake: a report of the Council on Science and Public Health. Arch Intern Med 2007;167:1460–8.

69. Asaria P, Chisholm D, Mathers C, et al. Chronic disease prevention: health effects and financial costs of strategies to reduce salt intake and control tobacco use. Lancet 2007;370:2044–53.

73. He FJ, MacGregor GA. Importance of salt in determining blood pressure in children: meta-analysis of controlled trials. Hypertension 2006;48:861–9.

SECTION V

Hemostasis and Thrombosis: From Nutritional Influences to Cardiovascular Events

CHAPTER 45

Risk Factors for Arterial Thrombosis

Giovanni de Gaetano, Romina di Giuseppe, &
Maria Benedetta Donati

John Paul II Center for High Technology Research and Education in Biomedical Sciences,
Catholic University, Campobasso, Italy

Introduction

Arterial thrombosis is responsible for heart attacks, stroke, and peripheral vascular disease. It usually affects individuals who already have developed atherosclerosis or narrowing of the arteries. The main known risk factors for arterial thrombosis include cigarette smoking, high blood pressure, increased levels of cholesterol, diabetes, increasing age, family history, saturated fat-rich diet, excessive body weight, and reduced physical activity. Nowadays, cardiovascular disease (CVD) is a leading cause of death among men and women in both developed and developing countries. In the latter, the high burden of CVD is attributable to the increasing incidence of atherosclerotic disease, due to urbanization, the relatively early age at which higher risk factor levels occur, the large size of population, and the high proportion of individuals who are middle aged. During the 1990s, about half of deaths due to CVD occurred in patients younger than 70 years in developing countries, as compared to about one-quarter in developed countries. Moreover, the projection of increase in ischemic heart disease (IHD) and cerebrovascular disease mortality in developing countries is estimated to be greater than in developed countries [1].

The association of any risk factor with coronary heart disease (CHD) may be similar across pop-ulations, but its prevalence may vary due to different population-attributable risk (PAR). In the INTERHEART study, a large international, case-control study, nine modifiable risk factors (Table 45.1) were found to explain more than 90% acute myocardial infarction (MI) in women and men, across all major ethnic groups [2]. In particular, all risk factors were significantly associated to acute MI, while alcohol, physical exercise, and fruit and vegetable consumption were inversely associated. The two most important risk factors for acute MI were smoking and abnormal lipids, followed by psychosocial factors, abdominal obesity, diabetes, and hypertension both in men and in women, even if their effect varied somewhat according to different regions of the world. Only smoking accounted for about 36% of PAR of acute MI (about 44% for men). Instead, avoiding smoking in combination with eating fruits and vegetables and practicing regular exercise was associated with 80% lower relative risk for MI. Other epidemiologic studies [3,4] also indicate that lifestyle and dietary modification reduced the risk of CHD in patients with coronary disease. Together, these observations add scientific evidence to the assumption that nutritional intervention greatly influences risk factors and natural history of CVD.

Mediterranean Diet (MD)

Prevention of arterial thrombotic disease has a high priority in developed countries. Daily intake of a

Nutritional and Metabolic Bases of Cardiovascular Disease, 1st edition.
Edited by Mario Mancini, José M. Ordovas, Gabriele Riccardi,
Paolo Rubba and Pasquale Strazzullo. © 2011 Blackwell Publishing Ltd.

Table 45.1 Modifiable risk factors for myocardial infarction in the Interheart Study.

Factors	Odds ratio	PAR (%)
Smoking	2.87	35.7
Increased ApoB/ApoA1	3.25	49.2
Hypertension (history)	1.91	17.9
Diabetes (history)	2.37	9.9
Abdominal obesity	1.12	20.1
Psychosocial factors	2.67	32.5
Daily fruits and vegetables	0.7	13.7*
Regular alcohol	0.91	6.7*
Regular physical activity	0.86	12.2*

*For the group without this factor.
Adapted from Yusuf et al. [2], with permission.

Table 45.2 Mediterranean diet score.

0 or 1 was assigned to each of nine components with the use of sex-specific median as cutoff.

Beneficial components (vegetables, legumes, fruits and nuts, cereal, and fish): above the median = 1

Detrimental components (meat, poultry, dairy products): below the median = 1

Ethanol: Moderate consumption ($\geq$5 g/day women <25 g, and = $\geq$10 g/day men <50 g) = 1

Lipid intake: ratio of monounsaturated to saturated lipids: above the median = 1

Ten-point total Mediterranean diet score ranged from 0 (minimal adherence) to 9 (maximal adherence).
Adapted from Trichopoulou et al. [10], with permission.

potentially anti-thrombotic diet may offer a convenient and effective way of CVD prevention.

The traditional Mediterranean diet (MD) is characterized by high intake of vegetables, legumes, fruits and nuts, cereals (in the past largely unrefined), and olive oil, a moderately high intake of fish, a low intake of saturated fat, and a low to moderate intake of dairy products (mostly in the form of cheese or yogurt) and of meat and poultry. A regular, moderate intake of ethanol, primarily in the form of wine—preferably during meals—completes the list [5] (see Chapter 10 and Chapter 5).

The Mediterranean Sea borders 18 countries and the diets vary from country to country. For example, the Italian MD is relatively moderate in olive oil and high in cereals, the Greek diet is rich in olive oil and fruits, and in Spain olive oil and fish are popular foods. Interest in MD derives originally from the Seven Countries Study, a milestone in epidemiologic research [6].

The positive health effects of the MD on CHD risk factors were also tested in several intervention studies. For 6 weeks, Finnish middle-aged men and women changed their usual diet to a Mediterranean type of diet, a change associated with more than 20% decrease in total cholesterol and low-density lipoprotein (LDL)-cholesterol and apoprotein B [7]. A southern Italy population changed its traditional MD to a diet rich in saturated fatty acids and cholesterol [8]. These dietary changes induced a significant increase of total cholesterol and

LDL-cholesterol. In another study, the substitution of dietary saturated fatty acids with monounsaturated fatty acid (MUFA) (oleic acid from olive oil) led to decreased plasma LDL-cholesterol concentrations [9]. In a large sample of the general Greek population, high adherence to the traditional MD was associated with a significant reduction in total mortality as well as of CHD and remarkably cancer mortality (Table 45.2) [10,11].

Mediterranean Diet Components

Despite the high complexity of its nutrient composition, two of the traditional components of the MD emerge as its principal foods, since they provide the higher percentage of energy and a lot of bioactive compounds: wine (alcohol) and virgin olive oil.

Alcohol and Cardiovascular Disease

Numerous epidemiologic studies suggest that CVD morbidity and mortality are inversely associated with light to moderate alcohol consumption (from a few drinks per week to one to three drinks per day), independent of age or smoking habits [12–15]. A meta-analysis of ecologic studies [13] reported an inverse association for wine in both men and women, a less strong association for spirits, but no association for beer. Several other studies gave similar results. Having been important in the early period of research on alcohol and cardiovascular risk, ecologic studies, however, suffer a number of limitations that do not allow us to take them into consideration today [13] (see Chapter 4).

In the Italian rural cohorts of the Seven Countries study, the lowest mortality from CVD occurred in the group of men who consumed an average of 77.8 g of alcohol a day, almost exclusivelywine [16]. A U- or J-shaped relationship between alcohol consumption and clinical events was indeed found in almost all studies, suggesting that nondrinkers or occasional drinkers have higher incidence and mortality rates than light or moderate drinkers, but similar or lower rates than heavy drinkers [17–21]. A meta-analysis of 34 prospective studies—including more than 1 million subjects and almost 100,000 deaths from any cause—investigated the relationship between alcohol dosing and all cause mortality, separately in men and women [20]. A J-shaped relationship between total mortality and alcohol intake was observed (Figure 45.1) [20]. In particular low levels of alcohol intake (one to two drinks per day for women and two to four drinks per day for men) were significantly associated with reduced mortality, while higher levels were associated with increased mortality.

Wine and Cardiovascular Disease

Mortality from CVD was reportedly lower in the French population even if they consumed a diet high in saturated fat [22]. The so-called "French paradox" was an attempt to explain this phenomenon assuming that in France regular red wine consumption would counteract the atherogenic effect of animal fats, thus lowering cardiovascular events and mortality [23]. More direct support to this hypothesis comes from four large prospective studies showing that in wine consumers cardiovascular and all-cause mortality risk is reduced more than in consumers of beer or spirits. In the Copenhagen City Heart Study [24], the risk of dying from CVD in a large population, followed for 10–12 years, reached a significant reduction in subjects drinking three to five drinks per day of wine (relative risk [RR], 0.44; 95% confidence interval [CI], 0.24–0.80) compared to subjects who never drank wine. The intake of the same amount of beer was associated with a smaller risk reduction (RR, 0.72; 95% CI, 0.61–0.88) while the intake of spirits was associated with a nonsignificant increased risk (RR, 1.35; 95% CI, 1.00–1.83). Wine intake

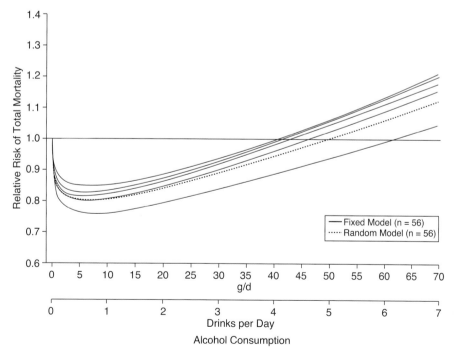

Figure 45.1 Examples of J-shaped curves showing the relative risk for all-cause death in relation to total alcohol intake. (Modified from Di Castelnuovo et al. (20), with permission.)

only was associated with a decreased risk of all-cause mortality. The same Danish group [19] reported that light alcohol drinkers (one to seven drinks per week) who avoided wine when compared with nondrinkers showed a slightly lower RR for all-cause death (RR, 0.90; 95% CI, 0.82–0.99) when compared with nondrinkers. The risk of death was even lower for light wine drinkers (RR, 0.76; 95% CI, 0.55–0.77). Heavy nonwine drinkers (>35 drinks/wk) showed a high risk of death when compared with heavy drinkers who included wine in their drinking habits. Moreover, mortality for both CHD and cancer in wine drinkers was significantly lower than in nonwine drinkers (RR, 0.76; 95% CI, 0.63–0.92 for light non-wine drinkers and RR 0.58; 95%CI 0.47-0.72 for wine drinkers). The reduction in CHD and all-cause death risk was independent of the level of wine intake.

Among 36,250 middle-aged healthy French men followed for 12 years, a significant higher reduction in the risk of CVD was found in subjects drinking up to 54 g of alcohol per day in the form of wine than in those drinking beer (39% vs. 26%). Furthermore only wine drinkers showed a significant 35% lower RR of all-cause mortality [25].

The British Regional Heart Study [26] followed 6,680 men for an average of 16.8 years: The greater protection against cardiovascular mortality conferred by wine as compared to beer (reference group) or spirits was only attenuated (RR, 0.71; 95% CI, 0.52–0.98 vs. 1.02; 95% CI, 0.83–1.25) when adjustment was done for common risk factors.

Wine and Cerebrovascular Disease

Evidence suggests that drinking wine is associated with a reduced risk of ischemic stroke but little or no protection against hemorrhagic stroke. However, in the cohort of the Copenhagen City Heart Study, weekly but not daily wine consumption was significantly associated with reduced risk of both ischemic and hemorrhagic stroke, but subjects drinking ≥42 units/wk had a 1.5-fold significant increase in risk [27].

From an Australian case-control study [28] including 331 matched pairs, only wine consumption lowered intracerebral hemorrhage risk. Both wine and spirits were associated with lower intracerebral hemorrhagic risk in men, while in women no significant association was found.

Mechanism(s) of Action of Alcohol

Alcohol affects several vascular and biochemical factors that have potential cardioprotective benefits. Induced changes in lipid profile are thought to represent a major mechanism to reduce the risk for CHD-related mortality and atherosclerosis [16–17,29]. However, other lipid-independent mechanisms may be important in contributing to reduce this risk.

Increase High-Density Lipoprotein Levels

Concentration of plasma high-density lipoprotein (HDL) and HDL3 mass decreased in temporary abstainers but not in moderate alcohol drinkers ($p \geq .05$) [30]. When the abstainers group restarted to drink, increased levels in HDL-cholesterol and HDL3 mass ($p \geq .05$), but no change in HDL2 mass was observed. In stratified and multivariate regression analyses [31], HDL-cholesterol levels increased with increased frequency of consumption of beer, wine, and spirits in a representative sample of the U.S. adult population. After adjustment for common factors, there were higher age-adjusted HDL-cholesterol levels with increasing quantities of alcohol consumed. In a study including 4,918 Spanish men and women aged 25–74 years, total alcohol intake was significantly associated to increased HDL-cholesterol in both sexes [32].

Antithrombotic Properties

An explanation for the "French paradox" [23] involved inhibition of platelet aggregation by alcohol, at consumption levels associated with reduced risk of CHD. Alcohol would act through inhibition of prostaglandin synthesis, like aspirin. Subsequent studies have shown that several polyphenols, contained in red wine, rather than alcohol, are able to inhibit platelet biosynthesis of thromboxane A2, a potent aggregation inducer and a vasoconstrictor [33–35]. Moderate alcohol consumption may also favorably affect fibrinogen concentration, tissue-type plasminogen activator, and plasminogen activator inhibitor [36], while a positive association between moderate alcohol intake and plasma concentration of endogenous tissue-type plasminogen activator (t-PA) was independent of HDL-cholesterol levels [37]. In a study conducted on

3,158 men aged 60–79 years without history of MI, stroke, or diabetes, a positive dose–response relationship was observed between total alcohol consumption and t-PA antigen and an inverse dose–response relationship between alcohol intake and fibrinogen levels [38].

Antiatherogenic Properties

Antiatherogenic properties of alcohol were described in animal and human studies. In a study on 1,676 men and 465 women undergoing coronary angiography [39], multivariate analyses showed that alcohol consumption was associated with lower percent of lumen narrowing in the main coronary vessels, suggesting that moderate alcohol consumption is independently associated with reduced coronary atherosclerosis.

Mechanism(s) of Action of Wine

Besides ethanol, (red) wine contains many substances such as phenols and tannins, which influence low-density lipoprotein oxidation, platelet aggregation, endothelial function, and smooth muscle cell proliferation [40]. It contains a wide variety of polyphenols, including phenolic acids, trihydroxy stilbenes (resveratrol) and flavonoids (catechin, epicatechin, and quercetin) [41]. Some of these molecules inhibit lipoprotein oxidation, promote nitric oxide formation by vascular endothelium, inhibit thromboxane A2 biosynthesis in platelets and leukotriene biosynthesis in neutrophils, and regulate lipoprotein production and secretion. These actions occur through the inhibition of various enzymes involved in cell signaling.

Antioxidant Properties

Atherosclerotic plaque formation reportedly involves lipoprotein oxidation inside arterial walls. Resveratrol attenuated indeed oxygenated LDL (oxLDL)-induced cytotoxicity, apoptotic features, generation of reactive oxygen species, and intracellular calcium accumulation [42].

A small group of patients undergoing percutaneous coronary interventions was randomized to red wine [250 ml/day] or control (abstinence from any alcoholic beverage). While the endothelium-dependent/independent dilation ratio significantly improved, after 2 months in both groups, wine

drinking show benefits only on parameters of oxidative stress [43].

The effects of wine consumption on antioxidant status were also investigated in a randomized controlled study on healthy volunteers [44]. Total plasma phenolic concentrations increased significantly after 2 weeks of daily moderate red wine consumption. The maximum concentrations of conjugated dienes and thiobarbituric acid-reactive substances in Cu-oxidized LDL were reduced, but HDL-cholesterol concentrations increased after red wine.

Antithrombotic Properties

Platelet aggregation plays a crucial role in atherosclerosis and the progression of coronary artery disease (CAD) [45]. Although alcohol inhibits by itself or potentiates platelet inhibitory drugs [46], red wine inhibits human platelet aggregation, possibly due to its polyphenolic compounds, resveratrol and quercetin having the greatest effects [47]. Aggregation of human platelets and the biosynthesis of thromboxane B2 are inhibited by red wine [48], while quercetin potentiates prostaglandin I2 by increasing levels of cyclic adenosine monophosphate (cAMP). In human volunteers, moderate red wine consumption decreased platelet aggregation [48] and plasma thromboxane B2 concentration [47]. As the mechanism of platelet inhibition by red wine polyphenols might be different from that of other platelet-inhibiting substances, the effect of its moderate consumption in the prevention of CAD might be additive to that of aspirin or other drugs. According to this hypothesis, Rotondo et al. [49,50] showed that trans-resveratrol further inhibited human platelet aggregation inhibited by aspirin. Trans-resveratrol also prevented polymorphonuclear (PMN) leukocyte aggregation and formation of mixed conjugates between PMN and platelets. Trans-resveratrol thus interferes with the release of inflammatory mediators by activated PMN and down-regulates adhesion-dependent thrombogenic PMN function, strengthening biological plausibility of the protective effect of red wine against CHD.

Tissue factor (TF) expression by endothelial and mononuclear (MN) cells from healthy donors, challenged *in vitro* by different stimuli, was inhibited by resveratrol or quercetin [51]. Both polyphenols strongly reduced TF mRNA in both cell types, by reducing nuclear binding activity of the transacting factor c-Rel/p65, induced by the agonists, a reduction dependent in turn upon inhibition of degradation of the c-Rel/p65 inhibitory protein Ikappa-Balpha. This is an additional molecular basis of the protective activity of red wine against CVD.

Gallic acid is a polyphenol structurally similar to salicylic acid, the major aspirin metabolite. Crescente et al. (personal communication, 2008) have lately found that this polyphenol shared with resveratrol and quercetin a similar platelet antioxidant activity, although gallic acid did not inhibit platelet aggregation and thromboxane biosynthesis. In interaction experiments, gallic acid, similarly to salicylic acid, blunted the inhibitory effect on platelet function of aspirin and the other two polyphenols. Molecular modeling studies suggested that all three polyphenols—like salicylate—formed stable complexes into COX-1 channel, with slightly different interaction geometries. The gallic acid–aspirin and polyphenol–polyphenol interactions at the platelet level might be relevant to the potential healthy value of the MD and of its possible interference with aspirin treatment.

Antiatherogenic Properties

In a study on apolipoprotein E (ApoE)–deficient mice [52], smaller atherosclerotic lesion areas and reduced susceptibility to oxidation of LDL were observed after either red wine or polyphenol chronic consumption, as compared with placebo. The susceptibility of LDL to aggregation was also reduced.

In an *in vivo* study on hypercholesterolemic rabbits, de-alcoholized or whole red wine showed a cardiovascular protective effect as red wine without affecting plasma lipid levels [53], a finding similar to that reported in hypercholesterolemic rats [54]. Human studies also suggest that the consumption of red wine [55] or alcohol-free red wine [56,57] leads to a significant increase in serum antioxidant activity and in the susceptibility of LDL to oxidation *in vivo*, limiting the extent of atheroma formation [57]. However, the results of large randomized clinical trials assessing the use of antioxidant therapies (mainly vitamin E) to reduce cardiovascular events were disappointing [58].

Olive Oil and Cardiovascular Disease

Most of the fat content of the MD is derived from a single component of the diet: the olive oil. This concept may be translated in a diet low in saturated fat and rich in MUFAs, in particular oleic acid.

Several epidemiologic studies provide an experimental basis supporting the beneficial effects of the MD, rich in olive oil, with regard to the reduction of CHD [59] (see Chapter 10).

The Seven Countries Study [6] first showed that the population of the Mediterranean island of Crete had the lowest rates of both CAD and cancer, suggesting a protective role against these chronic degenerative disease of low-saturated fat and high-oleic acid intake (olive oil), typical of the MD. The first strong clinical evidence in support to the health benefits of a Mediterranean-style diet derived from the Lyon Diet Heart Study [60], on patients recovering from an acute MI. The protective effects were attributed to higher intake of oleic acid and α-linolenic acid (ALA, 18:3, n-3) and lower intake of saturated fatty acids (SFAs) and linoleic acid (LA, 18:2, n-6), a conclusion supporting MUFAs as key components in the protective role of the MD. Olive oil reduced systolic and diastolic blood pressure in both normotensive and hypertensive individuals. More recently, MD was reported to be inversely associated with arterial blood pressure and olive oil intake by itself was inversely associated with both systolic and diastolic blood pressure. The modification in blood pressure by dietary olive oil was related to changes in the fatty acid composition of the cell membrane, which favorably affects its function [61].

Replacement of dietary SFAs with oleic acid from olive oil decreases plasma LDL concentrations, a possible contributory mechanism to the low incidence of CHD [62]. Oxidative modification of LDL is an important determinant in the development of atherosclerosis as it accelerates the uptake of LDL by macrophages, which starts the formation of a fatty streak. LDL may be protected against attacks of free radicals by plasma antioxidants. Lipoproteins enriched in MUFAs after long-term consumption of olive oil are less susceptible to oxidation as compared to particles enriched with PUFAs [63].

Several studies however raised the hypothesis that oleic acid alone cannot fully explain the healthy effect of olive oil. The differential effects of different oleic acid-rich oils on LDL oxidation were confirmed in normolipidemic subjects after the administration of virgin olive oil or high-oleic sunflower oil [64]. The protective effects of olive oil against CAD might therefore also be attributed to other components of the oil, in particular phenols. Oleuropein, hydroxytyrosol, and tyrosol, the major phenolic compounds of olive oil, are strong antioxidant and radical scavengers that may help to revert the imbalance between increased oxidative stress and impaired antioxidant defense that affects endothelial function, thus contributing to atherosclerotic disease progression.

Olive Oil and Hemostasis

Olive Oil and Platelets

A MUFA-rich diet decreases the urinary excretion of 11-dehydrothromboxane B2, a metabolite derived from TXA2, a potent inducer of platelet aggregation [65]. These results confirm early studies on healthy subjects [66] showing that an olive oil–rich diet lowered the sensitivity of platelets to collagen, while with a corn oil-enriched diet the threshold of aggregation to arachidonic acid was even raised.

The beneficial effects of MUFA-rich diets on platelets have been confirmed by a recent study [67]: Two levels of ingestion of MUFA (18% and 15% of the total supply of calories, respectively) with saturated fats (16%) were compared. Even if, in the short term, the effect of the elevated consumption was greater, after 16 weeks the results were identical at both levels of ingestion, keeping low platelet aggregation induced by arachidonic acid. Visioli's group observed and more recently confirmed [68] through experiments carried out during the postprandial phase that daily administration for seven weeks of 40 ml of virgin olive oil rich in phenolic compounds, compared with refined oil, was accompanied by lower TXB2 serum levels, confirming the influence of dietary polyphenols on platelet function and primary hemostasis.

Further links are suggested by the observation that a high-MUFA-rich diet reduces plasma levels of von Willebrand factor—a vessel wall component associated with the formation of platelet thrombus and an endothelial injury marker—in diabetic patients and healthy individuals [69,70, 72].

Olive Oil and Factor VII

Coagulation factor VII (FVII) is a key protein in thrombosis and a risk factor for CHD. FVII levels decrease after oleic acid-rich diets in respect to lauric and palmitic-rich diets, while no difference was observed when oleic and linolenic-rich diets were compared [71,72]. Meals rich in MUFA seem to have postprandial FVII responses lower than that observed after SFA-rich meals, similarly to that of PUFA or rapeseed oil-rich meals. Olive oil would promote lower postprandial FVII peaks after high fat meals than do SFA-rich dietary patterns [73].

Olive Oil and Tissue Factor

Tissue factor (TF) is a trans-membrane glycoprotein, expressed in the cells of arterial wall. The clotting activity in atheroma plaques increases in its presence, favoring the appearance of acute coronary syndrome. Tremoli et al. [74,75] observed that the amount and nature of fatty acids in the diet regulate TF expression, with the exception of PUFA that inhibited it. Diets such as the MUFA-rich MD lead to TF activity in circulating monocytes, while saturated fats raise basal levels of TF and even more post-prandially [76,77].

Tissue factor pathway inhibitor (TFPI) is an activated factor X–dependent inhibitor of TF-induced coagulation. The principal role of TFPI appears to be to inhibit small amounts of TF, which are probably essential for the maintenance of normal hemostatic balance.

In a randomized crossover study on the role of diets enriched with olive oil, sunflower oil, and rapeseed oil, no influence of dietary intervention on plasma TFPI levels was observed [78]. In contrast, the isocaloric replacement of a palm oil–enriched diet or a low-fat diet by an MD had been shown to reduce plasma TFPI [79].

In a more recent study [80], eicosapentaenoic/docosahexaenoic (EPA/DHA) induced a 15% increase in TFPI, while changes in markers of hemostasis and endothelial integrity did not reach statistical significance following consumption of either n-3 fatty acid diet. Although the decrease in plasma TFPI levels is difficult to interpret, it may reflect an increase in the protease on the endothelial surface, which would have a regulatory effect on thrombogenesis. The decrease in plasma TFPI levels could therefore be interpreted as a reduction in the protective effect of olive oil against thrombogenesis.

Olive Oil and Fibrinolysis

In the stabilization and progress of thrombus, fibrinolysis plays an important role as a mechanism regulated by the equilibrium between t-PA and its natural inhibitor PAI-1 (t-PA inhibitor type 1). The level of the latter substance rises with the ingestion of diets that are high in palmitic acid [71]. When the MD, rich in olive oil, was compared with a carbohydrate-rich, low-fat diet, levels of PAI-1 were reduced independently of the dietary cholesterol content in the diet [81]. These data were confirmed in a study on hypertensive patients under diet rich in virgin olive oil in which a reduction in PAI-1 plasma concentration was observed in comparison with soy oil [82]. Finally, a recent study conducted on healthy subjects showed that the administration of olive oil induced a lower postprandial response in PAI-1 and TF than the ingestion of high-palmitic sunflower oil and butter [83].

Conclusions

Arterial thrombosis is responsible for heart attacks, stroke, and peripheral vascular disease. Stroke is a major cause of disability worldwide. Prevention of arterial thrombosis is a crucial part of health care, the two main ways for preventing it being lifestyle changes and medication. Lifestyle changes have a major impact in reducing the risk of atherosclerosis, arterial thrombosis, and ischemic disease. Regular physical activity combined with a diet rich in fruit, vegetables, complex carbohydrates, monounsaturated fat, and fish, moderate alcohol consumption but poor salt, saturated fat, and simple sugars reduces the development of atherosclerosis and other chronic degenerative disease. The rates of vascular and total mortality are lower for people who drink low to moderate amounts of alcohol than for people who do not drink at all or drink heavily.

The cardioprotective nature of alcohol has been attributed to both its antithrombotic properties and its ability to increase HDL levels. Moreover, wine and especially red wine, due to its polyphenol content, might offer additional advantages and greater cardiovascular benefits than alcohol alone. In fact, polyphenols might reduce atherosclerosis by inhibiting lipoprotein oxidation and thrombosis independently of alcohol. Some believe this explains why France has a lower rate of CHD than the United Kingdom ("French paradox"). While it remains unclear whether red wine has any advantage over other forms of alcoholic beverages, grape juice contains the same polyphenol compounds as red wine and seems to produce the same biologic effects.

Like alcohol and red wine, olive oil, which is the main fat in the MD, exerts a wide range of anti-atherogenic effects and could contribute to explain the low rate of cardiovascular mortality in southern European Mediterranean countries, in comparison with other Western countries, despite a high prevalence of CHD risk factors [84]. Moreover, the combined effect of olive oil and red wine antioxidant polyphenols at nutritionally relevant concentrations inhibit endothelial adhesion molecule expression [85] and would provide beneficial postprandial effects on hemodynamics. These findings add new information on the favorable effect of some components of the MD, thus partially explaining its protection against atherosclerosis and thrombosis.

Acknowledgment

This chapter was prepared within the research program supported by the Italian Ministry of Research, decreto no. 1588.

Selected References

17. Corrao G, Bagnardi V, Zambon A, et al. A meta-analysis of alcohol consumption and the risk of 15 diseases. Prev Med 2004;38:613–9.

18. Gronbaek M, Di Castelnuovo A, Iacoviello L, et al. Wine, alcohol and cardiovascular risk: open issue. J Thromb Haemost 2004;2:2041–8.

32. Schroder H, Ferrandez O, Jimenez Conde J, et al. Cardiovascular risk profile and type of alcohol beverage

consumption: a population-based study. Ann Nutr Metab 2005;49:100–6.

67. Smith RD, Kelly CN, Fielding BA, et al. Long-term mo-nounsaturated fatty acid diets reduce platelet aggregation in healthy young subjects. Br J Nutr 2003;90:597–606.

83. Pacheco YM, López S, Bermúdez B, et al. Extra-virgin vs. refined olive oil on postprandial hemostatic mark-ers in healthy subjects. J Thromb Haemost 2006;4: 1421–2.

CHAPTER 46

Platelets, Leukocytes, and Vascular Wall Interactions in Cardiovascular Disease: Modulatory Effects of Dietary Polyphenols

Chiara Cerletti, Serenella Rotondo, & Giovanni de Gaetano
"John Paul II" Center for High Technology Research and Education in Biomedical Sciences, Catholic University, Campobasso, Italy

Introduction

Thrombosis—the most common cause of ischemic cardiovascular disease, such as myocardial infarction and stroke—is currently accepted as the late complication of atherosclerosis, a progressive inflammatory disease characterized by lipid infiltration in the wall of large arteries (atherosclerotic plaques). Platelet and leukocyte recruitment on endothelial cell constitutes an early mechanism of vascular inflammatory damage and consequent vessel occlusion [1]. During inflammation, signaling cascades result in activation of endothelial cells, platelets and leukocytes. The complex interaction between these vascular cells is influenced by both cell adhesion and production of soluble stimulatory or inhibitory molecules that alter cell function. The net effect of this cellular cross-talk on inflammation depends on the balance between inputs and can lead to either resolution and repair or perpetuation of inflammation, atherosclerosis and thrombosis [2].

In the first part of this chapter, we will briefly focus our attention on the mechanisms of vascular cell interactions, relevant for thrombosis and in-

flammation and their pathophysiological relevance, based on experimental and epidemiologic data. An excellent review paper has recently been published by Denisa Wagner and Paul S. Frenette on the vessel wall and its interactions [3]. We refer the reader back to this review for a more detailed description of vascular and blood cell adhesion mechanisms.

In the second part, we shall analyze available data on the interference of dietary polyphenols with the described cellular mechanisms, and discuss the biological plausibility of the beneficial effect of the Mediterranean diet (and of other polyphenol-rich diets) on cardiovascular disease.

Cell–Cell Interactions in Thrombosis

Adhesion of Platelets and Leukocytes to Endothelial Cells

More than 150 years ago leukocytes were already known to roll and adhere to blood vessel wall, an interaction that increased in inflammation [4]. Giulio Bizzozero in 1882 first described platelets as a new blood corpuscle, playing a relevant role in thrombosis and hemostasis, and observed that "every time when a vascular wall is damaged... arrest of white blood corpuscles represents a secondary phenomenon and may, perhaps, be caused by increased stickiness of blood platelets whereby the

Nutritional and Metabolic Bases of Cardiovascular Disease, 1st edition.
Edited by Mario Mancini, José M. Ordovas, Gabriele Riccardi, Paolo Rubba and Pasquale Strazzullo. © 2011 Blackwell Publishing Ltd.

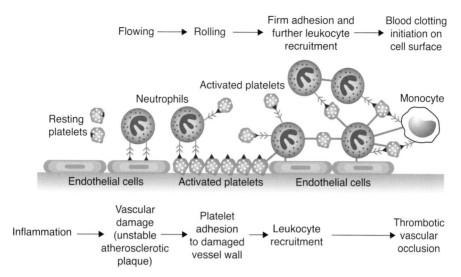

Figure 46.1 Schematic sequence of interactions between endothelial cells, platelets and leukocytes. (Reproduced from de Gaetano et al. [8], with permission.)

latter react with white blood corpuscles which have been brought in contact with the former by blood circulation" [5].

Many decades later, the modern version of intravital microscopy allowed the first quantitative observations of leukocyte rolling in the cheek pouch of hamsters and in mouse mesentery [6].

Platelet adhesion to and leukocyte rolling on endothelium are the initial stage of a multistep process leading to extravasation of white blood cells to sites of inflammation or infection, to platelet–leukocyte interaction and aggregation on a thrombogenic surface, and finally to vascular occlusion. Platelets may interact with endothelium even in the absence of any apparent morphological damage, but simply adhere to endothelium inflamed by different stimuli, such as infection, mechanic alteration, or ischemia and reperfusion or to endothelium located at lesion-prone sites, such as the carotid artery bifurcation. The recruitment of platelets and leukocytes at sites of vascular injury is a very rapid response and is mediated by the release of preformed components of the endothelium, including Weibel-Palade bodies and their major constituents, the von Willebrand factor's largest multimers and P-selectin; these are the most active promoters of platelet and leukocyte adhesion. P-selectin mediates both leukocyte and platelet adhesion and during secretion fuses with the endothelial plasma mem-

brane. The process of leukocyte rolling is initiated by P-selectin secretion and is concluded by leukocyte adhesion and transmigration to inflamed tissue [2,7,8].

Figure 46.1 depicts the schematic sequence of interactions between endothelial cells, platelets, and leukocytes flowing in blood that lead to vascular damage and thrombus formation.

On one hand, these events may favor the maintenance of vascular and tissue integrity, and on the other, they play a pathogenetic role in inflammatory and thrombotic disease. Recent data provide biological plausibility to the epidemiologic evidence of a significant association between leukocyte count and the incidence of coronary heart disease [9–13].

Sequence of Molecular Events: P-selectin – β-2 Integrin cross-Talk

P-selectin is a type-1 membrane glycoprotein with a C-type lectin domain, stored in the Weibel-Palade bodies of endothelial cells and in the α-granules of platelets [14], that recognizes specialized fucosylated sialoglycoconjugates, such as the tetrasaccharide sialyl Lewis X that decorate selected surface glycoproteins. P-selectin glycoprotein ligand-1 (PSGL-1), enriched at the very tip of leukocyte microvilli, plays a major role in the initial capture of leukocytes to the endothelium and controls rolling velocity and signal transduction, further contributing to leukocyte activation and expression of β2 integrins in their activated form.

Integrins are heterodimers formed by an α-chain and a β-chain, normally expressed in a closed low-affinity conformation on leukocytes, and upon activation result in increased affinity and avidity (strength of adhesiveness), leading to firm adhesion to endothelial intercellular adhesion molecule-1 (ICAM-1) and vascular cell adhesion molecule-1 (VCAM-1).

Leukocytes are recruited on activated platelets with molecular mechanisms similar to those just described, occurring at the site of vascular inflammation [7].

A variety of agonists can activate platelets, induce α-granule release and P-selectin expression on platelet surface: products of vascular damage (multimeric von Willebrand factor), subendothelial collagen, traces of thrombin, ADP, released by red cells or by activated platelets, platelet activating factor (PAF), or active products of the arachidonic acid metabolism, such as thromboxane A2, proteases, chemokines, or other inflammatory mediators, released by activated polymorphonuclear (PMN) leukocytes. Activated platelets within the circulation bind leukocytes, forming platelet-leukocyte conjugates, through P-selectin interaction with PSGL-1, a rapidly reversible tethering that induces in leukocytes an activating signal for β2-integrins. Tirosine kinases, mainly of the Src family, are involved and allow remodeling of cytoskeleton-β2-integrin linkages and clustering, which finally strengthens cell–cell adhesion. At variance with P-selectin involved in rolling, β2-integrins require functional up-regulation to become competent to bind their counter-receptors present not only on platelets, but also on other cells, such as endothelial cells or different classes of leukocytes, allowing multicellular interactions [7].

Other Adhesive Systems

In the past decade, two adhesive proteins, relevant for cell–cell interactions, have been described on platelets, CD40 and CD40 ligand (CD40L or CD154) [16]. CD40L is translocated to the platelet surface after activation and may interact with its counter-receptor CD40, present on platelets, on endothelial cells and monocytes/macrophages, thus facilitating platelet interaction with other

blood cells. The interaction CD40L-CD40 also up-regulates several functions in monocytes, such as chemokine and cytokine secretion, expression of the pro-coagulant tissue factor, up-regulation, and activation of adhesive receptors and proteases and differentiation of monocytes into macrophages. Different pathways are involved in CD40 signal transduction, such as activation of protein tyrosine kinases, phosphoinositide-3 kinase, and phospholipase Cγ2, followed by activation of specific transcription factors, such as nuclear factor-κB (NF-κB) [15].

Lately, SCUBE1 (signal peptide-CUB [complement C1r/C1s, Uegf, and Bmp1]-EGF (epidermal growth factor)-like domain-containing protein 1), a protein associated with platelet–endothelial interactions, virtually undetectable in healthy subjects, was reported as a marker of platelet activation during acute ischemic stroke [16]. SCUBE-1 from a novel family of proteins, is stored in platelet a-granules, translocated to the platelet surface upon thrombin activation, proteolytically released as small soluble fragments, and incorporated into thrombus.

Table 46.1 lists the major adhesion molecules involved in endothelium, platelet, and leukocyte interactions.

Soluble Adhesive Molecules

After cell surface expression, adhesive molecules, such as P-selectin, CD40L, and SCUBE1 from platelets, L-selectin from leukocytes or ICAM-1 and VCAM-1 from endothelium, are found in the circulation, as the result of proteolytic cleavage. Their biological activities as activators or inhibitors of cellular function are not completely clarified, but their increased circulating levels have been associated with a proinflammatory status or cardiovascular disease [17].

Functionally active products (and markers) of cell–cell interactions are also the transcellular metabolites of arachidonic acid, produced by cooperation between different cell types, such as the leukotrienes (LT) A4/C4 and lipoxins, or single cell products, such as LTB4 from leukocytes or thromboxane (Tx) B2 from platelets, produced in greater amount in to the presence or when adhered to different cell types [2,3,8].

Table 46.1 Major adhesion molecules in endothelium, platelet, and leukocyte interactions.

Molecule	Origin and expression	Function	Ligand
Selectins			
P-selectin	Stored in EC and platelet granules; expressed on cell surface on stimulation and released	Rolling of leukocytes on EC and platelets and of platelets on EC	PSGL-1
E-selectin	Induced by cytokines on EC	Rolling of leukocytes on EC	PSGL-1 ESL-1 CD44
L-selectin	Expressed on leukocytes	Secondary leukocyte recruitment	PSGL-1
Immunoglobulins			
ICAM-1	Up-regulated by cytokines on EC and leukocytes	Firm adhesion and transmigration of leukocytes	$\beta2$-integrins
ICAM-2	Constitutive on EC and platelets	Firm adhesion and transmigration of leukocytes; platelet adhesion to leukocytes	$\beta2$-integrins
VCAM-1	Up-regulated by cytokines on EC	Firm adhesion and transmigration of leukocytes	$\beta4$-integrins
PECAM-1	Constitutive on EC, platelets and leukocytes	Transmigration	PECAM-1
Integrins			
$\beta2$-integrins	Expressed on leukocytes; require activation	Firm adhesion to EC and platelets	ICAMs VCAM fibrinogen
$\beta3$-integrins	Expressed on platelets (αIIbβ3 or GpIIbIIIa) and on neutrophils/EC (αVβ3); require activation	Firm cell adhesion	Fibrinogen; extracellular matrix molecules
Tumor necrosis factor family			
CD40	Constitutive and expressed on EC,	Activates different EC, leukocyte,	CD40L
CD40L	leukocyte and platelet surface	and platelet function	CD40; αIIb β3 on platelets

Clinical and Epidemiological Evidence of Cell–Cell Interactions in Cardiovascular Disease

Despite the long-lasting discovery of the role of platelets in experimental thrombosis and the remarkable antithrombotic effect of antiplatelet drugs in ischemic disease, there is still little *direct* evidence of the role of platelets in the pathogenesis of vascular disease. This "platelet paradox" [18] mainly derives from the lack of a direct relationship between platelet number (and/or platelet function parameters) and number (and/or severity) of clinical vascular events: No evidence exists of reduced vascular risk in thrombocytopenic patients nor a proportional increase of ischemic risk following platelet transfusion.

In contrast, positive correlations between leukocyte count (neutrophil PMN, in particular) and risk of myocardial infarction or stroke have been suggested [11,12]. However, although leukocytosis has been associated with both acute thrombosis and atherosclerosis, until now no treatment reducing leukocyte function or number was shown effective in patients at high ischemic risk [13].

The hypothesis that leukocytes and platelets mutually interact and contribute to the development of thrombotic ischemic disease is taking more and more credit. Increased *in vivo* PMN activation and platelet–leukocyte interaction in different clinical manifestations of ischemic heart disease have been reported and an active role for these cells in the progression of vascular occlusion has been suggested. Platelet-leukocyte conjugates have been observed in peripheral blood from patients with unstable angina, stable coronary artery disease or mechanical heart valve replacement, as well as in patients with myeloproliferative disease [2]; their formation following percutaneous coronary interventions was considered a predictive index of acute re-occlusion [2,3,13,14]; moreover neutrophil activation by platelet P-selectin results in tissue factor expression and synthesis [19], a phenomenon inhibited *in vitro* and *ex vivo* by hydroxyurea in patients with myeloproliferative disease [20].

In the framework of a larger epidemiological study conducted by our group, platelet-leukocyte conjugates and their determinants were evaluated in citrated blood from 349 subjects (209 women, 16–92 years) randomly recruited from the general population [21]. *In vitro* platelet activation by ADP/collagen (but not by the inflammatory peptide fMLP or by LTB4) resulted in increased formation of platelet conjugates with PMN or monocytes, in parallel to platelet P-selectin and leukocyte CD11b expression. Mixed platelet–leukocyte conjugates and P-selectin expression were significantly associated with gender, age and platelet count. Among risk factors, a significant correlation was found between cell conjugates and glucose levels. This large study suggests that the presence and formation of platelet-leukocyte conjugates in whole blood from a large population reflects primary platelet–but not leukocyte–activation and varies with gender, age, platelet count, and blood glucose levels.

As with P-selectin, elevated plasma levels of CD40L have also been reported in patients at high cardiovascular risk (hypercholesterolemic, diabetic, etc.) [22]. In addition, elevated plasma concentrations of endothelial cell-derived adhesion molecules, including E-selectin, ICAM-1, and VCAM-1, are associated with coronary artery disease [17]. Whether the increase of soluble adhesive molecules is merely an epiphenomenal reflection of the inflammatory and thrombotic processes, or whether it directly contributes to acute coronary events remains to be established.

Modulation of Cell–Cell Interactions

Antiplatelet agents, such as dipyridamole, the thienopyridine clopidogrel, the anti-GpIIbIIIa abciximab, or the stable prostacyclin analogue iloprost, have been tested for their ability to modify platelet-leukocyte interactions. The control of cell–cell interactions is a new concept in pharmacology, including the modulation of cell signaling necessary for adhesive molecule expression and activation. Recently, heparins, and in particular low molecular weight heparins, have been shown to interfere with platelet-leukocyte (and tumor cell interactions) at the level of P-selectin-PSGL-1 adhesion [23]. We do not discuss in this chapter the effects of old or new drugs modulating cell–cell interaction [2,8], but focus our attention on the available information on the effects of natural or diet-derived polyphenols on cell function and interactions relevant to cardiovascular ischemic disease.

Dietary Polyphenols and Cell–Cell Interactions

Polyphenols constitute a large class of natural compounds that are widely distributed in fruit and vegetables of the human diet [24]. Epidemiologic studies suggest a protective relation between dietary intake of polyphenols and risk of cardiovascular disease [25–28]. A recent meta-analysis [29] reviewed the effectiveness of different flavonoid-rich sources on cardiovascular disease and found that chocolate or cocoa and tea may modulate important cardiovascular risk factors such as lipoproteins, blood pressure, and flow-mediated dilation. However, for other flavonoid sources, there were limited data from intervention trials with which to examine potential efficacy. It may be also pointed out that flavonoids constitute only a subclass, although relevant, of polyphenols which also include stilbenes, such as resveratrol, tannins, such as gallic/ellagic acid esters, and phenolic acids, which all together may contribute to the observed healthy effect of polyphenol-rich diet.

Experimental studies have tried to clarify the mechanisms through which these substances may exert their protective action. Polyphenols have been shown to be endowed with a large spectrum of biological activities which may interfere with the initiation and the progression of atherogenesis and thrombosis, first of all their antioxidant and radical scavenging properties.

Different polyphenols have also been shown to modulate cell functions involved in the process of thrombosis, such as vascular response, arachidonic acid metabolism in both platelets and leukocytes, platelet aggregation, and synthesis of prothrombotic and proinflammatory mediators, or to interfere with the expression and activation of genes that regulate adhesive functions and tissue factor activities in endothelial cells or leukocytes [30,31].

We have assembled many of the effects of polyphenols on mechanisms of interactions between platelets, leukocytes, and endothelial cells that play a pivotal role in early events in the pathogenesis of atherothrombosis.

For this purpose, we have included in Tables 46.2, 46.3, and 46.4 those intervention studies on *humans* given polyphenol-enriched sources and those *in vivo* or *in vitro* experimental models that tested the effect of dietary or pure phenols on vascular cell functions relevant for ischemic thrombotic disease.

Studies in Humans

Table 46.2 reports a summary of the intervention studies performed in human subjects, healthy or patients, listed according to the polyphenol source and the end-points tested.

Studies in Experimental *In Vivo* Models

Table 46.3 reports a summary of the *in vivo* experimental studies performed in different animal species and the effects of polyphenols (purified or of dietary origin) on different vascular and blood cells response related to ischemic disease.

Studies In Vitro

Table 46.4 reports a summary of the *in vitro* performed studies, testing the effect of polyphenols on cell-cell interaction and function relevant to thrombosis. Where indicated, also the possible molecular mechanism(s) hypothesized are reported.

Behind the expected differences among different compounds, dietary polyphenol intake, and cardio-

vascular protection appear to have favorable effects on cardiovascular protection in different settings.

However, there are several limitations of studies in humans mainly due to the inherent difficulty in ensuring compliance with dietary instructions, active product intake, and overall lifestyle in free-living persons. This is particularly important in dietary intervention studies where diet and exercise may modify the concentration of soluble mediators and inflammatory markers.

Results from studies in humans or in animal models may be difficult to compare because of differences in the design of intervention, such as duration or polyphenol composition, as well as in the biochemical and biological end-points. Furthermore, the comprehensive understanding of the protective effect of polyphenols is hindered by the lack of complete knowledge of their absorption, distribution, metabolism and excretion, heterogeneity of the biological activities of different subclasses as well as of their possible synergic activities *in vivo*. Few studies have investigated the effects of polyphenol metabolites formed in the body, such as deglycosylation during absorption or glucuronated, sulphated, methylated, and conjugated forms reaching the systemic circulation [24,65]. These conjugates are chemically distinct from their parent compounds, differing in size, polarity, and ionic form, and consequently different from the native compound for their biological effects [65].

Commercially available colonic metabolites of dietary polyphenols were shown to inhibit TRAP-induced platelet aggregation and P-selectin expression, at concentrations measured in plasma from human intervention studies [66].

In a model of first pass metabolism with cultured rat hepatocytes, the biological effect of flavonoids on endothelial cells was significantly decreased because of hepatic uptake or biotransformation [58]. Quercetin and its metabolites were able to inhibit VCAM-1, ICAM-1 and MCP-1 expression in stimulated HUVEC at concentrations (2–10 μM) achievable in plasma from a regular diet [67]. However, quercetin metabolites generally exhibited a reduced inhibitory activity, as compared to the parent aglycone. On the contrary, catechin metabolites, but not native catechin, inhibited the adhesion on monocytic cell U937 to interleukin (IL)-1β–stimulated HAEC [68].

Table 46.2 Intervention studies in humans with dietary phenols: effects on vascular cell function relevant for ischemic thrombotic disease.

Dietary intervention						
Diet/phenol	Dose (mg/day)	Time	Subjects (N)	Study design	Bioavailability	End-points and effects	Reference no.
Cocoa flavanols and procyanidins enriched tablets vs. placebo	234 flavanols and procyanidins	4 weeks	healthy adults (32)	Double-blind, random	Plasma catechins +81%, epicatechin +8%	ADP-induced platelet P-selectin ↓ Collagen- or ADP-induced aggregation ↓ F2 isoprostanes and TBARS =	32
Cocoa products with different amounts of flavanols	300, 600, 900 total flavanols	2–6 weeks	healthy subjects (12)	Double-blind, random	Not measured, but reportedly present in blood 2–6 hrs [34]	P-selectin, mixed aggregates in collagen-stimulated whole blood ↓ at 600–900 mg Leukocyte CD11b ↓ at all doses	33
Dark chocolate (40 g) flavonoid-rich vs. flavonoid-free	Total polyphenols ≈ to 620 epicatechin	Acute, tested at 2 hrs	heart transplant recipients (22)	Double-blind, random	Serum epicatechin levels	Vascular cold pressor test and endothelium-dependent coronary vasomotion improved, coronary artery diameter ↑ shear-dependent platelet adhesion ↓ TRAP and FRAP ↑, F2 isoprostane ↓	34
Dark chocolate (40 g) vs. white cholate (40 g)	74% vs. 4% cocoa	Acute, tested at 2 hrs	Healthy smokers (20)	Two parallel groups, random		Flow-mediated dilation ↑ up to 8 hrs shear-dependent platelet adhesion ↓ Total antioxidant status ↑ No effect of white chocolate	35,36
Four groups: Dealcoholised red wine (DWR) Cocoa beverage procyanidine-rich Water Caffeine-rich beverage	DWR: 2 mM total gallic acid ≈ Cocoa: 1 g epicatechins and oligomeric procyanidin	Acute, tested at 2 and 6 hrs	Healthy subjects (10 per group)	Each subject repeated the four different intakes		Unstimulated and stimulated platelet activation: DRW =; cocoa ↓; water =; caffeine ↑ response to epinephrine	37
Purple grape juice	7 ml/kg/day	2 weeks	Healthy subjects (20)	Before vs after juice	Plasma α-tocopherol levels ↑	Platelet function by ADP, collagen and PMA ↓; platelet superoxide ↓; platelet NO and plasma TRAP ↑	38

(Continued)

Table 46.2 (Continued)

Diet/phenol	Dietary intervention Dose (mg/day)	Time	Subjects (N)	Study design	Bioavailability	End-points and effects	Reference no.
Red wine vs. gin (30 g ethanol in 160 ml water/day)	576 vs very low polyphenols	4 weeks, 2 weeks wash-out	Healthy subjects (8)	crossover random	Plasma polyphenols levels	Monocyte adhesive molecules: red wine ↓ Monoc adhesion to TNFα-stimulated endoth cell: both intakes ↓	39
Red wine vs. before (30 g ethanol in 160 ml water/day)	576 polyphenols	4 weeks, 2 weeks wash-out	Healthy men (40)	crossover random	Plasma epicatechin gallate↑ after red wine	Monocyte adhesive molecules: ↓ Soluble endothelial adhesion molec: ↓ Monoc adhesion to endoth cell: ↓ Plasma fibrinogen and IL-1α: both intakes ↓	40
Red vs. white wine (20 g ethanol in 100 ml, twice daily)	200 vs 30 mg polyphenols x 2	4 weeks, 4 weeks wash-out	Healthy women (35)	Crossover random		Serum VCAM-1 & E-sel: ↓ red >white ICAM-1 & CD40L: ↓ only red Monocyte Mac-1, VLA-4, MCP-1: ↓ both Monocyte adhesion to endoth cells: ↓ red <white	41
Black tea vs. hot water	5 cups/day polyphenols content not specified	4 weeks (water first)	Subjects (22)	crossover random	24-h urine 4-O-methylgallic at the end of each week ↑	Soluble P-selectin: ↓ E-sel, ICAM-1, VCAM-1 = Coll- & ADP-induced aggregation =	42
Black tea (1.05 g extract in 250 ml water/day) vs. caffeinated tea (placebo)	6,4% flavonols	6 weeks, 4 weeks wash-out	Healthy non smoking men (37)	random double-blind	Measurement of caffeine in saliva for compliance	Platelet aggregates with monocytes or neutrophils: ↓ C reactive protein ↓ Soluble P-sel and plasma total antioxidant =	43
Tea or water, (450 ml acute, followed by 900 ml daily, chronic)	106 and 97 mg/dl, respectively, total flavonoids	Acute (2 hrs) and 4 weeks	CAD patients under aspirin (49)	crossover random	Plasma catechin ↑ after acute and chronic	No inhibitory effect on platelet aggregation, additional to aspirin	44
Flavanol-rich cocoa beverage vs. and combined to aspirin (81 mg)	897 mg/ml	Acute, tested at 2 and 6 hrs	Healthy subjects (16)	crossover random	Plasma epicatechin concentrations peaks at 2 hrs	Synergism with aspirin on platelet P-sel and GpIIbIIIa stimulated by ADP or epinephrine	45

≈: equivalents; TBARS: thiobarbituric acid-reactive substances; TRAP: total radical-reducing antioxidant potential; FRAP: ferric-reducing antioxidant potential; CAD: coronary artery disease.

Table 46.3 *In vivo* experimental models and effects of phenols on vascular cell functions relevant for ischemic disease.

Food or beverage	Administration Route, dose and time	Animal species	Phenols	Model, end-points, and effects	Ref. No.
Red wine or grape juice vs. white wine	i.v. (1.6 ml/kg) i.g. (4 ml/kg)	Dog	Polyphenols ↑ in red wine and grape juice vs. white wine	Coronary artery stenosis, platelet-mediated cyclic flow reduction (Folt's model) ↓	46
Purple grape and orange vs. grapefruit juice	i.v. and i.g. (2 and 10 ml/kg, respectively): acute 2 hr in dog; 7 days in monkey	Dog monkey	Grape juice contains: flavonols and antocyanidins; orange and grapefruit: flavanones and flavones	Dog coronary artery stenosis, platelet-mediated cyclic flow reduction (Folt's model) ↓ Whole blood collagen-induced platelet aggregation ↓ in grape and orange, not in grapefruit-treated animals (dog and monkey)	47
Red wine and alcohol-free red wine vs. white wine	8.4 ml/dl drinking water for 10 days	Rat	Polyphenolic concentration↑ in red vs. white wine	Bleeding time prolonged; experimental venous thrombosis ↓ platelet adhesion to fibrillar collagen ↓ plasma antioxidant activity ↑	48
Anthocyanins-rich or -free maize diet	8 weeks	Rat	Plasma and urine anthocyanins ↑	In vivo (coronary occlusion and reperfusion) and ex vivo (Langendorff) models of heart ischemia-reperfusion injury ↓	49
Alcohol-free red wine	In drinking water, for 1 or 5 months	Rat, fed normal or cholesterol-rich diet	Polyphenols content in lyophilized red wine	Aortic thrombosis: occlusion time longer platelet adhesion to fibrillar collagen ↓ Blood cholesterol levels, FVII or fibrinogen unaffected by wine	50
Red wine extracts or purified catechin (in alcohol), and alcohol	In drinking water for 12 weeks	Mouse, hypercholesterolemic ApoE-deficient	Catechin in plasma, urine and feces ↑	Blood thrombotic reactivity tested in a perfusion chamber model of experimental thrombosis ↓	51
Gallic acid	0.75–7.5 mg/kg, bolus and infusion (dose/hr) up to 3 hr	Normal and aged ApoE-deficient mouse	Platelet rolling and platelet-leukocyte rosettes over endothelium ↓ Single platelets deposition on endothelium =	52

i.v.: intravenous; ig: intragastric.

Table 46.4 *In vitro* studies on the effects of phenols in vascular and blood cell function and interactions relevant to thrombosis.

Cell type	Phenol	Cellular end-points and effects	Possible mechanism(s)	Ref. N
Endothelial cells from human umbilical vein (HUVEC)	flavanols (quercetin) and flavones (apigenin)	TNFα-induced VCAM-1, ICAM-1 and E-selectin expression ↓ PMN adhesion to stimulated HUVEC ↓	NF-κB transcription activation ↓	53
HUVEC	ethyl gallate	Il-1α- and TNFα-induced VCAM-1, ICAM-1 and E-selectin expression ↓ Leukocyte adhesion to stimulated HUVEC ↓	Cytokine-induced NF-κB translocation ↓	54
Human aortic endothelial cells Monocytic cell line U937	ginkgo biloba extracts (quercetin glucoside and other flavonoid glycosides)	TNFα-induced VCAM-1 and ICAM-1 expression ↓ U937 adhesion to human aortic endothelial cells ↓	NF-κB expression and activation ↓ TNFα-induced oxygen radicals production ↓	55
HUVEC THP-1 monocytes	flavones apigenin, luteolin, quercetin; catechin and epigallocatechin gallate ineffective	TNFα-induced VCAM-1 expression ↓ THP-1 adhesion to human aortic endothelial cells ↓	NF-κB nuclear translocation and DNA binding ↓	56
HUVEC THP-1 monocytes	epigallocatechin gallate and catechin	TNFα- or Il-1β- induced VCAM-1 (not ICAM-1 or E-selectin) expression ↓ TNFα-stimulated THP-1 adhesion to stimulated HUVEC ↓	NF-κB activation = Other transcription factors ↓	57
Human blood leukocytes and platelets; HL60 monocytes, P-selectin-transfected Chinese hamster ovary cell (CHO)	gallic acid	Leukocyte rolling over platelet monolayer = HL60 rolling over P-sel-CHO ↓ Leukocyte- endothelium and platelet-endothelium interactions =	Specific interaction with P-selectin	52
Human aortic endothelial cells (HAEC)	Soy flavones (apigenin), flavonols (quercetin and kaempferol)	TNFα-induced ICAM-1 and E-selectin (but not VCAM-1) expression ↓	No involvement of NF-κB; other cellular pathways	58
Human blood monocytes, HUVEC	soy isoflavones (genistein)	TNFα-simulated HUVEC- monocyte adhesion ↓ No effect on adhesive molecule (E-selectin, ICAM-1, VCAM-1 or PECAM-1)	Flow-dependent effect Activation of the nuclear transcription factor PPAR-γ	59
U937 or human blood monocytes, CD54-expressing HUVEC	equimolar mixture of genistein, daidzein, equol	U937 (or monocyte) adhesion to HUVEC ↓	Affinity of monocyte CD11a (receptor for CD54) ↓ Phytoestrogenic effect possible	60
Human PMN leukocytes and platelets	genistein, daidzein, equol	PMN homotypic aggregation ↓ PMN adhesion to thrombin-activated platelets ↓	Tyrosine protein phosphorylation ↓ Mac-1 activation ↓	61
Human saphenous vein endothelial cells (HSVEC), U937	resveratrol	TNFα-stimulated HSVEC - U937 adhesion ↓		62
Human PMN	resveratrol	Expression and activation of Mac-1 on stimulated (fMLP, C5a, orA23187) PMN ↓ PMN adhesion to thrombin-activated platelets ↓	Tyrosine protein phosphorylation ↓	63
Human blood platelet	quercetin, catechin	Collagen-induced CD40 ligand expression and ROS generation ↓ and synergistic effect of querc and cathec combination	CD40L expression related to platelet ROS generation ↓	64

Canali et al. [69] found that serum from volunteers who had ingested a single dose of red wine (5 ml/kg body weight) added to the culture medium of HUVEC, down-regulated the expression of genes for VCAM-1 and ICAM-1, but not of MCP-1. *In vitro* addition to these cells of the same wine sample, at alcohol concentrations corresponding to those measured in serum after red wine drinking, gave a different gene expression profile, resulting in up-regulation of VCAM-1, ICAM-1, and MCP-1. However, the serum phenol composition was not investigated in this study, but only the total phenol content. Direct transfer of *in vitro* observations to *in vivo* conclusions should, therefore, be made with caution, and identification and measurements of the physiologic polyphenol conjugates, as well as clarification of their biological activities, are a key prerequisite for a full understanding of the role of dietary polyphenols in human health.

Another point for future studies on biological effect of dietary phenols is the interaction between different polyphenols, as well as their interaction with drugs [70].

From an epidemiologic point of view, evidence of the beneficial cardiovascular effects of diets rich in polyphenols, mostly flavonoids, is quite large and consistent, although a recent meta-analysis has reached a negative conclusion [30]. Most of the trials available in the literature used flavonoid-rich products, rather than isolated flavonoids; thus, data are not sufficient to conclude that dietary flavonoids are the active agents in foods or beverages such as cocoa, tea, grape juice, wine, and soy, associated with decreased cardiovascular risk.

With the expected growth of interest in polyphenols, a better understanding of the role of these compounds in cardiovascular health is warranted and knowledge gaps must be clearly identified to help research advance in this promising scientific area.

Acknowledgments

We thank Maria Benedetta Donati for fruitful discussion. This work was partially supported by the Italian Ministry of Research (MIUR, Programma Triennale Ricerca, decreto 1588) and by the European Commission Sixth Framework programme (Food-CT-2005, FLORA project, contract No. 007130).

Selected References

3. Wagner DD, Frenette PS. The vessel wall and its interactions. Blood 2008;111:5271–81.
8. de Gaetano G, Donati MB, Cerletti C. Prevention of thrombosis and vascular inflammation: benefits and limitations of selective or combined COX-1, COX-2 and 5-LOX inhibitors. Trends Pharmacol Sci 2003;24:245–52.
19. Maugeri N, Brambilla M, Camera M, et al. Human polymorphonuclear leukocytes produce and express functional tissue factor upon stimulation. J Thromb Haemost 2006;4:1323–30.
51. Soulat T, Philippe C, Bal dit Sollier C, et al. Wine constituents inhibit thrombosis but not atherogenesis in C57BL/6 apolipoprotein E-deficient mice. Br J Nutr 2006;96:290–8.
67. Tribolo S, Lodi F, Connor C, et al. Comparative effects of quercetin and its predominant human metabolites on adhesion molecule expression in activated human vascular endothelial cells. Atherosclerosis 2008;197:50–6.

CHAPTER 47

Gene–Environment Interaction in the Molecular Regulation of Plasma Coagulation Proteins

Maurizio Margaglione,[1] *Elvira Grandone,*[2]
Matteo Nicola Dario Di Minno,[3] *& Giovanni Di Minno*[3]

[1] University of Foggia, IRCCS "Casa Sollievo della Sofferenza," S. Giovanni Rotondo, Foggia, Italy
[2] Unit of Thrombosis and Atherosclerosis, IRCCS "Casa Sollievo della Sofferenza,"
S. Giovanni Rotondo, Foggia, Italy
[3] Federico II University, Naples, Italy

Introduction

In Western Countries, ischemic complications of atherosclerosis, acute myocardial infarction, and ischemic stroke are the most common causes of morbidity and mortality [1]. An occlusive coronary thrombus on an ulcerated atherosclerotic plaque in the coronary arteries is the etiologic event in more than 90% of patients with Q-wave myocardial infarction [2]. The underlying abnormality in non-Q-wave myocardial infarction is often a ruptured atherosclerotic plaque, which acts as a nidus for the deposition and activation of platelets. In this case, thrombosis occurs but may not be totally occlusive, or an early spontaneous recanalization may happen. On the other hand, clinical trials show that prolonged treatment with antiplatelet drugs significantly reduces the recurrence of coronary ischemia. Thus, atherosclerosis is a necessary condition for myocardial infarction, but it is not sufficient in that it usually needs the occurrence of thrombosis.

The term "ischemic stroke" covers an array of different pathophysiological conditions. The atherosclerotic changes in the carotid and vertebrobasilar arteries resemble the atherosclerotic changes in the coronary arteries [3]. These lesions

may progress to local occlusion, but most often they do not become symptomatic until embolization to more distal arteries takes place. In the middle, anterior, and posterior cerebral arteries, the vessel wall and the lumen may be normal until the artery is suddenly occluded by an embolus derived from more proximal arterial lesions or from the heart [4]. Occlusion of the small penetrating arteries is thought to be due more often to degenerative vascular changes than to emboli, although other causes of infarction such as extracranial large-artery disease or cardioembolism are not uncommon [5]. Of these thrombotic events, only 25%–30% is prevented by the administration of antiplatelets drugs [6]. Because the rate of thrombotic disease increases progressively with aging, the risk for cardiovascular disease (CVD) and cerebrovascular disease is higher in the elderly [7,8]. Several coagulation (fibrinogen, factor VII, factor VIII) and fibrinolytic (tissue plasminogen activator [tPA]) factors rise with the increase of age, suggesting the hypothesis that a biochemical hypercoagulability and/or hypofibrinolysis in the elderly may constitute the basis for their increased thrombotic tendency [9–11]. On the other hand, an enhanced activity of coagulation enzymes has been reported in healthy men with age advancing up to 80 years [12,13] and a higher coagulation enzyme activity leading to discrete

Nutritional and Metabolic Bases of Cardiovascular Disease, 1st edition.
Edited by Mario Mancini, José M. Ordovas, Gabriele Riccardi,
Paolo Rubba and Pasquale Strazzullo. © 2011 Blackwell Publishing Ltd.

fibrin formation, and secondary hyperfibrinolysis was found in healthy centenarians without current or past thrombotic episodes [14]. These findings lend credence that hypercoagulability occurs as a consequence of the natural aging process.

Established Risk Factors

Several well-documented environmental variables modulate CHD risk. These include dietary fat, smoking, alcohol consumption, and lack of exercise [15]. In addition, personal conditions, such as overweight, diabetes mellitus, and arterial hypertension, are associated with a high risk for atherosclerosis and related ischemic complications [16] and are known to affect plasma levels of some acute-phase proteins. In recent years, epidemiologic studies have documented some hemostatic parameters whose abnormally high circulating levels may help identify subjects at risk for ischemic events. An increased risk for arterial thrombosis has been associated with high plasma levels of coagulation factors (fibrinogen, factor VII) [16–18], fibrinolytic parameters (tPA, plasminogen activator inhibitor-1 [PAI-1]),[19,20], and lipoproteins and apolipoproteins (low-density lipoprotein [LDL]-cholesterol, Lp(a), ApoB) [21,22]. Some of these, such as fibrinogen and PAI-1, are acute-phase proteins [23–25].

Coagulation and Inflammation

Inflammation plays a role in plaque formation, progression, and rupture [26–38]. Endothelial cells form a protective barrier preventing inflammatory cells from migrating into the vessel wall. However, perturbed endothelial cells express several adhesion molecules that bind leukocytes, which subsequently migrate into the subendothelial space with the aid of chemoattractant cytokines. In addition to inflammatory cells, perturbed endothelial cells leak in LDL-cholesterol, which is transformed in the vessel wall into oxidized LDL (oxLDL), a highly atherogenic molecule with proinflammatory properties. The inflammatory reaction results in vascular smooth muscle cell proliferation and migration to the site of lesion, and secretion from these cells contributes to the expansion of the extracellular matrix [29]. A thin cap separates the lipid core from the luminal blood, but production of collagen strengthens and stabilizes the fibrous cap. Macrophages produce matrix metalloproteinases (MMPs) that degrade collagen and inflammatory cytokines that influence the hemostatic activity of endothelial cells and play a role in weakening the fibrous cap resulting in plaque rupture [29] and initiation of thrombosis [30].

Searching for New Risk Factors

Geographical Puzzle

The development of arterial ischemia can only partly be accounted for by classic risk factors. In the 33 populations of the World Health Organization (WHO)/MONICA Core Study, the difference of mortality for coronary artery disease among populations was up to 20% correlated with the coexistance of hypertension, dyslipidemia, and smoking [30]. The risk for CVD and cerebrovascular ischemic disease is distributed differently throughout the world, that is, mortality for myocardial infarction is lower in southern than in northern European countries, in Japan than in North America [31–33]. Differences in lifestyle such as diet composition, smoking habits, stress, and obesity may reflect changes in incidence rate. In any case, changes in lifestyle only partially might explain these differences, suggesting that there are genetic determinants of the coronary artery and cerebrovascular disease.

Since there are many physiological and biochemical pathways involved in the development of arterial thrombosis and the human species is relatively old, with many population subdivisions and environmental changes, there are quite likely to be, on a worldwide scale, different mutations and gene combinations contributing to CVD and cerebrovascular disease. It was argued that large populations typically carry an array of alternative forms of genes that would never result in or contribute to something such as a new disease or trait if not coupled with the right environment or gene combination [34]. This concept implies that a genetic determinant increases the risk for a disease (e.g., by enhancing the plasma levels of a clotting protein, as do some polymorphisms), but it is neither necessary nor sufficient for disease expression, so-called "susceptibility locus." In other words, an allele at some locus makes it more likely that a person will become ill with a disease, but the presence of that allele is not the determining factor in disease expression. It merely lowers the threshold for the disease.

Genetic Exploration

In the last decade, genetic investigations have been carried out to better understand the pathogenesis of several diseases (e.g., cancer and metabolic diseases). Progress has also been made in our understanding of the mechanisms of genetic effects for CVDs. Observations that young individuals as well as families lacking major risk factors for thrombosis experienced thrombotic episodes fostered the search for inherited conditions predisposing to ischemic diseases [35–37]. The aggregation of ischemic disease in families and the observation that blood levels of entities considered as risk factors for CVD and cerebrovascular disease are genetically determined generated the hypothesis that the susceptibility to atherothrombotic disease could also be determined by genetic factors [38,39]. On the other hand, epidemiologic data available suggested that certain ethnic groups and specific subsets of population carried an increased risk for thrombotic cardiovascular episodes [37,40]. Genetic factors play a significant role in myocardial infarction and vascular risk factors [41]. The familial aggregation of coronary heart disease (CHD) can be in large part accounted for by clustering of CVD risk factors. It is well recognized that a history of parental CHD is associated with increased risk of myocardial ischemia [42]. The presence of coronary artery disease in a first-degree relative prior to age 55 years increases by tenfold the risk to other family members [43]. In several twin studies, most showed a strong genetic component in the pathogenesis of cardiovascular ischemia [44,45]. Although genetic factors appear to play a major role in determining the risk and development of myocardial ischemia, direct comparisons between coronary artery disease and stroke are difficult since the former is a fairly homogeneous entity and ischemic stroke is clinically and etiologically heterogeneous. By contrast with CHD, few important risk factors have been identified for ischemic stroke, and genetic factors, which seem to play a significant role in the pathogenesis of atherosclerosis, also contribute to this ischemic complication.

Aside from reported associations in small numbers of cases with Mendelian diseases, few studies have investigated the role of genetics in stroke. If genetic factors play a role in the etiology of stroke, one might expect epidemiologic studies to identify a family history of stroke as a significant risk factor. Several epidemiologic studies have examined this issue, with most being circumstantial and their results conflicting. It has been suggested that these discrepancies may be due to weakness in study design, ascertainment of family history, and inclusion of different subtypes of stroke. In the past, only four studies used modern statistical multivariate analysis to evaluate the extent to what standard risk factors played in determining stroke risk [46–49]. It is interesting to note that three of them, using multivariate statistical analysis and correction for age, did find a significant contribution of genetic factors to the development of stroke [40–43]. In parallel, a nearly fivefold increase in the prevalence of stroke among the monozygotic twin pairs compared with the dizygotic ones suggests that genetic factors may be involved in the pathogenesis of stroke [50]. Recently, a large prospective study conducted in the United Kingdom confirmed the existence of a link between a history of parental death from stroke and the risk of having stroke that appears to be independent of the established risk factors for cerebrovascular events [51].

Therefore, in addition to environmental risk factors, other important factors such as genetics and interaction with personal or environmental factors may account for a significant proportion of ischemic risk.

A strategy for identifying genes that influence cardiovascular and cerebrovascular risk is to ascertain genes that affect intermediate traits associated with atherosclerosis, for example, traits such as dyslipidemia, obesity, diabetes mellitus, and hypertension. Alternatively, phenotypes related to thrombosis, such as hypercoagulability and hypofibrinolysis, might be investigated in depth.

Gene–Environment Interaction

Gene–environment interaction implies that, in combination, the effect of the genotype and the environmental factor under study, deviates from the multiplicative effects of the factors. Some consistent examples of gene–environment interaction on

Table 47.1 Polymorphic markers and plasma levels of some predisposing factors: effect of different variables on the plasma levels of some predictors of ischemic heart disease.

Polymorphisms variable	Effect on plasma levels of the
Fibrinogen Bβ chain promoter	Up to 10% of interindividual variability. Effect of cigarette smoking and inflammation
Factor VII (Arg 353Gln)	Up to 30% of interindividual variability. Effect of triglycerides
PAI-1 (4G/5G)	Up to 26% of interindividual variability. Effect of triglycerides and inflammation
ApoE (ε2/ε4)	up to 17% of interindividual variability. Effect of sex hormones
MTHFR (C677T)	up to 30% of total plasma total homocysteine levels. Effect of folates and vitamin B_{12}

CHD risk exist. *ApoE* variants seem to play a role on CHD risk [52]. Moderate alcohol consumption has been shown to be cardioprotective, but the beneficial effect of moderate alcohol consumption appears to be modified by variation in the gene for alcohol dehydrogenase [53,54]. Triglycerides regulate plasma levels of PAI-1 and coagulation factor VII, as do folates for homocysteine. The presence of common molecular variations (polymorphisms) that confer sensitivity to the environmental factor clarifies this possibility (Table 47.1 and Figure 47.1). As a matter of fact, in addition to monitoring of variables difficult to be checked by alternative means (ApoE), studies on polymorphic markers have argued for fluctuations of some variables (fibrinogen, PAI-1, factor VII, MTHFR) as being the result of the interaction of some molecular variations with environmental factors.

Hunting for Genetic Risk Markers

Problems in defining gene variations or mutations that contribute to the propensity for common multifactorial, "complex," disorders, for example, myocardial infarction and ischemic stroke, are several. The genetic basis of complex diseases such as CHD and ischemic stroke very likely consists of several predisposing risk factors that can interact with environmental factors to produce the disease phenotype. Unlike single gene disorders where the relationship is essentially qualitative, complex disorders imply the involvement of many factors with variable and additive effects. A candidate gene or combination of genetic markers may be present in individuals, a single family, or populations that will not suffer from the target disease. In addition, based on the concept of the "selection by death," if genetic determinants play a role in determining arterial

thrombosis, why are they so much frequent? Most of the arterial ischemic disease develops late in life, after or during the reproductive years. A number of therapeutic strategies are now applied, allowing individuals who otherwise would suffer or die from arterial thrombosis to live and spread potentially deleterious genes to offsprings. Urbanization and "Westernized" lifestyle (diets, inactivity, pollution, stress) were not so prevalent in the past but are now represented in different degree throughout the world. Finally, it must be considered that a small contribution of any individual gene to the total incidence of the disorder needs a large sample, and hidden small biases in selection of patient and control groups could obscure positive data and make reproducibility difficult.

Understanding the role that functional gene polymorphisms play in cardiovascular risk and determining the levels of intermediate phenotypes (e.g. lipids) is essential to our understanding of the important metabolic pathways in the diseased and disease-free state. To address such polygenic structure is a challenge likely requiring simultaneous analysis of several risk factors, including genetic variants, in large study samples rich in phenotypes. Gene–gene and gene–environment interaction studies have recently attempted to answer this challenge by analyzing the interacting relations of putative risk loci [55–59]. The majority of these studies, however, use two to three genetic markers, thus failing to address the physiological entities or the underlying complex genetic profiles. The study of gene–environment interaction not only provides a useful means to improve our understanding of disease pathology at the molecular level but also allows for specific targeting of advice and therapies to high-risk subjects (those with a high-risk genotype in a high-risk environment).

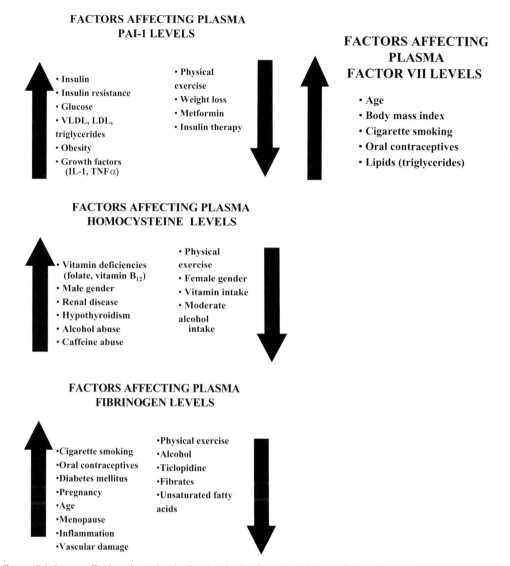

FACTORS AFFECTING PLASMA
PAI-1 LEVELS

• Insulin
• Insulin resistance
• Glucose
• VLDL, LDL, triglycerides
• Obesity
• Growth factors (IL-1, TNFα)

• Physical exercise
• Weight loss
• Metformin
• Insulin therapy

FACTORS AFFECTING
PLASMA
FACTOR VII LEVELS

• Age
• Body mass index
• Cigarette smoking
• Oral contraceptives
• Lipids (triglycerides)

FACTORS AFFECTING PLASMA
HOMOCYSTEINE LEVELS

• Vitamin deficiencies (folate, vitamin B$_{12}$)
• Male gender
• Renal disease
• Hypothyroidism
• Alcohol abuse
• Caffeine abuse

• Physical exercise
• Female gender
• Vitamin intake
• Moderate alcohol intake

FACTORS AFFECTING PLASMA
FIBRINOGEN LEVELS

•Cigarette smoking
•Oral contraceptives
•Diabetes mellitus
•Pregnancy
•Age
•Menopause
•Inflammation
•Vascular damage

•Physical exercise
•Alcohol
•Ticlopidine
•Fibrates
•Unsaturated fatty acids

Figure 47.1 Factors affecting plasma levels of major clotting factors involved in atherothrombosis.

Conclusions

Genetic factors that modulate the individual susceptibility to CVDs are common, functionally different forms of genes (polymorphisms), which are likely to have a modest effect at an individual level but because of their high frequency in the population can be associated with a high attributable risk. Environmental factors can modify the effects of a polymorphism, either by providing a necessary substrate for development of disease or by modulating the expression (effects) of the gene. The context

dependency (i.e., the importance of environmental [including nutritional] factors in influencing genetic risk) is now recognized. An allele may have a modest effect on risk in individuals who maintain a low environmental risk, but a major effect in a high-risk environment. There is now accumulating evidence that most of the susceptibility genes for common diseases do not have a primary etiological role in predisposition to disease. Rather, they act as response modifiers to exogenous factors such as stress, environment, disease, and drug intake. A better characterization of the interactions between environmental and genetic factors is a key issue in our understanding their role in the pathogenesis of multifactorial diseases such as myocardial infarction and ischemic stroke.

References

6. Davi G, Patrono C. Platelet activation and atherothrombosis. N Engl J Med 2007;357:2482–94.

15. Di Minno G, Grandone E, Margaglione M. Clinical relevance of polymorphic markers of arterial thrombosis. Thromb Haemost 1997;78(1):462–6.

16. Kannell WB. Bishop lecture: Contribution of the Framingham study to preventive cardiology. J.Am.Coll. Cardiol. 1990;15,206–211.

54. Younis J, Cooper JA, Miller GJ, et al. Genetic variation in alcohol dehydrogenase 1C and the beneficial effect of alcohol intake on coronary heart disease risk in the Second Northwick Park Heart Study. Atherosclerosis 2005; 180:225–32.

55. Ma DQ, Whitehead PL, Menold MM, et al. Identification of significant association and gene-gene interaction of GABA receptor subunit genes in autism. Am J Hum Genet 2005;77:377–88.

CHAPTER 48

Nutrition and Cardiovascular Disease: ω-3 PUFA

Elena Tremoli[1], Matteo Nicola Dario Di Minno[2], &
Giovanni Di Minno[2]
[1] University of Milan, Milan, Italy
[2] Federico II University, Naples, Italy

Introduction

Modern nutrition has emphasized health benefits of maintaining sufficient levels of the very-long-chain PUFA (i.e., C20 and C22) that belong to the ω-3 family. Such bioactive compounds, whose predominant sources are fish and vegetable oils, are not convertible and have very different biochemical roles. Linoleic acid (LA, ω-6) and α-linolenic acid (ALA, ω-3), with more than one double bond in their hydrocarbon backbone [1], are two of the main representative compounds of this class. Extreme nutritional deficiency of these fats results in a neuropathy that can be reversed with rapeseed oil or with other vegetable oils containing LA and ALA. Because they prevent deficiency symptoms and cannot be synthesized by humans (need to be supplied exogenously), they are defined as essential fatty acids (EFAs).

ω-3 PUFA: Biochemistry and Physiology

Recommended Intakes

In Europe, the suggested minimum requirement for LA is approximately 1% of energy intake, the minimum requirement for LNA being 0.2%–0.5% of en-

ergy intake [2,3]. In the United States, it is suggested that total PUFA intake should remain at 7% of energy intake and not exceed 10% [4]. In Japan [5], despite that the current dietary intake is approximately 26%, with a balanced intake of ω-6 and ω-3 PUFA, a gradual increased in the ratio, particularly in young persons, is observed. Hence, a more exhaustive nutritional education effort is necessary [6]. Several countries have recommended allowances not only for the absolute amount of PUFA, but also for a balanced intake of ω-6 and ω-3 PUFA. Adequate intake of ω-3 PUFAs is particularly important for women of childbearing age. An estimated 25 g of maternal DHA is required during pregnancy and lactation to support the development of the fetal and infant brain. Higher maternal intake in pregnancy may also reduce the risk of allergic disease in the offspring. However, a study of ω-6:ω-3 fatty acid ratios in umbilical cord blood showed only very weak direct associations with the onset of eczema and wheeze in infants [7]. Women of childbearing age are recommended to eat one or two portions of oily fish per week (about 0.4–0.8 g/day of ω-3 fats) but not more, given hypothetical concerns about toxic contaminants [2]. Accordingly, women before and during pregnancy and children younger than 16 years are advised by the U.K. government to avoid consumption of large predatory fish such as swordfish, which have accumulated high concentrations of mercury. For other adults, a maximum of four portions of oily fish per week are advised, including no more than one of swordfish, shark, etc [2].

Nutritional and Metabolic Bases of Cardiovascular Disease, 1st edition.
Edited by Mario Mancini, José M. Ordovas, Gabriele Riccardi,
Paolo Rubba and Pasquale Strazzullo. © 2011 Blackwell Publishing Ltd.

Metabolism

Within the human organism, the 18-carbon precursors ω-3 and ω-6 fatty acids are not inter-convertible and can be elongated and desaturated to more highly unsaturated members of their family, especially arachidonic acid (AA) and DHA. The liver is the primary site for EFA metabolism [8]. The first part of this pathway to AA and docosapen-taenoic acid (C22:5 ω-3 , DPA), respectively, takes place in the endoplasmic reticulum and consists of sequential alternating elongation and desaturation steps catalyzed by fatty acid elongase, Δ6- and Δ5-desaturase. The Δ6-desaturase is the rate-limiting step of the pathway. EFA in the plasma membranes serves as substrates for the enzyme cyclooxygenase (COX) and lipoxygenase (LOX) and are converted into a variety of very active, short-lived, hormone-like compounds referred to as "eicosanoids." The families of prostaglandins, leukotrienes, and related compounds are called eicosanoids because they are derived from 20-carbon EFAs that contain three, four, or five double bonds (AA, EPA, and DHA) and include prostaglandins (prostaglandin H [PGH], prostaglandin D [PGD], prostaglandin E [PGE], prostaglandin F [PGF]), prostacyclins (PGI), thromboxanes (TXA, TXB), and leukotrienes (LTA, LTB, LTC, LTD). In humans, AA is the most abundant precursor of this series. It is either derived from dietary LA or ingested as a dietary constituent. AA is esterified into the phospholipids of the cell membrane or other complex lipids. Since the concentration of free AA in the cell is very low, the biosynthesis of eicosanoids depends primarily upon its release from cellular stores by phospholipase A_2 (PLA_2). AA is the parent fatty acid of prostaglandins and thromboxanes of the two series, and the series four leukotrienes. In particular prostacyclin (PGI_2) is a potent vasodilator and antiplatelet agent; thromboxane A_2 (TXA_2) is a potent vasoconstrictor and pro-aggregating agent. Because of the increased amount of ω-6 fatty acids in the Western diet, eicosanoids from AA are formed in larger quantities than those formed from ω-3 fatty acids. EPA is the substrate for the series three prostanoids and the series five leukotrienes. Prostaglandins and thromboxanes of the three series exert a very limited proaggregatory and vaso-constrictive activity. In particular, while TXA_3 is

devoid of vasoconstrictor and proaggregating activities, PGI_3 exerts a vasodilator and antiplatelet effect.

Further prothrombotic and antithrombotic properties of ω-3 PUFA include lowering of plasma triglycerides; very-low-density lipoprotein (VLDL)-cholesterol; monocyte adhesion to endothelial cells; platelet-derived growth factor (PDGF) and LTB4; and enhancement of high-density lipoprotein (HDL)-cholesterol and of membrane fluidity [1]. From the precursors AA and EPA, the synthesis of prostaglandins is accomplished by COX (also called endoperoxide synthase, or fatty acid cyclooxygenase), a ubiquitous complex of microsomal enzymes. There are two isoforms of this enzyme: COX-1 and COX-2. The former is constitutively expressed in most cells (i.e., gastric mucosa, vasculature, glomeruli, and collecting ducts of the kidney) and is more concentrated on the endoplasmic reticulum. COX-2 is not constitutively present but may be induced at sites of inflammation, both in the endoplasmic reticulum and over the surface of the nucleus, by certain serum factors such as inflammatory cytokines (interleukin [IL]-1, IL-1β, IL-6, tumor necrosis factor [TNF]-α); growth factor (transforming growth factor (TGF)-β, endothelial growth factor [EGF]); tumor promoters (phorbol esters), and cyclic adenosine monophosphate (cAMP). Such expression is inhibited by glucocorticoids such as dexamethasone [9–11]. COX-2 oxidizes 18-carbon PUFA with much higher efficiency than COX-1 [12]. More in detail, DHA inhibits COX-1 [12]. Nonsteroid anti-inflammatory drugs compete directly (aspirin being the only one competing irreversibly) with arachidonate for binding to both the COX-1 and COX-2 site, thus inhibiting their activity [11].

Nutritional experiments and clinical studies [13,14] show that ingested EPA and DHA from fish or fish oil may replace AA in membrane phospholipids, especially platelets, erythrocytes, neutrophils, monocytes, and liver cells. The metabolites of EPA, DHA, and AA have competitive functions: At variance with AA, prostanoids and leukotrienes from EPA and DHA have antichemotactic, anti-inflammatory, and antivasoconstrictive properties. Since prostaglandins and thromboxanes of the three series exert a very limited proaggregatory and vasoconstrictive activity, AA is replaced by ingested EPA and DHA in membrane phospholipids, and this leads to a metabolic shift that in turn causes an antithrombotic state. The latter is due to a decrease in platelet aggregation, an increase in vasodilation, a decrease in whole blood viscosity, and an increase in bleeding time. In view of this, EPA and DHA are thought to be important in the treatment of thrombotic complications of arthrosclerosis, cancer, rheumatoid arthritis, psoriasis, and diseases of old age such as Alzheimer's and age-related macular degeneration [13–15].

Recently an alternative metabolic route for PUFA oxidation has been focused. *In vivo*, PUFA derived from membrane phospholipids can undergo auto-oxidation, generating a mixture of hydroperoxides, epoxides, and cyclic peroxides [16]. Of particular interest are the isoprostanes and epoxides of AA and of other PUFA. Isoprostanes of PUFA form a family of prostaglandin-related compounds, acting as autacoids. The urinary isoprostane index offers a method to estimate *in vivo* lipid peroxidation in various diseases. Epoxides of PUFA can be formed by autooxidation, by cytochrome P450, and possibly by the oxidative burst of inflammatory cells [17]. Epoxides of ALA are toxic, whereas epoxides of AA have a wide range of biological effects, in particular the 5,6-epoxide of AA is an excellent substrate of COX and thromboxane synthase, with vascular and renal effects [17].

ω-3 PUFAs and Prevention of CHD: Randomized Studies

In the early 1960 and 1970s, dietary advice to prevent recurrence of CHD was inconclusive. This was likely due to the small (approximately 500) number of subjecs examined. Moreover, in these studies, attempts to lower plasma cholesterol levels in survivors of MI were based on diets lower in fats or with high polyunsatuted/saturated ratios. Excessive consumption of foods containing ω-3 PUFAs increases total fat intake. In view of this, the intake of saturated fats was decreased and that of unsaturated was increased. Thus, the study design and the sample size may have been inadequate to address the issue [14]. In the 1980s, three retro-

spective studies [18–20] showed an inverse relation between fish consumption and CHD mortality. In parallel, fish fats containing EPA were shown to impair platelet aggregation and thromboxane formation, two major events in arterial thrombosis [21]. The combined data fostered the search for potential intenelationships between nutrition and thrombogenic factors.

The results of the large prospective Diet and Reinfarction Triad (DART) in the secondary prevention of MI [22] have further supported the possibility of such interrelationships. The DART study randomized 2,033 men who had recovered from a MI to advice to eat at least two portions (200–400 g) of oily fish per week, advice to reduce their total fat and saturated fat intake, or advice to increase their intake of cereal fiber. At 2 years, about 22% of patients who could not tolerate the recommended amount of fish took fish oils as a partial or total substitute. At this time, about 30% fewer people in the fish advice group died than those in other groups (9.3% vs. 12.8%; relative risk [RR], 0.71, 95% confidence interval [CI], 0.54–0.93), which was due to a reduction in CHD death (7.7% vs. 11.4%). There was no significant reduction in CHD events overall (CHD death or nonfatal MI) probably because the reduction in CHD death was counterbalanced by an increase in nonfatal MI. The equivalent weekly consumption of EPA was about 2.5 g (300 g of oily fish). The Lyon Heart study was a prospective, randomized single-blinded multicentric trial whose primary endpoints were death and nonfatal infarction [23]. Of the 600 survivors enlisted, half adopted a prudential diet and as many adopted a Mediterranean-type of diet, with more bread, vegetables, fish, fresh fruit, and olive oil (or margarine enriched in ALA for subjects who did not like olive oil). The subjects were analyzed for 5 years starting 6 months after the ischemic event. At the 2-year follow-up, there were 16 cardiovascular deaths in the control group and 3 in the experimental one. While no major effect was found on noncardiovascuiar mortality, the overall mortality was 20% in the control group and 8% in the experimental group. As with the DART study, the beneficial effect of this diet occurred early after randomization and was not associated with changes in plasma cholesterol or HDL-cholesterol levels. After correction for other factors, a surprisingly high (76%) reduction in the risk of cardiac death was found during the observation period. The protective effect of the experimental diet was associated with enhanced plasma levels of EPA and its parent fatty acid, ALA. In keeping with this, arachidonic acid was significantly reduced in subjects who had received the experimental diet. However, variables other than EPA were affected by a Mediterranean type of diet (experimental) in the Lyon Heart Study. The potent antioxidant substance, vitamin E, was significantly increased, while granulocyte count was lowered. Several retrospective and one prospective study have shown the association of high-normal white cell counts with cerebral thrombosis and reinfarction, the maximal association being found with granulocyte counts [24,25]. The combined data raise the possibility of thrombogenic mechanisms other than PUFAs in the cardioprotective effects of Mediterranean type of diets. Several authors have reported a variety of potential mechanisms of ω-3 PUFA (Table 48.1) that may be relevant to their antithrombotic potential. The Gissi Prevenzione trial [26] was a prospective, multicentric, open-labeled trial with a factorial design, in which 11,324 recent (<3 months) survivors of a first MI at age 50–80 years were randomly assigned to receive, in addition to the usual GISSI strategy (aspirin, β-blockers, nitrate, ACE-I,

statins), a supplementation of ω-3 PUFA (1 g/day corresponding to 850 mg of a mixture of EPA + DHA in a 1.0:1.4 ratio), vitamin E (300 mg/day), or the combination of ω-3 PUFA + vitamin E. The clinical assessment and food questionnaires were obtained at 6 months [6,12,18,30] and 42 months. Primary end-points were all-cause death, cardiovascular death, nonfatal MI, and stroke. While the treatment with vitamin E was not effective regarding event-free survival (293/2,828 in controls vs. 252/2,830, $p = .07$), the treatment with ω-3 PUFA significantly reduced the risk of cardiovascular disease (293/2,828 vs. 236/2,836, 10.4% two-way analysis, 15% four-way analysis, $p = .009$). The effect of the combination of PUFA + vitamin E (293/2,828 vs. 236/2,830, $p = .01$) was comparable to the ω-3 PUFA supplementation alone. When the data were stratified according to individual end-points, cardiovascular death (−30%), CHD death (−35%), total death (−20%), and sudden death (−45%) were all significantly reduced by the ω-3 PUFA supplementation. The 45% reduction in sudden death was not associated with changes in the use of drugs (e.g., antiplatelet agents, β-blockers, ACE inhibitors, or cholesterol-lowering agents) that may play a role in lowering the number of complex arrhythmias, thus the underlying mechanism remains elusive. On the other hand, in keeping with this, in

Table 48.1 Major dietary plant polyphenols and antioxidants.

Compound	Dietary source	Class/subclass/other
Apigenin	Parsley, artichoke, basil, celery, citrus fruit	Flavone
Caffeic acid	Red wine	Hydroxycinnamic acid
Chlorogenic acid	Coffee	Hydroxycinnamic acid
Daidzein	Soy milk, extract and nuts	Isoflavone
(−)-Epigallocathechin gallate (EGCG)	Green tea	Flavanol
Genistein	Soy milk, extract and nuts	Isoflavone
Hesperidin	Orange juice	Flavanone
Hydroxytyrosol	Extra virgin olive oil	Hydroxylated tyrosol
Kaempferol	Apples, onions, leeks, citrus fruits, grapes, red wine, tea	Flavonol
Luteolin	Celery, green pepper, perilla, camomile tea	Flavone
Lycopene	Tomatoes, tomato sauce	Carotenoid
Myricetin	Walnuts, grapes, berries, vegetables, wine	Flavonol
Oleuropein	Extra virgin olive oil	Tyrosol ester of elenolic acid
Pro-delphinidin B-2 3′-O-gallate	Green tea	Anthocyanin
Quercetin	Apples, onions	Flavonol
Resveratrol	Red wine, grapes, peanuts, soy	Stilbenes

79 patients with complex arrhythmias, ω-3 PUFA supplementation reduced the number of premature ventricular beats [27,28]; in 52 survivors of acute MI with left ventricular dysfunction, consumption of fish at least once a week was associated with marked effects on heart rate variability [29]; and in the Physicians' Health study, there was a strong inverse correlation between fish consumption and sudden death as well as total mortality [30,31]. Moreover, in the Nurses' Health Study (NHS), a 16-year cohort study in 84,688 female nurses, a higher consumption of fish and ω-3 PUFAs was associated with a 30% reduction in the risk of major coronary events. This reduction increased when the authors considered only fatal events (coronary deaths) [31]. Compared with women who seldom ate fish (less than once a month), those who ate fish weekly had an RR of CHD (CHD death or nonfatal MI) of 0.71 (95% CI, 0.58–0.87) and those who ate fish two to four times a week, had an RR of 0.69 (95% CI, 0.55–0.88). Eating fish appeared to have the greatest benefit in people at high risk of CHD. An antiarrhytmic/antifibrillatory effect of EPA is documented [32]. In 14 healthy volunteers, a one-month supplementation of a preparation of EPA and DHA superimposable to that employed in the GISSI Prevenzione study caused in parallel with increases in the plasma and platelet content of EPA and DHA, an impaired aggregation of platelets in response to collagen or ADP, which correlated ($p = .036$ and $.068$, respectively) to changes in the intracellular pH (pHi) of the Na^+/H^+ reverse transport [33]. In addition to platelet function, the latter mechanism is important as to lymphocyte function and blood pressure control [34,35]. The impaired aggregation was independent of thromboxane biosynthesis in that study. An additional explanation to elucidate the reduction of sudden death in the GISSI Prevenzione Study involves the fact that more than 80% of individuals were simultaneously receiving aspirin and of ω-3 PUFA. Since aspirin impairs thromboxane formation, a major mechanism of platelet activation and ω-3 PUFA impair ADP-induced aggregation, another important mechanism of platelet activation, sudden death prevention may well be the result of a more intensive anti-platelet treatment. Studies in other settings (coronary artery bypass graft, coronary stenting GISSI HF, etc) where the combination of an-

tiplatelet agents greatly reduced coronary deaths support this formulation.

In spite of mechanistic uncertainties, until the publication of the follow-up and of the DART-2 trial in 2003 [36,37], the evidence was that ω-3 from oily fish or supplements reduced the risks of fatal MI, sudden death, and overall mortality among people with existing disease [14]. DART-2 included 3,114 men with stable angina and tested the hypothesis that the main benefit of ω-3 fat was derived from its antiarrhythmic action in the presence of chronic disease. Surprisingly, DART-2 did not confirm this, showing an excess of sudden and total cardiac deaths. The excess was maximal in participants taking fish oil capsules rather than eating oily fish.

DART-2 is not the only study to show that ω-3 fat supplements have pro-arrhythmic as well as antiarrhythmic actions. A 2-year trial randomized 200 participants with an implantable cardioverter defibrillator and a recent episode of ventricular tachycardia or ventricular fibrillation to 1.3 g/day of ω-3 fats or placebo. The supplements did not prevent recurrent arrhythmia and appeared to be proarrhythmic in patients with ventricular tachycardia [38]. Since in the data obtained from the GISSI Prevenzione trial the evidence does support early protection against sudden death, it may be wise to make a distinction between patients with chronic disease, such as angina, and those with acute MI. However long term-term administration (3.9 years of follow-up) of 1 g/day ω-3 PUFA to a large population ($n = 3,494$) of patients with heart failure (HF), all receiving treatments of proven efficacy for chronic HF (ACE inhibitors, beta blockers, diuretics, digitalis, spironolactone) were effective in reducing all-cause mortality [adjusted HR (95.5% CI): 0.91 (0.833–0.998); p value: 0.041], and hospitalisations for cardiovascular reasons [adjusted HR (99% CI): 0.92 (0.849–0.999); p value 0.009]. The benefit was smaller than expected (RRR 7%–9% vs. assumed 15%), but it was supported by per-protocol analysis (RRR 12%–14%), and consistent across all the predefined subgroups. Major causes of death were worsening HF, 9.1% vs. 9.5% in the placebo ($n = 3,481$) group; presumed arrhythmia, 7.8% vs. 8.7% in the placebo group. No adverse events were noted (39). Finally, from studies on polygenic disorders, we have learned that by lowering the threshold and becoming a susceptibility gene, a polymorphism can lead to an effect assuming that it is present in the appropriate milieu [39]. The Lyon Heart Study has documented that nutrients may affect major determinants of myocardial ischemia such as fibrinogen or factor VII. However, the exent to what these and other hemostatic variables have been affected in studies devoted to dietary prevention of ischemia remains presently elusive.

ω-3 PUFAs and Prevention of Cardiovascular Death: Meta-analyses of Randomized Clinical Studies

A meta-analysis of 11 randomized clinical trials (RCTs) (duration 6–46 months) of ω-3 PUFA supplementation (nine trials) or advice to increase dietary fish intake (two trials) in patients with CHD first assessed a significant reduction in all-cause mortality (RR, 0.8; 95% CI. 0.7–0.9), fatal MI (RR, 0.7; 95% CI, 0.6–0.8), and sudden death (RR, 0.7; 95% CI, 0.6–0.9), but not nonfatal MI, with the fish/ ω-3 PUFA intervention [40]. However, the long-term benefits of eating fish were less clear. The DART study [36,37] did not find a long-term survival benefit in the fish-advice group after 10 years, but there was a less marked difference in fish consumption between groups at this time. On the other hand, one observational study in men without CHD at baseline found that eating oily fish was associated with a reduced CHD mortality while eating lean fish (e.g. plaice, cod, bream, perch, and pike) was not, suggesting that the type of fish is important [41]. Moreover, over the last months, a careful systematic meta-analysis that appeared in the *British Medical Journal (BMJ)* has drawn attention to uncertainties about some of the health benefits attributed to ω-3 fats. Of 15,159 titles and abstracts assessed, 48 RCTs (36,913 participants) and 41 cohort studies analysed, the pooled estimate showed no strong evidence of reduced risk of total mortality (RR, 0.87; 95% CI, 0.73–1.03) or combined cardiovascular events (RR, 0.95; 95% CI, 0.82–1.12) in participants taking additional ω-3 fats. The few studies at low risk of bias were more consistent, but they showed no effect of ω-3 on total mortality (RR, 0.98; 95% CI, 0.70–1.36) or cardiovascular events

(RR, 1.09; 95% CI, 0.87–1.37). When data from the subgroup of studies of long-chain ω-3 PUFAs were analysed separately, total mortality (RR, 0.86; 95% CI, 0.70–1.04; 138 events) and cardiovascular events (RR, 0.93; 95% CI, 0.79–1.11) were not clearly reduced. Accordingly, the authors concluded that the long-chain and shorter-chain ω-3 fats do not show a clear effect on total mortality, combined cardiovascular events, or cancer [42,43]. Neither RCTs nor cohort studies suggested increased risk of cancer with a higher intake of ω-3 PUFAs 3 (trials: RR, 1.07; 95% CI, 0.88–1.30; cohort studies: RR, 1.02; 95% CI, 0.87–1.19). Nor the claim that ω-3 PUFAs reduce the risk of cancer was not supported here or by another recent systematic review [44]. The findings of this meta-analysis differ from those of the systematic review by Bucher et al. [40], the latter being less comprehensive than the *BMJ* review [42,43]. The systematic review by Bucher et al. [40], did not include the DART 2 study [36,37]. The latter had the longest follow-up of all RCTs; it was the only RCT that specifically enrolled men treated for angina; moreover, in the latter, ω-3 PUFAs from oily fish had a different effect to fish oil supplements (but this was found not to explain the differences). Together, the two meta-analyses led to the concept that the effect of ω-3 PUFAs on cardiovascular disease is smaller than previously thought, and that its beneficial effect is limited to a specific group (patients after a MI or with heart failure).

Conclusions

Seventy-five years ago, long-chain ω-3 PUFAs were added to the list of essential nutrients [13]. Presently, while their use in childhood, lactation, and pregnancy is established, there are too few trials with adequate allocation concealment, as to the prevention of CHD, cancer, and other chronic disorders. Moreover, with respect to each health outcome analyzed, there are too few cohort studies in which the intake of ω-3 fat rather than total fish intake has been measured. Thus, newer more focused trials in the area are needed. To this end, two prerequisites deserve to be addressed:

a) either for geographic, nutritional, allergic, or economic reasons, not all communities have ready access to fish supplies. Significant issues deserve to be elucidated before plants can become commercially viable sources of ω-3 fatty acids. Microalgae are the primary producers of PUFA. Single-cell oils derived from fermentation of microalgae PUFA have promising biotechnological market both for feed and food, such as infant milk formulas with enriched DHA, and hens fed with microalgae to produce "OMEGA eggs." Unlike seafood, microalgal oils are cholesterol free and may help incorporate PUFA from other dietary sources. However, at present their cost of production is high. Crop plants may provide a much cheaper supply, provided they can be genetically engineered to synthesize sufficient concentrations of PUFA. Sequences encoding all major enzymes involved in microsomal PUFA biosynthesis have been cloned [13].

b) From studies on polygenic disorders, we have learned that by lowering the threshold and becoming a susceptibility gene, a polymorphism can lead to an effect assuming that it is present in the appropriate milieu [27]. Although nutrients affect major determinants of myocardial ischemia such as fib-rinogen and factor VII or PAI-1, the extent to what these and other hemostatic variables have been affected in studies devoted to dietary prevention of ischemia is elusive.

Selected References

2. Wang C, Chung M, Balk E, et al. Effects of omega-3 fatty acids on cardiovasculardisease. Rockville, MD: Agency for Health care Research and Quality; 2004.

13. Patil V, Gislerød HR. The importance of omega-3 fatty acids in diet. Current Sci 2006;90(7):908–9.

14. Di Minno G, Tufano A, Garofano T, Di Minno MND. Polyunsaturated fatty acids, thrombosis and vascular disease. Patophysiol Haemostasis Thrombosis 2002;32: 361–4.

38. Raitt MH, Connor WE, Morris C, et al. Fish oil supplementation and risk of ventricular tachycardia and ventricular fibrillation in patients with implantable defibrillators—randomized controlled trial. JAMA 2005;293: 2884–91.

42. Hooper L, Thompson RL, Harrison RA, et al. Risks and benefits of omega3 fats for mortality, cardiovascular disease and cancer: a systematic review. BMJ 2006;332: 752–5.

CHAPTER 49

Nutrition and Cardiovascular Disease: Homocysteine

Matteo Nicola Dario Di Minno[1], Elena Tremoli[2], &
Giovanni Di Minno[1]
[1]Federico II University, Naples, Italy
[2]University of Milan, Milan, Italy

Introduction

In the late 1960s McCully first suggested a link between homocysteine and vascular disease [1]. He observed that an infant with homocystinuria as a result of a rare condition of abnormal cobalamin metabolism exhibited widespread, severe arteriosclerosis indistinguishable from the lesions seen in cases of homocystinuria due to cystathionine β-synthase deficiency. Because hyperhomocysteinemia was common to these two metabolic disorders, McCully proposed that hyperhomocysteinemia results in arteriosclerotic disease. Seven years later, Wilcken and Wilcken showed that the concentration of homocysteine-cysteine mixed disulfide after a methionine load was slightly higher in coronary heart disease (CHD) patients than in age- and sex-matched controls [2]. This pioneering work has led to important studies [3,4] that allowed for the conclusion that both in men and women, elevations of plasma thCY are an independent graded risk factor for with CHD or cerebrovascular or peripheral vascular disease. In the following years, there has been a debate on whether thCY elevation is truly a risk factor or an epiphenomenon of atherosclerotic disease [5,6]. The debate has also been extended to those

studies that failed to show any relation between atherosclerotic vascular disease and homozygosity for the C677T mutation in the methylenetetrahydrofolate reductase (MTHFR) gene, which is associated with mild elevations of plasma thCY [7]. A meta-analysis in 1998 showed that the C677T mutation of the MTHFR gene is a weak risk factor for cardiovascular disease (CVD) [8]. This conclusion has been challenged on the basis of the different prevalence of this mutation in various ethnic groups [9]. Moreover, because folate and vitamins B_6 and B_{12} regulate HCY levels, the folate status of the population should have been taken into consideration while evaluating the link between HCY and CHD [10,11]. Finally, in an approach based on the concept of Mendelian randomization, the observed increase in risk of stroke among individuals homozygous for the MTHFR T allele is close to that predicted from the differences in thCY concentration conferred by this variant [12]. However, the relation between elevated plasma thCY and vascular disease is stronger in retrospective than in prospective studies [13]. Furthermore, major intervention studies showed that, while leading to a decrease in HCY levels, vitamin supplementation fails to have any significant effect on cardiovascular risk. In the following paragraphs, we discuss this complex issue, with emphasis on HCY metabolism and its regulation, animal models of disorders of HCY metabolism, thrombogenic mechanism(s) of HCY, and a critical review of the trials available.

Nutritional and Metabolic Bases of Cardiovascular Disease, 1st edition.
Edited by Mario Mancini, José M. Ordovas, Gabriele Riccardi,
Paolo Rubba and Pasquale Strazzullo. © 2011 Blackwell Publishing Ltd.

The Thrombogenic Mechanism of Homocysteine

Abnormalities of Platelet/Endothelial Cells

In homocystinuric patients as well as in nonhuman primates, platelet survival has been reported abnormally low [14,15]. In keeping with this, increased platelet *stickiness* was shown in the blood of homocystinuric patients and *in vitro* after the addition of homocysteine to plasma [14]. The latter has been challenged [15]. Increased platelet aggregation after HCY exposure has been documented. This concept has been challenged as well [14,15]. Discrepancies also exist about the effect of homocysteine thiolactone (HTL), the cyclic oxidation product of homocysteine, on platelet function. Early studies suggested that HTL had only a very small effect on platelet aggregation. However, at variance with the inactive salt (hydrochloride form), the free base of HTL fosters platelet aggregation. On the other hand, in synergism with other methyltransferase inhibitors, HTL inhibits platelet aggregation. A study that sheds light on such discrepancies is that of Stamler et al. [16]. Indeed, these authors have shown that homocysteine does not cause platelet aggregation. Instead, HCY increases platelet adhesion to endothelial cells (ECs) as a consequence of its toxic effect on the endothelium itself. ECs produce endothelium-derived relaxing factor (EDRF), which reacts with HCY to form 5 nitroso-homocysteine (SNOHO). The latter is a strong antiplatelet agent with a 5-minute half-life (for comparison, EDRF half-life is about 5–30 seconds). Therefore, in normal conditions, the toxicity of HCY is prevented by the formation of SNOHO. When HCY levels saturate the available amounts of EDRF, unmodified HCY becomes available, thus causing endothelial injury, with a consequent reduction of the EDRF production, followed by reduced formation of SNOHO and in turn of the antiplatelet potential. These data suggest a role for an oxidant stress in the risk of thrombosis related to elevated levels of HCY. In particular, the possibility that hydrogen peroxide is responsible for the cellular damage induced by HCY has been analyzed in detail by Starkebaum and Harlan [17]. Copper-catalyzed auto-oxidation of cysteine in alkaline media leads to the reduction of oxygen

and the generation of hydrogen peroxide. In view of this, Starkebaum and Harian showed that in a cell-free system, increasing concentrations of copper (1–50 M) increases HCY oxidation in a dose-dependent fashion. The addition of catalase to the system reduced oxygen consumption by nearly one half, thus suggesting that H_2O_2 was formed during the reaction. However, H_2O_2 did not accumulate in the presence of HCY, suggesting that HCY itself can scavenge H_2O_2. Interestingly, concentrations of 0.05–50 fM Cu_2 increased the rate of H_2O_2 formation, whereas at concentrations above 5 pM the formation of H_2O_2 was reduced, probably due to Cu catalysed reduction of H_2O_2 to water. The relationship between copper, HCY, and endothelial injury was further documented by the observation that a dose-dependent lysis of cultured bovine aortic endothelial cells occurred only when homocysteine (up to 5 mM) was added to endotelial cells in the presence of copper (2 pM). As for endothelial cells, the possibility has been explored that an oxidant stress may be involved in the platelet activation mediated by HCY. When severely increased in plasma (>100 pM/L), HCY can leak into the urine causing homocystinuria. In this severe form of hyperhomocysteinaemia, premature arteriosclerosis and arterial and venous thrombosis are common findings. Biochemical measurements of urinary metabolites and clinical trials with aspirin, indicate that enhanced biosynthesis of thromboxane A_2 (TXA_2) by platelet arachidonic acid is a major contributor to the risk of thrombosis associated with several risk factors [18]. We have previously reported [19] an abnormally high urinary excretion of 11-dehydrothromboxane B_2 and of 2,3-dinor-thromboxane B_2, major enzymatic derivatives of TXA_2 in 11 patients with homozygous cystathionine β-synthase deficiency (CBSD). The abnormally high excretion of this valuable index of in *vivo* platelet activation was independent of the presence of major cardiovascular risk factors. The possibility of a platelet origin for the abnormally high TXA_2 was suggested by the results of a cumulative inhibition of the excretion of thromboxane metabolites by 50 mg/day of aspirin. On the other hand, 500 mg of the antioxidant drug probucol resulted in a 40%–60% drop in the thromboxane metabolite excretion. Interestingly, the effects of probucol were not dependent on reduction of plasma cholesterol levels. Since oxidation of lipoproteins, which can induce platelet TXA_2 formation, is facilitated by homocysteine, inhibition of TXA_2 production by probucol is consistent with the possibility that oxidized lipoproteins contribute to an increased arachidonic acid metabolism in platelets of patients with CBSD. It is worth stressing that lipid peroxidation can be initiated not only by hydrogen peroxide, but also by superoxide and hydroxyl radicals, which can be generated during oxidation of thiols. Recently, an alternative metabolic route for arachidonic acid oxidation has been focused. *In vivo*, arachidonic acid derived from membrane phospholipids can undergo autooxidation, generating a mixture of hydroperoxides, epoxides, and cyclic peroxides [18]. Of particular intereset are the isoprostanes. They form a family of prostaglandin-related compounds acting as autacoids. Presently, the urinary isoprostane index provides a reliable method to estimate *in vivo* lipid peroxidation in various diseases. In addition, some of these isoprostanes are also able to cause activation of platelets and enhanced biosynthesis of TXA_2 linking in this manner *in vivo* oxidative stress and the risk of thrombosis associated with several risk factors. In subjects with homozygous homocystinuria due to CBS, we [20] have reported an abnormally high *in vivo* oxidative stress, as reflected by the excretion of major isoprostanes, leading to platelet activation. Similar results have been reported in patients with early-onset thrombosis and 677TT MTHFR genotype [21]. In the latter subjects, the abnormally high *in vivo* oxidative stress leading to an abnormally high TXA_2 biosynthesis is corrected by 5-methyl-tetrahydrofolate supplementation.

Abnormalities of Coagulation/ Fibrinolysis

Ex vivo data from patients with CBS indicate a variety of abnormaiities of the coagulation system, which suggest a hypercoagulable state in this setting [14,15]. Reduced levels of antithrombin (AT), factor VII, and protein C have been reported. In addition, *in vitro* studies provide a biochemical background for a hypercoagulable syndrome in hyperhomocysteinemia. Factor V activity and prothrombin activation have been shown to be increased by the addition of 0.5-10 mM HCY to cultured bovine aortic endothelial cells. While 8 hours were required to detect an increase in factor V activity in the presence of 10 mM HCY, 24–30 hours were needed at lower HCY concentrations (0.1 or 0.5 mM). These procoagulant effects may be consequent to changes in the activity of the natural anticoagulant protein C. A direct effect of HCY on protein C activation was subsequentiy shown [14]. Incubation of bovine or human umbilical vein cultured endothelial cells with 7.5–10 mM HCY for 6–9 hours inhibited protein C activation by 90%. This effect might be partially expiained by a competitive inhibition by HCY of the thrombomodulin–thrombin interaction. Hayashi et al. [22] provided additional insight into the mechanism by which HCY impairs thrombomodulin activity in HUVEC. They found a time- and dose-dependent inhibitory effect of HCY on thrombomodulin cofactor activity. Thrombomodulin activity, measured as protein C activation, was reduced to 5% or 10% of the baseline values after incubation with 10 mM HCY when the activity was determined on the cell surface or in whole cell extracts, respectively. Thus, their data suggest that the effect of HCY on thrombomoduhin activity is due to a reduction of the native thrombomodulin, which is followed by a compensatory increase in the expression of the thrombomodulin gene and of the total thrombomodulin level. Finally, in a cell-free system, they showed that HCY inhibits the binding of thrombomodulin to thrombin as the result of a decreased binding capacity of the reduced thrombomodulin. In addition, tissue factor (TF), a central protein of the extrinsic pathway of the coagulation, has been indicated as another potential target for the thrombogenic action of HCY [23]. Incubation of human umbilical vein endothelial cells with 10 mM HCY for 8 hours increased TF activity by sixfold. A clearcut concentration dependency of this effect (0.1–10 mM HCY) was also shown. HCY-induced TF activity was inhibited by N-ethylmaleimide, thus indicating that the sulphur group was instrumental in the observed phenomenon. Finally, the ability of HCY to induce TF mRNA, measured by a quantitative polymerase chain reaction technique, revealed an almost fourfold increase in the TF mRNA, when comparing HUVEC and fibroblasts after 3 hours of incubation with 10 mM HCY.

The effect of HCY on AT has been explored with emphasis on the interaction between AT and heparin-like glycosaminoglycans in porcine aortic endothelial cells [24]. The data show that the maximal AT-binding capacity to heparin sulphate is reduced to 30% of normal after a 24-hour incubation with 1 mM HCY. This effect is dependent on sulphydryl groups and appears to involve the generation of hydrogen peroxide, being prevented by catalase, but not by superoxide dismutase.

The interference of HCY with the fibrinolytic system has been addressed by Hajjar [25]. Treatment of cultured HUVEC with 1.5–7.5 mM HCY induced a 65% decrease in cellular binding sites for tissue plasminogen activator (tPA), and this was shown to be due to a reduction of the binding sites for tPA on the 40-kDa receptor protein. Interestingly, the receptor capacity to bind plasminogen was not altered, thus suggesting that the receptor had been altered only in the specific domain responsible for the binding of tPA, and that the COOH-terminal domain, which binds plasminogen, remains unmodified. Along the same line, Harpel et al. [26] also focused on the potential modulation of fibrinolysis by HCY addressing the interaction of plasmin modified fibrin and lipoprotein(a) [Lp(a)]. Because of its homology to kringle W of plasminogen, Lp(a) interferes with fibrinolysis by competing with plasminogen-binding sites. Harpel et al. showed that HCY enhances the binding of Lp(a) to fibrin, especially to plasmin-treated fibrin. This binding was inhibited by ε-aminocaproic acid, thus indicating lysine-binding site specificity, and was also increased by cysteine, glutathione, and N-acetylcysteine. Using gel electrophoresis and immunoblotting, the authors observed changes in the mobility of the apolipoprotein a [Apo(a)] moiety after exposure to HCY. They concluded that HCY alters the structure of Apo(a), possibly exposing additional binding sites for the fibrin surface. As a consequence, the thrombotic potential of Lp(a) is increased by HCY. Together these data show that elevated HCY levels result in increased oxidant stress, endothelial dysfunction, and a hypercoagulable state with increased thrombogenicity, all acting in combination to promote atherothrombosis [27].

Homocysteine and Cardiovascular Disease: Epidemiologic Evidence

Cross-sectional and case-control studies indicate an association between plasma concentrations of HCY and the extent of carotid, coronary, and peripheral vascular disease [28–30]. However, the variables measured in these studies are only surrogate measures of CVD. Recently, the whole area relating tHCY to CHD has been reviewed in detail [31].

Retrospective Studies

In a meta-analysis of 27 observational studies including about 4,000 subjects, hyperhomocysteinemia (defined as plasma HCY levels greater than the 90th or 95th percentile of levels in controls) was associated with an increased risk of atherosclerotic disease. An increase in basal total plasma HCY levels of 5 μmol/L was associated with 60% and 80% increased risk of CHD in men and women, respectively, similar to the effect of raising cholesterol by 0.5 μmol/L [4]. Subsequent observational studies have provided consistent support for the association between hyperhomocysteinemia and atherosclerotic vascular disease.

The European Concerted Action Project, which included 750 men and women with arterial vascular disease and 800 controls, showed that an increase in plasma HCY levels was an independent risk factor for CVD [32]. Subjects with total HCY levels more than 80th percentile had a 2.2-fold (95% confidence interval [CI], 1.6–2.9) increased risk for CVD compared with those with HCY levels less than the 80th percentile.

Prospective Studies

Findings from prospective cohort studies that evaluated the association between an increase in HCY levels and CVD have been inconsistent. Some of these studies reported a statistically significant positive association between elevated HCY and coronary heart disease (CHD) [33–36] and stroke [36,37]. In contrast, data from the Physicians' Health Study, a nested case-control study including 333 male patients and 333 controls (from a total population of 14,916 male patients) followed up for a mean of 7.5 years, failed to demonstrate any significant association between elevated HCY and risk for myocardial infarction (MI) and of CHD death (relative risk [RR], 1.7; 95% CI, 0.9–33.0, for subjects with more than 95th percentile versus less than 95th percentile of total HCY levels) [38]. No significant association between elevated HCY levels and risk of major coronary events or stroke emerged also from the Multiple Risk Factor Intervention Trial cohort [39], the Atherosclerosis Risk in Communities Study cohort [40], and the North Karelia Project [41]. Prolonged follow-up from the Physicians' Health Study also showed a lack of association between plasma HCY levels and risk for stroke and angina [42,43]. It is possible, however, that the U.S. attitude to fortify flour with folate may have been a confounder in these latter studies [44]. Subsequent meta-analysis of prospective observational studies of first events showed an association between hyperhomocysteinemia and elevated risk of CVD. An increase in plasma HCY levels by 25% (i.e., about 3 µmol/L) was associated with 11% and 19% excess risk for ischemic heart disease (IHD) and stroke, respectively, after correction for other cardiovascular risk factors [45]. However, bias may exist in this analysis, as the RRs associated with elevated HCY (by 3 µmol/L) were 1.49 (95% CI, 1.41–1.61) for IHD and 1.16 (95% CI, 0.99–1.37) for cerebrovascular accident (CVA) in retrospective studies, but 1.20 (95% CI, 1.12–1.30) for IHD, and 1.30 (95% CI, 1.11–1.52) for CVA for prospective studies. Furthermore, the number of strokes in these studies was relatively small. Similar results were obtained in a retrospective analysis of 16,849 patients for a 5 µmol/L increase in HCY [46]. Given the definite functional nature of the MTHFR single nucleotide polymorphism and its relationship to plasma HCY levels [47,48], it is possible to perform Mendelian randomization analyses of cohort studies. In a meta-analysis by Wald et al. [46], comparison of the high-risk TT genotype with other genotypes showed a 21% (95% CI, 6%–39%) increased risk of IHD and a nonsignificant 31% (95% CI, −20% to +215%) increased risk of stroke. A subsequent meta-analysis of 15,635 cases using Mendelian randomization showed that a 1.93 (range 1.38–2.47) µmol/L increase in HCY is associated with a 1.26 (95% CI, 1.14–1.40)-fold increase in CVA risk, close to the 1.20 (95% CI, 1.13–1.30)-fold increase in risk predicted on plasma levels alone [49]. Together, case-control studies and prospective studies support an association between elevated plasma HCY levels and increased cardiovascular risk [50]. However, whether lowering HCY levels by administration of folate and vitamins B_6 and B_{12} is associated with any significant decrease in vascular events in populations at risk remains the subject of ongoing debate.

Intervention Studies with Vitamins

Of a number of large prospective studies initiated to address this issue, involving a projected total of 52,000 subjects [51], three have recently been reported. In the first of these, the Vitamin Intervention for Stroke Prevention (VISP) study [52], 3,680 patients who had had a recent stroke were randomly assigned to treatment with folic acid, vitamin B_{12}, and vitamin B_6 at either high or low doses. In parallel with a dose-dependent reduction in HCY, there was no significant difference between the two groups in the rates of stroke (the primary end-point) or a composite of vascular outcomes (recurrent stroke, CHD event, or death) at the end of the 2-year follow-up period. However, this trial was limited by its low-dose, high-dose design, recruitment in the United States (where flour is folate fortified), vitamin B_{12} pretreatment, and low rates of stroke. A post hoc analysis that excluded those patients with low or very high vitamin B_{12} levels or with significant renal dysfunction showed a 21% benefit on major cardiovascular events ($p = .049$; adjusted for confounders $p = .056$) associated with vitamin B_{12} treatment [53]. The findings of two subsequent studies, the Norwegian Vitamin (NORVIT) trial [54] and the Heart Outcomes Prevention Evaluation (HOPE) 2 study [55], were consistent with those of VISP. NORVIT was a secondary prevention trial including 3,749 men and women with prior MI who were randomly assigned to one of four treatments administered once daily: folic acid, vitamin B_6, and vitamin B_{12} (group A); folic acid and vitamin B_{12} (group B); vitamin B_6 alone (group C); or placebo in addition to optimal cardiovascular drug care (group D). After a median follow-up of 40 months, combination vitamin treatment lowered mean total HCY levels by 27% and increased folate levels by 600%–700% in patients receiving folic acid plus vitamin B_{12}, but had no significant effect on the primary end-point (a composite of recurrent MI, stroke, and sudden death due to CHD). Event rates for the primary end-point were 18% in groups B through D. In the triple-therapy group (group A), the event rate was increased to 22% (95% CI, 0%–50%, $p = .05$) and for nonfatal MI by 30% ($p = .05$), countered by a nonsignificant 17% decrease ($p = .52$) in stroke. Overall, the event rate for the primary end-point with triple therapy (group A) compared with the other groups was increased by 20% (95% CI, 2%–41%). In NORVIT, a 14% increase in events ($p = .09$) was seen in the vitamin B_6 group (29% in a subgroup of smokers; $p = .05$), including increased rates of MI (19%; $p = .05$) and death (19%; $p = .11$). The HOPE 2 study involved 5,522 patients with vascular disease or diabetes treated daily with a combination of 2.5 mg of folic acid, 1 mg of vitamin B_{12}, and 50 mg of vitamin B_6 or placebo for an average of 5 years, recruited again mostly (70%) in the United States. Despite a substantial reduction in plasma HCY levels (3.2 μmol/L) in the combination vitamin group, there was no significant reduction in the risk of the primary end-point (a composite of death from cardiovascular causes, MI, and stroke), although there was a marginally significant 25% (95% CI, 3%–41%, $p = .03$) reduction in stroke in patients receiving vitamins compared with those receiving placebo [55]. A small increase in unstable angina admissions was noted with vitamin therapy. A Bayesian analysis of vitamin therapy using data from the NORVIT and HOPE 2 studies suggested that there is little effect of supplements on the rates of cardiovascular events, mortality, or MI, although there may be a beneficial effect on the rate of stroke [56]. In a smaller study ($n = 205$), treatment with the combination of folic acid, vitamin B_6, and vitamin B_{12} for 6 months was shown to significantly reduce the rate of restenosis (19.6% vs. 37.6% on placebo, $p = .01$) and the need for revascularization of the target lesion (10.8% vs. 22.3% on placebo, $p < .05$) after coronary angioplasty [57]. In an extension of this study, including 553 subjects who had undergone successful angioplasty of at least one significant stenosis, vitamin treatment was associated with a significant decrease in the incidence of the composite end-point of major adverse events (i.e., death, nonfatal MI, and need for repeat vascularization) after a mean follow-up of

11 months (RR, 0.68; 95% CI, 0.48–0.96, $p = .03$) [58]. Another study showed, however, that vitamin treatment might increase the rate of stenosis after coronary stenting [59]. Most recently, a meta-analysis of 12 randomized controlled studies of folic acid supplementation, including data from 16,958 subjects with preexisting vascular disease, showed that folic acid supplementation did not significantly reduce cardiovascular risk or all-cause mortality. The overall RRs for subjects treated with folic acid supplementation compared with controls were 0.95 (95% CI, 0.88–1.03) for CVD, 1.04 (95% CI, 0.92–1.17) for CHD, 0.86 (95% CI, 0.71–1.04) for stroke, and 0.96 (95% CI, 0.88–1.04) for all-cause mortality [60]. The disparity between evidence from epidemiologic and retrospective and prospective case-control studies and the results of these recent clinical trials could be due to inherent limitations in the observational studies. A wide range of conditions are known to increase plasma HCY levels [61] (Table 49.1). In addition, other cardiovascular risk factors such as smoking and elevated blood pressure are also associated with increased HCY levels [62]. Furthermore, individuals with preexisting atherosclerosis have higher HCY levels than those without [63]. Thus, it has been suggested by the HOPE 2 Investigators that HCY is a marker, rather than a cause, of vascular disease [55], and therefore, epidemiologic data could be the result of residual confounders. Given the confusing results to date, further trial evidence is required.

Intervention Studies with Lipid-Lowering Agents

Recent results indicating that some lipid-modifying agents, including nicotinic acid, colestipol, and fibrates, may cause elevated plasma total HCY levels have called attention to the issue [63–66]. The most likely mechanism for this increase is an alteration of creatine–creatinine metabolism and changes in methyl transfer [64]. In contrast, statins have no effect on plasma HCY concentrations [64]. Other agents commonly prescribed in patients with CVD affect HCY levels. In keeping with rises in creatinine, thiazide diuretics are associated with a 16% increase in plasma HCY [67]. An HCY-raising effect of metformin has been known since 1971,

Table 49.1 Determinants of homocysteine plasma levels.

Genetic
Transsulphuration defects

  Cystathionine β-synthase defect (chromosome 21):
  Homozygote: 1/340.000 born
  Heterozygote: 0.5% whole population
  Heterozygote mutation 844ins68: 10%–15% whole population in association with other risk factors

Remethylation defects

  5,10-methylenetetrahydrofolate reductase (MTHFR) defect:
  Homozygote: 1/3.350.000 born
  Heterozygote: 0.5% whole population
  Thermolabile variant of MTHFR C677T (50% activity):
  homozygote: 5%–20% whole population
  Methionine synthase defect A2756G
  Cobalamine/methylcobalamine conversion defect (cbl C,D,E,F,G)

Age/sex

  Increasing with age
  Male sex
  Menopause

Nutritional

  Folate $+$ vitamin B_{12} deficiency (elderly, pregnancy, malignancy)
  Vitamin B_6 deficiency
  Lifestyle: abnormal coffee and alcohol intake

Diseases

  Bowel: malabsorption of vitamin B_{12}
  Liver failure
  Renal failure and renal transplantation
  Psoriasis: folate reduction
  Lymphoblastic leukemia, malignancy
  Hipothyroidism
  Diabetes
  Arterial hypertension

Pharmacological

  Methotrexate: 5-methil-tetrahydrofolate reduction
  Estrogens: vitamin B_6 deficit
  Diuretics: interference with folate
  Anticonvulsants: (carbamazepine, isoniazide, fentoine):
  Interference with folate
  Folate antagonists
  Vitamin B_{12} antagonists (e.g., nitrate)
  Metformin
  Glitazones (some)
  Lipid-lowering drugs (colestipol, nicotinate, fibrates)

---

associated with a deficiency in vitamin B_{12} due to reduced uptake [68]. As a matter of fact, metformin reduces vitamin B_{12} levels by 10%–12% and folate by 8% and raises HCY by 13% [69]. The effects of metformin on HCY levels can be ameliorated through the use of calcium supplements [70]. More recently, a significant 20% increase in HCY has been described with rosiglitazone [70], whereas sulphonylureas have been shown to decrease HCY [65]. Forty-four combinations of metformin and glitazones are associated with varying effects with reduction in HCY seen with pioglitazone compared with rosiglitazone [71,72]. Antacids are also associated with reductions in acid-induced cobalamin release from food and hence secondary decreases in absorption. Both fenofibrate and bezafibrate have been shown to induce elevation in plasma levels of HCY [64]. In a direct comparative study, in which patients were randomized to treatment with fenofibrate or atorvastatin for 6 months (after an initial 6-week placebo runin period), fenofibrate induced a significant 35% increase in HCY levels (from 12.3 [3.9] μmol/L to 16.4 [4.6] μmol/L; $p < .0001$), whereas there was no significant change in the group receiving atorvastatin [73]. More recently, elevated plasma total HCY levels associated with treatment with fenofibrate were noted in both the Diabetes Atherosclerosis Intervention Study (DAIS) [74,75] and the Fenofibrate Intervention and Event Lowering in Diabetes (FIELD) trial [76]. In DAIS, in 418 patients with type 2 diabetes, treatment with fenofibrate 200 mg/day was associated with a 55% increase in plasma total HCY levels (from 11.5 [5.6] to 16.5 [10.7] μmol/L, $p < .001$). This increase was not related to changes in factors known to modulate plasma HCY levels, including serum levels of vitamin B_{12} and folate or renal dysfunction. Subsequent analysis showed that baseline, but not end-of-study, elevated plasma HCY levels decreased the beneficial effect of fenofibrate on angiographic determinants of focal coronary artery disease. Furthermore, HCY levels at the end of the study correlated negatively with coronary artery disease progression when data from all study patients were included in the analysis. In the fenofibrate group, there was no significant correlation between plasma total HCY levels and minimal lumen diameter, percent stenosis, or adverse clinical events. Thus, the DAIS Investigators concluded that the fenofibrate-mediated increase in

plasma total HCY levels observed did not attenuate the beneficial effects of fenofibrate on coronary artery disease or clinical events. FIELD included 9,795 patients with type 2 diabetes (78% without prior CVD) who were randomized to treatment with fenofibrate 200 mg/day or placebo following a 16-week runin period, comprising 4 weeks of dietary modification, 6 weeks of single-blind placebo, and 6 weeks of single-blind fenofibrate therapy. The mean duration of follow-up in the study was 5 years. At the end of the study, plasma HCY levels were on average 35% higher in the fenofibrate group than the placebo group (median concentrations 15.1 μmol/L vs. 11.2 μmol/L, $p < .001$). However, in a subset of fenofibrate-treated patients who were restudied after study completion, plasma HCY levels fell from a median of 15.0 μmol/L to 9.5 μmol/L, indicating that the effect of treatment was reversible [76]. This effect remains the subject of ongoing subgroup analyses by the FIELD Management Committee. Taken together, these findings indicate that although fenofibrate does appear to increase plasma total HCY levels, this effect does not attenuate or compromise the beneficial effects of treatment and is reversible following withdrawing of therapy.

Conclusions

Epidemiologic evidence and data from observational studies support an association between elevated HCY levels and increased risk of CVD. However, whether lowering HCY levels by administration of folate and vitamins B_6 and B_{12} is associated with any significant decrease in vascular events in populations at risk remains the subject of ongoing investigation. Of a number of large prospective studies initiated to address this issue, the three major studies that have reported to date have failed to show any significant effect of vitamin supplementation on cardiovascular risk. One of these studies (NORVIT) showed a trend for increased risk among patients who received folic acid plus vitamins B_{12} and B_6 [54]. Plasma HCY levels are increased by a wide range of factors. In addition, individuals with preexisting atherosclerosis have higher HCY levels than those without. These factors may have confounded the results of epidemiologic studies.

In addition, certain drugs may also increase HCY levels. Fibrates, nicotinic acid, and colestipol have been shown to increase HCY levels in clinical trials, suggesting the potential for attenuation of clinical benefit. However, evidence from key fibrate studies such as DAIS and FIELD failed to show any compromise in the beneficial effects of fenofibrate on CVD prevention [74,76]. Moreover, FIELD also showed that this effect on HCY was reversible following discontinuation of treatment. In conclusion, epidemiologic observations of an association between elevated HCY levels and cardiovascular risk do not prove the existence of a causal relation, as they may be subject to a number of confounders. Furthermore, clinical trials such as NORVIT, VISP, and HOPE 2 [52,54,55] showed that even though vitamin supplementation reduced HCY levels, there was no significant effect on cardiovascular risk. This is consistent with a recent meta-analysis that showed that folic acid supplementation was ineffective as a secondary prevention strategy for CVD [60]. Thus, HCY is likely to be a marker rather than a cause of CVD and such formulation does not provide support for routine screening for and treatment of elevated HCY to prevent CVD [56]. Data from ongoing studies are awaited to clarify this issue further.

Selected References

10. Selhub J. Homocysteine metabolism. Ann Rev Nutr 1999; 19:217–46.
15. Coppola A, Davi G, De Stefano V, Mancini FP, Cerbone AM, Di Minno G. Homocysteine, coagulation, platelet function, and thrombosis. Semin Thromb Hemost 2000; 26:243–54.
18. Davi G, Patrono C. Platelet activation and atherothrombosis. N Engl J Med 2007;357:2482–94.
49. Casas JP, Bautista LE, Smeeth L, et al. Homocysteine and stroke: evidence on a causal link from mendelian randomisation. Lancet 2005;365:224–32.
51. B-Vitamin Treatment Trialists' Collaboration. Homocysteine-lowering trials for prevention of cardiovascular events: a review of the design and power of the large randomized trials. Am Heart J 2006;151: 282–7.

SECTION VI
Nutrition, Metabolism, and the Aging Process

CHAPTER 50

Nutrients and Cellular Aging

Roberto Paternò[1] *& Francesco P. Mancini*[2]
[1] Federico II University, Naples, Italy
[2] University of Sannio, Benevento, Italy

Introduction

Aging, an unavoidable corollary of life, is a complex biological process associated with degenerative changes of organs and systems that lead to an increased vulnerability and a decreased ability of the organism to survive. Due to general improvement of healthcare conditions, most countries will be experiencing an increase of people older than 65 years, namely aged people. The continuing increase in life expectancy is one of humanity's most surprising achievement; in developing countries, life expectancy continues to increase at the rate of five or more hours per day [1] without even getting close to its limit [2].

The aging process at the organismal level could be a direct consequence of the aging process at the cellular level, although the biological links between the two processes are not understood, and there are normally aging cells in young or adult individuals. Therefore, whether cellular aging contributes to organismal aging is still controversial.

Nutrients

The multifactorial origin of aging depends on genetic and environmental contributions. Nutrition is one of the most influencing environmental factors and determines the fate of each living organism and of each living cell. Like most variables in biology, optimal nutrition follows a Gauss distribution in terms of adequate amounts of calories or contents of single components that favor a longer and

Nutritional and Metabolic Bases of Cardiovascular Disease, 1st edition.
Edited by Mario Mancini, José M. Ordovas, Gabriele Riccardi,
Paolo Rubba and Pasquale Strazzullo. © 2011 Blackwell Publishing Ltd.

healthier life. Therefore, either too little or too much is detrimental for health and longevity. Poor nutrition promotes many diseases such as metabolic and cardiovascular diseases (CVDs), as well as cancer.

Nutrients are classified as micronutrients and macronutrients.

Micronutrients

While macronutrients provide most of the calories and the building blocks of biological macromolecules, micronutrients are required for nearly all metabolic and developmental pathways and consist of approximately 40 essential compounds including minerals, vitamins, and other biochemicals. Unfortunately, in Western societies energy-dense and micronutrient-poor food is quite common [3]. When the intake of a micronutrient is below the Recommended Dietary Allowance (RDA), metabolic dysregulation may occur and degenerative diseases and accelerated aging may arise. These alterations are the consequence of the molecular and cellular damage induced by the insufficient ingestion of micronutrients. For example, an insufficient intake of folic acid can facilitate chromosome breaks [4]. Similarly, inadequate plasma levels of acetyl carnitine (ALC) and lipoic acid (LA) can accelerate mitochondrial decay, which is considered a major contributor to aging [5]. Carnitine is a carrier of fatty acids (FAs) from the cytoplasm into the mitochondrial matrix; LA is a mitochondrial coenzyme and potent antioxidant that induces a large number of antioxidant enzymes, like those of the glutathione biosynthetic pathway [6]. Aged mitochondria present with oxidatively damaged key enzymes; supplements of ALC and LA to old rats promote the synthesis of new enzymes, such as carnitine acyltransferase, that in turn partly restore mitochondrial function [7].

Magnesium is a divalent cation that is required by many enzymes to acquire full catalytic activity. Intakes of magnesium are below the Estimated Average Requirement (EAR) for large strata of the population, particularly the poor, the obese, the elderly, and teenagers [8,9]. In humans, magnesium deficiency is associated with hypertension, diabetes, metabolic syndrome, and some cancers such as colorectal cancer. It has been shown that magnesium deficiency provokes mitochondrial DNA damage, telomere shortening, cell-cycle arrest, and premature senescence in primary cultures of human cells, as well as damage to the DNA and cancer in the animal model [10]. Therefore, a magnesium supplementation should be considered in the case of deficiency, also considering that the risk of toxicity is very small.

Vitamin D is a cholesterol-derived compound that is formed in the skin during ultraviolet (UV) light exposure; it includes all those compounds that present the biological activity of cholecalciferol (vitamin D_3). Vitamin D_3 can also be introduced with food, especially with fish-liver oils, egg yolks, and butter. Smaller amounts of another form of vitamin D, called ergocalciferol (vitamin D_2), are present in foods of plant origin. Adequate levels of vitamin D promote the correct mineralization of bones by regulating the calcium–phosphorous metabolism and protecting from cancer (colon, breast, pancreas, and prostate) and CVDs [11]. Aged people often ingest less than the required amount of vitamin D through their diet so the vitamin D supplementation is a reasonable approach to reduce the risk for osteoporosis and metabolic bone disease [12]. Nevertheless, it has to be highlighted that in mouse models of aging, hypervitaminosis D showed traits of premature aging and the suppression of vitamin D reduced the premature aging-like features and extended lifespan [13]. However, the cellular and molecular mechanisms that underlie the protective effects of vitamin D with respect to degenerative diseases are largely unknown.

Among other micronutrients that can promote health and longevity by protecting cells from chromosomal breaks or other types of DNA damage, such as oxidative modifications, there are calcium, selenium, vitamin B_{12}, niacin, and choline. The increasing appreciation of DNA damage as a major event in the presence of dietary deficiencies suggests that it can be a relevant indicator to determine the EARs for better health and longevity.

Other micronutrients can retard cellular senescence by preventing mitochondrial decay. In particular, biotin, pantothenate, zinc, pyridoxine (vitamin B_6), riboflavin (vitamin B_2), iron, and copper take part in the biosynthesis of heme, which is an important component of complex IV in the mitochondrial electron transport chain [5]. The proper complement of complex IV reduces mitochondrial DNA damage, oxidant leakage, mitochondrial dysfunction, and cellular aging.

Iron is a transition metal that is crucial for the proper function of several key molecules in the organism including hemoglobin and myoglobin, mitochondrial complex IV, and several redox enzymes. In addition to its crucial role in the fundamental process of oxygen transport, iron is particularly important for the correct development of the brain, immune function, and neuromuscular physiology. Iron is the most abundant trace element in the body (4 g), but iron deficiency is the most frequent micronutrient deficiency in the world. Because of its massive presence in red blood cells, anemia is the principal marker of iron deficiency. Experimental data show that iron deficiency causes mitochondrial damage with consequent oxidative damage to DNA [14]. On the contrary, even if more data is needed on the age trend of iron concentrations in the brain, there is evidence that during aging, the total iron concentration is increased in some brain regions and the high concentrations of reactive iron can increase oxidative-stress–induced neuronal vulnerability [15].

Zinc is another transition metal that takes part in the formation of mitochondrial complex IV. In the human body, there are about 2–3 g of zinc, variously distributed in all tissues, with the highest amounts present in skeletal muscle, bone, skin, liver, and heart. The body does not store zinc and constant dietary intake is essential, since zinc deficiency causes a malfunction of the mitochondrial electron transport with consequent oxidative stress and damage to DNA, either involving single bases or provoking the breakage of an entire chromosome [16]. Not only does zinc deficiency damage

DNA, but it also decreases DNA repair, by inactivating the DNA base excision repair enzyme, and tumor suppression, by inactivating the p53 protein [16]. These combined effects may explain the association of zinc deficiency with cancer [17]. Indeed, basic protein motifs that allow the interaction of transcription factors with target genes promoters involve zinc atoms (zinc fingers) and more than 300 enzymes require zinc; hence, the vast majority of metabolic and signaling pathways depend on zinc availability because they involve zinc-requiring proteins.

Biotin is a vitamin that is required as a coenzyme for four important carboxylases: acetyl-coenzyme A (CoA) carboxylase, pyruvate carboxylase, propionyl-CoA carboxylase, and β-methylcrotonyl-CoA carboxylase. A clear relationship with premature senescence has been established for biotin deficiency in cultured human lung fibroblasts [18]. Biotin deficiency in the same system was also causing a decrease of heme content, release of oxidants, and DNA damage, all factors that can be crucial in the induction of the cellular aging mechanisms.

Macronutrients

Both exogenous lipids, which are contained in many foods, and endogenous lipids, which are produced by the liver, are a major source of energy for the body and accumulate in the white adipose tissue. Most important is the lipoprotein transport system that is responsible for carrying the hydrophobic exogenous and endogenous triglycerides through the aqueous plasma environment for delivery to the body cells.

In addition to this traditional well-recognized role, some dietary lipids are involved in the mitogenic control of several cells and, therefore, can influence the development and progression of colon, liver, and mammary carcinogenesis, as well as metastasis. Among other lipids, long-chain polyunsaturated FAs (PUFAs) have been implicated in carcinogenesis for a long time. However, it has been shown that ω-3 long-chain PUFAs inhibits cancer and carcinogenesis in various experimental settings, such as chemically induced colon carcinogenesis in rats and colon tumor growth and metastasis in nude mice implanted with HT29 colon tumor cell line [19,20]. On the other hand, caution must

be exerted because a high intake of dietary lipids has been associated with an increased incidence of colon and breast cancer. This is an explicative example of the possible subtle differences that can exist between different members (long-chain PUFA, other PUFA, or saturated FAs) of the same family of molecules (lipids) when looking at their biological effects. Indeed, different long-chain PUFAs can have opposite effects on cancer growth, and different FAs are incorporated into the cell membranes depending in a large part on the dietary FA intake. Phospholipids of the membrane bilayers are cleaved at position 2 by phospholipase A2, following a signaling cascade that is initiated by specific stimuli. When arachidonic acid (AA) is generated from phospholipids containing ω-6 PUFAs or eicosapentaenoic acid (EPA) is generated from phospholipids containing ω-3 PUFAs, the eicosanoid metabolism is activated. This is centered on the activity of a few key enzymes, cyclooxygenase (COX), lipoxygenase (LOX), and epoxygenase. COX catalyzes the conversion of AA into prostaglandin D2, prostaglandin F2α, prostacyclin, prostaglandin E2 (PGE2), and thromboxane A2. 5-LOX accelerates the production of the 4-series leukotrienes and 5-hydroxylated eicosapentaenoate from AA. Likewise, 12- and 15-LOX catalyze the transformation of AA into 12- and 15-hydroxylated eicosapentaenoate products. EPA, the ω-3 PUFA present in fish oil, gives origin to analogous compounds with an additional double bond. However, this relatively small chemical difference has been shown to bring about major biological consequences: the proinflammatory and oncogenic properties of the AA derivatives are much more potent than those of the EPA metabolites. This fact provides a rationale for the relative protective role of fish oils on cancer and explains the protection against cancer development provided by aspirin and other COX inhibitors.

It is most likely that, by influencing inflammatory and oncogenic pathways, long-chain PUFAs are also important regulators of the aging process both at the organismal and at the cellular level.

An additional point about dietary FAs must be taken into account: although the possible beneficial effects of the derivatives of dietary ω-3 PUFAs, PUFAs, on the whole, are more susceptible to oxidative damage than saturated FAs (SFAs). Therefore, by eating large amounts of PUFAs, more PUFAs will be incorporated into the cell membranes, and PUFA-rich cell membranes will undergo greater injuries and functional impairment in the event of oxidative stress. This is why dietary monounsaturated FAs (MUFAs) and oleic acid in the first place could provide a beneficial compromise between the risks carried by saturated fats and the high tendency of PUFAs to oxidation. Dietary recommendations should, therefore, encourage the consumption of olive oil for its high content of the MUFA oleic acid, fish and fish derivatives for their high content of ω-3 PUFA, and the large amounts of antioxidant-rich fruit and vegetables, when consuming other PUFA.

Proteins are absorbed in the intestine as free amino acids. Dietary amino acids are important for the generation of new tissues (in the growing organism, during pregnancy, or during tissue regeneration), for producing secretions with high protein content, and for the maintenance of the body steady state that requires a continuous cellular and molecular turnover. At the cellular level, the proper turnover of damaged cellular proteins is a crucial mechanism that retards cellular aging. Proteasome is the major cellular machinery devoted to degrade unnecessary or damaged nuclear and cytoplasmic proteins by proteolysis. Hence, this large protein complex is closely related to aging. Its proteolytic activity declines with aging, leading to the accumulation of modified toxic protein such as the oxidized proteins detected in aging brain [21]. This, in turn, can induce cell injury or premature cell death by apoptosis or necrosis [22].

Protein synthesis may also play a role in aging. It is well known that a relevant age-related decline of the total protein synthesis takes place in rat, but it is not clear whether this reduction of protein synthesis is a beneficial adaptation to reduced mitochondrial function and energy production, as a consequence of aging, or directly contributes to the aging. Recent studies in somatic nematode tissues suggest that the reduction of protein synthesis extends lifespan [23].

A major mechanism that relates dietary carbohydrates and cellular aging is that persistently elevated blood glucose levels result in the covalent modification of proteins and this phenomenon increases with age and promotes cellular aging [24,25]. Dysregulation of glucose metabolism is favored by a diet containing too many carbohydrates, especially simple refined sugars. Glycated proteins, together with other similarly modified macromolecules, are called advanced glycation end-products (AGEs), and AGE is a specially well-suited acronym because of the association of AGEs with age-related pathologies.

Nutrients and Macroautophagy

Dietary amino acids can also trigger a specific process that plays an essential role in controlling the aging of mammalian cells: macroautophagy. In this process, cellular membranes sequester portions of the cytoplasm within vacuoles, vacuoles fuse with lysosomes, and cytoplasmic matter is degraded by lysosomal acid hydrolases. Macroautophagy, which is highly conserved in almost all lower plants and animals and also in higher species, is an important physiological function that allows the ongoing molecular turnover within the living cell. It is also a mechanism to provide the nutritionally deprived cell with essential elements, particularly a sufficient level of amino acids to sustain protein synthesis during starvation [26]. Macroautophagy decreases in the aging cell and contributes itself to cellular aging. This functional decline is documented by a reduced formation of autophagic vacuoles and a retarded fusion of vacuoles with lysosomes. Consequently, an inefficient turnover of intracellular components and a partial derangement of the signaling pathways take place and favor the aging process [27]. If protein intake can influence macroautophagy and macroautophagy can influence cell aging, then the dietary proteins can influence cell aging. In particular, a careful caloric and protein restriction can stimulate macroautophagic activity and consequently prevent or retard cellular aging. However, the optimal protein intake is the one that keeps the macroautophagic mechanism active but prevents a negative nitrogen balance and loss of the lean mass. Needless to say, physical exercise or an active lifestyle must always go along with any choice of nutritional pattern. In this way, protein requirement is kept at a relatively high level by the sustained demand of exercised skeletal muscles and the risk of protein waste is reduced. Generally, only a few amino acids regulate autophagosome formation and they vary depending on different cells and tissues. It has been shown that only leucine is able to inhibit macroautophagy in skeletal and cardiac miocytes, while more than one amino acid is necessary to produce the same effects in liver cells [28]. In rat hepatocytes, at least eight amino acids (leucine, glutamine, tyrosine, phenylalanine, proline methionine, histidine, and tryptophan) co-operate to suppress autophagic proteolysis [28].

Although the regulation of protein metabolism by amino acid levels has been known for quite a while, the molecular details of this mechanism have begun to be elucidated only more recently. A first step to understanding any cellular response to any stimulus is to identify the molecular sensors and their location. A wealth of experimental data point to a cell membrane receptor; recently, dipeptidyl peptidase IV (DPPIV) has been identified by mass spectrometry sequencing as a putative leucine receptor [29]. Upon binding of leucine, DPPIV could elicit an inhibitory control of different intracellular signaling pathways, including mitogen-activated protein kinase (MAPK) and class III phosphatidyl-inositol 3-phosphate pathways, which are involved in promoting the formation of the autophagic vacuole. The MAPK signal pathways are among the major pathways involved in regulating cellular responses to genotoxic stress, and in particular, activation of extracellular signal-regulated kinases (ERKs) has been primarily implicated in cell proliferation and survival, whereas activation of c-Jun NH2-terminal kinases (JNKs) and p38 MAPKs has been involved in growth arrest and apoptosis. The balance between the survival (ERK) and the death (JNK e p38) signaling pathways is critical in determining cellular survival in aging process [30]. Although leucine can activate DPPIV, which is constitutively expressed in liver, kidney, and intestine, the lack of expression this peptidase in skeletal muscle excludes the possibility that this protein could be a general receptor for leucine. There is enough evidence to support the thesis that several amino acid sensing mechanisms coexist and cooperate to the regulatory action of the amino acids. Alternatively, the amino acid receptors could be expressed selectively, depending on the cell type and function.

A possible influence of glucose on macroautophagy has also been claimed. However, a clear relationship with inhibition of autophagy has emerged only for insulin, which is anyway strictly regulated by glycemia.

Interestingly, vitamin C and other antioxidants such as vitamin E and green tea polyphenols (cat-echin and epigallocatechin-3-gallate) have demonstrated a macroautophagy stimulating activity [29]. These findings provide an additional mechanism by which antioxidants exert their antiaging effect. They not only prevent oxidative damage to cellular structures, particularly proteins, but also favor the recycling of damaged cellular components by inducing their destruction by macroautophagy.

Calorie Restriction and Cellular Aging

The title of the famous bestseller by Ancel and Margaret Keys *Eat Well and Stay Well* from the middle of the last century nowadays should be modified due to the accumulating evidence that a moderate caloric restriction, not causing starvation, is a potent inducer of longevity in different organisms, from yeast to mammals. These days, Keys would have probably titled his book Eat Well and Less and Stay Well for a Longer Time.

It has been known for a long time that calorie restriction (CR) extends lifespan, but how this happens has been fully obscure until recently. Since the first observation that CR significantly extended the lifespan of rodents [31], the same observation has been reproduced in a wide range of organisms, including yeast, spiders, worms, fish, mice, rats, and according to emerging data, also nonhuman primates [32–34].

In the last few years, some molecular pathways that link reduced calorie intake to the aging process have been identified. CR prevents many of the changes in gene expression and transcription-factor activity that normally occur with aging, including basal elevations in expression of heat-shock proteins [35,36] and attenuation of stress-induced Hsp70 expression [37]. CR increases the ability of rodents to withstand a wide range of physiological stresses, improves thermotolerance, and reduces heat-induced cellular damage in aged rats [38].

Important observations were already available about the reduced incidence of several diseases in different calorie-restricted experimental animals. Diabetes, kidney disease, several cancers, and autoimmune diseases develop less frequently in animals on a low-calorie diet. Moreover, the evolution of some neurodegenerative diseases, such as Alzheimer's and Parkinson's disease, was retarded

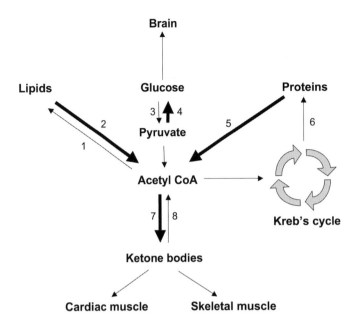

Figure 50.1 Metabolic changes during fasting and calorie restriction (CR). Solid arrows indicate increases due to fasting or CR. Thin arrows indicate down-regulation due to fasting or CR. (1 = fatty acids synthesis; 2 = β-oxidation; 3 = glycolysis; 4 = neoglucogenesis; 5 = amino acid degradation; 6 = amino acid synthesis; 7 = ketogenesis; 8 = ketolysis.)

and characterized by CR [39]. Although aging is a multifactorial process, a leading hypothesis about CR and life extension originates from the oxidative theory of aging, which identifies oxidative damage to DNA, RNA, protein, and lipids as the culprit of a progressive decline of cellular functions and consequently of the whole organism vitality. The possibility that reduced calorie intake might lower the production of ROS as a direct consequence of a slower metabolism has been largely abandoned when a reduction of the metabolic rate was not observed in calorie-restricted animals. Alternative hypotheses predict that either a more efficient mitochondrial electron transport chain or a more efficient removal of ROS, by enzymatic means such as superoxide dismutase (SOD), or both, may be responsible for the lower levels of oxidative damage to cells in the presence of a low-calorie intake. Another working hypothesis is that protein turnover and, therefore, the removal of damaged proteins are accelerated during periods of limited food supply, due to the attempt of the organism to extract energy from sources that are alternative to glucose and fats. In this condition, the accumulation of aberrant, nonfunctioning damaged proteins is abolished and consequent harmful aging effects in the cell are avoided [40]. This mechanism refers back to the macroautophagy discussed in the previous paragraph.

CR is also associated with a reduced formation of AGEs, thus limiting their negative effects on cellular aging. Although neoglucogenesis is stimulated during CR, the amounts of the newly formed glucose are never exceedingly and particularly committed to energetic needs of brain, while skeletal and cardiac muscle shift to lipid oxidation and ketone bodies utilization. A full picture of the metabolic changes occurring during CR is depicted in Figure 50.1.

More recently, the elucidation of a pathway that prolongs lifespan of the single cell and the whole organism provides additional molecular bases to the positive effects of CR on longevity. The yeast *SIR2* gene, a member of the sirtuin/Sir2 family of NAD+-dependent deacetylases, prolongs life of yeast mother cells and is crucial to the formation of spores, the special long-surviving form of yeast cell. The *SIR2* ortholog, *SIR2-1*, also prolongs lifespan of *C. elegans*, and a similar action is played by the homolog *SIR2p* in the protozoan *Leishmania* [41,42]. It has also been demonstrated that these genes mediate life-prolonging effects of CR in *Saccaromyces cerevisiae* and *Drosophila melanogaster* [43]. More interestingly, it has been shown in mice that the mammalian ortholog of *SIR2*, *SIRT1*, is induced by CR and in turn can induce peroxisome-proliferator-activated receptor-γ

Table 50.1 Major dietary plant polyphenols and antioxidants.

Compound	Dietary Source	Class/Subclass/Other
Apigenin	Parsley, artichoke, basil, celery, citrus fruit	Flavone
Caffeic acid	Red wine	Hydroxycinnamic acid
Chlorogenic acid	Coffee	Hydroxycinnamic acid
Daidzein	Soy milk, extract and nuts	Isoflavone
(−)-Epigallocathechin gallate (EGCG)	Green tea	Flavonol
Genistein	Soy milk, extract and nuts	Isoflavone
Hesperidin	Orange juice	Flavanone
Hydroxytyrosol	Extra virgin olive oil	Hydroxylated tyrosol
Kaempferol	Apples, onions, leeks, citrus fruits, grapes, red wine, tea	Flavonol
Luteolin	Celery, green pepper, perilla, camomile tea	Flavone
Lycopene	Tomatoes, tomato sauce	Carotenoid
Myricetin	Walnuts, grapes, berries, vegetables, wine	Flavonol
Oleuropein	Extra virgin olive oil	Tyrosol ester of elenolic acid
Pro-delphinidin B-2 3'-O-gallate	Green tea	Anthocyanin
Quercetin	Apples, onions	Flavonol
Resveratrol	Red wine, grapes, peanuts, soy	Stilbenes

coactivator 1α (PGC-1α). The latter stimulate mitochondrial biogenesis that is associated with longer lifespan [44]. Moreover, *SIRT1* represses the activity of p53, consequently inhibits apoptosis, and therefore, is a good candidate to be a longevity gene in mammals [45]. Based on this evidence, apoptosis may limit mammalian lifespan; thus, inhibiting apoptosis could be the secret for long life. However, it is more complicated than that, because apoptosis is an important mechanism to eliminate damaged cells, especially in the aging organism.

There are several changes in old cells promoting apoptosis: increased Fas expression in lymphocytes, decreased Bcl-2 in lymphocytes, decreased telomere length, decreased Hsp72, decreased mitochondrial function, and increased tumor necrosis factor receptor I and II (TNFR I and TNFR II) [46]. The consequent increase in apoptosis could lead to cell loss as in neuronal degeneration as Alzheimer's and Parkinson's diseases. On the other hand, a decrease of apoptosis induces loss of phenotypic fidelity of somatic cells, which can induce the age-related increase in cancer incidence.

In conclusion, there is more to understand in order to clarify the overall strategy that long-lived organisms adopt to gain longevity and avoid malignancies and other degenerative diseases.

Resveratrol, a Paradigmatic Dietary Polyphenol with Pleiotropic Effects

A huge number of phenolic compounds can be ingested with diet and most of them derive from plants (the most relevant in biology are reported in Table 50.1). Numerous biological activities have been attributed to these substances, many of which have potential health-promoting effects in several species, including humans. A major distinction among dietary phenols considers flavonoid and non-flavonoid compounds. Flavonoids have a general structure reported in Figure 50.2. Among non-flavonoid components stilbenes are an

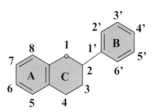

Figure 50.2 General structure of flavonoids. The three phenolic rings are indicated as A, B, and C. Biochemical activity of flavonoids and their metabolites depend on their chemical structure and the relative position of the functional groups.

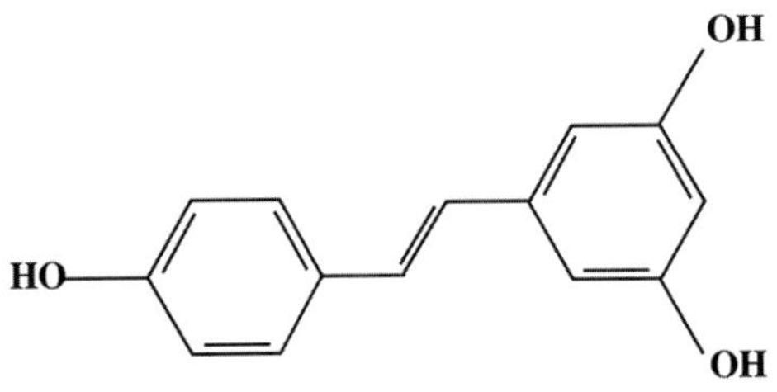

Figure 50.3 Chemical structure of the trans-resveratrol (3,4′,5′ trihydroxistilbene, molecular weight = 228). The two phenolic rings are linked by an ethenic bridge.

Table 50.2 Biological activities of trans-resveratrol.*

- Antioxidant
- Inhibition of lipid peroxidation
- Regulation of lipid metabolism
- Regulation of transcription factors
- Inhibition of platelet aggregation
- Phytoestrogenic activity
- Copper chelation
- Anti-inflammatory activity
- Vasodilating activity
- Pro-apoptotic activity
- Anti-cancer activity
- Regulation of kinases

*These activities have been demonstrated *in vitro* or in experimental models (isolated organs, laboratory animals).

important class of plant phenols and include resveratrol. Resveratrol is a phytoalexin that plants produce to fight infections, especially from yeasts. Besides other nondietary vegetable sources, resveratrol has been identified in peanuts, groundnuts, and grapevines. Therefore, the most important dietary source of resveratrol can be red wine in those people that use to drink regularly such beverage during meals. Its polyphenolic structure (Figure 50.3) provides the molecule with a powerful antioxidant capacity [47]. On these bases, it was speculated that moderate wine consumption might contribute to the beneficial effects of the Mediterranean diet, and it was suggested that resveratrol could be a key factor of the "French paradox," i.e., the unusually low incidence of CVD compared to the high intake of saturated fats. Interestingly, there is a relatively high frequency of uncomplicated obesity in Mediterranean countries such as Italy [48,49], and red wine is commonly present on Italian tables. However, it is important to keep in mind that a glass of red wine contains less than 1% of the resveratrol given to the mice in the experimental studies. Since these potential benefits of resveratrol became appreciated, the number of studies about resveratrol has increased exponentially, and a wealth of biological effects have been attributed to resveratrol (Table 50.2). Besides all of these activities that altogether can attain a protective effect on degenerative disease and CVD in particular, a new burst of interest in this molecule has been generated by the report that resveratrol administration to mice counteracted the negative effects of a high-calorie diet on health and survival but did not prevent obesity [50]. However, a tenfold higher dose of resveratrol did protect mice against diet-induced obesity, improved mitochondrial function and insulin sensitivity in high-fat fed mice, and these metabolic

effects have been associated with the activation of SIRT1 [51]. Indeed, in an earlier study, resveratrol was recognized as the most potent enhancer of human SIRT1 activity *in vitro* among 20,000 screened molecules. Therefore, resveratrol could mimic calorie restriction in humans, thus delaying aging and age-related diseases such as cardiovascular diseases, cancer, and neurodegeneration. In addition, resveratrol exhibits an anti-proliferative, pro-apoptotic action via inhibition of the mitogen-activated protein kinase, the nuclear factor-κB and the PI3K/AKT pathways [47,52]. Furthermore, resveratrol is considered a phytoestrogen because of its striking similarity to the synthetic estrogen, diethylstilbestrol, and its ability to interfere with some steroid activities [47].

A schematic of the pathway going from CR to prolonged lifespan and the site of action of plant polyphenols is reproduced in Figure 50.4.

In conclusion, several intracellular pathways have been elucidated that point to the control of cellular aging by nutrients; however, the relationship between cellular and organismal aging is still controversial.

Since micronutrients are required for most metabolic and developmental pathways and macronutrients provide energy and the building blocks of biological macromolecules, too little or too much of both of them is detrimental for health and longevity.

The best-characterized inducer of longevity, at both the cellular and the organismal level, is CR

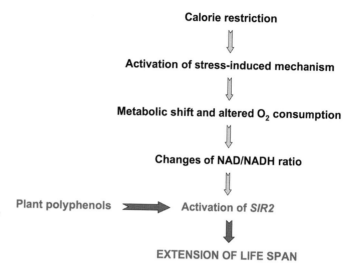

Figure 50.4 A schematic of the pathway going from calorie restriction to prolonged life span. The site of action of plant polyphenols is also indicated.

without undernutrition, which promotes longevity in different organisms, from yeast to mammals. Among several mechanisms hypothesized to explain the effect on longevity, CR prevents many of the changes in gene expression and transcription factor activity that occur with aging, induces a more efficient mitochondrial electron transport chain, and determines a more thorough removal of ROS, which, in turn, results in lower levels of oxidative damage to cells. CR also stimulates mitochondrial biogenesis, which is associated with a longer lifespan, and macroautopahgy, which is an evolutionary conserved function that retards cellular aging by eliminating damaged cellular components. Finally, the abundance of natural antioxidant-rich foods in the diet holds the promise to retard cellular aging and promote longevity.

Selected References

4. Fenech M. The Genome Health Clinic and Genome Health Nutrigenomics concepts: diagnosis and nutritional treatment of genome and epigenome damage on an individual basis. Mutagenesis 2005;20:255–69.

5. Ames BN. Low micronutrient intake may accelerate the degenerative diseases of aging through allocation of scarce micronutrients by triage. Proc Natl Acad Sci USA 2006;103:17589–94.

15. Zecca L, Youdim MB, Rieder P, et al. Iron, Brain ageing and neurodegenerative disorders. Nat Rev Neurosci 2004; 5:863–73.

18. Atamna H, Newberry J, Erlitzki E, et al. Biotin deficiency inhibits heme synthesis and impairs mitochondria in human lung fibroblasts. J Nutr 2007;137:25–30.

44. Guarente L. Mitochondria-A nexus for aging, calorie restriction, and sirtuins? Cell 2008;132:171.

CHAPTER 51

Interaction between Diet and Genes on Longevity

Annibale Alessandro Puca[1], *Chiara Viviani Anselmi*[1], *&*
Thomas Perls[2]

[1] IRCCS Multimedica, Milan, Italy
[2] Boston University Medical Center, Boston, MA, USA

Introduction

Aging is a multifactor and complex process regulated by stochastic interactions (random damage to vital molecules), extrinsic interventions (diet and calorie restriction), and intrinsic/genetic alterations. A number of centenarian (people 100 years or older) studies exploit the strong selection of favorable genotypes in exceptionally aged individuals to study candidate genes and to perform genome-wide analyses. Replications of observed associations of genotypes with longevity, coupled with functional studies to define mechanisms whereby specific genotypes influence lifespan-associated phenotypes, are essential for delineating true positive genetic findings. Such findings could potentially lead to preventive and therapeutic interventions for several age-related diseases that cause significant morbidity and mortality among older people.

Lipoprotein-Related Candidate Genes and Longevity

Numerous genes have been identified that are either positively or negatively selected in the centenarian population as a consequence of a demographic selection. The *microsomal triglyceride trans-fer protein (MTP)* gene has been suggested as such a gene given findings in linkage and association studies of centenarian samples and its strategic role in lipid transport. Studies in isolated hepatocytes have shown that MTP is important during several steps in the assembly and secretion of apolipoprotein B (ApoB)–containing lipoproteins from the human liver and intestine [1].

Later, MTP also determines the maturation of the nascent lipid particle by taking part in the final lipidation process, which probably involves fusion between the primordial particle and a preformed lipid droplet ("second step"). Also, a common functional G/T polymorphism has been detected 493 base pairs upstream from the transcriptional start point that influences low-density lipoprotein (LDL) levels [2]. The G variant appears to bind two or three nuclear proteins that do not bind to the T variant. Moreover, subjects homozygous for the *MTP* −493T allele had a lower LDL-cholesterol concentration in plasma [2]. This common genetic variation of the *MTP* promoter is likely to have important implications for cardiovascular diseases (CVDs). Specifically, coronary artery disease (CAD) and other vasculopathies attributed to unfavorable lipid profiles account for a large percentage of human mortality. For these reasons, common polymorphisms that influence lipid metabolism should be candidates for association studies in oldest old samples. In this respect, the −493T variant showed a lower frequency in centenarians compared to young controls [3,4]. Also, Barzilai et al. [5] reported that lipoprotein

Nutritional and Metabolic Bases of Cardiovascular Disease, 1st edition.
Edited by Mario Mancini, José M. Ordovas, Gabriele Riccardi,
Paolo Rubba and Pasquale Strazzullo. © 2011 Blackwell Publishing Ltd.

particle sizes are increased in centenarians and their offspring and suggested that this "trait" would increase the likelihood of attaining exceptional longevity.

Interestingly, for many years *Allium sativum* (garlic) has been proposed to possess therapeutic features. The effects of garlic on serum lipid levels and on atherosclerosis have been investigated extensively [6,7]. Recent studies conducted by Marie Lin et al. [8] have shown that long-term dietary supplementation of fresh garlic may expert a lipid lowering effect partly through reducing intestinal *MTP* gene expression, thus suppressing the assembly and secretion of chylomicrons from intestine to the blood circulation. Future research aimed at identifying the active components and elucidating the molecular mechanism of garlic induced changes in *MTP* gene expression and lipoprotein production should yield novel therapeutic measures for prevention and treatment of hyperlipidemia. These data in conjunction with a discovered functional polymorphism in the promoter of the *MTP* gene (−493G/T) suggest the importance of modest differences in MTP levels in influencing lipoprotein metabolism and associated disease risks.

Barzilai et al. noted an approximately three-fold increased frequency of homozygosity (valine-valine, VV) of a common functional variant (I405V) in the *cholesterol ester transfer protein (CETP)* gene and decreased CETP levels among Ashkenazi Jewish centenarians and their children [5]. CETP mediates the transfer of cholesterol esters (CEs) from high-density lipoprotein (HDL) to lipoproteins containing ApoB. These data suggested that high HDL-cholesterol (HDL-C) levels are associated with longer life, according to a previous study by Glueck et al. [9].

Another gene, *Apolipoprotein C3*, encodes proteins involved in lipoprotein metabolism and thus favorable alleles showing increases in allele frequencies among older subjects should be associated with a favorable lipoprotein profile. Specifically, APOC3 is a major component of very-low-density lipoproteins and chylomicron remnants; it is also a minor component of HDL [10]. *In vitro* it has been shown to inhibit the activity of lipoprotein lipase, resulting in delayed triglyceride (TG) clearance from plasma [11]. Several studies have shown that various single nucleotide polymorphisms (SNPs) of the *APOC3*

gene either within the promoter region, in particular the T-455C variant polymorphism in the insulin response element, or in the gene, are associated with elevated TG levels and ApoC-III concentrations [12] and represent an independent susceptibility factor for CAD, particularly in the presence of metabolic syndrome [13]. Furthermore, Atzmon et al. noted a APOC3 genotype associated with low levels of APOC3 and longer lifespan [14]. In this study of 66 polymorphisms belonging to 33 candidate genes, the *APOC3* -641CC genotype was overrepresented with increasing age, thus providing evidence that this polymorphism provides a selective advantage for survival to exceptional old age [14].

Fatty Acids and Aging

Interestingly, Olivieri et al. found that the phenotypic effects of the *APOC3* polymorphism are modified by dietary long-chain *n*-3 polyunsaturated fatty acids (PUFAs) [15]. Briefly, the consumption of PUFAs contained in fish and particularly in fish oil has also been described to affect serum ApoC-III concentrations through a mechanism similar to that exerted by lipid-lowering medications, which involves the activation of a specific nuclear receptor, peroxisome proliferator-activated receptor-α (PPARα) [16]. In fact, *ApoC-III* is one of the target genes trascriptionally down-regulated by PPARα activation, thus contributing to the lipid and lipoprotein-lowering properties of fish or fish oil intake [16]. Humphries et al. [17] reported that the *APOC3* C-1100T polymorphism affects the consistency and magnitude of changes in plasma cholesterol in response to a diet rich in polyunsaturated fats. In a study by Lopez-Miranda et al. [18], the SstI[1] restriction site, which arises from a cytosine-to-guanine substitution in the 3' untranslated region of *APOC-III* gene, was shown to be associated with the changes in total cholesterol and LDL-C induced by a diet rich in monounsaturated fatty acids (MUFAs). In particular, the "SstI polymorphism" distinguishes between two alleles S1 and

---

[1]SstI is a restriction endonuclease that cuts double-stranded DNA. This enzyme makes two incisions, one through each of the sugar-phosphate backbones (i.e., each strand) of the double helix without damaging the nitrogenous bases.

S2. The S2 allele has been associated with elevated triacylglycerol, cholesterol, and ApoC-III concentrations. The same SNP was also reported to interact with smoking in determining plasma lipid responses to dietary changes [19]. Recently, Brown et al. [20] demonstrated that a diet low in saturated fat was associated with lower concentrations of Apo B, total cholesterol, and LDL-C ("beneficial lipid profile") only among individuals homozygous for *APOC3* promoter polymorphisms[2]. Specifically, the hypolipidemic properties on *n*-3 PUFAs have been pharmacologically exploited to reduce CAD risk and fish oil capsules are now recognized as useful medications in TG-associated dyslipidemia [21]. Puca et al. [22] reviewed the role of lipids and lipid-associated cell activities in the predisposition to longevity from lower eukaryotes to humans. Briefly, high amounts of phospholipid PUFAs are thought to impair lifespan due to an increase in the susceptibility of membranes to lipid peroxidation and its damaging effect on cellular molecules. Several studies have highlighted the role of membrane lipids in membrane fluidity and permeability, which in turn are influenced by three types of fatty acid (FA) residues present in the membrane; saturated FA (SFA), MUFA, and PUFAs. Precisely, PUFAs can be of the "*omega*" or the "*n*" series and can be further distinguished by two distinct families, *omega*-6 (*n*-6) and *omega*-3 (*n*-3). While PUFA precursors (C18:2 *n*-6 and C18:3 *n*-3) are acquired only with diet, SFAs are also endogenous, derived from the activity of elongase enzymes, and are transformed into MUFA by *delta*-9 desaturase (C16:0 and C18:0 to C16:1 *n*-7 and C18:1 *n*-9, respectively) [23]. Kumar et al. showed that *delta*-9 desaturase activity and consequent MUFA production decreases in older individuals [24]. These concepts have been summarized in the "membrane pacemaker theory of aging," which states that high

membrane fluidity and low membrane peroxidizability are the optimal membrane conditions for promoting longevity.

The membrane pacemaker theory of aging emerged from the study of the relationship between body mass and metabolic rate of mammals and birds, where small birds and mammals have higher mass-specific metabolic rates than large ones [25,26]. The theory proposes that the membrane-associated activities (maintenance of the plasmalemmal Na^+ gradient and mitochondrial H^+ gradient) are significant and dominant components of the basal metabolic rate (BMR); highly polyunsaturated membranes have distinctive physical properties that cause the proteins in the membranes to have a high molecular activity and thus result in higher rates of metabolic activities of cells, tissues and consequently the whole animal. A link between metabolic rate (MR) and lifespan was suggested about a hundred years ago and later elaborated into the "rate of living theory." Membranes that have different FA compositions will differ dramatically in their susceptibility to oxidative damage and this in turn may be related to lifespan variation [27]. The susceptibility of membrane lipids to oxidative alterations is related to two inherent properties, the chemical reactivity of the FAs composing the membrane bilayers and the cellular activities involved in membrane redox reactions. The first property is the peroxidizability of lipids caused by the unsaturation and conjugation of FA double bindings. The second property relates to reactive species production as a majority of subcellular and cellular membranes participate in such activities [28]. More recently, Else and Hulbert [29] proposed that the life-extending action of calorie restriction's ability to modify the FA composition of the membrane supports the membrane pacemaker hypothesis of aging.

Oxidatively modified proteins from reactive oxygen- or nitrogen-derived species have been shown to accumulate in aged tissues [30]. For example, many oxidatively modified proteins are the result of byproducts such as reactive aldehydes caused by the lipid peroxidation process. Kikugawa et al. [28] characterized protein damage caused by oxidized lipids and cross-linked proteins derived from lipid hydroperoxides. Lucas and Szweda [31] reported the formation of reactive aldehyde,

---

[2]The mechanism by which this fatty acid acts on ApoC-III production is not completely clear because the in vitro demonstration of PPARα receptors activation as a necessary step to lower apolipoprotein synthesis has recently been contradicted by the results of a study on PPARα-deficient mice. In this respect, n-3 fatty acids may interfere with ApoC-III gene transcription and may be mediated to some extent by insulin or by nuclear factors operating on the "APOC3 insulin responsive element" on the gene promoter (Dallongeville et al.).

4-hydroxy-2-nonenal (HNE) compounds in membrane proteins. These compounds potentiate oxidative damage to membranes and mitochondrial DNA in liver and brain [32]. Lipid peroxidation is an oxidative process initiated by reactive species, including O_2, singlet oxygen, and free radicals in which unstable FAs, due to their conjugated double bond structure, undergo oxidative modification. Another interesting aspect to lipid peroxiation's role in aging and age-related diseases is that transition metals, which are known to increase with age, are required for oxygen activation and the generation of free radicals [33]. A search for documentation on increased lipid peroxidation during aging resulted in consistent findings that lipids are indeed more oxidized with older age. For example, using the quantity of exhaled pentane as a marker for oxidized lipids, Matsuo et al. [34] gave convincing evidence from longitudinal measurements of *in vivo* lipid peroxidation from rats over the course of their life spans. In the same study, these investigators also were able to show that calorie-restricted (CR) rats produced much less pentane throughout their life, indicating the suppressive action of CR on lipid peroxidation. In another approach, Pepe et al. [35], found age-related changes of PUFA that correlated with cardiac mitochondrial lipid composition. A lot of evidence attributes increased lipid peroxidation during aging to several factors including increased oxidative stress due to reduced antioxidant levels, increased production of reactive species including reactive aldehydes, and increased pro-oxidant transition metals.

FA composition also changes with aging. An interesting shift occurs in the FA profile toward the reduction of lipid peroxidation by replacing more oxidizable fatty acids with less oxidizable and more stable fatty acids [36,37]. More specifically, highly peroxidizable very long-chained PUFAs, such as arachidonic (20:4), docosapentanoic (22:5), or docosahexanoic (22:6) acids, are replaced with FAs having fewer, less oxidizable double bonds, such as linoleic (18:2), and linolenic (18:3) acids; yet, these PUFAs are able to maintain a stable membrane structure [36].

The "membrane pacemaker theory of aging" emphasizes the damage caused to membrane fatty acids for a number of reasons. The first is that membrane fatty acids are located at the primary site of reactive oxygen species (ROS) production (the mitochondrial membrane) and are in such close proximity that no antioxidant defense system is able to prevent their peroxidation. The second is that lipid peroxidation is an autocatalytic (and thus self-propagating) chain reaction that once initiated will continue unless stopped by antioxidant mechanisms. The third reason is that many of the products of lipid peroxidation are very reactive molecules themselves and are thus harmful to other molecules. The aldehydes produced by lipid peroxidation include hydroxynonenal (HNE, from *n*-6 PUFA) and hydroxyhexenal (HHE, from *n*-3 PUFA) and it has been proposed that much of the cellular and subcellular damage associated with oxidative stress is attributable to the deleterious actions of these peroxidation products. Indeed, HNE decreases mitochondrial membrane fluidity [38] and HNE and HHE inhibit the mitochondrial adenine nucleotide translocase [39]. Hydroxyhexenal is a potent inducer of the mitochondrial permeability transition [40] and hydroxynonenal at high concentrations is cytotoxic, while at intermediate concentrations it inhibits DNA and protein synthesis and stops cell growth [41]. HNE stimulates mild uncoupling of mitochondria through the "uncoupling proteins" (UCP1, UCP2, and UCP3) and the adenine nucleotide translocase [42]. The consequence is that the whole loop might act as a negative feedback homeostatic system limiting mitochondrial ROS production.

In summary, the "mitochondrial theory" hypothesizes that mitochondria are a critical component of aging. This theory is particularly meaningful when one considers possible interventions and antioxidant strategies.

Calorie Restriction

The only treatment that extends lifespan in a wide range of species is dietary calorie restriction (CR). It is one of the most examined aspects of aging and there are several excellent reviews [43–45]. It has been most studied in rats and mice where it extends both mean and maximum lifespan. Within limits, the degree of life extension is linearly related to the degree of dietary CR and is not dependent on the age at which it is imposed [44]. CR exerts its effects by both slowing the intrinsic rate of aging and suppressing pathogenesis [46]. Interestingly, in CR animals, both membrane potential and mitochondrial uncoupling were shown to be modulated in an effort to protect mitochondrial integrity [44].

CR can exert its effects very rapidly. In a series of nutritional-shift experiments where groups of *Drosophila melanogaster* were shifted between full diets and restricted diets at various times during their adult life, mortality rates changed within two days of the dietary shift [47]. The connection between CR and the "mitochondrial free radical theory of aging" has been brought about by numerous investigations describing a lower mitochondrial free radical generation rate in calorie restricted animals compared with *ad libitum*-fed animals [48,49].

The consensus is that CR exerts diverse aging modulating actions via multiple mechanisms including redox-responsive transcription factors and gene expression involved in both physiological and pathological processes. As proposed by the "oxidative stress theory of aging" [50], if oxidative stress, the cause of redox imbalance, interrupts cellular homeostatic mechanisms thereby contributing to aging, any intervention that suppresses oxidative stress would exhibit an aging-attenuating effect. Since mitochondria are considered a hub of oxidative stress, and because of their high oxygen consumption, they have been the subject of many studies on oxidative damage [51] and its attenuation by CR [46,49].

In this respect, normal oxygen consumption by mitochondria inevitably results in the production of oxygen free radicals, which in turn damage important biological molecules and the accumulation of this damage is manifest as aging. Moreover, the "rate of living" and "oxidative stress" theories of aging can be theoretically integrated by supposing that higher levels of ROS are generated by a higher metabolic rate [49,52]. Free radicals are molecules capable of independent existence that contain one or more unpaired electrons[3]. The "theory of mitochondrial aging" predicts that the mitochon-drial DNA's (mtDNA) proximity to the cell's major source of free radicals renders it particularly susceptible to oxidative insults and thereby increases the rate of mtDNA mutations, leading to an aggravation of aerobic respiration dysfunction (mtDNA encodes proteins of the respiratory chain). The consequent decrease of electron transfer leads to further production of ROS, thus establishing a vicious cycle of oxidative stress and energetic decline, which is suspected to be one of the principal causes of aging [53].

Since it was proposed that CR worked, at least in part, by decreasing oxidative stress [49], several studies have shown that moderate CR leads to lower oxidative damage to cellular macromolecules. In accordance, many investigations have consistently reported reduced levels of mutagenic oxidative modifications in mtDNA after long term CR [54]. In particular measurement of *in vitro* ROS production, such as the rate of mitochondrial H_2O_2 production is reduced [49,54,55]. That the rate of *in vivo* lipid peroxidation is also decreased by calorie-restriction is demonstrated from its effects on ethane and pentane exhalation [34,56] as well as the urinary excretion of aldehydes [57].

However, there also have been studies indicating, at least in some instances, that oxidative stress is not an important factor in the occurrence of senescence. Orr et al. [58] reported that the life span of long lived *Drosophila melanogaster* is not increased by the overexpression of the following antioxidant enzymes: CuZn-superoxide dismutase, Mn-superoxide dismutase, thioredoxin reductase, and catalase. Also Van Remmen et al. [59] found that in mice deficient in Mn-superoxide dismutase the increased oxidative stress/damage does not affect life span and other sensitive parameters. Thus, it remains an open question whether CR's ability to attenuate oxidative damage plays a major role in life extending action. This view has been challenged because of findings that show that the restriction of a specific dietary component without a decrease in caloric intake can result in life extension.

---

[3]An important free radical in biological systems is the superoxide radical, $O_2 \cdot -$, which is produced as a by-product of normal mitochondrial respiration. One electron reduction of O_2 to form the superoxide anion ($O_2 \cdot -$) and dismutation of $O_2 \cdot -$ to yield hydrogen peroxide (H_2O_2) occurs during mitochondrial respiration. Mitochondria are also involved in the generation of nitric oxide (NO) via the nitric oxide synthase (NOS) reaction. $O_2 \cdot -$ and NO· react to form another oxidant, peroxynitrite (ONOO-), which represents a potential source for the more powerful and aggressive hydroxyl radical (·OH).

In particular, *SIRT1*, the mammalian ortholog of the *SIR2* gene that mediates the life extending effect of CR in yeast [60], is a key regulator of cell defenses and survival in mammals in response to stress. Specifically, Sir2 (silent information regulator 2) is a nicotinamide adenine dinucleotide (NAD)–dependent deacetylase that is required for longevity due to CR in the budding yeast *Saccharomyces cerevisiae* and in the fruit fly *Drosophila melanogaster* [61]. In mammals, CR induces a complex pattern of physiological and behavioral changes, such as a reduction in blood glucose, triglycerides, and growth factors, and an increase in movement and foraging activity [62]. At this regard, Chen et al. [63] suggested that a parameter of mammalian calorie restriction, up-regulation of physical activity, requires the gene that codes for *Sirt1*. The molecular mechanism for this increase in physical activity is not known. It is possible that CR triggers changes in brain regions that govern physical activity and that Sirt1 is a regulator of this pathway. Interestingly, Sirt1 mediates other effects of CR in mammals, such as the extension of life span. Particularly, Sirt1 governs adipogenesis and fat mobilization from white adipose tissues (WATs). Overexpressing Sirt1 in adipocytes lessens adipogenesis, whereas knocking down Sirt1 enhances it [64]. Moreover, adipogenesis from WATs of Sirt1$^{+/-}$ mice is compromised under food limitation. In fact, Sirt1 controls adipogenesis by binding to PPARγ, an essential regulator of WAT. Sirt1 promotes insulin secretion from pancreatic β cells by directly binding to the promoter of the *mitochondrial uncoupling protein gene 2* (UCP2) and repressing expression [65]. In these respects, Sirt1 is involved in fat storage, insulin secretion and glucose homeostasis thus modulating at least some major aging pathways.

In mammals, CR elicits a complex pattern of physiological and behavioral changes that are linked to longer and healthier life: increased physical activity that might be related to foraging, decreased body weight, body fat, blood glucose, insulin, triglyceride, and cholesterol, and increased insulin sensitivity and glucose tolerance [66]. These effects are opposite to what is observed with accelerated aging: increased body fat especially in the visceral area and peripheral tissues such as liver and skeletal muscle, increased insulin resistance, and elevated cholesterol [67,68]. Gene expression data from calorie restricted animals demonstrate changes related to oxidative stress including up-regulation of redox-sensitive and pro-inflammatory genes such as interleukin (IL)-2, IL-6, and tumor necrosis factor-α (TNF-α) [69]. The biochemical analyses of the anti-inflammatory action of CR on various transcriptional factors such as nuclear factor-κB (NF-κB), activator protein-1 (AP-1), and PPARs were reported recently [70,71]. Kim et al. found that the age-related activation of NF-κB is enhanced by degradation of its subunits, IκB, allowing NF-κB to translocate into the nucleus during aging [70]. The increase in inflammatory gene expression strongly suggests deregulated cellular signaling pathways, making the organism more vulnerable to other insults [72]. Thus, Chung et al. proposed the "molecular inflammation hypothesis of aging" [73]. This hypothesis identifies the age-related inflammatory process as a possible molecular cross-talk mechanism that bridges biological and pathological processes. The anti-inflammatory action of CR can be attributed more likely to its ability to suppress age-related oxidative stress than to a chronically elevated glucocorticoid level, which is potentially deleterious to the organism [74].

In order to understand the mechanisms for the wide range of beneficial biological effects of CR, "*Hormesis*" has been suggested as a major explanation by considering CR as a low-intensity stressor [75]. Specifically, all living systems have the intrinsic ability to respond, to counteract and to adapt to the external and internal sources of disturbances. "*Hormesis*" represents mild stress induced stimulation of protective mechanisms in cells and organisms resulting in biologically beneficial effects. Single or multiple exposures to low doses of otherwise detrimental environmental agents, such as irradiation, food limitation, heat stress, antibiotics, pesticides, hypergravity, ROS, and other free radicals may have a variety of longevity-extending effects [76]. These potential beneficial actions may include increased longevity, retardation of senescent deterioration, retardation of age-associated diseases, and enhanced coping with intense stress. In this regard, Puca et al. [22] found an increase of endogenous trans fatty acids in long-living descendants compared to age-matched controls, pointing to an increase basal radical stress as key determinant of longevity. The concept of "hormesis," by providing mechanistic explanations for the apparently paradoxical and nonlinear effects of potentially damaging agents, has given rise to new lines of investigation in anti-aging research [77,78].

In conclusion, we have discussed the major findings that links diet and the genes that influence longevity, from lower organisms to primates. It emerges the importance of CR in modulating the longevity genes and its ability of diminish the deleterious effect of reactive species on aging. It is tempting to speculate that in a near future we will able to modulate important life-span markers, such as serum lipoproteins by intervening with diet based on patient's genetic profile.

Selected References

4. Puca AA, Daly MJ, Brewster SJ, et al. A genome-wide scan for linkage to human exceptional longevity identifies a locus on chromosome 4. Proc Natl Acad Sci USA 2001; 98:10505–8.

22. Puca AA, Chatgilialoglu C, Ferreri C. Lipid metabolism and diet: possible mechanisms of slow aging. Int J Biochem Cell Biol 2008;40:324–33.

61. Greer EL, Brunet A. Signaling networks in aging. J Cell Sci 2008;121:407–12.

62. Easlon E, Tsang F, Dilova I, et al. The dihydrolipoamide acetyltransferase is a novel metabolic longevity factor and is required for calorie restriction-mediated life span extension. J Biol Chem 2007;282:6161–71.

75. Masoro EJ. Hormesis and the antiaging action of dietary restriction. Exp Gerontol 1998;33:61–6.

CHAPTER 52

The Role of Diet on Cognitive Decline and Dementia

Alfredo Postiglione & Giovanni Gallotta
Dementia Study Center, Federico II University and ASL Napoli 1, Naples, Italy

Introduction

Age-related cognitive decline is not uniform. Some abilities, such as vocabulary and general knowledge, can remain stable until very old age, while attention, executive functions, and memory abilities start to decline in middle adulthood and progress until death [1]. However, it is difficult to understand whether the patterns of cognitive decline reported in many studies are attributable to normal aging or to pathological conditions very frequent in old age, such as cardiovascular disease, diabetes mellitus, and depression, which are known to be independently associated with impaired cognitive performance. The passage from a "normal" age-related cognitive pattern to pathological cognitive decline is progressive with the elderly person shifting to self-reported memory complaints, mild cognitive impairment (MCI), and overt dementia, in most cases AD.

The maintenance of cognitive function with aging is a major determinant of quality of life in older age and there is increasing evidence indicating a role for lifestyle factors in successful brain aging. Many epidemiologic studies provide evidence that dietary patterns may play a role with both beneficial and detrimental influences to age-related cognitive decline and dementia risk [2]. Studies have focused on the association between AD and homocysteine-related vitamins (B vitamins), antioxidant nutrients (vitamin E and C, carotenoids, flavonoids, enzymatic factors), and dietary lipids, especially those present in fish [3]. However, when evaluating these studies, it should always be taken into consideration that AD is a chronic disease with a long latency period before being clinically manifest, and therefore, it is very difficult to have studies for enough time and in large enough samples to be able to observe the influence of dietary habits on cognitive decline and risk of dementia. Moreover, prospective and controlled trials should include at baseline subjects in their adulthood, since elderly people are often at nutritional risk not only because of alterations in smell and taste, impaired digestion, absorption, or utilization of nutrients due to chronic disease or drug-nutrient interactions, but also as a result of various physical, socioeconomic, and behavioral factors. Therefore, since cross-sectional studies cannot determine whether an observed relation is a cause or effect of a disease process, only prospective studies are able to provide a correct temporal relation for a cause–effect interpretation of diet and dementia association.

Macronutrients and Micronutrients in Relation to Age-Related Cognitive Decline and Dementia

Dietary Fats

Among the macronutrients, FAs may play an important role in modulating the risk of cognitive decline and dementia with the degree of saturation and the position of the first double bond being

Nutritional and Metabolic Bases of Cardiovascular Disease, 1st edition. Edited by Mario Mancini, José M. Ordovas, Gabriele Riccardi, Paolo Rubba and Pasquale Strazzullo. © 2011 Blackwell Publishing Ltd.

the most critical factors. FAs can be categorized as saturated FAs (SFAs) and unsaturated FAs. SFAs are present in products such as meat, diary products, cookies, and pastries. Monounsaturated FAs (MUFAs) are present in olive oil. Polyunsaturated FAs (PUFAs) comprise two classes: the n-6 class (i.e., linoleic acid [18:2n6] and arachidonic acid [20:4n6]) and the n-3 class (i.e., linolenic acid [18:3n-3], eicosapentaenoic acid [EPA,20:5n-3], and docosahexaenoic acid [DHA,22:6n-3]). DHA is formed from linolenic acid, an essential FA that must be obtained from the diet, but is present also in fatty fish or fish oil. Fatty fish are the primary source of n-3 PUFA, while vegetable oils are the main source of n-6 PUFA. PUFAs have an important role in neuronal membrane phospholipids and are essential for brain development and functioning. FAs with multiple bonds increase fluidity to cell membranes with each double bond conferring a 37-degree angle to the carbon chain. Moreover, n-3 (omega-3) PUFAs have an anti-inflammatory capability by modulating cytokine activity, neurotrophin, expression, and antiapoptotic pathways [4,5]. In experimental animal studies, a diet low in n-3 PUFA induces cognitive decline and neuroinflammation and increases neuropathology.

In the EVA study, higher levels of n-3 PUFA in erythrocyte membranes were associated with reduced risk of cognitive decline over 3 years; however, higher levels of n-6 FA were associated with increased risk [6]. In the Framingham study, subjects with the highest levels of plasma phosphatidylcholine DHA presented a 47% reduction in the risk of developing all-cause dementia, but not AD [7]. In the Chicago Health and Aging Project (CHAP), subjects with high dietary intake of SFA had a two to three times higher risk of incident AD and a faster rate of cognitive decline [8,9]. The Italian Longitudinal Study on Aging (ILSA) found that high MUFA and PUFA energy intakes, though not studied independently, were associated with better cognitive performance among elderly people aged 65–84 years [10]. In the Three-City cohort study, regular use of n-3 FA was associated with a decreased risk of borderline significance for all-cause dementia, while regular consumption of n-6 FA not compensated by consumption of n-3 rich oils was associated with an increased risk of demen-

tia. However, in this study the effects of n-3 PUFA appear influenced by the presence of apolipoprotein E4 (ApoE4) phenotype, since the beneficial effects of fruits, vegetables, and fish were present only among the ApoE4 noncarriers [11]. In the Washington Heights-Inwood Columbia Aging Project (WHICAP) study, higher fat intake was associated with double the risk of AD but only among participants who were ApoE4 carriers [12]. Similar results were observed in a Finnish study, in which high SFA intake was associated with increased risk of dementia, while moderate intake of PUFA with reduced risk, especially among ApoE4 carriers [13].

Few RCTs have been carried out to determine whether supplementation with n-3 PUFA would prevent cognitive decline and dementia, but results are still limited. Freund-Levy et al. [14] recently found no significant benefit of 6 months of supplementation with 1.7 g of DHA and 0.6 g of EPA per day in patients with AD on tests of cognitive function as compared to placebo. When all subgroups were continued on n-3 PUFA supplementation for a further 6 months, a stop in cognitive decline was observed in those with MCI, who previously received placebo. Kotani et al. [15] reported that supplementation with 120 mg of arachidonic acid and 120 mg of DHA versus olive oil placebo for 90 days gives a significant benefit only in subjects with MCI, but not in those who were already affected by AD.

A recent review by Fotuhi [16] summarized the results in seven studies published from 1997 to 2008 that focused on the association between n-3 PUFA and risk of AD. Three showed that fish consumption was associated with a statistically significant reduced risk of AD [11,17,18], but three did not find any association [7,19,20] and one showed higher serum PUFA in those who developed dementia [21]. Two other studies [22,23], described in the National Institutes of Health (NIH) statement [24], did not find any association. The NIH statement concluded that there was no consistent association between PUFA, as estimated by dietary history of fish consumption, and incident AD. On the other hand, the same review by Fotuhi [16] included three studies evaluating the association with cognitive decline and concluded that long-chain n-3 PUFA favor the slowing of cognitive decline [6,25,26]. The role of Mediterranean diet and risk of AD and cognitive decline has also been investigated. A high compliance to the Mediterranean diet was associated with significant lower risk of progressing from MCI to AD [27] and of incident AD, especially if combined with high levels of physical activity [28]. Two cohort studies [28,29] found that a good adherence to the Mediterranean diet may be associated with less cognitive decline in later life. There are also new reports [30,31] suggesting that high intake of fruits and vegetables may protect against cognitive decline and incident dementia.

In conclusion, high dietary intakes of SFA were probably associated with increased risk of incident AD, while high intakes of PUFA, as fish consumption, and MUFA seem to have a beneficial effect against cognitive decline and dementia. More studies need to be performed to investigate the beneficial effects of PUFA supplementation in the prevention of cognitive decline and AD, since no definitive randomized study has yet been performed [24,32].

B Vitamins

Five cohort studies examined the association between B vitamins or berries and development of AD [33–37]. When based on measured serum folate levels, it seems that low folate levels are associated with increased risk of AD [36,37], while this association was never found for vitamin B_{12}. However, there is no consistent evidence between folate and vitamin B_{12}, based on estimated intake or plasma levels of these factors and cognitive decline [24].

Folate, vitamin B_{12}, and vitamin B_6 are co-factors in the methylation of homocysteine (Hcy). High plasma levels of Hcy (>14 μmol/L) are neurotoxic and may have a direct role on cognitive decline. Hcy itself, and folate and vitamin B_{12} deficiency, can disturb methyl-action and/or redox potentials promoting calcium influx, amyloid and tau protein accumulation, apoptosis, and neuronal death. Seven prospective studies, reviewed by the IANA Task Force [4], examined plasma levels of Hcy and B vitamins in relation to incident AD. In the Kungsholmen Project, persons with low levels of vitamin B_{12} (≤150 pmol/L) or folate (≤10 nmol/L) had twice the risk of developing AD compared with people with normal vitamin levels. In the Baltimore Longitudinal Study of Aging, higher intake of folate, vitamin E, and vitamin B_6 was associated in-

dividually with decreased risk of dementia. In the WHICAP study, the highest quartile of total folate intake was related to a lower risk of AD, while vitamin B_{12} and B_6 levels were not related to the risk of AD. High levels of Hcy were not related to decline in memory score over time. In the Conselice Study of Brain Aging, high levels of Hcy and low folate concentrations were independently associated with dementia and AD, while no significant relation was found for vitamin B_{12}. In the Framingham study, there was no association with serum B vitamins, while Hcy was associated with higher risk of AD. In the CHAP study, no association was found between folate and vitamin B_{12} intake and incident AD. It is probable that elevated plasma Hcy concentration might be implicated with the risk of dementia, but it is unclear whether it is associated with cognitive decline, since most of the studies identified in the NIH report did not find any association between Hcy levels and cognitive decline [24]. However, it should be reminded that plasma Hcy levels rise with age, renal insufficiency, use of coffee and tobacco, and sequelae of heavy alcohol use.

This association has raised pharmacological interest, as Hcy can be lowered by folic acid and vitamin B_{12} supplementation, suggesting that this supplementation could lower the risk of dementia. Durga et al. [38] found that folic acid supplementation significantly improved memory, sensorimotor speed, and information processing speed. Other studies did not find any beneficial effects of folate and vitamin intake on the risk of developing AD [4].

Antioxidants and Other Vitamins

Antioxidants, such as vitamins E (tocopherol), C (ascorbic acid), carotenes, polyphenols (flavonoids), and enzymatic cofactors of superoxide dismutase and glutathione peroxidase (zinc, selenium, manganese) are able to reduce neuronal damage and death from oxidative reactions by inhibiting the generation of reactive oxygen species (ROS), apoptosis, and beta-amyloid toxicity or deposition. There is also evidence that dietary intake of antioxidants is associated with low risk of stroke, and therefore, cerebrovascular disease could be a link between dietary antioxidant vitamins and AD. Polyphenolic compounds (plant polyphenols

[PPs]) found in plants may have a direct effect on cell signaling, growth, and differentiation. Studies in animal models have found that PPs reduce neuroinflammation and stimulate the activity of phosphatidylinositol-3 kinase (PI3K) with improved neuronal survival and memory. Since the production of ROS may be involved in cognitive decline, research has explored how antioxidants in foods and supplementations can affect cognitive decline and dementia [39,40].

Data from prospective studies are conflicting. Seven studies examined the effect on cognitive decline of food intake of antioxidant nutrients [41–47] and five [41–45] observed a statistically significant inverse association. Alternatively, in the WHICAP study [46] and in the Honolulu-Asia Aging Study [47], food intake of beta-carotene, vitamin E, and vitamin C was not associated with the risk of incident AD. In a recent report from the Cache County Study, high antioxidant intake from food and supplement sources of vitamin C, vitamin E, and carotene was able to delay cognitive decline in elderly [48]. In two recently published RCT studies, vitamin E supplementations (2,000 IU/day and 600 IU/day) had no effect on progression to AD among persons with MCI [49] or among healthy older women [50]. A possible explanation of the discrepancies among food and supplement sources of antioxidant nutrients may be that vitamin E supplementation consists of alpha-tocopherol, which decreases the absorption of γ-tocopherol, which has anti-inflammatory effects and is a major scavenger of reactive nitrogen species. Therefore, the beneficial effects could derive from other forms of tocopherol or by a combination of more forms. In the EVA study [51], low levels of lycopene and zeaxanthin were associated with poor cognitive function, while in the MacArthur Studies of Successful Aging [52] high levels of beta-carotene were inversely associated with cognitive decline in those who were ApoE4 carriers. Also in the EVA study, the greatest decline in cognition was associated with the lowest plasma selenium concentration at baseline [53]. In the Duke Established Populations for Epidemiologic Studies of the Elderly (EPESE) [54], subjects under antioxidant supplements (vitamins C, E, and A, selenium, and zinc) had a lower risk of cognitive decline than nonusers. Akbaraly et al. found that decreases in plasma selenium after

9 years of follow-up were associated with cognitive decline, but no association was observed after 2 years [4].

The recent NIH statement concluded that there is little evidence suggesting the beneficial protective effect of vitamins E and C, beta-carotene, and flavonoids on reducing the risk of AD and cognitive decline [24]. The results of the published studies on antioxidant nutrients and cognitive decline or dementia may suggest the use of a balanced combination of several antioxidants in order to have a beneficial prevention of incident AD. However, since it is difficult to isolate the specific effect of each nutrient, extensive epidemiologic and RCTs are still needed before to recommend the effective and optimal supplementation, also taking into consideration that treatment with vitamins E and A may even increase mortality [55].

Alcohol

Alcohol is a neurotoxin and exposure to intoxicating doses can result in neuronal mitochondrial dysfunction and degeneration in rats. On the other hands, alcohol consumption increases high-density lipoprotein, decreases platelet adhesiveness, and improves endothelial function. Wine contains flavonoids as antioxidant that is not present in beer and spirit.

In the Nurses' Health Study [56], elderly women drinking less than 15 g/day of alcohol had a relative risk of cognitive impairment of 0.81 (95% confidence interval [CI]: 0.70–0.93) compared to nonalcohol drinkers. In contrast, women consuming more alcohol (15–30 g/day) presented no significant improvements in cognitive functions relative to those consuming no alcohol. In the Cardiovascular Health Study [57], persons consuming one to six drinks per week had a low risk of dementia and/or AD as compared to those consuming no alcohol (odds ratio [OR], 0.46; 95% CI: 0.27–0.77). Increasing alcohol decreased or reversed the benefit: OR, 0.69; 95% CI: 0.37–1.31 for those drinking 7 to 13 drinks per week and OR 1.22, 95% CI: 0.60–2.49 for those consuming 14 or more drinks per week. Contrary to what commonly believed, the type of alcohol beverage does not seem important [56,57]. A recently published review [58] examined the association between alcohol use and the development of AD in nine prospective community cohort studies published from 2002 to 2006. All drinkers combined had a lower risk of AD compared to nondrinkers. Light to moderate drinkers also had a lower risk of AD compared to nondrinkers, but heavy/excessive drinkers showed no difference in risk compared to nondrinkers. The authors concluded that light to moderate alcohol use in late life was associated with lower risk of AD. The NIH statement [24], after the examination of the review by Anstey [58] and the identification of other studies on the association between alcohol use and cognitive decline published since 2006 [59–63], concluded that the association between alcohol use and cognitive decline is inconsistent. All reviewers noted that results of all studies are complicated by variation in the type of beverage used, in the criteria for measuring and categorizing quantity, in the possibility that former drinkers may have stopped drinking for health problems that predispose to cognitive impairment. In the absence of RCTs on alcohol effects, no recommendation could be made. Those who drink should be moderate drinkers (three servings per day), but those who do not drink should not be encouraged to drink.

Plasma Insulin, Dietary Glucose, and Cognition

Insulin resistance (IR) and/or hyperinsulinemia result in brain injury, compromise cognitive function, and could increase neuropathologic progression of AD. IR is associated with the development of age-related diseases including hypertension, coronary heart disease, stroke, cancer, and type 2 diabetes mellitus. IR and hyperinsulinemia increase systemic inflammatory responses and oxidative stress leading to increased central nervous system (CNS) inflammation; increased proinflammatory cytokine levels can down-regulate PI3K with subsequent caspase activation. Therefore, it seems possible that IR promotes amyloid-beta deposition and neuroinflammation with subsequent cognitive deterioration and AD [4].

In the Nurses' Health Study [64], women without a diagnosis of diabetes but in the highest quartile for C-peptide levels had significantly higher odds of cognitive impairment 10 years later as compared to women in the lowest quartile (OR, 3.2; 95% CI: 1.3–7.8). In the WHICAP study [65], among 683 persons with mean age of 76.2 years followed

for a median of 5.4 years, the risk of AD was higher in the highest quartile of insulin levels (OR 1.7; CI 95%: 1.0–2.7) as compared to those in the lowest quartile. The association of IR and risk of dementia was even higher when only nondiabetic persons were included. In the Atherosclerosis Risk in Community (ARIC) cohort [66], IR was associated with lower verbal learning, recent memory, speed, sustained visual spatial skills, and associative learning, as well as mental agility. The review by Biessel et al. [67] examined 11 studies, where the incidence of dementia was compared between subjects with and without diabetes mellitus. The authors concluded that patients with diabetes mellitus have an increased risk of AD and those with an ApoE$_4$ allele doubled the relative risk. The meta-analysis study by Lu et al. [68] supported a similar association between diabetes mellitus and increased risk of AD. In the Cardiovascular Health Study, the OR for developing AD in subjects with both diabetes mellitus and ApoE$_4$ allele was 4.99 (95% CI: 2.70–9.20) [69]. In the Kungsholmen Project, the hazard ratio of incident AD for subjects with borderline diabetes mellitus was 1.87 (95% CI: 1.11–3.14) and for nondiagnosed diabetes mellitus 3.29 (95% CI: 1.20–9.01) [70].

The reviews by Cukierman [71] and by Lu [68] concluded that diabetics are more likely than nondiabetic subjects to develop a cognitive decline. Also, the NIH statement concluded that there are mixed data linking diabetes mellitus with a rapid rate of cognitive decline and that a number of studies have identified declines in selective cognitive function, such as Digit Symbol Substitution (DSST), word fluency (WF), and delayed recall on auditory verbal learning test, but the specific affected domain has varied across studies [24].

On the possible association between the metabolic syndrome and the risk of incident AD, the NIH statement concluded that the metabolic syndrome is not associated with a higher risk of AD, but with a modestly increased risk of cognitive decline in studies with subjects younger than 80 years. This relationship is not any more valid in persons older than 85 years [24].

While chronic dietary habits that lead to IR, oxidative stress, and inflammation are associated with poorer cognitive function and risk of dementia, even circadian glycemic fluctuation in normal individuals and in those with type 2 diabetes mellitus may compromise cognitive function. A number of studies have shown positive effects on cognitive functions when providing glucose as a drink or after the ingestion of a breakfast compared with the fasting state. During a period of intense cognitive demand, normal persons tend to have a decrease in blood glucose, suggesting a direct relation between cognitive performance, systemic glycemia, and brain glucose utilization [72]. A study by Nilsson et al. [73] observed that subjects with higher glucose tolerance performed better in the cognitive tests, exploring working memory, and selective attention, after a breakfast with low-glycemic index (GI) compared to a breakfast with high GI and suggest that cognitive functions are enhanced by avoiding a sharp decline in blood glucose concentrations and by maintaining a higher glycemia in the late postprandial period. Therefore, a low-GI diet seems preferable in the prevention of the risk of cognitive decline.

In patients with type 2 diabetes mellitus, the ingestion of a high-GI food causes a decline in cognitive functions, such as delayed verbal memory [74]. These studies suggest that raising blood glucose levels into an optimal range improves cognition in healthy elderly adults and in those with cognitive decline. However, excessively high blood glucose levels, as observed in patients with type 2 diabetes mellitus, may be associated with cognitive dysfunction due to higher and prolonged elevations in blood glucose levels. The food-induced cognitive decrements observed in patients with type 2 diabetes mellitus are associated with elevation in blood glucose levels and could be reduced by the consumption of low-GI carbohydrate foods, such as pasta [5].

A number of studies have shown that poor glucose regulation is associated with impaired cognition and this is more frequent in older people, who tend to have worst glucoregulation. Elderly persons with poorest glucose regulation performed the worst in several tests (i.e., working memory and executive functions) [65]. Also, higher glycosylated hemoglobin levels were associated with poorest performance in paragraph recall [72]. Decline in verbal memory has been observed in elderly people with worse glucoregulation and in those with type 2 diabetes. At least three studies have shown

that improvement of glucose regulation following drug treatment leads to cognitive improvements, such as mental agility, processing speed, modified cue recall, and nonverbal reasoning [75–77]. There is clear evidence that impaired glucose regulation is associated with impaired cognition, in particular episodic memory. This impairment is minimal in young people but increases in older people who may have other aging processes with secondary reduction in brain function. Few studies suggest that drug treatments that improve glucose regulation also produce cognitive improvements in diabetic patients.

Conclusion

Prevalence of dementia, in particular AD, will increase dramatically in coming years. This neurodegenerative disease causes disability and dependency and is responsible for enormous burden on caregivers, health care, and economic resources. All these aspects make brain health an important public issue and a target for prevention, since there is evidence that cognitive decline and dementia can be prevented, especially through population-wide approaches. A diet rich in fatty fish, fruits, and vegetables with moderate alcohol consumption is able to prevent and control also many cardiovascular risk factors, such as hypertension, hyperlipidemia, and diabetes mellitus and, therefore, reduces the occurrence of coronary heart disease, stroke, and vascular-related dementia. Since in AD cardiovascular risk factors seem to play an important role in the development or worsening of the disease, from a public health perspective, actions for brain health may have issues similar to those contained in the prevention of stroke and heart disease. In fact, except for a few cases of genetic familial origin, the majority of patients with stroke, heart disease, and dementia arise from the progression of social, environmental, and behavioral conditions, as outlined in Figure 52.1, providing the opportunity to change all these events by using specific public health interventions [78]. New studies should investigate whether a healthy diet that is able to prevent cognitive decline and dementia has beneficial effects directly on brain aging or whether these effects are mediated through the prevention and control of classic cardiovascular risk factors, such

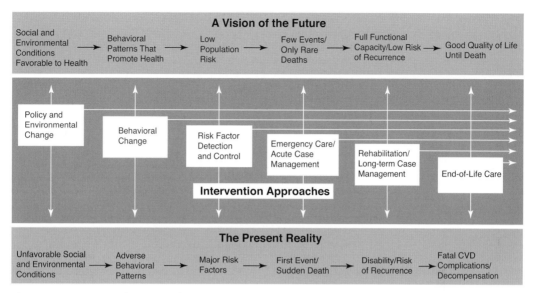

Figure 52.1 Promotion on brain health [78], as an action of a public health action plan to prevent heart disease and stroke. Available at http://www.cdc.gov/dhdsp/library/action_plan/index.htm.

as hypertension, hyperlipidemia, diabetes mellitus, smoking, and hyperhomocysteinemia. While it is reasonable to encourage the consumption of adequate fatty fish and foods rich in vitamins and antioxidant nutrients as a part of general dietary recommendations, no data suggest to supplement the diet with additional pharmacological treatment and further RCTs need to be performed to answer this question.

Selected References

1. Singer T, Verhaeghen P, Ghisletta P, Linderberger U, Baltes PB. The fate of cognition in very old age: Six-year longitudinal findings in the Berlin Aging Study (BASE). Psychol Aging 2003;18:318–31.

2. Volicer L. Editorial: clinical neurosciences in the journal of health and aging. J Nutr Health Aging 2008;12:125–6.

11. Barberger-Gateau P, Raffaitin C, Letenneur L, Berr C, Tzourio C, Dartigues JF, Alperovitch A. Dietary patterns and risk of dementia. The Three-City cohort study. Neurology 2007;69:1921–30.

17. Barberger-Gateau P, Letenneur L, Deschamps V, Peres K, Dartigues JF, Renaud S. Fish, meat, and risk of dementia: cohort study. BMJ 2002;325:932–3.

36. Ravaglia G, Forti P, Maioli F, Martelli M, Servadei L, Brunetti N, Porcellini E, Licastro F. Homocysteine and folate as risk factors for dementia and Alzheimer disease. Am J Clin Nutr 2005;82:636–43.

CHAPTER 53

Neurovascular Protection in Old Age

Jean-Marc Bugnicourt[1] *& Jean-Marc Chillon*[2]

[1]Service de Neurologie, and Laboratoire de Neurosciences Fonctionnelles et Pathologies
Université d'Amiens, Amiens, France
[2]INSERM, ERI12, and University of Picardie Jules Verne, Amiens, France

Introduction

Neurovascular protection in old age is a large topic that can include various items such as healthy aging, stroke primary, and secondary prevention, cerebrovascular diseases (CeVDs), and dementia as well as Alzheimer's disease (AD). In this chapter, we mainly consider cognitive impairments associated with CeVD. We first briefly define vascular cognitive impairments and then consider its prevention against putative risks factors such as arterial hypertension, lipidemic abnormalities, atherosclerosis, and hyperhomocysteinemia. Early detection is essential for prevention of cognitive decline. Nevertheless, whenever possible, we present evidences for the benefit of prevention in old age.

Cognitive Impairments Associated with Cerebrovascular Disease

Vascular dementia (VD) is the second cause of dementia after AD. However, there is now increasing evidence of overlapping between these two dementias with increased levels of amyloid plaques and neurofibrillary tangles in hypertensive subjects and numerous vascular pathology associated with AD. Furthermore, CeVD may play an important role in determining the presence and severity of the clinical symptoms of AD. It is now increasingly recognized that dementia in the elderly is a continuum

Nutritional and Metabolic Bases of Cardiovascular Disease, 1st edition.
Edited by Mario Mancini, José M. Ordovas, Gabriele Riccardi,
Paolo Rubba and Pasquale Strazzullo. © 2011 Blackwell Publishing Ltd.

of pathologies, with pure AD and VD representing the two extremes and mixed dementia (AD with CeVD) in between [1].

The initial concept of multi-infarct dementia has been considerably extended considering that clinically important cognitive impairments associated with vascular disease frequently do not fulfill traditional criteria for dementia [2]. The consequences on diagnostic criteria for vascular cognitive impairments are beyond the scope of this review, and as defined by others, we use the term *vascular cognitive impairment* to refer to all forms of mild to severe cognitive impairment associated with and presumed to be caused by CeVD [2]. Cognitive impairment may be related to stroke, multiple cortical infarcts, multiple subcortical infarcts, silent infarcts, strategic infarcts, small-vessel disease with white matter lesions, and lacunae [3]. This may be even more important with old age. Poststroke cognitive decline seems more frequent and the ability in the activities of daily living worsens relatively more after stroke in older than younger subjects [4].

The pathophysiological mechanisms of vascular cognitive impairments highlight the potential role of cardiovascular risk factors, genetic predisposition, lifestyle, and age [5]. In the following section, we consider management of hypertension, hypercholesterolemia, and hyperhomocysteinemia, emphasizing treatments that are more suitable in old age and their impact on cognitive functions. We also consider lifestyle with avoidance of smoking, nutrition, and exercise.

Hypertension and Vascular Cognitive Impairment in the Elderly

Hypertension and Dementia

It is well acknowledged that arterial hypertension is a major risk factor for stroke. However, if the benefits of blood pressure lowering in patients with CeVD extend across age-groups, the absolute benefits appear greater among those younger than 65 years [6]. Thus, it may be necessary to be cautious before starting aggressive antihypertensive therapies in the elderly [7]. In fact patients with long-standing hypertension associated with small-vessel disease may have adverse effects on cerebral perfusion and hence on cognitive function with aggressive antihypertensive treatment [7]. This is emphasized by a recent review of the effects of blood pressure reduction on cognitive function based on pooled data from clinical trials [8]. Antihypertensive treatment reduced decline in global cortical function and memory but not in subcortical executive function and learning capacity [8]. Furthermore, a subgroup meta-analysis of seven clinical trials that enrolled 1,670 very old subjects (older than 80 years) showed that active antihypertensive therapy significantly reduced stroke, but there was no treatment benefit for cardiovascular death and a nonsignificant relative excess of death from all causes [9]. In another meta-analysis of outcome trials, it was suggested that use of antihypertensive treatment to prevent stroke is justified in older patients whose systolic pressure is 160 mm Hg or higher [10]. Absolute benefit was larger in men, in patients 70 years or older and in those with previous cardiovascular complications or wider pulse pressure [10].

Antihypertensive Treatments and Dementia

Considering now the consequences of antihypertensive treatments on cognitive function, beneficial effects may also depend on the level of blood pressure or on the class of antihypertensive drugs used. A study showed that treatment of moderate hypertension in 65- to 74-year-old patients with a diuretic, a β-blocker, or placebo has no influence on cognitive function [11]. In contrast, in the double-blind placebo-controlled Systolic Hypertension in Europe (Syst-Eur) trial, antihypertensive treatment, starting with the calcium channel blocker nitrendipine as first-line medication, combined or replaced with the angiotensin-converting enzyme inhibitor enalapril (second-line medication) and hydrochlorothiazide (third-line medication) in elderly, was associated with a lower incidence of dementia [12]. If 1,000 hypertensive patients were treated with antihypertensive drugs for 5 years, 19 cases of dementia might be prevented [12].

Another trial, the Scandinavian Multi-Infarct Dementia Trial failed to show a significant effect of nimodipine on cognitive, social, or global assessments in patients defined as affected by multi-infarct dementia [13]. However, a post hoc analysis suggested that nimodipine may have a favorable effect in the subgroup of patients affected by subcortical (small-vessel) VD [14]. This was later confirmed by an ad hoc designed trial showing that in patients affected by subcortical VD, nimodipine may be of some benefit [15].

A beneficial effect of calcium channel blocker on cognitive function may not be simply related to a decrease in blood pressure but other properties of calcium channel blocker such as antioxidative properties and a decrease in capillary wall damage may be involved. Other antihypertensive drugs of interest may be drugs targeting the renin-angiotensin system. The perindopril-based blood pressure–lowering therapy has shown that blood pressure decrease even in the normotensive range decreases the risk of stroke recurrence in patients with previous CeVD [16]. An analysis of the pre-specified secondary outcomes of long-term disability and dependency indicated that a blood-pressure lowering therapy involving perindopril for all participants and indapamide for slightly more than half reduced the odds of long-term disability and dependency by one-fifth [17]. This benefit was due mainly to a reduction in recurrent stroke [17]. A substudy protocol of the Hypertension in the Very Elderly (HYVET) trial assessing cognitive decline and dementia incidence (HYVET-COG) is currently underway. As PROGRESS, treatment is based on the association of perindopril and indapamide with the difference that in HYVET indapamide is the first-line therapy and perindopril the second-line therapy. Another difference is that HYVET study incorporates patients older than 80 years with sustained sitting systolic blood pressure 160–219 mm Hg and diastolic blood pressure 90–109 mm Hg [18]. Contrary to PROGRESS, previous CeVD was not a criterion for patient's inclusion. Results of the pilot study for HYVET indicates a reduction in stroke and stroke mortality but with the possibility of excess death with active treatment [18].

Hypercholesterolemia and Vascular Cognitive Impairment in the Elderly

As mentioned above, AD and CeVDs are currently recognized as coexisting processes that contribute to the expression of dementia. This overlap between the two disorders is partly explained by the fact that vascular risk factors as hypertension, history of stroke, diabetes mellitus, and hypercholesterolemia are all associated with a high risk of AD. Several studies suggest a connection between cholesterol metabolism and susceptibility to AD/dementia. However, the relationship between serum total cholesterol, use of statins, and cognitive function in the elderly remains unclear.

Cholesterol is an essential component of brain cell membranes and has a crucial role in development and maintenance of neuronal plasticity and function. Cholesterol also influences the activity of the enzymes involved in the metabolism of the amyloid precursor protein (APP) and in the production of β-amyloid (Aβ). A high-cholesterol environment may favor activity of β and γ secretases. Gamma secretase increases Aβ production and results in amyloidogenic products that aggregate as extracellular plaques, whereas cleavage by α secretase results in nonamyloidogenic or soluble APP. The relationship between cholesterol and Aβ production and metabolism remains unclear. In animal studies, dietary cholesterol accelerates Aβ deposition in the brain [19]. In contrast, *in vitro* studies have shown that a high-cholesterol environment results in reduced production of soluble APP [20].

Hypercholesterolemia and Dementia

The role of dyslipidemia in the development of cognitive impairment/dementia remains unclear.

The few studies that have examined the association between serum lipid levels and cognitive function report conflicting results. If we consider longitudinal studies, high cholesterol levels have been associated with both an increased [21] or a decreased [22] risk of cognitive impairment, AD, or VD. Other studies with long follow-ups showed no association: the Hisayama study [23], the Framingham cohort [24], and the Honolulu-Asia Aging Study [25] found no difference in total serum cholesterol (TC) between subjects with AD, VD, or nondemented subjects. Possible explanations for this heterogeneity of results may be the use of single measure of serum lipids, the restriction of the study population to men or whites or the brief follow-up. Another possible explanation is that TC was assessed in midlife or late life. Indeed, the risk of dementia/AD seems to be linked to high midlife TC, whereas late-life TC has a less clear significance. In the CAIDE study (Cardiovascular Risk Factors, Aging and Dementia), Solomon suggested that the significance of TC levels may change over time from risk factor to risk marker [26]. According to this hypothesis, high midlife TC may be associated with poorer later-life cognition. In contrast, decreasing TC levels in late life may reflect incipient dementing processes, such as decreasing nutrition years before onset of symptoms. Thus, late life decreasing TC levels would be a consequence rather than a cause of dementia. High midlife TC is also a major modifiable risk factor for ischemic stroke and might influence late-life cognition by increasing vascular pathologies, which have been associated with cognitive impairment. In this view, Reitz et al. reported an association between high TC and VD [27].

In older age, studies on TC and dementia have short follow-ups and led to unclear conclusions regarding their potential association. Solomon [26] and Reitz [27] showed no association, whereas in an 18-year longitudinal study, in 70-year-old subjects, Mielke reported an association between the highest quartile of TC and a lower risk of dementia [28]. However, the author concluded that high TC in late life may be an indicator of better health status, and this association was seen only in nonsmokers. Another potential explanation is mortality bias; older patients with the highest total cholesterol levels may have had an increased risk of mortality and, therefore, had less risk to develop dementia over the course of the study.

Statins and Dementia

Several experimental studies on the effects of statins on dementia showed an increased activity of α secretase and decreased concentrations of extracellular Aβ [29] and raise the possibility that statins may lower the incident rate of AD. However, the outcome of studies relating plasma lipid-lowering treatment to cognitive functions has also been conflicting. Whereas early case-control studies suggested that statins may delay the onset of AD [30], the most recent prospective studies did not find any significant decrease in dementia incidence among statins users [31]. However, despite these controversial results, statins may be beneficial for cognition in nondemented subjects, by acting through changes in both serum and brain cholesterol. Among the three major components of the chemical structure of statins, the variable side-chain determines the solubility across the blood–brain barrier (BBB). Lipophilic statins can cross into the brain readily, while hydrophilic statins do not. An unresolved question is whether the statins need to cross the BBB to exert a beneficial effect in the CNS. Moreover, besides their lipid-lowering effect, statins have many other pleiotropic properties potentially important for brain health such as inhibition of platelet aggregation, improvement of endothelial function, and inhibition of proinflammatory factors [32].

Recently, Panza reported that the risk of AD is reduced in patients who received statins therapy in midlife [21]. In contrast, two randomized controlled trials examining the cognitive effects of statins found no significant differences on cognitive outcomes [33,34]. However, cognitive outcomes were the secondary end-point and not the main objective of these trials and the sample sizes were not powered to respond to this question. Finally, another study conducted in older age failed to show a significant association between statins and cognitive outcomes [27].

Statins therapy is associated with a reduction in the risk of stroke in patients with coronary artery disease. Moreover, the Women's Health Study, a prospective cohort study of 27,937 apparently healthy women, reported a strong association between the risk of ischemic stroke and both TC and low-density lipoprotein-cholesterol (LDL-C) levels [35]. In a recent meta-analysis of more than 90,000 patients, statins therapy reduces the risk of

first stroke by 21% placebo, and this reduction was largely accounted for by LDL-C reduction following treatment [36]. In contrast, in older patients, the effects of statins on stroke risk reduction in patients with coronary artery disease seem unfavorable. In a post hoc analysis of the PROspective Study of Pravastatin in the Elderly at Risk (PROSPER) trial, no significant reduction in stroke risk was found between patients with pravastatin 40 mg daily and placebo [34]. In secondary stroke prevention, the Stroke Prevention by Aggressive Reduction in Cholesterol Levels (SPARCL) study showed a 16% risk reduction of fatal and nonfatal stroke with atorvastatin 80 mg daily versus placebo [37]. The fact that patients in the atorvastatin group experienced fewer ischemic strokes regardless of the severity categories, compared to patients randomized to placebo, might reduce the risk of VD. This may be of interest as, even in older age, high doses of statins have an excellent safety profile. However, in a previous study including patients from the PROSPER cohort and evaluating the effect of pravastatin on the progression of brain white matter lesions, no difference was seen between the two groups [38]. The results of this study indicates that this statin, but perhaps not all, does not prevent cerebral small-vessel disease, an important cause of cognitive decline.

In conclusion, despite accumulating controversial research, recent findings provide argument for the involvement of cholesterol in both AD and VD. As a major modifiable vascular risk factor, cholesterol may contribute in setting up early foundations for developing late-onset AD and stroke risk, suggesting early statins therapy in prevention of dementia. However, disturbed cholesterol metabolism might just reflect the neurodegenerative process long before clinical symptoms develop.

Homocysteine and Vascular Cognitive Impairment in the Elderly

Hyperhomocysteinemia and Dementia

Homocysteine is a non-protein-forming, sulfur-containing amino acid, formed upon demethylation of methionine. The total homocysteine level in plasma or serum is a sensitive indicator of vitamin B_{12} and folate deficiencies. Several studies have shown that elevated plasma levels of homocysteine are associated with VD and AD [39]. Homocysteine may be involved in VD and AD because of its direct neurotoxicity [40] or as a risk factor for cardiovascular disease (CVD) [41]. Indeed, homocysteine is a strong predictor of stroke in middle-aged men [42] and contributes to the risk of silent brain infarction in elderly people [43].

Plasma levels of homocysteine are elevated in the elderly, possibly following a decrease in cystathionine synthase activity [44] or a decrease in vitamins (folate, vitamin B_{12}, and vitamin B_6) status and intake [45]. Thus, it is tempting to conclude that homocysteine may be linked to cognitive impairments in the elderly. Numerous studies have shown a link between elevated serum concentrations of homocysteine and/or reduced folic acid or vitamin B_{12} levels and cognitive impairment in the elderly [46].

Vitamins Supplementation and Dementia

The interest in homocysteine as a contributor of cognitive impairment is due to the fact that it is a modifiable risk factor. In Western populations, daily supplementation with 0.5–5.0 mg folic acid and 0.5 mg vitamin B_{12} would be expected to decrease blood homocysteine concentrations by about one-quarter to one-third [47]. However, most of the studies on vitamins (B_{12} and/or B_6) and/or folate supplementation and cognitive functions in elderly subjects are disappointing. One study found that patients with mild to moderate dementia and elevated plasma homocysteine levels improved clinically with increased test scores after vitamins supplements, while severely demented patients and patients with normal plasma homocysteine levels did not improve [48]. Two studies reported an improvement in language function, one study in patients with cognitive impairment [49] and one study in older subjects free of significant cognitive impairment [50]. It is possible that most of the studies failed to indicate an effect of supplementation with vitamins or folate on cognitive function in elderly subjects following irreversible or vitamin-independent neurocognitive decline or an insufficient dose or duration of vitamin supplementation.

Metabolic Syndrome, Diabetes, Obesity, Lifestyle, and Vascular Cognitive Impairment in the Elderly

Metabolic Syndrome and Dementia

As indicated in various chapters of this book, metabolic syndrome (MS) consists of an association of factors such as obesity, glucose intolerance, hypertension, low plasma high-density lipoprotein-cholesterol and high plasma triglycerides that have been identified as risk factors for stroke. Several studies indicate that MS is associated with an increased risk of cognitive disorders [51]. This association is present in a stroke-free population, suggesting that the MS is a determinant of neuroaging [51]. Part of the impact of MS on cognition may be linked to inflammation. One study has shown that MS contributes to cognitive impairment in the elderly with a high level of inflammation [52]. It has already been shown that inflammation may play a role in cognitive impairment, as serum markers of inflammation are associated with cognitive decline in well-functioning elderly people [53]. This suggests a potential impact of anti-inflammatory drugs on cognitive function. A randomized clinical trial has shown that daily aspirin improves or stabilize declines in cognition among patient with multi-infarct dementia [54]. However, aspirin is also an antiplatelet drug and impact of the treatment on cognition may be due to this effect.

Diabetes and Dementia

Impaired cognitive function has been frequently reported in diabetic patients. Following the studies, changes in cognitive function with diabetes may affect only elderly white women [55] and/or concern essentially psychomotor speed, processing speed and verbal episodic memory [56]. Furthermore, diabetes in midlife may be linked to dementia more than three decades later in the very old survivors in a male cohort [57]. Finally, both diabetes and impaired glucose tolerance in the elderly are associated with mildly impaired cognitive function [58]. Diabetes may induce dementia by disrupting aminergic neurotransmitter pathways, by affecting transport of nutrient across the BBB and by altering the cerebral circulation and the vascular tissues [56]. Other potential mechanisms may be a central neuropathy similar to the peripheral neuropathy observed in diabetes [56] or insulin resistance [59].

One interesting point is the impact of diabetes treatment on cognitive function. As indicate in a review from 2005, most studies suggest that better glycemic control improves cognition at least in people with mild diabetes. In people with severe diabetes, there is no benefit of treatment, possibly following permanent brain damage [60].

Obesity and Dementia

Obesity and overweight have been found to be independent risk factors for CVD. It has been shown that the relative risk of stroke increases with the body mass index [61]. However, few studies have considered the impact of obesity or overweight on cognitive function. Two studies have shown a relation between obesity and cognitive deficit in men only [62,63]. Adverse effects of obesity on cognitive function were independent and cumulative with the effects of hypertension [62]. Furthermore, the gender specific results for obesity but not for diabetes suggest that the underlying mechanisms linking them to cognition may be different [63]. The central obesity prevalent in men may explain the gender specificity.

Lifestyle and Dementia

The link between the MS, obesity, diabetes, glucose intolerance, and cognitive function suggests that a healthy lifestyle may be of benefit for cognitive function in the elderly. A healthy lifestyle may decrease the risk of CeVD and thus of vascular dementia. Moderate physical activity reduces the risk of stroke in men [64]. Furthermore, vigorous exercise in adulthood confers protection from stroke in later life [65]. Similarly, smoking cessation decreases the risk of stroke particularly in light smokers [66]. As summarized in a recent review, physical activity has also an impact on cognition. Fitness level at baseline predicts higher levels of cognitive performance 5–8 years later [67]. Another recent review indicates that lifestyle modification with particularly an increased physical activity and a change in food intake can impact on cognitive and mental health even in later life [68]. Limiting caloric intake and restricting the consumption of saturated fat prevent CVD and exerts strong effects on the brain [68]. Specific food compounds, such as nutritional antioxidants,

may decrease the vulnerability of the brain to inflammation and oxidative stress [68]. However, this lifestyle change may sometimes be difficult to implement in patients, especially for the elderly with cognitive deficits. The higher cognitive processes such as decision making and prospective memory required for the initiation and maintenance of new behaviors may be altered in old subjects [68].

Treatments and Vascular Cognitive Impairment in the Elderly

Stroke Prevention

Considering the impact of stroke on vascular dementia, stroke prevention, and especially secondary stroke prevention is of interest to maintain cognition in old age. Controls of hypertension, hypercholesterolemia, and diabetes have already been mentioned above. Another important point in stroke secondary prevention is antithrombotic or anticoagulant therapies. A meta-analysis of randomized trials of antiplatelet therapy has shown that antiplatelet drugs are protective in most type of patients at increased risk of occlusive vascular events including ischemic stroke [69]. Furthermore, the effects of anticoagulant prophylaxis with warfarin in preventing stroke in the practice settings was equivalent to that in randomized trials even if patients in practice settings were older and sicker [70]. However, side effects of anticoagulant misused, especially hemorrhage, and treatment's mistake in elderly people may contribute to a negative attitude of physicians toward antithrombotic drugs in secondary stroke prevention in the elderly.

Estrogens and Cognitive Function

Estrogens have vasoprotective activity attributed to beneficial effects on lipid metabolism and direct actions on the vasculature. These findings may explain the protective effects of estrogens against age-related disorders including AD and stroke [71]. However, the Women's Health Initiative Memory Study has shown that estrogens had an adverse effect on cognition which was greater among women with lower cognitive function at initiation of treatment [72]. Estrogen therapy alone and estrogen plus progestin did not improve cognitive function and even increased the risk of dementia or mild cognitive impairment among women between 65 and 79 years of age at study entry [73].

Other Treatments and Vascular Dementia

Numerous trials have been performed in VD and the results have generally been disappointing and no drug treatment as been approved for the treatment of VD by the European regulatory agencies [74]. In a recent review, Pantoni has observed that some drugs (nicergoline, memantine, posatirelin, propentofylline, and pentoxifylline) may show limited benefits in VD [74]. Part of the disappointing results observed may be due to the enrolment of patients with heterogeneous subtypes of VD, small sample size, and the use of inadequate cognitive tests more related to AD than to VD [74].

Drugs of potential interest for treatment of VD are the cholinesterase inhibitors approved in USA and Europe for AD. Galantamine has shown significant benefits in cognition, activities of daily living, behavior, and global function in patients with probable VD or AD combined with CeVD [75]. Another study indicates that galantamine is effective for improving cognition in patients with VD. However, the improvement in activities of daily living was similar with galantamine to that observed with placebo [76]. Cognitive improvement with galantamine was greater than with placebo for all subtypes of cerebrovascular lesions except in subjects with VD due to single strategic infarcts or in subjects with recent onset of VD. This may be consecutive to spontaneous improvement related to the natural history of recovery after stroke [76]. Finally, in a recent meta-analysis of randomized controlled trials (published and unpublished data), Kavirajan and

Schneider reported that cholinesterase inhibitors and memantine produce small benefits in cognition. The clinical significance for patients with mild to moderate VD is uncertain and the data do not support a widespread use of these drugs in VD [77]. However, subgroups of patients that may benefit of the treatments may be identified with individual analyses. Finally, this meta-analysis also pointed out the challenges in designing clinical trials for VD with heterogeneity in patients, the choice of diagnostic imaging methods, and the possibility that AD coexist with VD explaining part of the beneficial effects observed. Furthermore, most of the trials were of 6 months in duration, as for the AD trial, a duration that may have been too brief to assess the effectiveness of the treatments [77].

Selected References

3. van der Flier WM, van Straaten EC, Barkhof F, et al. Small vessel disease and general cognitive function in nondisabled elderly: the LADIS study. Stroke 2005 Oct; 36(10):2116–20.
8. Birns J, Morris R, Donaldson N, et al. The effects of blood pressure reduction on cognitive function: a review of effects based on pooled data from clinical trials. J Hypertens 2006 Oct;24(10):1907–14.
26. Solomon A, Kareholt I, Ngandu T, et al. Serum cholesterol changes after midlife and late-life cognition: twenty-one-year follow-up study. Neurology 2007 Mar 6;68(10): 751–6.
46. Mooijaart SP, Gussekloo J, Frolich M, et al. Homocysteine, vitamin B-12, and folic acid and the risk of cognitive decline in old age: the Leiden 85-Plus study. Am J Clin Nutr 2005 Oct;82(4):866–71.
67. Kramer AF, Colcombe SJ, McAuley E, et al. Fitness, aging and neurocognitive function. Neurobiol Aging 2005 Dec; 26 Suppl 1:124–7.

CHAPTER 54

Cardiovascular Risk Factors and Their Treatment in the Oldest Old

Kay-Tee Khaw

University of Cambridge, Cambridge, U.K.

Introduction

The current phenomenon of aging of the population is unprecedented in human history, with many more people living to old age. For example, in the United Kingdom, by 2040 those older than 65 years will constitute about one-quarter of the population; those older than 75 years, 12%; and those older than 85 years, 5% of the total population, with comparable figures in most industrialized countries [1]. Maintaining the health of the older population is a huge public health challenge. Cardiovascular diseases (CVDs) are now not only the leading cause of mortality worldwide both in developed and in developing countries but also a leading cause of disability in later life. The major CVDs are stroke and coronary heart disease, but CVDs also encompass such conditions as aortic aneurysms, peripheral vascular disease, and contribute to clinical conditions including cardiac failure, renal vascular disease, vascular dementia, and retinal disease. The aims of CVD prevention in later life must consider not just mortality reduction but prevention of disability and improving quality of life.

There are now dozens of risk factors documented for CVD including inflammatory factors, hemostatic factors, endogenous hormone levels, and factors involved in glucose and homocysteine metabolism, as well as many behavioral factors including diet, physical activity, and psychosocial stress. Nevertheless, the classical CVD risk factors—raised blood pressure, raised blood cholesterol levels, and cigarette smoking habit—remain paramount and their role in the etiology of cardiovascular disease is supported by overwhelming evidence. Though the relationship of these risk factors with specific CVD end-points may vary (e.g., blood pressure is more strongly related to stroke and cholesterol to coronary heart disease), raised blood pressure and raised blood cholesterol levels are still the only CVD risk factors for which randomized trials of reduction have unequivocally and consistently demonstrated reduction in CVD end-points, and these are the two risk factors that are the main focus of this chapter.

Despite the wealth of evidence, there is still some debate about the value of cardiovascular risk factor reduction in older populations. Older people may differ from the young in many ways. Physiologic measures such as blood pressure and cholesterol may be markers of different pathophysiologic processes in older people: for example low blood pressure in older people may reflect cardiac decompensation and low body mass index may reflect loss of muscle mass rather than lower body fat percentage. Selective mortality of those with high levels of risk factors may mean that older people are resistant survivors. Older people are a heterogeneous group and successive birth cohorts may have very different experiences during their life course, different survival patterns, and health characteristics.

Part of the debate arises from the paucity of evidence on the role of CVD risk factors in the oldest old, as many early observational studies and trials of risk factor reduction omitted older people. We,

Nutritional and Metabolic Bases of Cardiovascular Disease, 1st edition.
Edited by Mario Mancini, José M. Ordovas, Gabriele Riccardi,
Paolo Rubba and Pasquale Strazzullo. © 2011 Blackwell Publishing Ltd.

therefore, need empirical evidence that CVD risk factors still predict health outcomes in the oldest old, and more importantly, that reduction of these risk factors will improve health outcomes relevant in this older population. In recent years, there has been increasing recognition of the need to include older people in trials. Though definitions of the oldest old vary, one definition generally accepted is those 75 years and older. Though studies have not always reported age-specific data for the oldest age-groups but for all age-groups, more studies have now included older people.

Blood Pressure and Cardiovascular Disease

A systematic review [2] of 61 prospective observational studies of blood pressure and mortality in one million adults with no previous vascular disease recorded at baseline emphasized that while the observed relative risk for CVD associated with a given difference in blood pressure was lower in older compared to younger people (e.g., for each 20 mm Hg lower systolic blood pressure, stroke risk was 33% lower in those aged 80–89 years but 62% lower in those aged 50–59 years), the absolute risk difference was in fact substantially greater in older people since their absolute rates of CVD were higher.

In contrast, very similar relative risk reductions in older and younger people associated with blood pressure lowering medication have been observed in trials. The Blood Pressure Lowering Treatment Triallists' Collaboration conducted meta-analyses to quantify the relative risk reductions achieved with different regimens to lower blood pressure in two age groups, younger than 65 years and 65 years or older [3]. In 31 trials with 190,606 participants, the meta-analyses showed no clear difference between age-groups in the effects of lowering blood pressure or any difference between the effects of different drug classes on major cardiovascular events. Meta-regressions also showed no difference in effects between those younger than 65 years and 65 years or older for major cardiovascular events. For every 5 mm Hg reduction in systolic blood pressure, there was an estimated 11.9% reduction in major cardiovascular events in those older than 65 years and 9.1% in those 64 years or older. The authors concluded that reduction of blood pressure

produces benefits in all age groups. As Staessen et al. in an accompanying commentary emphasized [4], since the absolute risk of cardiovascular events is higher in older than younger people for a similar relative risk reduction in blood pressure, far fewer patient years of treatment are needed to prevent one major cardiovascular event in an elderly person.

While most comparisons of treatment in older people have used 65 years as a cut-point for the older age-group, the target age-group in the HYVET trial was specifically the very old, 80 years or older. This trial of treatment of hypertension with a diuretic (indapamide) plus angiotensin-converting enzyme inhibitor (perindopril), if required, affirmed the benefits of blood pressure reduction in the very old (80 years or older) [5]. Lowering systolic hypertension (=160 mm Hg) or diastolic hypertension (90–109 mm Hg) to below 150 mm Hg systolic and 80 mm Hg diastolic reduced stroke incidence by 30%, cardiovascular death rates by 23% and cardiac failure by 64% with fewer serious adverse events in the active treatment group. Thus, the evidence clearly demonstrates the benefits of blood pressure reduction for prevention of adverse clinical sequelae, in those with hypertension, even in the very old.

Cholesterol and Cardiovascular Disease

A meta-analysis of 61 prospective studies on 900,000 adults, mostly in western Europe or North America, reported that 1 mmol/L lower total cholesterol was associated with 54%, 35%, and 17% lower coronary heart disease mortality at ages 40–49, 50–69, and 70–89 years, respectively [6]. However, cholesterol concentrations were not strongly related to stroke risk and at older ages (70–89 years) and particularly in those with systolic blood pressure over about 145 mm Hg, total cholesterol was in fact negatively related to hemorrhagic and total stroke mortality.

Nevertheless, and somewhat paradoxically, a review of trials of cholesterol reduction with statin therapy estimated not only substantial reductions in coronary heart disease incidence associated with approximately 1mmol/l average lowering of low-density lipoprotein (LDL)-cholesterol concentrations (12% reduction in all cause mortality, 19%

reduction in coronary mortality) but also 17% reduction in fatal or non-fatal stroke and, overall, 21% in any major vascular event [7]. The absolute benefit related to the absolute risk of events, such that older people at greater absolute risk would have greatest absolute benefits. Although only 4 of the 14 trials reviewed included participants older than 75 years, this age-group also showed significantly lower (18%) major vascular event rate per mmol/L LDL-cholesterol reduction, or about 3% absolute rate reduction (19.7% vs. 16.8% event rate) over 5 years. This overview concluded that the evidence reinforced the need to consider statin treatment to reduce LDL-cholesterol in all patients at high risk of any type of major vascular event.

Adverse effects of treatment are of particular importance in the oldest old in whom, arguably quality of life is as important as extending survival, and who may also be more sensitive to side effects of medication. Rare but clinically important adverse effects of statins are peripheral neuropathy and myopathy. Not all trials report these adverse effects consistently nor have the power to look at elderly groups specifically. Additionally, there is substantial patient selection for trials. However, the Health Protection Study, one of the largest with 20,536 patients randomized to 40 mg simvastatin or placebo, reported very similar proportions (approximately 33%) in active or placebo groups with unexplained muscle pain and weakness and only 0.5% in either active or placebo groups discontinued medication because of muscle symptoms.

Smoking and Cardiovascular Disease

Although there are no randomized trials of smoking cessation on CVD outcomes in the oldest old, the adverse effects of cigarette smoking on health at all ages has been conclusively demonstrated and there is little doubt about the benefits of stopping smoking.

The Coronary Artery Surgery Study (CASS) reported that the relative risk of myocardial infarction or death in those who continued smoking compared to those who stopped was 2.9 in those aged 70–74 years and 1.5 for those aged 55–59 years. Based on 40 and then 50 years of follow-up from the British Doctors Study, Doll [8,9] compared survival of cigarette smokers who stopped smoking at different ages with that of nonsmokers and with that of those who continued to smoke. Those who stopped at around 60 years gained about 3 years of life expectancy compared with those who continued. Even those who stopped at 65–74 years of age (mean age 71 years) had age-specific mortality rates beyond age 75 years appreciably lower than those who continued.

Other Risk Factors

Many other risk factors have been implicated in CVD risk in younger cohorts, and it is likely that they also have effects at older ages. For example, diabetes, glucose intolerance, or hyperinsulinemia is an important risk factor for coronary heart disease in men and women older than 65 years [10,11]. However, for most risk factors, there is still a paucity of data in older persons in their relation to cardiovascular risk and even less data on the effectiveness of risk factor reduction. Indeed recent trials on reduction of some of these risk factors not specifically in the elderly, such as the Action to Control Cardiovascular Risk in Diabetes Study Group (ACCORD) trial, with targeted strict control of blood glucose or folate supplementation targeted at homocysteine metabolism have not shown encouraging results [11–14]. Thus, while individuals may be identified at increased cardiovascular risk because of higher levels of the newer risk factors, evidence suggests that most benefit would derive from control of the classical risk factors blood pressure and lipids in these high-risk groups.

Who to Treat? Absolute Cardiovascular Disease Risk

There is, therefore, little doubt from the large body of observational and trial evidence that control of high blood pressure and raised cholesterol will reduce CVD risk even in the oldest old. The question then arises of who should have pharmacologic treatment. The treatment of cardiovascular risk factors and identifying those who would most benefit from pharmacologic interventions has moved from treatment of individual risk factors at fixed thresholds to treatment based on absolute CVD risk [15]. These thresholds have been variously set at 30% or

20% risk of CVD or 5-10% CVD mortality over the next 10 years [16,17]. The proportion of people aged over 75 years who are likely to fall within this high risk category will vary according to the prevailing CVD rates in different communities and the prevalence of other risk factors However, since absolute rates of CVD rise sharply with increasing age, most people aged over 75 are likely to be eligible for treatment based on their age alone irrespective of risk factor levels. Notwithstanding the continuous relationship between risk factor level and CVD risk, most clinicians would probably prefer to be cautious, avoiding polypharmacy and minimizing medication use in the elderly where possible and err on the side of prudence in terms of treatment. As guidelines recognize [16], there is still a need to consider and take into account individual patient preferences and values when balancing the magnitude of potential benefits and costs when considering pharmacologic interventions in people older than 75 years.

Population-Based Approach: Reduction of Risk Factor Levels in the Community as a Whole

In most communities, mean levels of risk factors such as blood pressure and cholesterol and hence, prevalence of hypertension and hypercholesterolemia increase with increasing age. This, coupled with the observation that most people over age 75 would be considered at high cardiovascular risk has led to consideration of the potential impact of lifestyle factors in addition to smoking habit in reducing cardiovascular risk in the general community. Many communities have been documented in which blood pressure and cholesterol levels do not rise with age and where CVD rates are low. While not the main focus of this chapter, a brief summary considers lifestyle factors that may contribute to lowering cardiovascular risk in the oldest old.

Nutrition

High dietary sodium intake is related to higher blood pressure levels and in particular, the rise of blood pressure with increasing age. The InterSalt Study of 52 communities worldwide estimated that a reduction of 100 mmol sodium daily is associated with a 5–10 mm Hg systolic blood pressure decrease; the lower the average sodium intake in communities, the lower the rise of blood pressure with age [18]. Older persons appear to be more sensitive to the blood pressure–raising effects of sodium [19,20]. Trials confirm these effects; a trial of modest reduction of salt intake from 10 to 5 g daily in elderly men 60–78 years of age reported blood pressure reduced by 7 mm Hg (systolic) and 3 mm Hg (diastolic); similar changes were observed in normotensive and hypertensive participants [21]. Other nutritional factors that have been reported to be associated with lower blood pressure levels include high potassium, calcium, magnesium, and dietary figer intake (generally from fruit and vegetables) and low fat intakes, and some of these have also been related to subsequent CVD events [22,23].

Long-term lifestyle intervention trials with clinical CVD end-points are difficult to conduct for reasons of feasibility and compliance; a randomized trial of a potassium enriched salt or regular salt to enrich dietary potassium and reduce sodium intake, with 1,981 veterans in a veteran retirement home reported not only a 41% reduction in CVD mortality in the experimental group but also that the people in the experimental group spent significantly less in patient care for CVD than did the control group [24].

The role of high dietary saturated fat in coronary heart disease is supported by a wealth of clinical, laboratory, and epidemiologic evidence. The Women's Health Initiative did not find any differences in CVD end-points in postmenopausal women randomized to a lower fat diet. However, in this trial the polyunsaturated to saturated fat ratio was unchanged, and trials which have demonstrated reduction in CVD have generally increased the polyunsaturated to saturated fat ratio, or changed other types of fat in the diet. The Lyon secondary prevention trial of a Mediterranean α-linolenic acid–rich diet reported a 70% reduction in mortality [25]. A review of the literature suggested that several dietary components including fish, nuts, dark chocolate, fruit, and vegetables and moderate alcohol intake might be associated with substantial cardiovascular benefits [26].

Physical Activity

Physical activity is beneficially related to both blood pressure and blood lipid levels, as well as heart disease and stroke, and increasing evidence suggests that even moderate levels such as walking appear protective for CVD as well as death in older men and women [27–29].

Just as individual preferences and effect on quality of life must be important factors when considering treatment of blood pressure and cholesterol in the oldest old, so also must these be taken into account for lifestyle recommendations. What evidence there is suggests that relatively modest differences in health behaviors such as not smoking, high fruit and vegetable intake, moderate physical activity, and moderate alcohol consumption may not only influence CVD risk in the elderly, but as important may be beneficially related to quality of life, as assessed for example by physical functional health [30–32].

Conclusions

There is now increasing evidence that the classical CVD risk factors—raised blood pressure, raised blood cholesterol, and cigarette smoking—predict subsequent CVD even in the oldest old. Increasing trial evidence also indicates that reduction of blood pressure reduces CVD incidence; although fewer data are available for cholesterol lowering in older people, available evidence using statins also indicates benefits for both ischemic heart disease and stroke. The absolute benefits of risk factor reduction are larger in the older people who have higher CVD rates, although decisions to treat rest on judgments of the individual risk benefit balance. The prevalence of elevated risk factors levels increases with age; primary prevention or reduction of elevated risk factor levels in the general population through lifestyle changes such as reduction of dietary sodium and saturated fat and increasing fruit and vegetable intake has been shown to be feasible and effective. Although there still a paucity of evidence in older persons, it is likely that the other risk factors documented in younger cohorts will have effects in the elderly and offer future possibilities for interventions. The elderly are not a homogenous group, and it is likely that different cohorts of the elderly with very different early and middle life experiences will differ in the relative importance of risk factors such that continuing evidence is required. In the interim, the profound international variation and secular trends in risk factor levels and CVD rates even at older ages together indicate substantial potential for prevention of a large proportion of CVD in the elderly.

Selected References

5. Beckett NS, Peters R, Fletcher AE, et al. Treatment of hypertension in patients 80 years of age or older. N Engl J Med 2008;358(18):1887–98.

6. Lewington S, Whitlock G, Clarke R, et al. Blood cholesterol and vascular mortality by age, sex, and blood pressure: a meta-analysis of individual data from 61 prospective studies with 55,000 vascular deaths. Lancet 2007; 370(9602):1829–39.

14. Bazzano LA, Reynolds K, Holder KN, et al. Effect of folic acid supplementation on risk of cardiovascular diseases: a meta-analysis of randomized controlled trials. JAMA 2006;296(22):2720–6.

20. Khaw KT, Bingham S, Welch A, et al. Blood pressure and urinary sodium in men and women: the Norfolk Cohort of the European Prospective Investigation into Cancer (EPIC-Norfolk). Am J Clin Nutr 2004;80(5): 1397–1403.

30. Khaw KT, Wareham N, Bingham S, et al. Combined impact of health behaviours and mortality in men and women: the EPIC-Norfolk prospective population study. PLoS Med 2008;5(1):e12.

CHAPTER 55

Nutrition and Lifespan in Developing Countries

Arun Chockalingam

Simon Fraser University, Burnaby, BC, Canada

Demographic transition

Over the last 60 to 70 years, the global demography has changed. The world as a whole is transitioning from a high-fertility, high-mortality state to a low-fertility, low mortality state [1]. The rate at which this demographic transition occurs varies from country to country. However, the phenomenon is uniform all over the world. Other factors that play a major role in increased life expectancy are infant mortality, mortality in people younger than 5 years, and maternal mortality [2]. Thus, the life expectancy of the population has increased in every country and every region of the world [1], but the countries are at different stages of demographic transition.

In stage one (pre-industrial society), death rates and birth rates are high and roughly in balance. In stage two (developing countries), the death rates drop rapidly due to improvements in food supply and sanitation, which increase lifespan and reduce disease. These changes usually occur as a result of improvements in farming techniques, access to technology, basic healthcare, and education. Without a corresponding fall in birth rates, this produces an imbalance, and the countries in this stage experience a large increase in population. In stage three, birth rates fall because of access to contraception, increases in wages, urbanization, a reduction in subsistence agriculture, an increase in the status and education of women, a reduction in the

Nutritional and Metabolic Bases of Cardiovascular Disease, 1st edition.
Edited by Mario Mancini, José M. Ordovas, Gabriele Riccardi,
Paolo Rubba and Pasquale Strazzullo. © 2011 Blackwell Publishing Ltd.

value of children's work, an increase in parental investment in the education of children, and other social changes. Population growth begins to level off. During stage four, there are both low birth rates and low death rates. Death rates may remain consistently low or increase slightly due to increases in lifestyle diseases due to low exercise levels and high obesity and an aging population in developed countries. Life expectancy, thus, has increased in every continent, as can be seen from Table 55.1.

Many countries such as China, Brazil, India, and Thailand have passed through the demographic transition very quickly due to fast social and economic change, just in the past 25–30 years due to globalization. Some countries, particularly African countries, appear to be stalled in the second stage because of stagnant development and the effect of HIV/AIDS. This is evident from Table 55.1 where only sub-Saharan African countries did not have a steady increase in life expectancy that was similar to any other region of the world.

Epidemiologic Transition

"Epidemiologic transition" refers to relatively constant patterns of changes in patterns of disease as societies develop. Scholars in population changes and public health [4,5] have studied the disease pattern along with changing socioeconomic, cultural, and economic patterns. However, the modern concepts and theory behind epidemiologic transition were postulated by Omran [6]. The epidemiologic transition parallels the demographic transition and advancement in technology. Omran explained

Table 55.1 Life Expectancy 1950–2005 [3].

Region of the world	Life expectancy (yr)		
	1950	1985	2005
Asia (excluding Middle East)	42	60	67
Central America and Caribbean	50	65	72
Europe	67	73	74
Middle East and North Africa	42	60	67
North America	68	75	78
Oceania	64	70	74
South America	53	63	71
Sub-Saharan Africa	38	49	46

epidemiologic transition into periods with differing mortality patterns and disease levels. He classified these periods/phases as "age of pestilence and famine," which includes high mortality related to very poor health conditions, epidemics, and famine; "age of receding pandemics (early and late phase)," which has a progressive decline in mortality as epidemics become less frequent; and "age of degenerative and man-made diseases," in which we see further decline in mortality, increase in life expectancy, and the predominance of chronic noncommunicable diseases [6].

The transition from the age of pestilence and famine (predominantly infectious diseases) to the age of degenerative and man-made diseases is well explained by major categories of diseases determinants [6]. They are as follows: *Ecobiologic determinants* of mortality deal with disease agents, the level of hostility in the environment, and the resistance of the host. *Socioeconomic, political, and cultural determinants* involve standards of living, health habits, and hygiene and nutrition. *Medical and public health determinants* are specific measures of prevention and cure to deal with disease.

While the Western world has reached the age of degenerative and man-made disease, whereby it has overcome the troubles due to much of infectious diseases, many of the developing countries face the double burden of both infectious and degenerative chronic diseases [7]. According to World Health Organization (WHO) classification [8], average low- and middle-income countries share a 36% burden of group 1 diseases (communicable/infectious, maternal and perinatal conditions, and nutritional dis-

orders), 54% burden of group 2 (chronic noncommunicable diseases), and a 10% burden of group 3 diseases (injuries). In contrast, high-income countries record their burden of diseases as group 1, 7%; group 2, 87%; and group 3, 6%.

Globalization and Growing Epidemic of Chronic Diseases in Developing Countries

As the globalization progresses, many of the developing countries are readily adopting the Western lifestyle—taking fast food and processed food rich in fat and carbohydrates, less consumption of fruits and vegetable, and less physical activity [9]. Globalization has multiple consequences and a probable impact on health status [10]. For example, global transnational trade of tobacco and alcohol not only provides increased marketing for the exporting countries but also harms the health of importing nations. Many governments in the developing world balance their books with support from tobacco companies' grants, and hence, their policies become skewed. The net effect is deteriorated health of their citizens [11].

Due to globalization coupled with reduction in communicable diseases, economic growth in developing countries has increased life expectancy. As a consequence, many people are living longer and are susceptible to chronic diseases such as cardiovascular and cancer [12]. Furthermore, obesity has increased, exercise has decreased, and adverse dietary changes including a greater reliance on animal fats are seen [7,13]. The growing rate of cardiovascular disease (CVD) incidence in countries such as Russia has shown a reversal in longevity. For example, the life expectancy in Russia in 1988 was 64.6 years, and in a short period of 6 years, it declined to 57.6 years in 1994 [13]. In the absence of epidemiologic data and surveillance, it is difficult to identify the cause for such a decline. However, epidemiologists speculate that this downturn could be attributable to deteriorating diet, more smoking, and political and economic turmoil.

Nutrition Transition

As we saw above in the demographic transition, the major shifts in fertility and mortality patterns

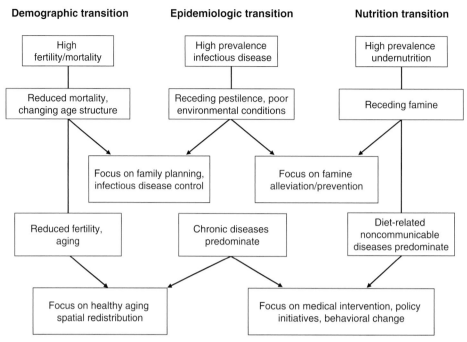

Figure 55.1 Stage of health, nutritional, and demographic change. (Reproduced from Popkin BM. Public Health Nutr 2002;5:93–103, with permission.)

have a direct correlation to shifts in diet, physical activity, and body composition. The concept of "nutrition transition" focuses on large shifts in the structure of diet. As the world moves toward globalization, it is evident that that there is a significant growth in urban living. In turn, urban living is linked to large changes in diet and body composition showing a direct correlation to high levels of obesity in developing countries (and, of course, developed countries). Popkin [14] defined nutrition transition through five broad patterns, namely: (a) hunting and gathering food, (b) famine, (c) receding famine, (d) degenerative diseases, and (e) behavioral changes. Interestingly, these five patterns have strong relations to Omron's hypothesis [6] on epidemiologic transition (Figures 55.1 and 55.2).

New Trends in Global Diet

Global availability of inexpensive vegetable oils and fats has resulted in significantly increased fat consumption among developing nations [15]. As incomes rise and urbanization increases, generally, diets high in complex carbohydrates and fiber are replaced by more varied diets with higher contents of

fats, saturated fats, and sugars [16,17]. Fat-rich diets, especially of animal origin, have been regarded as richer and more flavorful and often tend to be varied [18]. Until just after World War II, the majority of fats consumed were animal fats, milk, butter, and meat. In the last few decades, we have seen a revolution in the production of oilseed-based fats. Technological breakthroughs in the development of high-yield oilseeds and in the refining of high-quality vegetable oils resulted in lower cost of baking and frying as compared to animal fats [19]. During this era, world demand for vegetable fats was propelled by health concerns for animal fats and cholesterol. At the same time, economic incentives and political initiatives fueled the produced substantial levels of vegetable fats both in developed and developing countries, particularly in southern Asia (palm oils) and Latin America (soybean oil) [20]. Between 1991 and 1997, the production of vegetable oils increased from 60 million to 71 million metric tons [21]. The production and export of vegetable oils are promoted through direct subsidies, credit guarantees, food aid, and market development programs [21].

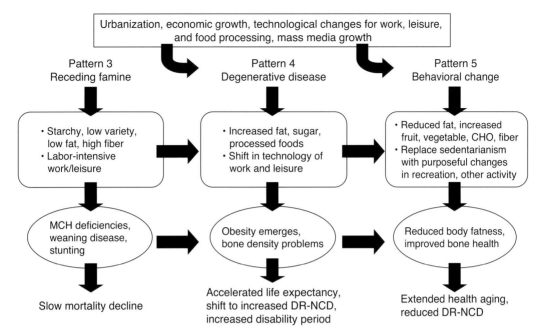

Figure 55.2 Stages of nutrition transition. (Reproduced from Popkin BM. Public Health Nutr 2002;5:93–103, with permission.)

Incomes and Diet Structure

Approximately three decades ago, the global diet structure was directly related to the gross national product (GNP) per capita, with high GNP levels being associated with greater energy coming from animal and vegetable fats and sugars [17]. Over time, the income–diet relationship has changed significantly, fat consumption is not as dependent on GNP, and access to high-fat diets has increased for low-income countries. The differences can be accounted for by significant increases in vegetable fat consumption across both low- and high-income countries. The availability of vegetable fats is currently independent of income and accounts for a great proportion of dietary energy, whereas the relationship between the availability of animal fats and income is currently less substantial than in the past [22].

Urbanization and Increased Consumption of Fast Food

There are large differences in the diets of people living in rural areas and those in urban areas particularly in lower income countries [23]. Urban diets characteristically contain larger amounts of su-

perior and milled grains, polished grains, high-fat and high-sugar foods, animal products, processed foods, and foods prepared outside the home (fast foods) [24]. Urbanization is linked to greater consumption of fats and sweeteners in lower income areas [23].

Impact on Child Health

The reduction of malnutrition in developing countries has been paralleled with increased obesity rates in children [25]. Levels of childhood obesity in low-income countries are nearing the levels of childhood obesity in the United States [25]. The relationship between rates of obesity in low- to middle-income countries and income are typically positively correlated, although increasingly this relationship is being found to be inverse, with higher rates of childhood obesity now being seen in the poor in comparison to the rich [26].

Malnutrition to Overnutrition

As mentioned earlier, the rate of obesity in low-income countries is on the rise, which can be linked to economic and nutrition transition. Malnutrition is frequent in low-income countries. There exists evidence for malnutrition early in life as a risk factor for chronic disease and obesity in adulthood [27]. It is suggested that excess body fat buildup can result from metabolic and hormonal changes triggered by malnutrition.

Health Policy

The changes in nutrition and demographics in the developed world have created a whole new set of challenges for policy makers. Noncommunicable diseases and obesity are substantial problems for policy makers and need to be brought to the forefront. The millennium development goals fall short in this area, as noncommunicable diseases are absent from the goals [28]. The shift internationally from communicable diseases to noncommunicable diseases has resulted in significant burden for developing countries from chronic disease [29]. This burden resulting from increases in chronic disease is coupled with the burden of malnutrition, which remains a serious issue for developing countries. A recent WHO report [30] calls for action against chronic noncommunicable diseases (CNCDs), such as cardiovascular conditions (heart disease and stroke), some cancers, chronic lung diseases, and type 2 diabetes mellitus. which reached epidemic proportion worldwide. These conditions account for 60% of all deaths worldwide, and about 80% of chronic disease deaths occur in low- and middle-income countries. What is even more alarming is that CNCDs account for 44% of premature deaths worldwide [31]. In addition to human toll, CNCDs have an enormous negative economic impact [32]. The economic boom enjoyed by globalizations in the world's most populous countries such as China and India could be neutralized in the next 10 years due to CNCDs, as these two countries are projected to lose as much as $558 billion and $237 billion, respectively [32].

Several thought leaders from both developed and developing countries came to a consensus on this growing epidemic and issued a new Grand Challenge in chronic noncommunicable diseases [33]. They called for research needed to address top 20 policy and research priorities in six different goal areas: raise public awareness; enhance economic, legal and environmental policies; modify risk factors; engage business and community; mitigate health impacts of poverty and urbanization; and reorientate health systems.

Nutrition, Food Security, and International Trade Policy in Light of Globalization

A healthy diet is a critical determinant of a healthy life. Research over the past half century has clearly demonstrated that individuals that consume an energy-balanced diet that is low in fat, particularly saturated fat, and high in complex carbohydrates, particularly those from fruits and vegetables, are healthier, consume less health services, and in general enjoy a higher quality of life with increased longevity. This is true even for those of advanced age [34].

The challenge of producing healthy food for the world's more than 6 billion people is immense. This is made more complex by the planet's limited land mass, its increasing population, and our life expectancy. In addition, as more and more arable lands are converted to housing, the ecology and environment on which agriculture depends are gradually being destroyed [35].

Significant improvements in the areas of food security and nutritional status have been made. Technology can increase the production of food, through such means as soil enrichment or genetically modifying grains and vegetables that produce high-volume, high-energy crops. Both of these approaches exact a high price, however. Despite the greater availability of these technologies, there is an increasing distrust of their safety and potential degradation of the environment on the part of the public. Enriching the soil through increased use of chemicals is perceived to have a potential to harm human health. This influences political decisions and policies about the acceptance of this food technology [35]. For example, countries that use genetically modified seed run the risk of growing crops that are unmarketable to other countries. These policies affect the low- and middle-income countries. The benefits and concerns of food technology must be carefully assessed before its adoption for wide use in a country.

Unfortunately, experience to date with the mass production and global distribution of some foods has had in many instances a negative impact because the food has been unhealthy or culturally insensitive (e.g., many fast foods). In addition, the growing concentration of food production and distribution by fewer and fewer multinational conglomerates threatens to displace local production capacity and creates great dependency and precludes choice. In North America, the growing popularity of organically grown and produced food stuff is indicative of the increasing public reaction against the developments in food technologies.

It is important that developing food technologies targeted at increasing food production also aims to improve nutritional status. The technologies need to be designed to produce foods with a nutrient content consistent with decreasing the risk of developing chronic diseases. For example, biotechnology is currently focusing on producing foods with a healthy lipid profile and increased antioxidant content. Technologies should also aim at producing a more varied food supply to replace the monocomponent diets currently ingested in a great part of the world.

Modern food technology offers great potential for developing food items that comply well with expert recommendations (less saturated fat, salt, sugar) and are at the same time tasty and affordable. This potential should be tapped, not only in countries with established market economies where such developments have started, but also in low- and middle-income countries.

However, the technology to increasing food production to increase nutritional status will not necessarily lead to the redress of food security where profound inequities exist and where distribution and access by those in need may not be improved. It is critical that programs and policies ensure that any potential benefits that may results from the incorporation of food technology to increase food production and nutrition value ensure that all populations of the world benefit from these developments [35].

Nutrition Policy for Aging Population in Developing Countries

With increasing elderly populations in developing countries, new issues for policy makers arise. Issues of both undernutrition and overnutrition exist in low-income countries affecting the functional status of the elderly. With an aging population of both malnourished and overweight individuals, high rates of disability and illness will be consequences [36]. Policy development is needed to fully understand the effect nutrition transition has on the elderly in low-income countries.

Selected References

29. World Health Organization. Diet, nutrition and the prevention of chronic diseases. Report of a joint WHO/FAO Expert consultation. Geneva: WHO; 2003.

31. Lopez Ad, Mathers CD, Ezzati M, et al. (eds). *Global Burden of Disease and Risk Factors*. Washington, DC: Oxford University Press and World Bank; 2006.

32. Adeyi O, Smith O, Robles S. Public policy and the challenge of chronic non-communicable diseases. Washington, DC: World Bank; 2007.

33. Daar A, Singer PA, Prasad DL, et al. Grand challenges in chronic non-communicable diseases: The top 20 policy and research priorities for conditions such as diabetes, stroke and heart disease. Nature 2007;450:494–6.

34. Knoops KTB, de Groot LC, Kromhout D, et al. Mediterranean diet, lifestyle factors, and 10-year mortality in elderly European men and women. J Am Med Assoc 2004; 292:1433–9.

Index

Note: Italicized *f*'s and *t*'s refer to figures and tables.